Nutrition & Wellness for Life

Dorothy F. West, Ph.D.

Food and Nutrition Author and Educator

Publisher
The Goodheart-Willcox Company, Inc.
Tinley Park, Illinois
www.g-w.com

The Goodheart-Willcox Company, Inc. Brand Disclaimer: Brand names, company names, and illustrations for products and services included in this text are provided for educational purposes only and do not represent or imply endorsement or recommendation by the author or the publisher.

The Goodheart-Willcox Company, Inc. Safety Notice: The reader is expressly advised to carefully read, understand, and apply all safety precautions and warnings described in this book or that might also be indicated in undertaking the activities and exercises described herein to minimize risk of personal injury or injury to others. Common sense and good judgment should also be exercised and applied to help avoid all potential hazards. The reader should always refer to the appropriate manufacturer's technical information, directions, and recommendations; then proceed with care to follow specific equipment operating instructions. The reader should understand these notices and cautions are not exhaustive.

The publisher makes no warranty or representation whatsoever, either expressed or implied, including but not limited to equipment, procedures, and applications described or referred to herein, their quality, performance, merchantability, or fitness for a particular purpose. The publisher assumes no responsibility for any changes, errors, or omissions in this book. The publisher specifically disclaims any liability whatsoever, including any direct, indirect, incidental, consequential, special, or exemplary damages resulting, in whole or in part, from the reader's use or reliance upon the information, instructions, procedures, warnings, cautions, applications, or other matter contained in this book. The publisher assumes no responsibility for the activities of the reader.

The Goodheart-Willcox Company, Inc. Internet Disclaimer: The Internet listings provided in this text link to additional resource information. Every attempt has been made to ensure these sites offer accurate, informative, safe, and appropriate information. However, Goodheart-Willcox Publisher has no control over these websites. The publisher makes no representation whatsoever, either expressed or implied, regarding the content of these websites. Because many websites contain links to other sites (some of which may be inappropriate), the publisher urges teachers to review all websites before students use them. Note that Internet sites may be temporarily or permanently inaccessible by the time readers attempt to use them.

 The Career Clusters icons are being used with permission of the States' Career Clusters Initiative

Library of Congress Cataloging-in-Publication Data

West, Dorothy F.
  Nutrition & wellness for life / Dorothy F. West.
    p. cm.
  Rev. ed. of: Nutrition, food, and fitness. c2006.
  Includes index.
  ISBN 978-1-60525-446-3
  1. Nutrition. 2. Physical fitness-Nutritional aspects. 3. Health.
  I. West, Dorothy F. Nutrition, food, and fitness. II. Title.
  III. Title: Nutrition and wellness for life.
  RA784.W48 2012
  613.2-dc22
                                                    2011010625

Front cover image: Shutterstock Images LLC
Back cover image: © Masterfile Corporation

Introduction

Nutrition & Wellness for Life stresses the crucial roles nutritious diet and daily physical activity play in health throughout the life span. The text will help you understand how your decisions affect your state of wellness at the various stages of the life cycle.

The body's need for various nutrients may be greater at some stages of the life cycle. This text helps you understand the sources and functions of the nutrients your body requires for a lifetime of optimal health. You will learn how to achieve healthy weight and body composition by balancing energy. The text also discusses the health consequences and possible causes of abnormal eating and exercise patterns.

Nutrition & Wellness for Life explores strategies for staying physically active through the life span. It covers the special needs of the competitive athlete. The text also discusses the relationship between social and mental health and your nutrition and activity. You will learn to recognize sources of stress and healthy strategies for reducing their impact on your total wellness.

Healthy eating requires planning and preparation. The text discusses safe food handling as well as healthy menu planning and food preparation techniques. It also explores considerations when selecting various nutrition and wellness products and services.

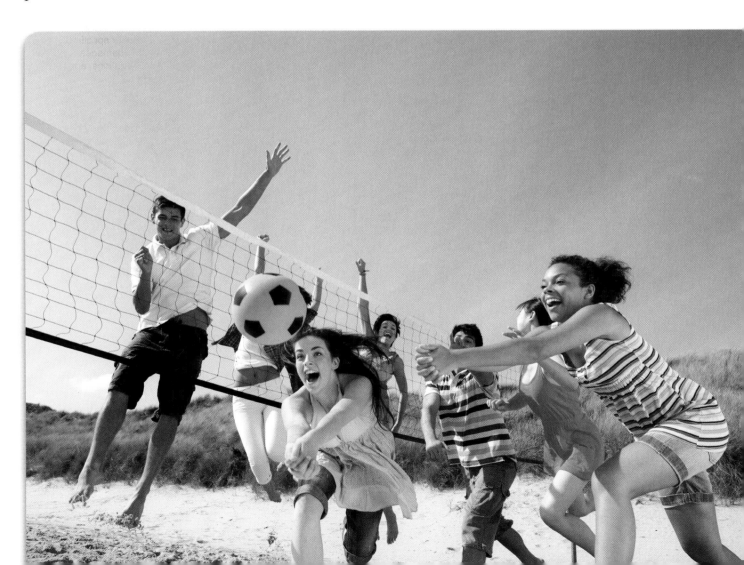

About the Author

Dorothy West attended Pennsylvania State University where she earned a bachelor's degree in dietetics and master's degree in teacher education with an emphasis on family and consumer sciences. Dorothy received her doctorate in teacher education with an emphasis on home economics secondary education and family resource management from Michigan State University. She stayed on to serve as an associate professor in the Department of Family and Child Ecology. She has developed and taught courses on curriculum, evaluation, and strategies for teaching nutrition at the secondary level. Dorothy played an active role in writing nutrition curriculum for the Michigan State Department of Education.

Dorothy has taught in the Netherlands, Okinawa, and England. She served as Chairperson of the Social Sciences Department at the LCC International University in Lithuania and taught foods courses at Kodaikanal International School in India. She played a role in the development of the International Baccalaureate (IB) middle school food technology curriculum materials. During her career, Dorothy has been active in membership and leadership roles with the Michigan Association of Family and Consumer Sciences (MAFCS) and American Association of Family and Consumer Sciences (AAFCS).

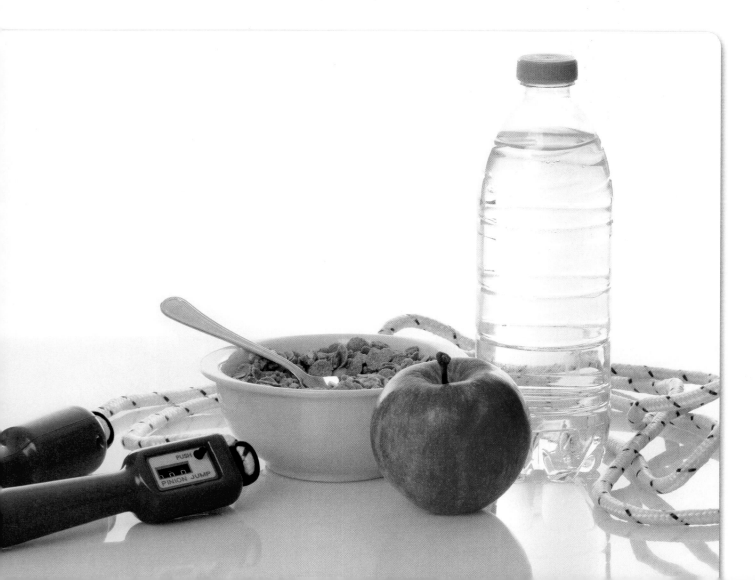

Acknowledgments

The author and Goodheart-Willcox Publisher would like to thank the following professionals who provided valuable input:

Contributing Author

Martha Dunn-Strohecker, Ph.D., CFCS
Author of Family and Consumer Sciences Textbooks and Faculty Member, North Shore Community College
Marblehead, Massachusetts

Reviewers

Carol Byrd-Bredbenner, Ph.D., R.D.
Nutrition Professor and Specialist
Chair, Family and Consumer Sciences
Rutgers, The State University of New Jersey
New Brunswick, New Jersey

Barb Hancock-Henley
Educational Specialist, Family and Consumer Sciences
Henrico County Public Schools
Highland Springs, Virginia

Lee Ann Napier
Culinary Arts Instructor
Scott County High School
Georgetown, Kentucky

Carol Newman
Family and Consumer Sciences Instructor
Northeast High School
Pasadena, Maryland

Janice Sullivan
Family and Consumer Sciences Instructor
Southington High School
Southington, Connecticut

LuAnn L. Soliah, Ph.D., R.D.
Professor and Director of Dietetics Program
Baylor University
Waco, Texas

Healthy Cooking Techniques and Recipes

Brief how-to's explain six different healthy cooking techniques

Part One
Food Habits: A Lifestyle Choice

Chapter 1 Making Wellness a Lifestyle
Chapter 2 Factors Affecting Food Choices
Chapter 3 How Nutrients Become You
Chapter 4 Nutrition Guidelines

22

Grilling

Grilling is a popular preparation method used to cook many types of foods including meats, fish, poultry, fruits, and vegetables. Today, you might find pineapple spears and hearts of romaine grilling alongside steak.

Grilling uses high heat to cook foods. The heat source is located below the food. Food is placed on a grate over the heat source. As the food cooks, juices and fat drip onto the heat source creating smoke. The smoke imparts a unique flavor to the food. Grilling is a healthy cooking method because fat is able to drip away from the food.

Successful grilling begins with a preheated grill. When foods are placed on a cool grill, they are more likely to stick or tear. A hot grill is also necessary to create the grill marks that are the trademark of properly grilled foods. Before food is placed on the grill, it must be clean. Use a wire brush to clean the grate and help prevent sticking. Brush the food with a light coating of oil before placing on the grill to avoid sticking and tearing. Always place the "good" side of the food on the grill first. Be sure not to move the food until the grill marks have formed. Use long tongs or a spatula—not a fork—to turn foods. A fork punctures the food allowing juices to escape and food to dry out.

Grilling is not appropriate for tougher cuts of meat. These cuts require long cooking at lower temperatures to become tender.

Grilled Peach Salad (6 servings)

Ingredients

- 1½ tablespoons vegetable oil
- 4 firm, ripe peaches
- 1 ounce Parmesan cheese, large shred
- 3 tablespoons pine nuts, toasted
- 4 ounces baby lettuce
- ¼ cup balsamic vinaigrette

Directions

1. Preheat grill to medium heat.
2. Halve and pit unpeeled peaches. Cut each half into 3 wedges and lightly brush with oil.
3. Place pine nuts on a sheet pan in a 300°F oven for 10 minutes until lightly browned. Shake pan after about 5 minutes to ensure even browning.
4. Place wedges on grill. Cook for about 2 minutes on each side.
5. Arrange 4 wedges on a bed of lettuce. Sprinkle with grated cheese and pine nuts. Drizzle with vinaigrette.

Part Six
Making Informed Choices

Chapter 20 Keeping Food Safe
Chapter 21 Meal Management
Chapter 22 Become an Informed Consumer

466

Poaching

Poaching is a food preparation method that uses gentle heat and liquid to cook food. This method is favored for delicate foods such as fish. The poaching liquid is often flavored to enhance the taste of the food being cooked. For example, a mixture of onions, carrots, and celery called *mirepoix* is often added. Other seasonings such as herbs, spices, vinegar, or lemon juice can be added to the poaching liquid as well. There are two ways to poach foods—shallow or deep poaching. Food is fully submerged in the liquid when using deep-poaching method. Shallow poaching uses only enough liquid to cover the food about halfway.

To poach properly, the temperature of the poaching liquid must be maintained between 160°F and 180°F. If you do not have a thermometer, use visual cues to maintain the appropriate temperature. Poaching liquid should barely move with small bubbles breaking the surface occasionally. If the poaching liquid becomes too hot, the food may disintegrate or become tough and rubbery. The fish is gently simmered until the flesh is opaque and flaky. The cooking liquid can be reduced and served as a sauce to accompany the fish.

Poaching is often used on foods such as fish, chicken, or eggs. It is a healthy cooking method because no fat is needed and the natural flavors and nutrients of the food are preserved.

Poached Salmon (6 servings)

Ingredients

- 1 tablespoon canola oil
- ½ cup onion, chopped
- ½ cup carrots, chopped
- ½ cup celery, chopped
- 4 cups water
- 1 lemon, sliced
- salt and pepper to taste
- 1½ pounds salmon fillets

Directions

1. In a large skillet, heat the oil and sauté the onions, carrots, and celery for 5 minutes. Add the water, lemon slices, and salt and pepper to the skillet. Let the mixture simmer for 5 additional minutes.
2. Place the salmon in liquid. Lower the heat and cook gently for about 15 minutes or until flesh is opaque and flaky. Cooking liquid should not be allowed to simmer or boil.
3. Remove salmon from the skillet carefully with a slotted spoon or spatula and serve hot.

467

Recipe examples incorporate the featured cooking technique

Chapter Openers

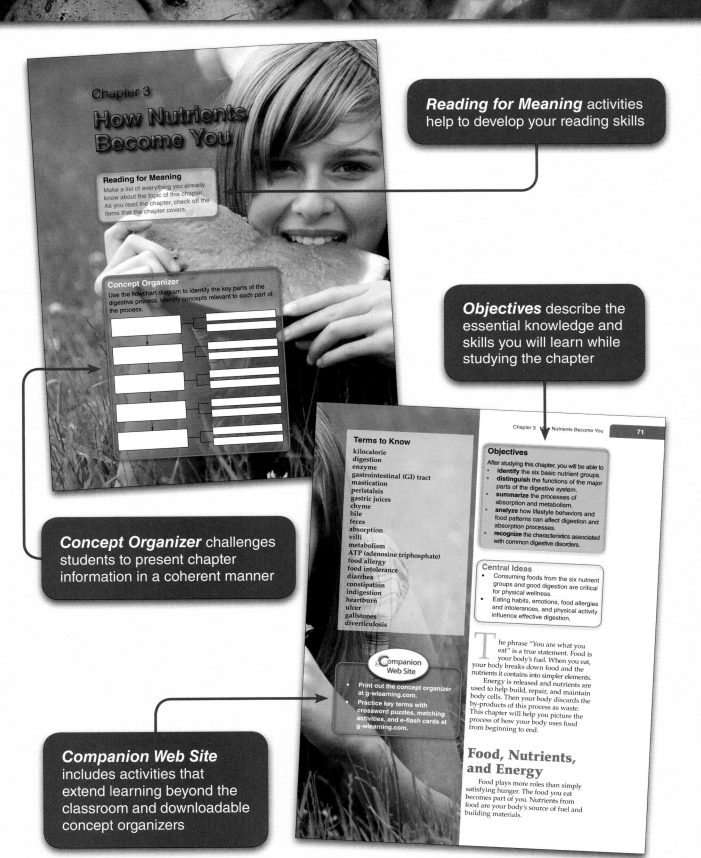

Reading for Meaning activities help to develop your reading skills

Objectives describe the essential knowledge and skills you will learn while studying the chapter

Concept Organizer challenges students to present chapter information in a coherent manner

Companion Web Site includes activities that extend learning beyond the classroom and downloadable concept organizers

Chapter 3

How Nutrients Become You

Reading for Meaning
Make a list of everything you already know about the topic of this chapter. As you read the chapter, check off the items that the chapter covers.

Concept Organizer
Use the flowchart diagram to identify the key parts of the digestive process. Identify concepts relevant to each part of the process.

Chapter 3   How Nutrients Become You   71

Terms to Know

kilocalorie
digestion
enzyme
gastrointestinal (GI) tract
mastication
peristalsis
gastric juices
chyme
bile
feces
absorption
villi
metabolism
ATP (adenosine triphosphate)
food allergy
food intolerance
diarrhea
constipation
indigestion
heartburn
ulcer
gallstones
diverticulosis

Companion Web Site
- Print out the concept organizer at g-wlearning.com.
- Practice key terms with crossword puzzles, matching activities, and e-flash cards at g-wlearning.com.

Objectives
After studying this chapter, you will be able to
- **identify** the six basic nutrient groups.
- **distinguish** the functions of the major parts of the digestive system.
- **summarize** the processes of absorption and metabolism.
- **analyze** how lifestyle behaviors and food patterns can affect digestion and absorption processes.
- **recognize** the characteristics associated with common digestive disorders.

Central Ideas
- Consuming foods from the six nutrient groups and good digestion are critical for physical wellness.
- Eating habits, emotions, food allergies and intolerances, and physical activity influence effective digestion.

The phrase "You are what you eat" is a true statement. Food is your body's fuel. When you eat, your body breaks down food and the nutrients it contains into simpler elements. Energy is released and nutrients are used to help build, repair, and maintain body cells. Then your body discards the by-products of this process as waste. This chapter will help you picture the process of how your body uses food from beginning to end.

Food, Nutrients, and Energy

Food plays more roles than simply satisfying hunger. The food you eat becomes part of you. Nutrients from food are your body's source of fuel and building materials.

Chapter Features

8

Chapter 17 Maintaining Positive Social and Mental Health **407**

Characteristics of Positive Mental and Social Health

Positive mental and social health may be reflected in someone who

- maintains a positive self-image
- respects and takes good care of self
- finds pleasure in life; is happy and active most of the time
- shows awareness of personal thoughts and feelings and can express them in positive ways
- works to meet daily problems and challenges
- is not afraid to face problems and is willing to seek help when crises arise
- plans for achieving future goals
- enjoys humor and can laugh at self
- knows how to end personal relationships that are hurtful
- shows interest in learning and growing from mistakes and can accept criticism
- tolerates frustration without undue anger
- works well in group situations
- continues to work with an individual or group even when his or her ideas are rejected
- develops talents and abilities to their fullest
- enjoys positive interpersonal relations with people of both sexes
- genuinely likes people and shows interest in meeting new people
- considers the needs and rights of others when expressing personal needs and rights
- respects differences in appearances, race, religion, interests, and abilities

17-10 People who display many of these characteristics tend to have positive views of themselves and strong relationships with others.

Mentally healthy people are likely to view life's challenges as opportunities for growth. When an event occurs, they identify the issues involved. They think clearly about their goals. Then they search for solutions to resolve the problem. If a situation becomes too overwhelming, mentally healthy people are not afraid to ask others for help.

Self-Concept and Mental Health

Your **self-concept** is the idea you have about yourself. It is how you see your behavior in relation to other people and tasks. Part of having good mental health is having a positive self-concept. You have a realistic view of

Extend Your Knowledge

Community Programs to Support Social and Mental Health

Develop a proposal for a community-based program to promote better social or mental health among the residents in the community. State the overall goal of the program. Give reasons why this program is needed and how it will achieve the goal. Provide a brief description of how the program would operate, who would oversee it, and the population served by it. Estimate the cost to start and maintain the program for one year. Find two references from literature or professionals in the field to support your program goals and cost estimates.

Colorful charts amplify concepts presented in the text.

Extend Your Knowledge feature encourages you to seek more facts on one or more chapter topics

Wellness Tips suggest ways to promote health and fitness in your life

---

430 Part Five Other Aspects of Wellness

Extend Your Knowledge

Personality, Stress, and Health

Research the relationship between personality types and stress responses. Ask the school counselor for references identifying literature on personality types. How does personality type affect the risk of health problems? Summarize your findings with a poster presentation.

Managing Stress

You cannot avoid all stress. However, you can learn to manage it. Most healthy, productive people search for ways to manage the stress in their lives. Stress management provides them with opportunities for personal growth. Viewing stress as positive allows people the chance to be creative. Learning how to adapt to negative stress helps people rationally deal with the changes that occur throughout life.

You can use a number of techniques to help you manage stress. Begin by learning to recognize the signs of stress. Rely on available

support systems. Learn how to relax and use positive self-talk.

The key is to choose the methods that most easily fit into your lifestyle. Combine a variety of methods for greatest effects on total health. Be sensitive to other techniques that seem to help you relax.

At the very least, learning how to lessen the negative effects of stress can help you enjoy life more. At best, you can reduce your risks of disease and improve your state of wellness.

Recognize Signs of Stress

Identifying the warning signs of stress in your life is an important first step in stress management. Your emotions, behaviors, and physical health may all give you clues that negative stress is starting to take a toll. Frustration, irritability, and depression are common emotional signs of distress. Withdrawing from friends, grinding your teeth, and forgetting details are behaviors that may warn you of negative stress. Headaches, upset stomach, and fatigue are health indicators that you may have too much stress in your life.

You can learn to read your body's stress signals through biofeedback. **Biofeedback** is a technique of focusing on involuntary bodily processes in order to control them. Using biofeedback involves being aware of such conditions as your breath and pulse rates. Hard breathing or a rapid pulse rate may be a sign of distress. When you realize you are breathing hard or your pulse is racing, you will know you may be under stress. Then you can make a conscious effort to relax and bring your breathing and pulse back to normal levels. Through biofeedback, you may be able to avoid a headache or calm a nervous stomach caused by stress.

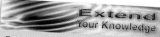

Wellness Tip

Laughter—Medicine for Stress

Have you ever noticed how good you feel after a good, hearty laugh? Research shows that laughter is an excellent source of stress relief. Not only does a hearty laugh reduce levels of stress hormones like *adrenaline*, it also increases beneficial hormones like *endorphins*. The next time you feel stressed or frustrated, laugh about the situation instead of worrying over it, watch a funny movie or your favorite cartoon, read a joke book, or join some friends for an evening of fun and laughter.

Chapter Features

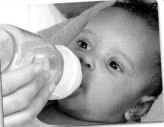

an increased volume of body fluids to support their developing babies. Lactating women need fluids to produce breast milk. People on high-protein diets require extra water to rid their bodies of the waste products of protein metabolism. A buildup of these waste products can cause kidney damage.

Older adults have the same need for fluids as young adults. The thirst mechanism of older adults can change and fluid intake can be affected. Some older adults choose to limit water intake if they have urinary incontinence problems. This requires medical treatment to avoid dehydration. Adequate fluid intake is necessary for continued good health through the aging years.

10-4 Infants need more water per unit of body weight than children and adults.

Math Link

Making Conversions

According to the Dietary Reference Intakes for water, the AI for 14- to 18-year-old males is 3.3 liters per day and 2.3 liters per day for females in this age range. Liters (L) and milliliters (mL) are metric system units used to measure volume. The following are common U.S. and metric system conversions:

1 L = 1000 mL
30 mL = 1 fl. oz.
8 fl. oz. = 1 cup
4 cups = 1 quart

1. Convert the AIs for 14- to 18-year-old males and females from liters to fluid ounces. (round up to one decimal)
2. Convert the fluid ounces to cups for both groups.

Supplying the Body's Water Needs

Drinking liquids generally supplies the greatest amount of fluids. Of course, plain water is a pure source of this vital nutrient. However, milk, soft drinks, juices, broth, tea, and other liquids also have high water content.

You may be surprised to learn foods supply almost as much of your daily water needs as liquids. Most foods contain some water. Some foods are higher in water content than others. As an example, summer squash is 96 percent water, whereas orange juice is only 87 percent water. Even foods that look solid are a source of water. For instance, bread is 36 percent water. Butter and margarine contain water, but cooking oils and meat fats do not, **10-5**.

Roughly 12 percent of your water needs are met through metabolism. When carbohydrates, fats, and proteins are broken down in the body, some water is released. Your body can then use this water in other chemical reactions.

Career boxes explore the education requirements and job outlook for various careers in the nutrition and wellness industries

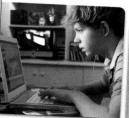

13-5   Students need to balance time spent in sedentary study with time spent in physical activity.

Education & Training

Sports Nutrition Consultant

Sports nutrition consultants work under contract with healthcare facilities or in their own private practice. They perform nutrition screenings for their clients and offer advice on diet-related concerns related to sports nutrition. Some work for wellness programs, sports teams, and coaches.

Education: Sports nutrition consultants need at least a bachelor's degree. Licensure, certification, or registration requirements vary by state.

Job Outlook: Applicants with specialized training, an advanced degree, or certifications beyond the particular state's minimum requirement should enjoy the best job opportunities. Employment is expected to increase.

Losing Excess Body Fat

People who are overweight due to excess body fat would improve their health by reducing their fat stores. Creating an energy imbalance is required for weight loss. Numerous strategies for accomplishing this goal are promoted in books and magazines. Some of these strategies are safe and effective, others are dangerous. Knowing some basic information can help overweight people make sound weight-management decisions.

People should consider several factors when thinking about beginning a weight-loss program. One factor is health status. Women should not try to lose weight during pregnancy. Nutritious foods and a minimum weight gain are required to ensure the health of a developing fetus. People who are ill should avoid restricting calories to lose weight. The body needs an adequate supply of nutrients to restore health.

Meeting these nutrient needs is difficult when calories are severely restricted.

Age is another issue to keep in mind when considering a plan to reduce body fat. Weight loss is not recommended for children and teens who are still growing. Losing weight could permanently stunt their growth. The recommendation for children and teens is to hold weight steady and grow into it. If a child is extremely obese, then health care supervision is needed.

People need to evaluate their motivation and body structure when considering weight loss. The main goal of weight management is good health. People who try extreme weight-loss methods to achieve an unrealistically slim appearance may put their health at risk. Remember, weight above a standard range is a health risk only if it is due to excess body fat. Weight due to muscle mass is not a cause for concern and does not indicate a need for weight loss.

Math Links provide opportunities to develop related math skills

important not to wait for the thirst begin consuming liquids. Older need to make a point of drinking they do not feel thirsty.

the body may lose a fair amount of fluid before signaling thirst. When the body either loses or takes in too much water, fluid imbalances result.

Replacing lost water is important in athletic performance. Athletic performance levels decline after a 3 percent loss in water weight. When water is lost from working muscles, blood volume decreases. The heart must pump harder to supply the same amount of energy. Mental concentration is affected as fluid losses increase. Some clear signs of dehydration are fatigue and lack of energy. Other symptoms may include dizziness, headache,

Effects of Water Loss

Because fluids make up a high percentage of your body weight, when you lose water, you also lose weight. Someone who wants to drop a few pounds may think this is good news. However, the weight you want to lose is fat, not water. Water weight is quickly regained when body fluids are replenished.

Even a small percentage weight drop due to water loss will make you feel uncomfortable. When you lose two percent of body weight in fluids, you will become aware of the sensation of thirst. Both the brain and the stomach play a role in making you aware there is a water imbalance. If you do not replace water losses, you may become dehydrated. **Dehydration** is a state in which the body contains a lower-than-normal amount of body fluids.

When dehydration occurs, the body takes steps to help conserve water. Hormones signal the kidneys to decrease urine output. Sweat production also declines. As the volume of fluid in the bloodstream drops, the concentration of sodium in the blood increases. The kidneys respond to the higher blood sodium level by retaining more water. These water-conserving efforts cannot prevent all fluid losses from the body. If fluids are not replaced, the damaging effects of dehydration will begin to take their toll.

Some older adults do not always recognize the thirst sensation. In cases such as

Case Study: Losing the Hydration Game

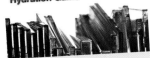

Taryn is a 15-year-old girl who lives in Denver, Colorado—also known as the "Mile High City." Taryn loves to spend many hours playing basketball outside in the summer months. It is hot, sunny, and dry in the summer. There is a water fountain in a building near the basketball court, but she does not bother to take the time to drink. Her friends tell her to bring a water bottle with her. She usually forgets the water and thinks it is not that important anyway. Sometimes she remembers on her way to the game and buys a can of soda from a vending machine.

Taryn is often disappointed with her game. She finds that she runs out of energy by mid-game and often gets a headache. She wants to improve so that she can make the high school team next year.

Case Review

1. What do you think is contributing to Taryn's disappointing performance on the basketball court?

2. Why do you think Taryn believes that water is not important?

Case Studies illustrate chapter concepts with real-life scenarios and follow-up questions

Chapter Review

Reading Summary reviews chapter content

Review Learning challenges your recall of content

Critical Thinking employs the higher level thinking skills

Reading Summary

Minerals are inorganic elements that can be divided into two classes. The macrominerals, or major minerals, include calcium, phosphorus, magnesium, sulfur, sodium, potassium, and chloride. The microminerals, or trace minerals, include iron, zinc, iodine, fluoride, selenium, copper, chromium, manganese, and molybdenum.

Although you need only small quantities of minerals, getting the right amounts is a key to good health. Without adequate intakes, deficiency symptoms can occur. At the same time, you need to avoid mineral excesses, which can be toxic.

Each mineral plays specific roles in the body. The vital functions of minerals include becoming part of body tissues. Many minerals help enzymes do their jobs. Some minerals help nerves work and muscles contract. Minerals also promote growth and control acid-base balance in the body. They help maintain fluid balance, too.

Minerals are widely found throughout the food supply. Selecting fresh and wholesome foods is preferred over the use of supplements. A health problem, such as osteoporosis, may require the use of a supplement. Choose a variety of plant and animal foods. Limit your use of highly processed foods. Eat the recommended daily amounts from each group in MyPlate. Following this basic nutrition advice should provide you with most of your mineral needs.

Review Learning

1. True or false. Because they are needed in larger amounts, macrominerals are more important for health than microminerals.
2. Where is nearly all the calcium in the body stored?
3. Which group from MyPlate is the primary source of calcium?
4. Give two reasons women are at greater risk than men for developing osteoporosis.
5. What is the relationship of meeting adequate phosphorus needs to good health?
6. What are five dietary sources of magnesium?
7. Where are high concentrations of sulfur found in the body?
8. What process helps equalize the fluid balance inside and outside of body cells?
9. What is the pH of a neutral substance, such as water?
10. What minerals are contributed by salt, and what is the primary source of

---

18. Name two microminerals other than iron, zinc, iodine, fluoride, and selenium and give a function of each.
19. What are three factors that affect the mineral content of plant foods?
20. True or false. An excess of some minerals can interfere with the absorption of others.

Critical Thinking

21. **Identify evidence.** What evidence can you give about whether it is better to eat whole, fresh foods or take supplements for minerals that may be lacking in the diet?
22. **Analyze behavior.** What human behaviors are detrimental to absorption of essential minerals?

Applying Your Knowledge

23. **Menu plan.** Write a one-day menu that meets the RDA for calcium for a friend who refuses to drink milk. Your friend is not lactose-intolerant and likes cheese and other dairy products.
24. **Showcase display.** Create a showcase display titled "Tracking the Sodium in Your Diet." Mount labels illustrating the high sodium content of popular snack foods and convenience products. Beside each label, identify the sodium content of a low-sodium alternative. Include information on how to read the Nutrition Facts panel to determine foods that are low in sodium.
25. **Mineral brochure.** Prepare a brochure describing factors that increase and decrease mineral absorption and availability. Share your brochures at school.
26. **Food technique.** Select one of the techniques for choosing, preparing, and/or storing foods carefully to maximize the mineral content of your diet. Implement the technique in your personal life. Share the change you have made with the class.

Technology Connections

27. **Prepare a PSA.** Select one of the minerals discussed in this chapter. Research the health benefits associated with consumption of that mineral. Using the information from your research, write and video-record a public service announcement (PSA) promoting the benefits and sources of the mineral you selected.
28. **Sodium quiz.** Sodium intake is a controllable risk factor for high blood pressure. Take *The Scoop on Sodium* quiz on the American Heart Association Web site to test your knowledge about sodium and your health.
29. **Electronic presentation.** Research recommendations for teens on the use and selection of mineral supplements on the National Institutes for Health Web site. Prepare an electronic presentation to communicate what you learn with others.

---

30. **Calcium quiz.** Take the *Calcium Quiz* on the Dairy Council of California Web site to assess your calcium intake. Complete the section on goals for increasing or maintaining calcium in your diet and print them off as a reminder.

Academic Connections

31. **Science.** With the help of the science department, use litmus paper to identify the pH of 10 food items and record your findings in a chart. Then investigate why eating foods that are acidic does not drastically affect the pH of your digestive tract. Share what you learn in a brief oral report.
32. **Speech.** Working in pairs, role-play a discussion between two people—one loves fruits and vegetables and the other does not. The fruit and vegetable lover must convince the other person to try new foods rich in minerals and vitamins.
33. **Math.** Keep a one-day food diary of all the food and beverages you consume. Include amounts of any salt added to your food at the table. Use food labels, appendix C, or Internet nutrient analysis to determine the total milligrams of sodium consumed. The *Dietary Guidelines* recommendation is not to exceed 2,300 milligrams of sodium in one day. Calculate your intake as a percent of the recommended maximum intake of 2,300 milligrams.
34. **History.** Learn about the history of iodine. Who discovered it? Was that person searching for an essential mineral when he or she discovered iodine? Write a brief paper summarizing your findings.
35. **Science.** Use a reliable anatomy and physiology resource to investigate the urinary system's role in regulating fluid-electrolyte balance in humans. Write a brief summary describing the role of the various system organs.

Workplace Applications

Interpersonal Skills

Presume you are a dietitian. Your interpersonal skills—your ability to listen, speak, and empathize—are a great asset in working with clients. Lilly is your latest client. She was recently diagnosed with osteoporosis. In addition to the medicine her doctor prescribed, Lilly was instructed to seek nutrition counseling about ways to increase the calcium in her diet. What calcium-rich foods would you recommend to Lilly? How much should she have daily?

Technology Connections encourages exploration of chapter concepts using various technologies

Workplace Applications relate chapter content to the work setting

Applying Your Knowledge actively engages you in the learning process

Academic Connections activities strengthen skills in core areas, such as history, math, science, and social studies

Appendixes

Appendix A

Career Planning

Appendix A: Career Planning outlines choosing a career, finding meaningful employment, succeeding on the job, making a job change, and entrepreneurship

Appendix B

Eating Well with Canada's Food Guide

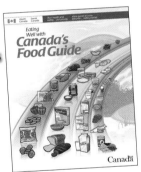

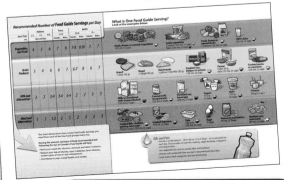

Appendix B: Eating Well with Canada's Food Guide identifies and promotes healthy eating for consumers

Appendix C

Dietary Reference Intakes

Appendix C: Dietary Reference Intakes includes current Recommended Dietary Allowances and Adequate Intakes, and Tolerable Upper Intakes Levels for vitamins and minerals

Appendixes

Appendix D: Nutritive Value of Foods is a comprehensive list of foods and their nutrient content

Appendix E: Exchange Lists for Meal Planning classifies foods into groups of similar nutrient and caloric content

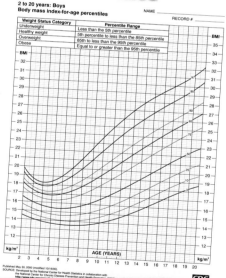

Appendix F: Body Mass Index-for-Age Percentiles graph weight status

Contents

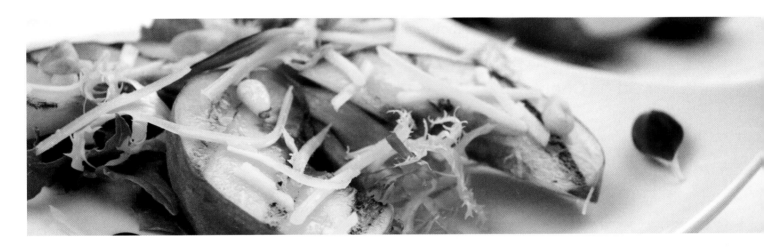

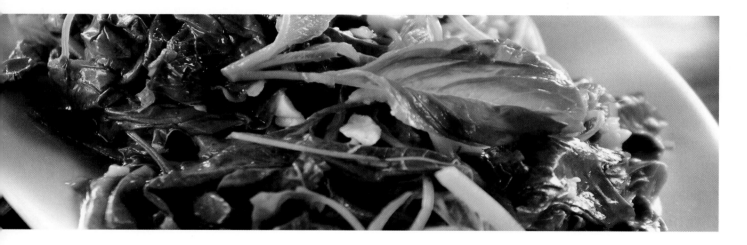

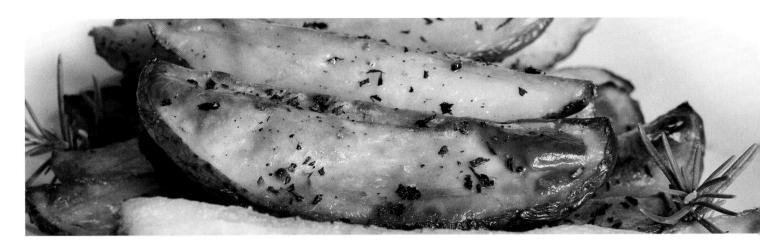

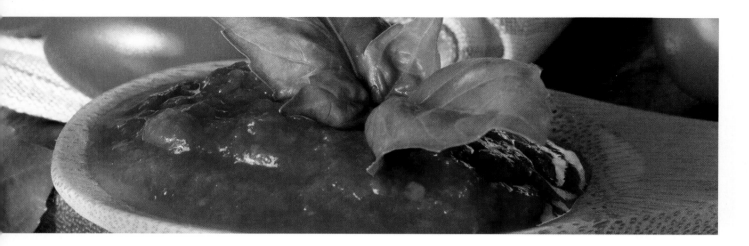

Chapter 18   Stress and Wellness   420

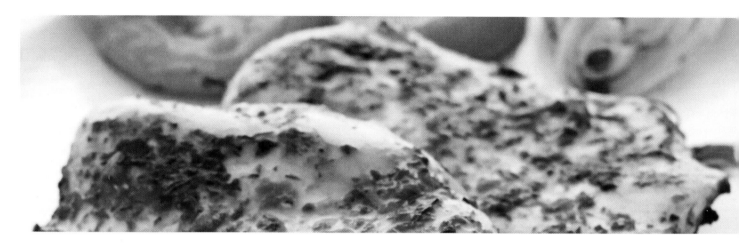

Chapter 19   Drug and Supplement Use and Your Health   440

Part Six
Making Informed Choices   466

Chapter 20   Keeping Food Safe   468

Chapter 21   Meal Management   490

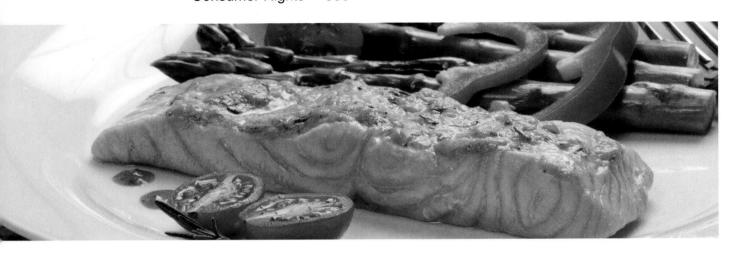

Features

Part Content

Wellness Tip

Featured Careers

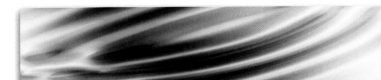

Extend Your Knowledge

Case Study

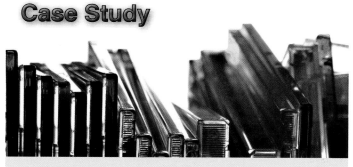

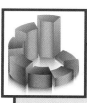

Math Link

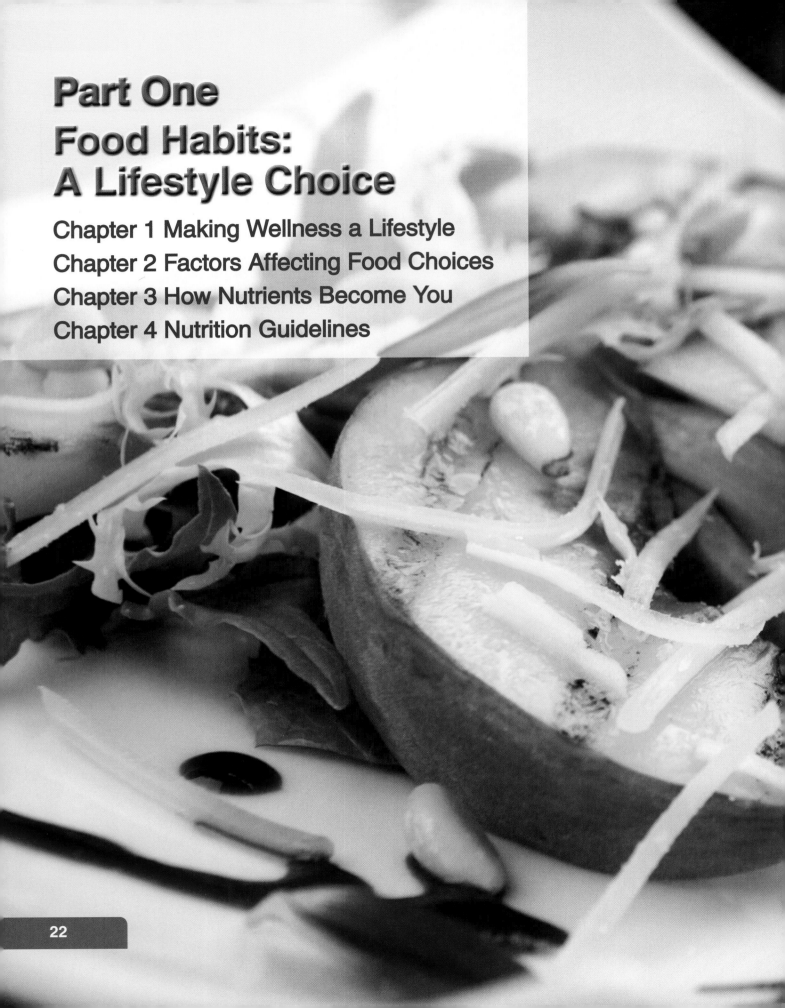

Part One
Food Habits:
A Lifestyle Choice

Grilling

Grilling is a popular preparation method used to cook many types of foods including meats, fish, poultry, fruits, and vegetables. Today, you might find pineapple spears and hearts of romaine grilling alongside steak.

Grilling uses high heat to cook foods. The heat source is located below the food. Food is placed on a grate over the heat source. As the food cooks, juices and fat drip onto the heat source creating smoke. The smoke imparts a unique flavor to the food. Grilling is a healthy cooking method because fat is able to drip away from the food.

Successful grilling begins with a preheated grill. When foods are placed on a cool grill, they are more likely to stick or tear. A hot grill is also necessary to create the grill marks that are the trademark of properly grilled foods. Before food is placed on the grill, it must be clean. Use a wire brush to clean the grate and help prevent sticking. Brush the food with a light coating of oil before placing on the grill to avoid sticking and tearing. Always place the "good" side of the food on the grill first. Be sure not to move the food until the grill marks have formed. Use long tongs or a spatula—not a fork—to turn foods. A fork punctures the food allowing juices to escape and food to dry out.

Grilling is not appropriate for tougher cuts of meat. These cuts require long cooking at lower temperatures to become tender.

Grilled Peach Salad (6 servings)

Ingredients

- 1½ tablespoons vegetable oil
- 4 firm, ripe peaches
- 1 ounce Parmesan cheese, large shred
- 3 tablespoons pine nuts, toasted
- 4 ounces baby lettuce
- ¼ cup balsamic vinaigrette

Directions

1. Preheat grill to medium heat.
2. Halve and pit unpeeled peaches. Cut each half into 3 wedges and lightly brush with oil.
3. Place pine nuts on a sheet pan in a 300°F oven for 10 minutes until lightly browned. Shake pan after about 5 minutes to ensure even browning.
4. Place wedges on grill. Cook for about 2 minutes on each side.
5. Arrange 4 wedges on a bed of lettuce. Sprinkle with grated cheese and pine nuts. Drizzle with vinaigrette.

Chapter 1
Making Wellness a Lifestyle

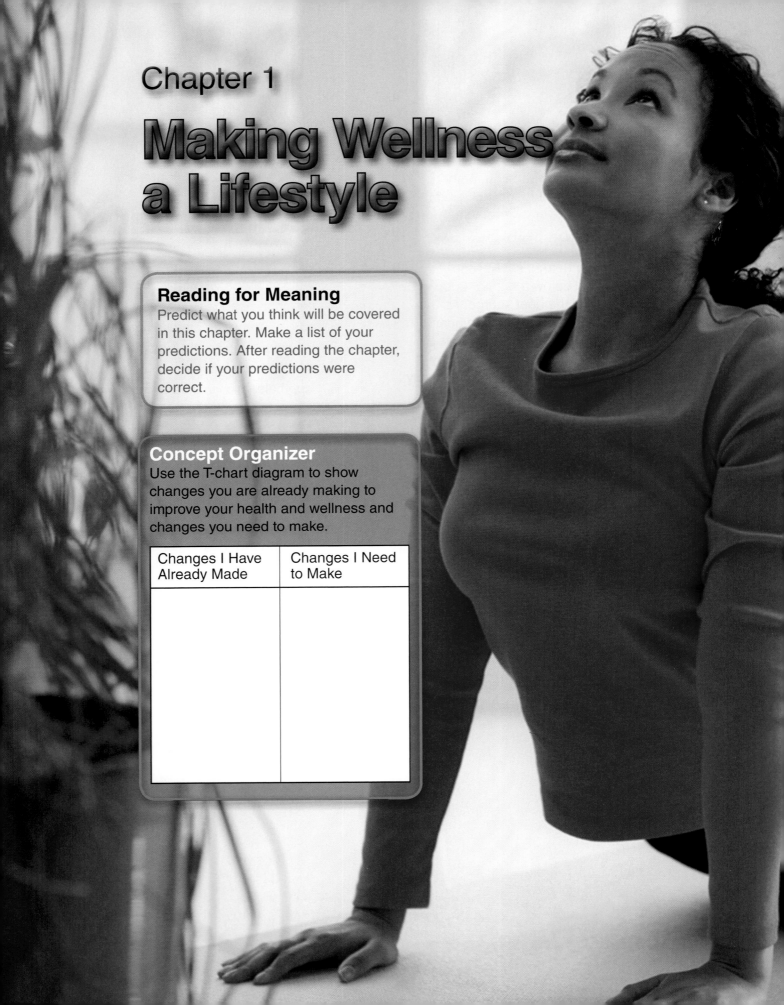

Reading for Meaning
Predict what you think will be covered in this chapter. Make a list of your predictions. After reading the chapter, decide if your predictions were correct.

Concept Organizer
Use the T-chart diagram to show changes you are already making to improve your health and wellness and changes you need to make.

Changes I Have Already Made	Changes I Need to Make

Terms to Know

wellness
quality of life
premature death
optimum health
physical health
stress
mental health
social health
holistic medicine
risk factor
environmental quality
diagnosis
diet
peer pressure
nutrition
nutrient
scientific method
hypothesis
theory
life expectancy

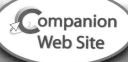

Companion Web Site

- **Print out the concept organizer at g-wlearning.com.**
- **Practice key terms with crossword puzzles, matching activities, and e-flash cards at g-wlearning.com.**

Objectives

After studying this chapter, you will be able to

- **summarize** how physical, mental, and social aspects of wellness affect quality of life over the lifespan.
- **recall** factors that contribute to disease.
- **distinguish** those factors that affect wellness over which you have control.
- **judge** how your lifestyle choices affect your health now and in the future.
- **implement** a behavior-change contract to improve your health.
- **evaluate** the importance of nutrition research for making healthy food choices.
- **understand** why the use of the scientific process is important when conducting nutrition research.

Central Ideas

- Total wellness involves your physical health, mental health, and social health throughout life.
- You can choose healthful behaviors such as eating right, staying fit, and managing stress to help meet your wellness goals.

You make choices every day that affect how you feel, think, and act. You decide what you will eat and when you will sleep. You choose how physically active you will be, too. Your actions affect who you are now and the person you will become. You are responsible for making decisions that benefit your health.

How healthy will you be 10 years from now? You could be healthier and in better physical shape than you are now! Choosing behaviors that promote health can have lifelong benefits. You can take steps to feel just as fit at age 50 as you do at age 15.

What Is Wellness?

Wellness is the state of being in good health. Wellness is often associated with quality of life. **Quality of life** refers to a person's satisfaction with his or her looks, lifestyle, and responses to daily events. When people are in good health, they have a desire to stay fit and live a healthful lifestyle. They are energetic and have an enthusiastic outlook. They are able to successfully meet the challenges of each day. When people are not in good health, life's events can become harder to manage. This causes a decrease in quality of life.

Most people want to continually improve their quality of life as they grow and mature. Trying to achieve a high level of wellness is one way to improve quality of life.

The Wellness Continuum

You can use a continuum to define your personal state of wellness. Premature death is at one end of the continuum and optimum health is at the other. **Premature death** is death that occurs due to lifestyle behaviors that lead to a fatal accident or the formation of an avoidable disease. **Optimum health** is a state of wellness characterized by peak physical, mental, and social well-being, **1-1**.

Your health status determines your place along the wellness continuum. Being free from illness and having much energy indicate that you have a high level of physical wellness. If you are able to cope with life's challenges and maintain stable relationships, you exhibit mental and social wellness, too. This means you probably fall near the optimum health end of the continuum. A short-term decline in any of these areas may temporarily move you toward the other end of the continuum. However, the key is your overall state of health most of the time. This is your wellness point.

If you are already at optimum health, you will want to find out how to maintain this state of wellness. If you are not at optimum health, you can learn how to change your lifestyle to move toward that goal. The key to achieving wellness rests with you. No one can force you to change. Moving toward optimum health happens because you want change to happen.

Once you begin taking steps to improve your health, you will start to notice the benefits. You might feel stronger and more alert. You may begin to feel better about yourself. Maybe you will find it easier to cope with the daily problems of life. Perhaps you will feel more satisfied with your performance at home, school, work, and play. You may begin to experience better relationships

Wellness Continuum	
Premature Death	**Optimum Health**
Low energy level	High energy level
Frequent illness	Infrequent illness and quick recovery from illness
Inferior stress management skills	Superior stress management skills
Poor social relationships	Excellent social relationships

1-1 Evaluate your physical, mental, and social health to determine where you fall along the wellness continuum.

with family members and friends. You may notice additional benefits of wellness in the future. Having optimum health will help you face the challenges of parenthood, career changes, and other aspects of active adult living.

Aspects of Wellness

Wellness means much more than not being sick. It also means more than eating healthful foods and being physically fit. There are three major components of wellness—physical, mental, and social health. Each contributes to your total sense of wellness in special ways. Together they affect how you look, feel, and act.

Physical Health

Physical health refers to the fitness of your body. It requires numerous body parts to work in harmony.

A number of factors can harm your physical health. For instance, getting too little rest will reduce your energy for exercising and doing chores. Eating too much or too fast may upset your stomach. Lack of physical activity, poor sanitation, and reckless actions can also keep your body below peak performance level. Too much stress can negatively impact your physical health. **Stress** is the inner agitation you feel in response to change. Tobacco and alcohol and other drugs can harm physical health, too. Choosing lifestyle behaviors that avoid these factors will help you stay in good physical health, **1-2**.

Health care professionals use medicine, physical therapy, diet, and surgery to care for the physical health of their patients. They keep informed on research about alternative treatments, such as the use of herbs and nutrient supplements. As the costs of health care

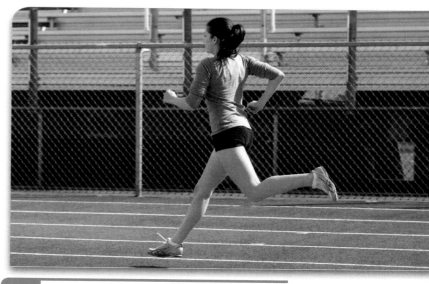

1-2 Getting regular exercise is an important requirement for maintaining good physical health.

services rise, people are becoming more interested in learning how to prevent disease. Doctors often suggest that patients combine medical care with lifestyle changes. You will read more about making lifestyle changes later in this chapter.

Mental Health

Have you ever felt stressed, depressed, and emotionally exhausted? These feelings may be related to your current state of mental health. **Mental health** has to do with the way you feel about yourself, your life, and the people around you. People with good mental health generally like themselves for who they are. They express positive attitudes and work to keep a balance in all aspects of their lives—socially, physically, spiritually, and emotionally. They tend to act according to a set of socially acceptable values. They may also hold beliefs that help them see their relationship to a larger universe. When problems arise, mentally healthy people seek ways to resolve problems.

Irrational fears, anxiety, and depression may be signs of a mental health problem, **1-3**. If you are concerned

Signs of Teen Mental Health Problems

- Becomes moody
- Withdraws from social activities and friends
- Is overactive and jumpy
- Acts and feels tired
- Worries about personal health problems
- Becomes aggressive with friends and family
- Loses concentration in class and does worse academically
- Has difficulty making decisions
- Feels life is too hard

1-3   A teen who is exhibiting these warning signs may need help.

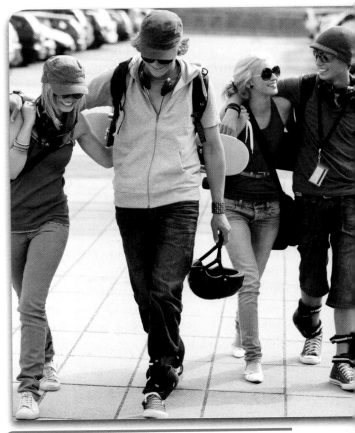

1-4   Positive interactions with friends contribute to a sense of social health.

about your mental health, you should talk to a trusted adult. Share concerns and problems with parents, teachers, counselors, or clergy persons. These people may be able to help you better understand who you are and what you want to become. Building effective communication and problem-solving skills can go a long way toward helping you improve your mental health.

Social Health

Social health describes the way you get along with other people. Friends and family members help enrich your life. Social health can be negatively affected when disagreements occur and problems arise. Learning to resolve conflicts with others is an important skill that can help you achieve and maintain good social health, **1-4**.

Social health is related to an understanding and acceptance of roles. People have different role expectations for sons, daughters, husbands, wives, mothers, fathers, girlfriends, boyfriends, teachers, students, employers, and employees. You may want to analyze your roles for possible conflicts. For instance, you may be expected to be a

follower in your role as an employee. However, you may be expected to be a leader in your role as team captain. Learning appropriate ways to act in each role can contribute to your social wellness.

Social health affects a person's outlook on life and his or her personal state of wellness. For example, a teen on a first date might become so nervous that he gets an upset stomach. A student who worries about being accepted among friends may find it hard to fall asleep at night.

Building social skills allows you to improve your social health. One such skill is learning how to use good communication to resolve conflicts with others. Seeking and lending support to people who need your help is another important social skill.

Building a positive self-image will also help you improve your relationships. Developing these skills will help you reach optimum social health. Reaching this optimum level means you can work, play, and interact with others cooperatively. Optimum social health contributes to your state of physical and mental health, too.

Learning how people develop physically, mentally, and socially can positively affect your sense of wellness. You may feel reassured in knowing you are normal in your growth patterns.

Holistic Approach to Wellness

Holistic medicine is an approach to health care that focuses on all aspects of patient care—physical, mental, and social. It evolved because many medical doctors saw links among physical, mental, and social health. Treatment programs and medicine may not be enough to cure a physical illness. The effect of physical treatment can depend on mental and social health. Low self-esteem or loneliness can reduce a person's desire to get better. These factors can also delay the healing process by impairing the function of the body's immune system. The trend is for health care professionals to work in teams when a sickness occurs. This provides greater insight for understanding the various components of how best to help a patient. Specialists, consultants, and mental health professionals work with each other to understand the various aspects of treatment to improve patient health.

A holistic approach to wellness is well-rounded. You need to be aware of your physical, mental, and social health needs. You must manage time, money, and other resources to address your needs in all these areas. If you spend

all your time working out, you may end up neglecting relationships. This would cause your social health to suffer at the expense of your physical health. If you spend all your money going out with friends, you may feel anxious because you cannot pay back the money you borrowed from your parents to buy new sports equipment. Your state of mental health may be reduced in favor of your social health. Taking a holistic approach to wellness means making choices that fit together to promote all facets of health, **1-5**.

Factors That Affect Wellness

Why is it important to recognize the impact of health-related decisions in the teen years? The reason is your present actions and attitudes are shaping the person you will be in the future. Habits are hard to change once established. This is true for good habits as well as bad habits. Once you take on an unhealthful behavior, you are more

A Holistic Approach to Wellness

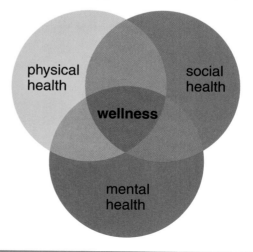

1-5 Physical health, mental health, and social health all contribute to a total sense of wellness.

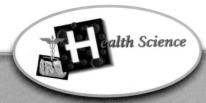

Health Science

Health Educators

Health educators encourage healthy lifestyles and wellness. They work with people to encourage behaviors that can prevent diseases, injuries, and other health problems. They cover such health-related topics as proper nutrition, exercise and fitness, avoiding sexually transmitted infections (STIs), and the habits and behaviors necessary to avoid illness. Health educators must be able to assess the needs of each group and tailor their educational programs to them. For example, programs for teens would vary greatly from programs for older adults because of the age and needs of each group.

Education: Entry-level positions generally require a bachelor's degree from a health education program. Courses in psychology, human development, and a foreign language are helpful. Experiences with internships or volunteer opportunities can make applicants more appealing to employers. A master's degree is generally required to work in public health.

Job Outlook: The demand will remain high. Due to the rising cost of health care and the need for people to learn how to live healthy lives, career opportunities for health educators will continue to increase.

likely to repeat it. Likewise, once you choose a healthful behavior, you can easily make it a regular part of your life.

Because you are responsible for making many decisions, you have much control over your personal state of wellness. You can engage in activities that lead to the decline of your health. You can also follow practices that help ensure good health.

Improving your odds for a long and healthy life requires an understanding of the consequences of poor choices. It also involves recognizing wise choices. Learning

about exercise, health care, and which foods best nourish your body will aid you in making wise choices.

Factors That Contribute to Disease

A **risk factor** is a characteristic or behavior that influences a person's chance of being injured or getting a disease. Researchers identify risk factors by studying the traits and actions of large groups of people. Then the researchers determine what effects these traits and behaviors have on the people's health.

Certain lifestyle habits, environmental conditions, and health care limitations are known to be risk factors you can control. Hereditary factors affect your risk of disease, too. Genetic research continues to explore ways to help people avoid or delay the onset of inherited diseases. However, heredity continues to be a factor that alerts people to their risk factors for specific diseases. Knowing your risk factors can encourage early prevention.

Unhealthful Lifestyle Choices

Heart disease, cancer, and stroke are three major causes of death among adults in the United States. The Centers for Disease Control and Prevention (CDC) estimate lifestyle choices account for about half the factors contributing to these diseases. One example of a lifestyle choice is a decision about smoking. Smoking is a risk factor for cancer and heart disease. If you choose to smoke, you are at increased risk of getting these diseases. On the other hand, choosing not to smoke lessens your chances of getting these diseases. Arming yourself with knowledge and the confidence to make healthful choices will help you avoid the pressure of peers and ad campaigns that tempt you to smoke.

Other lifestyle choices include decisions about the foods you eat, stress management, and exercise. You should avoid choices in each of these areas that increase your risk of disease. Eating large amounts of fast foods that are high in fats, refined sugars, and salt supplies your body with many calories, but little else that it needs for proper growth and development. Excess calories contribute to overweight, which increases the risk for many diseases. Failing to manage your time can increase your stress level, which can negatively affect your health. Spending little time being active or participating in sports can contribute to weight problems and other health risks.

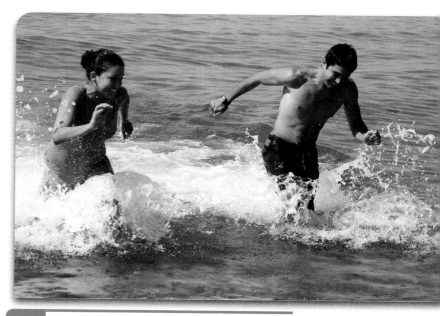

1-6 A high-quality environment that provides fresh air and clean water poses few health risks.

Poor Environmental Quality

Have you noticed when your classroom is hot and stuffy, your concentration on learning decreases? While your health may be not in danger, your learning ability may be slowed down. This is one example of how environmental factors affect quality of life.

About one-fifth of the risk factors that contribute to leading causes of death are related to poor environmental quality. **Environmental quality** refers to the state of the physical world around you. It relates to the safety of the water you drink, the air you breathe, and the food you eat. It also pertains to your exposure to the elements, **1- 6**.

Pollutants in water and air and contaminants in food decrease the quality of the environment. For example, consuming food that is improperly refrigerated can cause severe sickness. In countries where food, water, and shelter are scarce or unsafe, the quality of life is greatly reduced.

Some jobs require people to assume greater environmental health risks than others. You may want to think about the safety of the work environment as you evaluate career choices. Compare the job of an urban construction worker with that of a sales representative. What environmental risk factors can you identify in each job? Jobs that require the use of heavy equipment and exposure to dangerous conditions add risk to health and safety.

Inadequate Health Care

Inadequate health care is a factor that contributes to your health risk. Medicine is not an exact science. Doctors cannot always assess symptoms and test results to easily reach a correct diagnosis. A **diagnosis** is the identification of a disease. Failing to diagnose, or recognize, a disease early enough can interfere with effective treatment. Some health care facilities lack the specialists or equipment needed to treat certain diseases. Sometimes facilities are not managed well or treatments are not given properly.

Inadequate health care is not always the fault of medical professionals. Patients sometimes interfere with the quality of their health care. Some patients fail to get regular checkups, which are needed to help physicians evaluate and maintain patients' health. Other patients do not seek medical care soon enough when they are experiencing symptoms. Some patients may delay seeing a doctor due to a lack of health insurance or inability to pay. Others may hesitate out of fear.

Even when patients go to a physician, they can lessen the effectiveness of their care. They might not share important information with the physician. They might fail to follow the physician's advice. When you are a patient, you have a responsibility to play an active role in your medical care.

Heredity

Twenty-five percent of the factors that contribute to leading causes of death are hereditary. Inheriting these factors is beyond your control. Genes you received from your parents determine your body structure and other physical traits. Genes can also affect your likelihood of developing certain diseases, **1-7**.

Tracing your family's health history may provide vital information for you to manage your wellness. With this knowledge, you and your medical doctor can create a plan to keep you healthy. It may include lifestyle changes and more frequent visits with the doctor. There may be specific tests to detect the early onset of a known familial disease. For example, if your family health history includes type 2 diabetes, you may be at an increased risk for this disease. Being aware of this risk factor allows you to exert some control over it. You can eat healthy, get plenty of

Math Link

Calculating Percentages

Health-care professionals track and study surgical errors in order to improve their processes. This information is used to find ways to reduce errors during surgery. One process improvement that resulted was the use of a checklist of identifications, equipment used, and procedures completed before, during, and after surgery. The checklist was used to improve accuracy and patient care. One large hospital, that performs 500 surgeries each year, noticed the number of reported surgical errors decreased from five in 2009 to one in 2010.

1. Compute the decrease in surgical error rates. (Be careful with your decimals.)
2. If there were two errors next year, what would the error rate be?

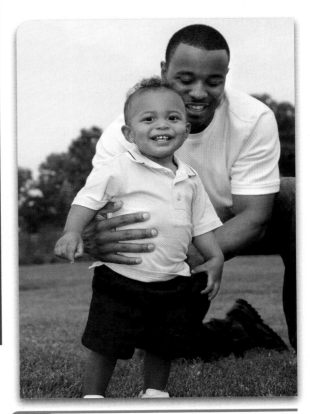

1-7 Some factors that affect health are inherited from parents.

exercise, and maintain a healthy body weight. Taking these steps may help you prevent type 2 diabetes.

You cannot change who your biological parents are. Likewise, you cannot change the genes you inherit from them. However, you can keep yourself in good physical condition. This helps you avert the influence of genetic risk factors. It also improves your body's ability to handle diseases if they do develop.

Health-Promoting Choices

Studies show you have much control over the factors that influence your health. Health care experts have identified certain behaviors that make a difference in a person's quality of life and wellness level. By choosing these behaviors regularly, you can promote good health and perhaps lengthen your life.

Choose a Healthful Lifestyle

Because you can control your lifestyle choices, you can also control some of your risks for disease. Your diet is a lifestyle factor that has a strong correlation with many diseases. **Diet** refers to all the foods and beverages you consume. You have a large amount of control over your diet. For example, you can choose to eat a diet rich in fruits, vegetables, and whole grain products. This choice helps reduce your risk of some cancers and leaves you feeling alert and active.

Choosing to become physically fit is also considered a lifestyle choice. Researchers find that physically fit people often feel better about themselves and their relationships with others. Exercise is required for becoming physically fit. The benefits of becoming physically fit are clear— improved health and wellness, better weight management, reduced risks of

Case Study: A Healthier Lifestyle Choice

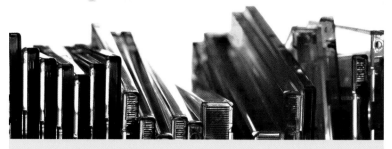

Raj is 16 years old. His 41-year-old father is currently receiving medical treatment for heart disease. Raj's father has smoked cigarettes since he was 14. Raj's 40-year-old mother is healthy, but she loves to cook the curried rice and chicken she enjoyed as a child. She loves making Indian desserts, too. She is now about 40 pounds (18.1 kg) overweight. Raj decided he wants his life to be different. He wants to be more physically active than his parents and is hoping to avoid health problems. His heredity factors place him at increased risk for acquiring heart disease.

Case Review

1. How do Raj's ideas about quality of life compare with those of his parents?

2. What lifestyle choices can Raj make now to reduce the risk for future heart and weight problems?

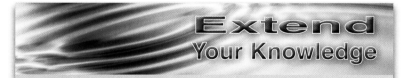

The Effects of Lifestyle Choices on Health

Develop 10 interview questions about personal lifestyle choices. Include questions about topics such as foods typically eaten, number of meals eaten each day, daily activity level, quality of daily environment, availability of medical services, family health history, and other lifestyle choices that affect health and wellness. Use your questions to interview an adult over age 70. Consider which factors contributed to this individual's long life and which may have reduced his or her quality of life. Report your conclusions to the class.

certain diseases, and other mental and social health benefits.

The earlier you begin making healthful lifestyle choices, the more you decrease your risk of early disease.

Health experts recommend adopting the following practices into your lifestyle:

- Provide your body with fuel throughout the day by eating three or more regularly spaced meals, including breakfast, **1-8**.
- Supply your body with needed nutrients to support health, growth, and development.
- Sleep eight to nine hours each night.
- Maintain a healthy weight.
- Stay active. Accumulate at least 60 minutes of physical activity most days of the week to help improve physical, social, and mental health.
- Do not smoke.
- Avoid drinking alcoholic beverages.
- Do not use street drugs.
- Carefully follow your physician's instructions when using prescription drugs.

Throughout this book, you will read about the impact of each of these practices on health. Although these behaviors may sound simple, many people fail to follow them. Instead, they develop poor health habits. This may occur for a number of reasons. Some people take good health for granted. Perhaps they feel they are strong enough to withstand the strain of poor health habits. Others do not notice the slow toll such habits take on their health. For instance, frequently eating high-calorie desserts and snack foods in place of fruits and vegetables deprives your body of needed nutrients. However, you may not notice the gradual decrease in energy level and other health effects caused by this eating habit.

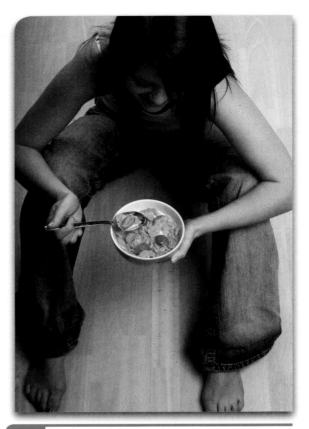

1-8 Choosing balanced meals helps young adults reduce their risks of early disease.

Another reason people form poor health habits is they fail to realize how addictive some behaviors can be. Perhaps you have heard someone say, "I can quit drinking alcohol whenever I want." This person may not realize how physically and emotionally dependent on alcohol he or she has become. Most people need professional services to overcome addictions.

Resist Negative Peer Pressure

Peer pressure can play a role in the development of health habits. **Peer pressure** is the influence people in your age and social group have on your behavior. The desire to be accepted leads many teens to try activities their peers encourage. This can often be good, such as when friends invite one another to become involved with a sport. However, peer pressure is negative when it encourages people to pursue activities that can endanger their health. Teens who urge their friends to smoke cigarettes, drink alcohol, or drive recklessly are using negative peer pressure. Negative peer pressure may play a role in making accidents and suicide the leading causes of death among teens.

You can stand up against negative peer pressure and still come out a winner. Combating negative peer pressure requires self-confidence. You need to believe in your ability to evaluate the effect a choice will have on your health. You also need to be strong enough to say no to what you consider to be a poor choice. Be aware that people who have trouble resisting negative peer pressure may admire you for doing so, **1-9**.

Improve Your Environment

You can do your share to make your environment a healthful one. Carpool or take public transportation to avoid polluting the air with car exhaust. Use cleaning products that do not pollute water supplies with harmful chemical wastes. Handle food carefully to avoid contamination that can cause illness. These are just a few of the many steps you can take to improve the quality of your environment.

Besides these personal efforts, you can work with others to improve the environmental quality of your area. Contact local industries about

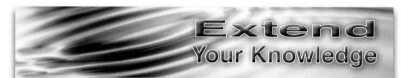

Extend Your Knowledge

Locate Community Wellness Resources

Complete an investigative inquiry about a health club, health care clinic, wellness center, or other community facility concerned with the health of citizens. Write a brief description stating who is encouraged to use this resource and how much it costs. Also, specify what services the center or agency provides and the expected benefits of participation. Place your description, and any brochures you may gather, in a notebook to create a community wellness resource directory.

Avoiding Negative Peer Pressure

- Demonstrate confidence in your decision and do not be embarrassed.
- Remember your personal goals and show respect for your personal limits to avoid being influenced negatively.
- Spend time with people who share your values for health and wellness. Avoid situations where peer pressure may tempt you to make harmful choices.
- Consider the consequences if you gave in to negative peer pressure.
- Role-play your response to a peer-pressure situation. Practice using firm, confident statements. Consider using humor, flattery, challenges, or topic changes to avoid undesirable situations.
- Talk to a trusted family member or friend about the situations and temptations with which you are struggling.
- Know what is important to you and what you hope to accomplish. This will help you build confidence to make positive choices.

1-9   Prepare possible responses to peer pressure before you find yourself in an uncomfortable situation.

the efforts they are making to reduce their impact on the environment. Write to government officials if you have concerns about the quality of the air or water in your community. Talk with your employer about the benefits of creating a work environment that surpasses federal health and safety standards. These steps can help promote the health of many people.

Choose Quality Health Care

Choosing quality health care will help you reduce health risks. The first step is to select a physician who has a reputation for providing quality care services. Choose facilities that can meet your needs and are approved by your health care provider. See your doctor for regular checkups. Seek your doctor's advice when you first notice a health problem. Research has shown that early detection of health problems is the best way to prevent serious illness. When you visit your doctor, describe your symptoms completely and accurately. Ask questions to be sure you understand your symptoms and treatment, **1-10**.

Making a Change

Changing one behavior can affect all aspects of your health. Knowing this can increase your motivation to make positive changes. For instance, you may have heard eating breakfast can help you concentrate better in school (mental health). However, this may not be enough to encourage you to eat breakfast. Eating breakfast can also help you maintain a healthy weight (physical health). It can moderate mood swings and help you interact more positively with others, too (social health). Knowing these added benefits may be just the incentive you need to start eating breakfast.

Questions Your Doctor Can Answer
What is causing these symptoms?
How long will the symptoms last?
Are these symptoms normal for someone in my age range?
What are my options for treatment?
What are the possible risks and side effects associated with prescribed medications or treatments?

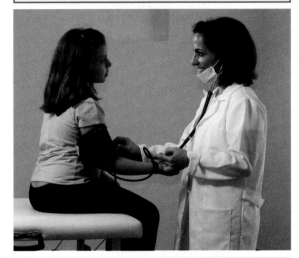

1-10 Patients should feel free to ask their doctors questions.

Although you may be motivated to improve your health, you may not know how to start. Answering the questions in Figure **1-11** can help you pinpoint areas where you might improve.

Once you have identified an area, set a goal for improvement. Then make a behavior-change contract to help you achieve your goal. Write your goal at the top of a sheet of paper. Then set up a chart. In the first column of the chart, list specific steps you will take to reach the goal. For instance, suppose your goal is to improve your diet. You might list steps such as "Eat breakfast daily" and "Drink no more than one soft drink daily." List the days of the week across the top of the chart. Each day you complete a listed step, give yourself a check. This allows you to see the progress you are making toward your goal.

It will take time for you to notice most physical, mental, and social health benefits of a lifestyle change. Follow the listed steps and keep your chart for at least three weeks. After that time, evaluate the results of your efforts. Ask yourself what factors helped you complete steps you marked with a check. Then ask yourself what kept you from completing those steps left unchecked. For instance, you might notice that eating breakfast on weekends is easier because you have more time in the morning. You might find that limiting your soft drink consumption on weekends is hard when you are socializing with friends.

Your evaluation will help you set new goals and plan steps for achieving them. Try to consistently reach your goal for a period of six weeks. After this time, you will have formed a new habit that will be an ongoing part of your wellness lifestyle. Achieving optimum health is a lifelong process of consciously evaluating daily lifestyle choices.

Seeing positive results in one lifestyle area can affect your desire to change other areas. For instance, if you improve your eating habits, you are likely to have more energy. This may increase your willingness to begin an exercise program or join a sports team.

Your confidence that good health practices will improve your state of wellness will help you follow such practices. However, not all your daily choices will be in the best interest of your health. Everyone skips a meal or overeats snack foods once in a while. Little harm is done unless you start making such choices on a regular basis.

Assess Your Lifestyle Choices

Do you
- avoid the use of tobacco?
- avoid the use of alcohol and street drugs?
- regularly eat a nutritious diet, including breakfast?
- manage your weight?
- get daily physical activity to maintain fitness?
- manage stress effectively?
- get enough sleep?
- carefully follow the instructions on medicine labels?
- wear protective clothing when participating in sports and fitness activities?
- avoid taking unnecessary risks?
- avoid unsafe sexual practices?
- take appropriate safety precautions when using equipment and machinery?
- enthusiastically participate in school and community activities?

1-11 If you can answer "yes" to most of these questions, you are making lifestyle choices that promote good health.

Nutrition and Wellness

One factor that has been shown to have a big impact on wellness is nutrition. **Nutrition** is the sum of the processes by which a person takes in and uses food substances. There has been widespread growth in the study of nutrition in recent years. Scientists once thought foods contained just a few basic nutrients. **Nutrients** are the basic components of food that nourish the body. Today, scientists know of over 45 nutrients needed in the diet, **1-12**.

Growth in nutrition science is linked to growth in the field of epidemiology. *Epidemiology* is a branch of science that studies the incidence of disease in a population. After World War II, epidemiologists began exploring factors related to heart disease, cancer,

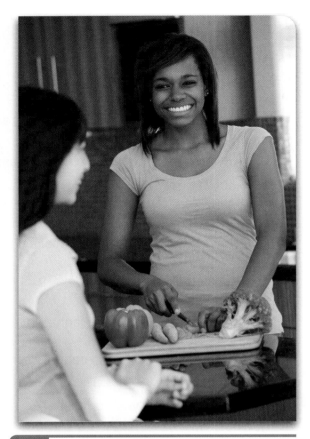

1-12 Eating food provides the body with needed nutrients.

and viral infections. One factor that interested them was diet. They conducted studies to learn how eating patterns of large groups of people related to certain disease patterns.

Sometimes nutrition studies involve comparing the effects of various food choices. For instance, researchers might want to compare the health of people who eat meat with those who do not. They might compare the health effects of high-fiber diets with low-fiber diets. Researchers can also compare diet and lifestyle patterns among cultures.

What have researchers learned from all their nutrition studies? They have learned that eating specific foods cannot cause or prevent certain diseases. However, they have found that following certain eating patterns tends to increase or decrease a person's

chances of illness. For instance, studies have shown that eating sugar does not cause diabetes. Nevertheless, eating a diet high in simple sugars can increase a person's risk of becoming overweight. This, in turn, can increase his or her risk of developing type 2 diabetes.

Nutrition scientists continue to research the roles food components play in the human body. They use research methods to discover answers to questions about the links between diet and health. As a student of nutrition, you will use tools similar to those used by scientists. Correct use of these tools will help you understand and apply information covered in this text.

In your future, you may find yourself eligible to participate in a nutrition or medically based research project. *Clinical studies* use accepted research methods with human subjects. The studies often focus on new methods of screening, prevention, diagnosis, or treatment for the improvement of health. New therapy methods may be tested. For example, a clinical study may focus on the role of exercise in preventing type 2 diabetes for people who have a family history of the disease. The study may be designed to learn more about how to treat the condition. Other studies focus on measuring safety factors and possible side effects. Clinical studies use scientific methods to gather and analyze data.

Using the Scientific Method to Study Nutrition and Wellness

One tool that scientists and dietitians use is the scientific method. The **scientific method** is the process researchers use to find answers to their questions. Once the question is determined, the researcher states the hypothesis. A **hypothesis** is a suggested answer to a scientific question. It can be tested and verified. An experiment is devised to test the hypothesis to determine if it is true, **1-13**.

The following example illustrates the use of the scientific method. A researcher becomes aware of statistics showing men do not tend to live as long as women. This prompts her to raise the question: Why do males have a shorter life expectancy than females? The researcher begins observing males and females. Through these observations, she notes that men seem to exercise less than women. This causes her to form a hypothesis. The researcher's hypothesis states: Men do not live as long as women because

men do not exercise as much as women. The researcher then compares the life spans of men and women who do the same amount of exercise. Suppose this test revealed that men who exercise as much as women have the same life expectancy as women. This would indicate the hypothesis is true. Conversely, suppose the testing revealed that men who exercise as much as women still have a shorter life expectancy. This would indicate the hypothesis is false.

If other researchers have conducted many experiments and reached the same conclusion, a theory forms. A **theory** is a principle that tries to explain something that happens in nature. Although it is based on evidence, a theory is not a fact. It still requires further testing.

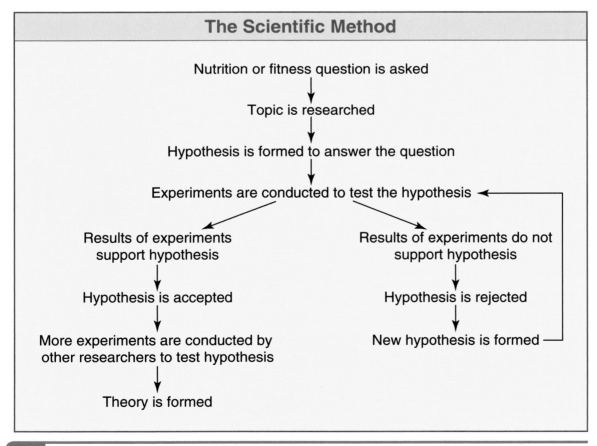

The Scientific Method

Nutrition or fitness question is asked
↓
Topic is researched
↓
Hypothesis is formed to answer the question
↓
Experiments are conducted to test the hypothesis

Results of experiments support hypothesis
↓
Hypothesis is accepted
↓
More experiments are conducted by other researchers to test hypothesis
↓
Theory is formed

Results of experiments do not support hypothesis
↓
Hypothesis is rejected
↓
New hypothesis is formed

1-13 Through the scientific method, researchers are able to test and verify possible answers to their questions.

There are still many unanswered questions about diet, disease, and health. Addressing the following questions helps researchers choose which food science, nutrition, and physical fitness topics to study:

- How is current technology affecting these areas?
- What gaps of knowledge currently exist related to the problems identified?
- How many people will be affected by learning about the information?

- Are resources available (money, time, staff, other resources) to do the research?
- How can current technology be used to advance research?
- Where will the study take place and who will participate?
- Are the rights of people protected, and is the physical environment left unharmed?

Evaluating Research Reports

You can learn about some of the latest findings and recommendations for improving your wellness level. Television and radio newscasts often include brief reports about the results of health and nutrition studies. Information is covered in greater detail in newspaper and magazine articles. Professional journals present more technical information. Hundreds of health and nutrition Web sites on the Internet provide a wealth of data.

As you evaluate information, keep a number of points in mind. Identify the audience to which the report is directed. Is the information intended to update professionals or pique consumer interest? Be aware of who is relaying the information. Is it a media reporter or a health or nutrition professional? Take note of the size and length of the study. Did it involve eight people observed for three weeks or 8,000 people observed for three years? Keep in mind that many experiments are conducted to prove or disprove a theory. Not all experiments will yield the same results. A single study is not a sufficient basis for recommending changes in behavior.

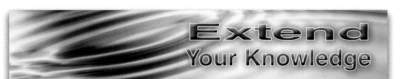

Consider Becoming a Participant in a Clinical Study

Researchers look for people who qualify to participate in clinical studies. Usually, anyone who meets the specific criteria of the study can enroll. Federal agencies have strict guidelines regarding the determination of eligibility for research studies, especially as related to children and other special populations.

Most institutions that run clinical studies have an Institutional Review Board (IRB). This group is given the responsibility for reviewing and approving a study. Research procedures are examined to assure safety for the participants.

Some clinical studies simply ask the participant to fill out a survey regarding specific health problems, food consumption patterns, or exercise patterns. More intensive research may require more of your time and involve physiological testing. Volunteering to participate in a clinical research study is a way to contribute to the understanding of human diseases and the development of new drugs, devices, and procedures.

There is a lot to consider before deciding to get involved. The individual must evaluate the benefits and the risks. Visit the National Institutes of Health Web site to find the benefits and risks of participating in clinical studies. Is there someone you know who is involved in a clinical research study? Would you ever consider participating in a study?

Healthful Living in the United States

Studies show many people in the United States are not following the most healthful eating and physical activity patterns. Studies also show nutritional problems tend to increase as income levels decrease. A number of health and fitness problems are affecting the nation's state of wellness.

- Among youth, the percent overweight has more than doubled in the last 20 years. Now, 17 to 18 percent of youth ages 12 to 19 are obese. Approximately one-third of youth are overweight or obese.
- Among adults, an estimated 65 percent of U.S. adults are overweight. Nearly 30 percent of adults are considered obese.
- About one-third of the people in the United States eat an inadequate diet.
- Popular lifestyles include less and less physical activity, **1-14**.

Wellness Tip

Private Pep Talk

Manage your stress with a pep talk. Instead of thinking "I'll never be able to figure this out," say to yourself "I have the skills to solve this problem." In general, if you would not say it to someone else, do not say it to yourself.

- Important nutrients are missing from the diets of some groups of people, such as teens and older adults.
- Fat, cholesterol, sodium, and sugar intake are higher than recommended.

These problems arise for several reasons. Some people do not have enough money to acquire adequate nutrition. Others lack the information, desire, or skills needed to select a nutritious diet. Some people may not know they need to make changes. Still others simply choose to ignore current nutrition recommendations.

One reason some people give for disregarding nutrition recommendations is nutrition messages may appear unclear or contradictory. Findings from one study seem to dispute the findings from another study. One source says to eat more fiber. Another reference focuses on the importance of protein. Sports books say one thing; diet books say another; and advertisements say something else. Even government nutrition guidelines change periodically. What is a health-conscious person supposed to believe as he or she tries to make wise lifestyle choices?

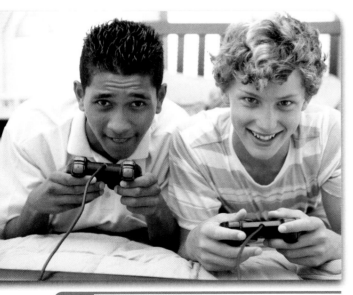

1-14 Many people fail to balance sedentary work and leisure activities with physical activity.

Education can help you sort out conflicting messages. Learning the scientific method and studying about functions and food sources of nutrients will help you assess media reports. Asking questions will also help you evaluate nutrition information. Finding out who conducted a study and how it was conducted can help you decide whether the results are valid.

Recent nutrition studies have uncovered convincing information that supports the need for improved eating habits. Researchers have found that people who eat high-fat diets, especially the harmful fats, are more likely to have heart disease. Identifying this link helped researchers discover that eating a low-fat diet can reduce the risk of heart disease. As people became aware of these findings, they began to change their eating habits. Food manufacturers now produce a wide selection of reduced-fat foods for consumers. For example, you can find low-fat hotdogs, nonfat muffins, and fat-free soups in the supermarkets and restaurants. Consumers are now buying and eating reduced-fat or nonfat products more than ever before. However, on the average, consumers are now eating more total calories and are more likely to be overweight. These factors have kept the overall risk of weight-related diseases from decreasing.

One result of improved nutrition research, expanding food technology, and the increased availability of quality food, is an increase in life expectancy in the United States over the last 100 years. **Life expectancy** is the average length of life of people living in the same environment. Life expectancy in the United States is about 77 years. With improved health, life expectancy tends to increase. Together, healthy people make a healthy nation. Following nutrition and physical activity guidelines will help you and your family maintain good health. In so doing, you contribute to the health of the nation.

Reading Summary

Wellness involves being in good physical, mental, and social health. People can define their personal states of wellness as points on a continuum between premature death and optimum health.

A number of factors can negatively affect wellness by contributing to disease. Most of these factors are unhealthful lifestyle choices, over which you have control. Poor environmental quality, inadequate health care, and heredity can contribute to disease, too. You can counteract these factors by making health-promoting choices. Choose a healthful lifestyle and resist peer pressure to engage in unhealthful behaviors. Work to improve the quality of your environment and seek health care when you need it. You can set and work toward goals for improving behaviors that affect your health.

Nutrition and daily physical activity are two factors that have been shown to have a big impact on health. Experts use the scientific method to find answers to their questions about these factors. Their findings have led many people to change their lifestyle habits. However, a number of nutrition and fitness concerns still exist in the United States. With education, skills, and motivation, people can eat better and exercise more to maintain better health.

Review Learning

1. Describe the characteristics of people functioning at the various extreme points on the wellness continuum.
2. Provide an example of how physical, mental, and social health interrelate.
3. List common symptoms that may appear when there are mental health problems.
4. What are two social skills that can help teens improve their social health?
5. Why is it important to choose health-promoting lifestyle patterns during the teen years? during the adult years?
6. For reducing the risk of disease, which risk factors are considered controllable and which are not?
7. Name the three major causes of death among adults in the United States.
8. List five lifestyle practices that health experts recommend people adopt.
9. Describe what is included in a behavior-change contract for achieving a goal for personal improvement.
10. Explain the difference between a hypothesis and a theory.
11. What are two factors that have contributed to health and wellness problems in the United States?
12. If obesity is a national health problem in the United States, how does this affect the nation as a whole?

Critical Thinking

13. **Draw conclusions.** Think about where you currently fit along the wellness continuum. Draw conclusions about ways you can improve your physical, mental, and social health to achieve optimum wellness.

14. **Predict consequences.** If people in the United States continue along the current path of eating and fitness patterns, predict the consequences of these behaviors on life expectancy for future generations.

Applying Your Knowledge

15. **Wellness continuum.** In class activity: Label one end of the room "Premature Death" and the other end of the room "Optimum Health." Stand between the two points to indicate where you place yourself on the wellness continuum. Explain to the class why you chose to stand where you did.

16. **Conduct an interview.** To learn more about the effects mental and social health can have on physical health, interview a health care professional. Summarize your findings in a written report.

17. **Discussion.** In pairs, discuss your response to the statement: If it's fun, it can't be a healthful lifestyle choice. List 10 activities that are both fun and healthful.

18. **Create a poster.** Contact local community health agencies to gather quantities of health information brochures. Use these to develop a "Wellness Information Corner" in your classroom. Make posters inviting students throughout your school to take advantage of this resource area.

19. **Career research.** Refer to the Occupational Outlook Handbook online to prepare a report detailing a position description and future needs for clinical dietitians in the United States and in other countries.

Technology Connections

20. **Wellness directory.** Create a list of Internet Web sites that offer information on wellness. Rate each site for accuracy and usability of information and credibility of source. Prepare a list and add it to the wellness resource directory suggested in the chapter.

21. **Life expectancy calculations.** Find a life expectancy calculator online to learn about which factors and lifestyle choices add years to life. Complete the questionnaire and analyze the results. Identify your major health risk areas and suggest methods for changing risky behaviors into health-promoting behaviors.

22. **Chart health risks.** Using computer software, prepare a chart which describes factors that add risk to health and factors that reduce risks to health and wellness. Evaluate the potential health risks for quality of life over the life span.

23. **Electronic presentation.** Prepare an electronic presentation showing the life expectancy rates comparing at least four other countries. Use the Internet to locate data. Illustrate your data by selecting at least one country with shorter and one with longer life expectancy rates. Hypothesize why you believe average life expectancies vary from country to country.

Academic Connections

24. **Writing.** Write and present a play on methods teens could use to avoid negative peer pressure.

25. **Literature.** Identify short stories about teens who made poor choices that had negative consequences in their lives. Describe the choice that was made and the outcomes. Suggest ways to help change the situation so the outcomes are more positive.

26. **Social studies.** Research to find current legislation related to nutrition or wellness issues. Select one issue and write a brief summary to share with the class. Include your opinion of the legislation in the summary.

27. **Science.** Contact the state department of public health or a community hospital for a health and wellness lifestyle questionnaire. Complete your answers to the questionnaire. Identify the top three lifestyle changes that would probably provide the greatest benefits to your health.

28. **Math.** In 2006, the share of young adults 18 to 24 years old who never smoked was 70.2%, according to the Centers for Disease Control and Prevention. In 1965, far fewer could make that claim—only 47.6%. Calculate the percentage increase in nonsmokers among members of this age group during that 41-year span.

Workplace Applications

Settings Goals

Most employers value employees that can set and achieve reasonable, attainable goals. Here are a few things you need to know about goals. Goals should

- be specific and positive
- be measurable
- have a target deadline (either short-term—several months, or long-term—several years)

Think about your personal wellness and how it relates to you as an employee. In writing: set a goal for changing one aspect of personal wellness, determine how you will measure achievement of this goal, and identify a deadline for meeting this goal.

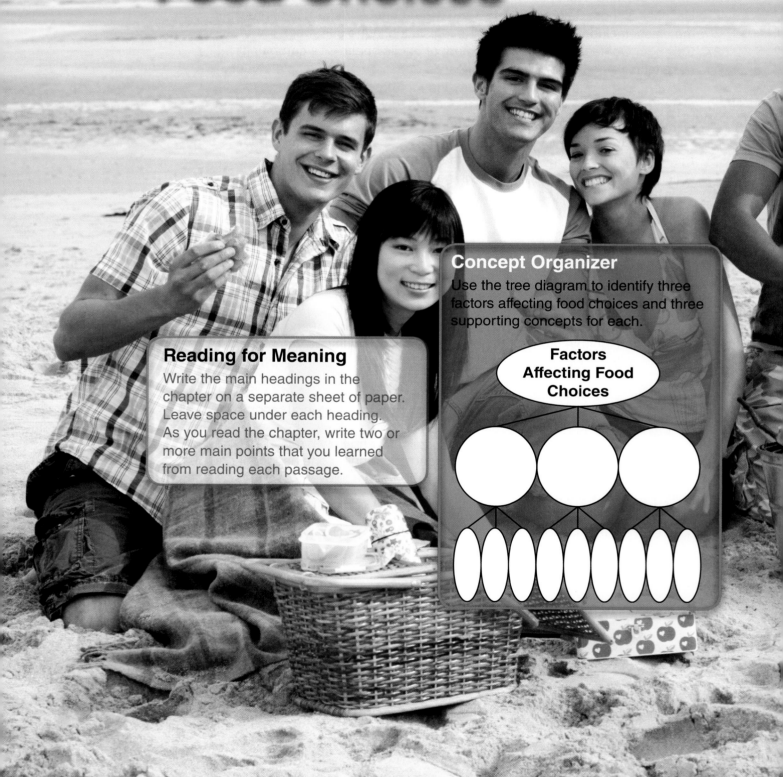

Chapter 2
Factors Affecting Food Choices

Reading for Meaning

Write the main headings in the chapter on a separate sheet of paper. Leave space under each heading. As you read the chapter, write two or more main points that you learned from reading each passage.

Concept Organizer

Use the tree diagram to identify three factors affecting food choices and three supporting concepts for each.

Factors Affecting Food Choices

Terms to Know

culture
ethnic food
soul food
food norm
food taboo
kosher food
value
status food
staple food
technology
food biotechnology
aseptic packaging

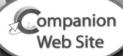

Companion Web Site

- **Print out the concept organizer at g-wlearning.com.**
- **Practice key terms with crossword puzzles, matching activities, and e-flash cards at g-wlearning.com.**

Objectives

After studying this chapter, you will be able to
- **explain** how culture influences people's eating patterns.
- **evaluate** the social influence of family and friends on people's eating patterns.
- **analyze** the effect of emotions on the way people eat.
- **relate** how agricultural resources, technology, economic factors, and politics affect the availability of food.
- **analyze** the effects of global and local events and conditions on food choices and consumer practices.

Central Ideas
- People choose foods for many factors that go beyond the need of satisfying hunger.
- Family and friends play major roles in determining what, where, and when you eat.

What people eat says a lot about them. Food tells a story about where people live, what they do, and what they hold to be important. Food reflects people's history and affects their future. In fact, one way to find out about a group of people is to study their daily food habits.

What factors affect people's food choices? When choosing food, you probably think about what tastes good. However, you may not realize all the other factors that affect people's daily food choices. Where you live and the people around you affect the foods you choose to eat. The resources available to you and your experiences with food are also likely to shape your food choices.

Food Is a Reflection of Culture

You may have had the experience of guessing where someone comes from by the way he or she speaks. Similarly, you might be able to guess where people come from by some of the foods they eat. Like speech patterns, food habits are a reflection of culture. **Culture** refers to the beliefs and social customs of a group of people. It affects all aspects of your life, from where you live to how you dress.

What foods people serve for a meal is an example of cultural influence. Insects are a sweet delicacy in some cultures. However, people seldom serve them for meals in the United States. Families in the United States are far more likely to serve barbecued chicken, lasagna, or even moo shu pork than insects. Clearly, food practices vary from culture to culture.

While changes in culture appear minor from one year to the next, culture is never static. Culture changes over time as new ideas are introduced. For instance, in recent years much information about health and fitness has been introduced. This information has caused people in the United States to become more health conscious. Many aspects of culture have reflected this change. Today, people are more likely to spend their time in health clubs than people in the past. They are more likely to spend their money on exercise equipment. They are also more likely to eat special low-fat foods.

Ask your grandparents how often they ate low-fat yogurt and fat-free cookies when they were children. Did they ever go to a health-food store during their childhood? The difference between their responses and that of youth today reflects a change in culture.

What factors have helped shape your culture? Family members, friends, and other people who are close to you help pass along culture. Schools, religious organizations, and the media are also key influences.

Historical Influences

Have you ever researched your family tree? A family tree shows family relationships from one generation to the next. The diagram of a tree is used to identify parents, grandparents, and other relatives from past generations. Detailed information, such as a health history and places of birth, is included on the tree. Many people in the United States have roots based in other cultures. Maybe your ancestors came from Europe, Africa, Asia, or Latin America. When people came to the United States from these lands, they brought many foods and food customs with them.

When early settlers came to America, they found a vast amount of land. The climate was moderate and the soil was fertile. The settlers brought with them wheat, barley, oats, and rye. They found these grains grew well in this new land. They also brought fruits, vegetables, and herbs from their homelands. Figs, dates, broccoli, carrots, mint, and parsley are among the many foods these immigrants brought to America.

Many foods were being grown in America before the first settlers arrived. Native Americans grew corn, beans, potatoes, sweet potatoes, tomatoes, squash, chili peppers, and pumpkins. The settlers combined these foods with foods from their homelands to create a variety of dishes. These dishes are now part of America's diverse cuisine, **2-1**.

Ethnic Influences

Some of the foods you choose to eat may be based on your ethnic group. Groups of people who share common blood ties, land ties, or racial and religious similarities are called ethnic groups. What pulls group members together is their shared beliefs and group norms. Members of ethnic groups also share food traditions. **Ethnic foods** are foods that are typical of a given racial, national, or religious culture. For instance, **soul food** is traditional food of the African American ethnic group. Soul food includes such dishes as chitterlings, collard greens, and ham hocks. Sharing common foods helps build a sense of ethnic pride.

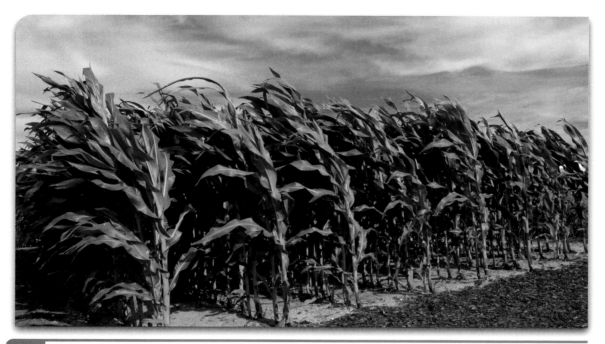

2-1 Native Americans were growing corn before the first settlers arrived. Today, the United States is the leading corn-producing nation.

Ethnic groups have **food norms**, or typical standards and patterns related to food and eating behaviors. For example, most meals among the Pennsylvania Dutch include something sweet and something sour. The Pennsylvania Dutch often serve pickles or pepper cabbage as the sour element of a meal. Then they serve a sweet dessert at the end of the meal.

Some ethnic groups have special ways of selecting, buying, cooking, serving, eating, and storing foods. Group members take pride in these unique food habits. Many Italian cooks shop for food every day to get the freshest ingredients. Some Indian cooks prepare foods in a special oven called a *tandoor*. The British serve tea with cookies or sandwiches as a light meal in the late afternoon. These customs are ways of expressing deep-rooted ties to a common heritage.

Ethnic food traditions help build bonds of togetherness. Many ethnic groups serve special foods on certain days of the year to build positive emotions. The Japanese traditionally eat black beans on New Year's Day for good health and fortune for the new year. Jewish people eat apples and honey as part of their New Year celebration so the coming year will be sweet. What foods are part of your family's ethnic tradition?

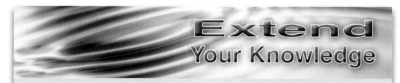

What Can You Learn from Your Family Tree?

A family tree shows relationships of ancestors and descendants in one family. Draw your family tree placing your name on the trunk of the tree and your parents' names on the lower branches. Include all your grandparents on higher branches. Go back in your history as far as possible. Family trees often include birth dates and places of birth. Age and cause of death can be noted for each person. The tree will help you learn about your cultural heritage and potential inherited health issues.

You can recognize many ethnic foods by their ingredients, seasonings, and preparation methods. Ethnic ingredients are usually plentiful in the region from which the foods come. For instance, corn and beans grow well in Mexico. Therefore, many Mexican dishes feature corn and beans. Many ethnic cuisines get their characteristic flavors from a few typical seasonings. Spanish dishes are often flavored with onions, garlic, and olive oil. Middle Eastern foods are often seasoned with saffron, cumin, and ginger. Certain cooking methods also typify some ethnic cuisines. Chinese dishes are often stir-fried or steamed.

Today in the United States, people seem to have a growing interest in and taste for ethnic foods. Specialty stores, farmers' markets, and supermarkets are beginning to carry more of the foods used in ethnic menus. Chinese, Mexican, Greek, and Thai are just a few of the many types of ethnic restaurants listed in the Yellow Pages, **2-2**. Many communities hold ethnic festivals, which allow visitors to try national specialties.

Throughout this century, many more international visitors, immigrants, and refugees are likely to come to the United States. A growing number of people from the United States will travel internationally for business, study, and recreation. This is likely to expand the range of ethnic foods available to you as you make food choices. Being willing to experience new tastes by trying different ethnic dishes will add variety to your diet.

Food Taboos

In most ethnic groups, social customs prohibit the use of certain edible resources as food. Such customs are called **food taboos**. Many people in the United States enjoy eating beef.

Hindus living in India and other parts of the world, however, have a food taboo against eating beef. Their culture considers cows to be sacred. People in some Asian countries cannot understand why people in the United States do not savor dog stew. In the United States, there is a food taboo against eating dog meat.

No single diet pattern is acceptable to all people. People learn feelings about food through cultural experiences. What tastes good depends largely on what you were taught to believe tastes good.

Regional Influences

You may choose to eat some foods because they are popular in your region. Each region of the United States features some distinctive types of foods. This is

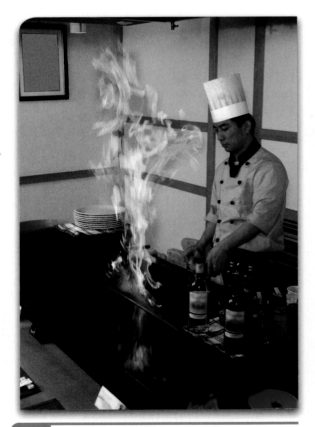

2-2 Ethnic restaurants give people a chance to sample the flavors of another culture.

because each region reflects different ethnic heritages and each heritage is typified by different foods. For instance, the Southwest has a large Mexican-American population. The tortillas, tacos, and tamales that are popular in the Southwest reflect this heritage. Many Asian people helped settle the Pacific Coast. They contributed rice dishes and the stir-fry cooking method to the cuisine of this region, **2-3**.

Religious Influences

Religious beliefs have influenced people's food choices for centuries. Certain religious groups have rules regarding what members may or may not eat. For example, many Orthodox Jews follow dietary laws based on their interpretation of the Old Testament. These laws forbid the eating of pork and shellfish. They also specify meat and dairy foods may not be stored, prepared, or eaten together. Foods prepared according to these laws are called **kosher foods**.

Many other religions also have restrictions regarding food and drink. For instance, Muslims fast during the days of the ninth month of their calendar year. Seventh-Day Adventists eat a vegetarian diet. They abstain from drinking alcohol, tea, and coffee because of their drug effects on the body.

Some members of religious groups view food customs as strict commandments. Others observe the customs to help keep traditions alive for future generations.

Case Study: Future Food Taboo?

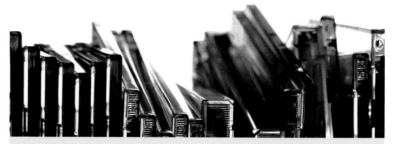

In Japan, whale hunting is a tradition that dates back hundreds of years. Whale meat was once an important and common family food. Now, whale dishes are mostly found in restaurants or the meat is canned and sold in supermarkets. Whale is not as popular as it once was, but it is still enjoyed by some people. The Japanese whaling ships catch primarily minke whales and lesser amounts of fin whales. Environmentalist groups and others oppose the practice of killing whales. Their concerns focus on the harpooning methods used to kill whales and the threat to the number of minke whales in the sea.

Case Review

1. Do you think eating whale meat will become a food taboo? Why?

2. Name several common taboos that can be found in your family or community of friends. How do you think they became taboos? Will attitudes toward the taboo ever change? Why?

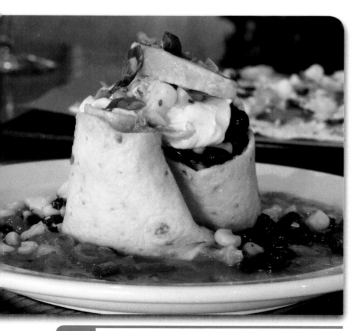

2-3   Burritos are a popular Southwestern dish that reflects Mexican influences.

Social Influences on Food Choices

Have you noticed that food seems to taste better when you share it with people you know and like? Food often plays a role in social relationships with family members and friends. These people may influence the foods you choose to eat.

Family

The family is a major influence on the diets of young eaters. You no doubt formed many of your beliefs about food when you were much younger. By watching your family members, you learned about table manners and how to eat certain foods. You learned about food traditions for holidays, birthdays, and other special occasions. You probably also adopted some of the food likes and dislikes of your family members, **2-4**.

Like culture, families change over time. Years ago, most households had two parents—a father who went off to work and a mother who stayed home. The mother was usually responsible for preparing food. Dinner was often served as soon as the father came home from work. Families have changed in many ways during the last century. The following changes have led to new trends in what, how, and when families eat:

- *More households are headed by working single parents.* A working single parent is likely to have only a limited amount of time for meal preparation. Families today often rely on prepared foods to help save time. Meal preparation tasks may be shared among family members. The evening meal may be eaten later because preparation cannot begin until one or more family members arrive home.

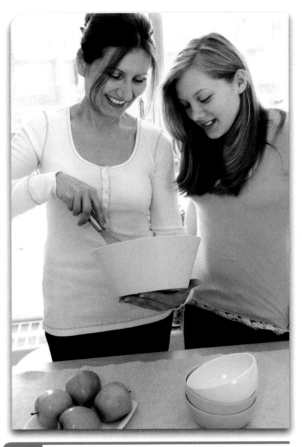

2-4 Families teach children about traditional foods for special occasions

- *Many dual-worker families have more income at their disposal.* Dual-worker families may be able to afford to buy more timesaving kitchen appliances and ready-made food products. They might have enough money to eat out more often. They might have sufficient means to hire someone to help with food preparation tasks, too. Dual-worker families have hectic schedules and eating times may vary from day-to-day. Family members sometimes find themselves eating meals on the run or preparing individual servings. Very few family meals may be shared together throughout the week.
- *The average family size is smaller.* Manufacturers are offering many food products in smaller portion sizes to better suit smaller households.

- *Family members are increasingly mobile.* Working family members may commute to their jobs. Children and teens are frequently involved in a variety of activities. Busy schedules often keep family members from eating meals together. Many family members are in the habit of serving themselves whenever they are hungry.

Values make a difference in the kinds of changes seen in family food behaviors. **Values** are beliefs and attitudes that are important to people. Traditions, such as making special foods and eating together, are important values in many families. Such traditions can bring family members closer emotionally and socially. This is probably why some families make a point to eat together at least once a day.

Friends

Your friends and peers play a major role in determining what, where, and when you eat. Have you noticed that your friends like many of the same foods you like? Popular foods for teens include pizza, tacos, hamburgers, French fries, milk shakes, and soft drinks. Specific favorites may vary from one region of the country to another. However, some foods seem to be popular among teens everywhere.

Anywhere people gather you are likely to see food. Students eat lunch together in the school cafeteria. Fans eat hot dogs, popcorn, and nachos at sporting events, **2-5**. Friends enjoy sharing snacks and meals together at one of the more than 300 fast-food chains. Movie theaters, parties, church gatherings, and shopping malls are all places where people meet with friends and enjoy food.

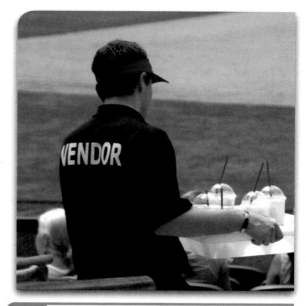

2-5 Food is available almost anywhere people gather.

Just as friends eat together almost anywhere, they also eat together almost anytime. Jogging partners may share breakfast after an early morning run. Neighbors may meet for midmorning coffee and rolls. Business associates often gather for lunch to discuss company decisions. A group of classmates may search the cupboards for an after-school snack. Couples and families enjoy sharing dinner in the evening at home and in restaurants. Teenagers may raid the refrigerator for a late-night study break.

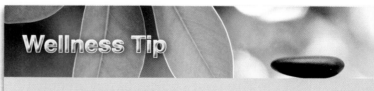

Wellness Tip

Eating Out, Plan Ahead

To eat healthfully when eating out, plan ahead. Look at menus online and choose healthful foods from all food groups. Select foods that are baked, braised, broiled, grilled, steamed, or poached. For a lighter meal, order a child-size portion or an appetizer. Planning ahead and knowing what's available can help you stick to your healthy eating plan.

When serving food to friends at a social event, people often choose foods that help create a festive mood. Certain foods add special meaning to social events. Thanksgiving turkey and wedding cake are popular examples.

When people serve food to friends, they want to serve foods their friends will like. Sometimes foods that people perceive as being popular are not the most healthful. For instance, adults may serve cake and cookies at a card party. Teens may serve chips and soda to a group of friends. These foods are high in calories, fat, and sugar and low in other nutrients.

You do not have to stop serving snack foods that are low in nutrients. However, you might want to offer your friends some healthful snacks, too. Fresh fruits or vegetables with a low-fat dip make tasty, healthful alternatives to high-fat, high-calorie snacks.

Peers affect eating behaviors as well as food choices. Teens commonly worry about body weight, complexion problems, and the impressions they make on others. Some teens try new eating behaviors that are reported to address these problems. Fad dieting is one such behavior that is popular among teens.

When choosing eating behaviors, just as when choosing foods, you need to keep health in mind. For instance, choosing to follow a fad diet to lose weight can be harmful. Fad diets often severely limit calories. Someone who restricts calorie intake during the teen years can inhibit his or her growth.

Are your choices based on nutrition knowledge or the influence of your peers? Examine how much your friends influence your eating behaviors and food choices. Think about the extent to which they affect when, where, and what you eat. Ask yourself if you tend to eat after school or in the evenings because you are with your friends.

Evaluate whether you order popcorn at the movies or hot dogs at a basketball game because your friends are doing so. Do you find yourself ordering a cheese and sausage pizza because that is what your friends like? Becoming aware of how others affect the quality of your diet can help you improve your overall health.

The Status of Foods

Sometimes people choose foods to tell a story about their social status. *Social status* is identified by a person's position in the community. Power and wealth influence social status.

Some foods are called *status foods*. **Status foods** are foods that have a social impact on others. Status foods are often served at special occasions to influence or impress important people. Caviar is a traditional status food served at social events of the rich and famous. Caviar is an expensive delicacy consisting of the unfertilized eggs (roe) of sturgeon fish and prepared in a salt solution, **2-6**. Classic caviar comes

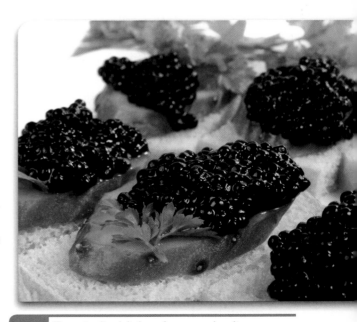

2-6   Due to its high price, caviar is a status food.

primarily from Iran or Russia and is harvested by commercial fishermen working in the Caspian Sea. Is caviar a status food for you? What foods do you know to be status foods?

The status of a food often affects its cost but has little to do with its nutritional quality. For instance, filet mignon is a high-status food; hamburger is not. Filet mignon has no more nutritional value than hamburger, yet it costs about six times more.

Over time, the status level of foods can change. A low-status food can become a high-status food. For example, quinoa (pronounced KEEN-wah) is a grain that might be considered a low-status food in Peru where it is widely used. The Inca called the grain *quinoa*, meaning "mother grain" in their language. The grain is a good source of quality protein, higher than many other common grains used in cereals and baking. The grain dates back over 5,000 years. The tiny seed is no bigger than a mustard seed. The grain can be used in making hot cereals, pancakes, muffins, breads, cookies, or other baked products. Now, quinoa is being marketed in the United States as an exotic, new grain. Often found only in specialty stores, it may be viewed as a high-status food to some people.

Media

The media is a strong social influence on food choices. People may choose to prepare foods in a way described in a newspaper or magazine or on a television program. They often choose the brand name of the foods identified in the recipe. They may choose to buy foods reported to have certain health benefits.

The media carry food advertisements. Television commercials have an especially strong impact on people's food choices. Commercials are designed to acquaint you with products. After you hear or see an ad over and over, you are more likely to buy the product.

Research shows that children in the United States view an average of 25,629 commercials a year. Children become socialized to want the foods they see advertised. More than half of the commercials are for foods high in calories, sugar, fat, and salt. Eating such foods instead of fresh fruits, vegetables, and whole grain cereals can harm children's health.

The effects of commercials on people's eating behaviors are hard to escape. The media portray young, thin people as the ideal of beauty. This entices some people to go on weight-loss diets to achieve the ideal. It is best to consult a dietitian or doctor before starting any diet.

Emotions Affect Food Choices

People use food to do more than satisfy physical hunger. Many people choose to eat or avoid certain foods for emotional reasons. For example, suppose you ate a hot dog for lunch and later in the day you felt terribly sick. This may lead you to form a mental connection between hot dogs and illness. You may think, "Hot dogs make me sick, and I never want to eat one again!" Such an emotional response can outweigh hunger pangs and nutrition knowledge in its effect on your food choices, **2-7**.

Mental Connections with Foods and Eating Patterns

Food/Eating Pattern	Mental Connection
Luncheon salads	Femininity
Meat and potatoes	Masculinity
Carving meats	Strength, authority
Expensive foods	Status, elegance
Sharing food	Trust, friendship, hospitality
Giving food as a gift	Custom, affection
Snacking	Amusement, camaraderie
Family dining	Security
Formal dining	Tradition, ritual
Eating alone	Independence, loneliness, punishment
Refusal to eat	Sacrifice, retaliation
Overeating	Anxiety, greed, frustration, lack of self-control
Fad dieting	Insecurity, vanity, popularity

2-7 Emotional factors cause some people to form mental connections with certain foods and eating patterns. What foods create emotional responses for you?

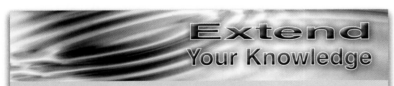

Extend Your Knowledge

What Makes a Food Masculine or Feminine to Eat?

Find five teens and five older adults who are willing to respond to your food survey. Using a list of foods you assembled, ask each group to identify which foods are considered masculine and which are feminine. Prepare your lists and check their responses. Which foods are identified as masculine and feminine? Does age of the respondent make a difference in his or her attitude toward foods? Summarize your survey results and form a hypothesis. Write a short article for the school or local press.

Emotional Responses to Food

Food evokes many emotional responses. People develop most of their emotional reactions toward foods in early life. For some people, food creates feelings of good luck and happiness. For others, food produces feelings of frustration or disgust. Play a word association game with a friend to learn more about your emotional response to food. What feelings come to mind when you hear the words *chocolate*, *liver*, *spinach*, and *ice cream*?

You learn some emotional responses to food in the context of family, school, community, religion, and the media. In other words, your culture affects how you will react to the food presented to you.

Some emotional responses to food may be associated with gender. Research has shown that some people connect maleness with hardy foods, such as steak and potatoes. Similarly, some people link femaleness with dainty foods, such as parfaits and quiches.

Using Food to Deal with Emotions

Food not only evokes emotions, it can also be used to express emotions. Many people offer food as a symbol of love and caring. People show concern by taking food to neighbors and friends who have an illness or death in the family.

People often choose to eat certain foods to help meet emotional needs. For instance, a chocolate bar may cheer you up when you are depressed. Your grandmother's recipe for macaroni and cheese may comfort you when you are feeling lonely. A double scoop of ice cream might be just what you need to celebrate a good report card.

Chicken noodle soup may nourish your emotions as well as your body when you have a cold.

Frustration can lead some people to eat more or less food than their bodies need. Other people use food to help them deal with fears. Both types of people use the pleasure of eating to avoid thoughts that are annoying or scary. Have you ever found yourself wanting to snack heavily before a big event in your life? If so, you may have been associating food with emotional comfort.

Some feelings related to food can be harmful. Some teens and young adults, mainly girls, starve themselves to be very thin. This pattern of eating is grounded in emotions and requires the help of professional counselors. People must examine the way they use food to help put eating behaviors into a healthy perspective.

Food Used for Rewards or Punishment

Foods can be used to manipulate behaviors. For instance, parents may use food to change a child's behavior. If parents want to encourage a child to do something, they may give a special treat. Cookies, ice cream, and candy are popular rewards for good behavior, **2-8**.

People who have been rewarded with food as children may continue to reward themselves with food as adults. They may select food rewards even when they are not hungry. Following this learned pattern of behavior can lead to weight management problems.

Sometimes parents take foods away from children as a punishment. For instance, a parent may withhold dessert when a child misbehaves at the dinner table. This can cause some children to develop negative emotions toward food and eating. Some children carry such negative associations into their adult years.

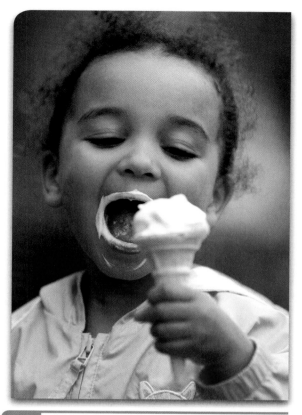

2-8 Using well-liked foods to reward children may establish poor eating patterns.

Case Study: Teaching Eating Behavior

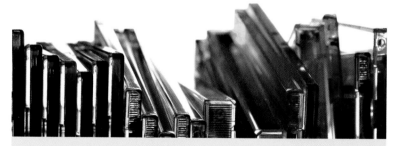

Jenny is a hyperactive two-year-old child. When the family goes to a restaurant, Jenny can be very loud and has a hard time sitting still. Her parents give her lollipops to keep her quiet. At home, they tell her that if she eats her dinner, she can have a special treat of chocolate chip cookies.

Case Review

1. What is Jenny learning from these experiences?

2. How do you think the parents' behaviors will impact Jenny's life as an adult?

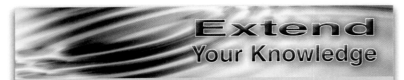

Umami—A New Basic Taste?

Umami—the fifth basic taste—is somewhat new to Western culture, but has been understood in Asian culture for centuries. Umami is a savory, meaty taste that results from glutamate. Glutamates occur naturally in some foods such as mushrooms, aged cheeses, tomatoes, seafood, and seaweed. Monosodium glutamate (MSG) is a flavor additive that also produces umami taste. Research to learn more about how umami impacts other ingredients in a dish. Next time you are eating your favorite dish, consider whether umami is a contributing factor in the flavor.

Individual Preferences Affect Food Choices

You choose to eat many foods simply because you like them. What causes you to like some foods more than others? Your emotions are one

Math Link

Calculating Snack Percentages

Carlos was working as a helper in a preschool classroom. He noticed when a group of 10 children were served apple slices, 9 out of 10 children ate their entire snack. The next day the same 10 children were served pear slices; only 6 out of 10 ate all their snack.

- What was the difference in the percentage of the class that ate their apple snack compared to those that ate their pear snack?

factor. You are likely to prefer foods that you associate with positive emotions, such as comfort and caring. However, you are apt to dislike foods that you associate with negative feelings, such as guilt and fear.

Your genes are partly responsible for your food preferences. You were born with personal preferences for certain tastes and smells. Everyone has taste buds that sense the tastes of sweet, salty, sour, bitter, and umami. Just how you perceive each of these tastes is part of your unique makeup. For instance, one person might wince in pain from the heat he or she feels when eating a jalapeño pepper. Another person may hardly notice the heat when eating one of these peppers. This difference in taste perception is due to genetics. It helps explain why members of the same family who have the same background often prefer the same foods. If your taste preferences are different from other members of your family, you may have inherited a different set of genes.

Although genes play an important role in determining taste preferences, your experiences with food affect your preferences, too. Suppose someone offers you a choice between fried grasshoppers and a hamburger. If you have eaten hamburgers but never tried grasshoppers, you are more likely to choose the hamburger. Someone from China, where fried grasshoppers are a delicacy, might be more likely to choose the grasshoppers. People simply prefer what is familiar to them, 2-9.

The Influences of Agriculture, Technology, Economics, and Politics

Sometimes you have control over what is available to eat and sometimes you do not. When you buy food, you have control over what is in your cupboards. However, you have little control over what foods are available in the grocery store. Factors that can affect what foods are sold in stores include agriculture, technology, economics, and politics.

Most people in the United States have many foods available to them. This is not the case for many people throughout the world. In poor countries, agriculture, technology, economics, and politics affect more than the variety of foods available. These factors can affect whether there is food available at all.

Agriculture and Land Use

Food production is plentiful when important resources are available to grow crops. These resources include
• fertile soil
• adequate water supply
• favorable climate
• technical knowledge
• human energy

The availability of these five resources differs greatly among regions throughout the world. Crops need fertile soil in which their roots can take hold. Fertile soil supplies the nutrients plants need to grow. In some regions, the soil quality is too poor to support crop growth.

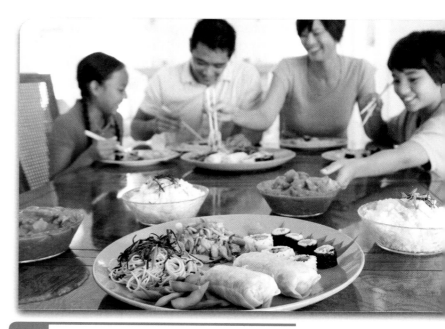

2-9 Most people prefer to eat foods that are familiar to them.

Quality of soil varies from area to area in the United States and throughout the world. The typical diet of a region usually is based on the foods that grow well there. For example, soil quality in the Andes Mountains of South America is too poor to support many types of crops. However, such hardy crops as potatoes grow well there, yielding large amounts in a small amount of acreage.

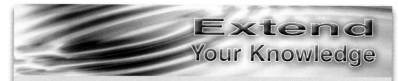

Extend Your Knowledge

Food and Agriculture Organization (FAO)

Many private and government agencies work to end global hunger. Some specialize in short-term crisis relief. Others work on long-term solutions, such as improving farming methods. The Food and Agriculture Organization (FAO) is an international organization that focuses on increasing crop yields in developing nations. FAO is also concerned with the fair distribution of food to rural people. FAO is part of the United Nations system.

Therefore, potatoes are a staple food in the countries through which the Andes extend, including Chile, Peru, and Bolivia. A staple food is a mainstay food in the diet. A **staple food** supplies a large portion of the calories people need to maintain health.

In Asia, rice grows well and is a staple food in the diet. Western Europe and the United States have conditions favorable for growing wheat. Bread made with wheat flour is a mainstay in the diets of these regions. Corn grows well in South American soil. Therefore, South American people eat many corn-based foods. Rye is a staple crop in Russia and northern Europe. This grain is used to make the hardy breads typical of this region, **2-10**.

Water availability affects food availability. Experts predict lack of fresh water will be one of the most serious concerns in this century. Rainfall is not always plentiful enough to fill the rivers and streams. Watering crops to increase yields creates a heavy draw on underground water supplies. Thus, water resources are at risk of being depleted.

Climate refers to the average temperatures and rainfall in a region. Different crops grow best in different climates. For instance, citrus fruits require warm temperatures for an extended time. Apples, on the other hand, cannot withstand long periods of warm weather. That is why most oranges come from warm regions such as Florida, Israel, and Spain. Apples tend to grow well in cooler regions such as Washington, Oregon, and Russia. Wherever the weather can sustain plant life, people can raise some type of food.

Technical knowledge is specialized information. It helps farmers get the most from their land. Through experience and scientific study, farmers have learned ways to increase crop production. They have discovered what nutrients crops need to grow. This helped them develop planting techniques and chemical fertilizers that replenish the soil with those nutrients. Farmers have determined how much water crops require, and have installed elaborate watering systems to provide it. They have identified what weeds and insects are damaging to plants. This has enabled them to take steps to control these pests.

Human energy is needed to plant seeds and harvest crops. In areas where the other four resources are available, a few people can produce an abundant food supply. When the other resources are scarce, however, many people may be needed to grow only small amounts of food. In the midwestern United States, the soil is fertile and an ample amount

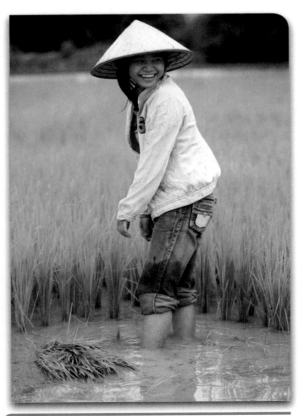

2-10 The climate in Laos is suitable for growing rice. Therefore, rice is a staple food in the diets of the Lao.

of rain falls each year. The climate is suitable for growing crops such as corn, wheat, and soybeans. Farmers in this area are able to take advantage of the latest information about the most productive farming methods. These factors allow a midwestern farmer to produce enough grain to feed thousands of people per year.

Consider the contrast presented by a farmer in a country such as Afghanistan. Much of the land is covered by mountains or desert, making it difficult to farm. Although some areas have fertile soil, rainfall is insufficient to support crop growth. Many farmers lack access to current technical knowledge. They are also unable to obtain high-quality seeds, modern machinery, and chemicals to help stimulate plant growth and control insects. In Afghanistan, many farmers barely produce enough food to feed their families.

Technology

Shoppers in the United States often find New Zealand kiwifruit and Mexican mangoes in the produce section of the supermarket. With the help of science and technology, and transportation resources, foods from many lands are as close as the local grocery store.

In the last 75 to 100 years, many changes in technology and agriculture have influenced how food gets from farm to table. **Technology** is the application of a certain body of knowledge. Modern farming machinery, faster food-processing systems, and rapid transportation are all examples of technological advances. The invention of new foods and food-handling processes has increased the food supply, **2-11**.

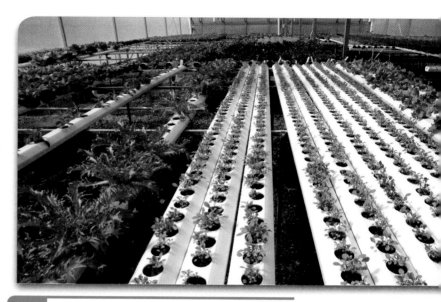

2-11 Technological advances such as hydroponic greenhouses helped increase the food supply.

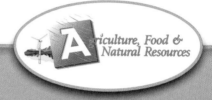
Agriculture, Food & Natural Resources

Food Technologist

Food technologists work in the food processing industry, universities, and government. They generally work in product development—applying the findings from food science research to improve the selection, preservation, processing, packaging, and distribution of food.

Education: Most jobs require a bachelor's degree, but a master's or doctorate degree is usually a requirement for university research positions. Relevant coursework includes life and physical sciences, such as cell and molecular biology, microbiology, and inorganic and organic chemistry.

Job Outlook: The demand for new food products and safety measures will drive the job growth for food technologists. Food research is expected to increase because of heightened public awareness of diet, health, food safety, and *biosecurity*—preventing the introduction of infectious agents into herds of animals. Advances in biotechnology and nanotechnology should also spur demand, as food technologists apply these technologies to testing and monitoring food safety.

New foods are being developed more rapidly with modern food biotechnology. **Food biotechnology** uses knowledge of plant science and genetics to develop plants and animals with specific desirable traits while eliminating traits that are not wanted. Genes that carry the desirable trait are moved from one plant to another. Genes are units in every cell that control an organism's inherited traits. For centuries, farmers have worked to breed desirable qualities into plants and animals. Food biotechnology increases the speed and accuracy of this process. The new plants may be more resistant to factors such as disease, pest, or drought. These factors reduce yields or require use of chemicals or other resources to fight. By reducing or eliminating these factors, more food can be produced on less land using fewer chemicals, and less water or other resources. Some food biotechnology focuses on enhancing the nutritional content of a food. For example, researchers have developed corn with higher concentrations of specific protein components and more healthful cooking oils.

The use of biotech foods has caused controversy in some groups and countries around the world. The safety of biotech foods concerns some consumers. Food biotechnology that is well regulated poses little threat to people or the environment. Experts point out that biotech foods are just as safe as traditional foods. Developers must consult with the FDA before they can introduce a new biotech food. This process takes several years. It ensures these products pass FDA's food safety assessment.

Many of the discoveries and advances in food biotechnology begin in USDA research centers. The USDA also oversees field trials and large-scale production of biotech plants and animals, **2-12**. The Environmental

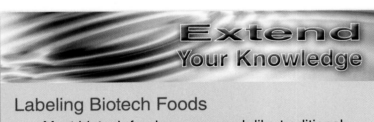

Labeling Biotech Foods

Most biotech foods are so much like traditional foods that special labels are not needed. However, labels are required for the following:

- food that causes an allergic reaction in some people
- food whose nutrient content is changed (for example, a bioengineered carrot with more vitamin A)
- food for which an issue exists regarding how the food is used or consequences of its use
- food that is new to the diet

New foods introduced to the public always require labeling. It does not matter whether the food is the result of biotechnology or traditional crossbreeding methods. Visit the FDA Web site to learn more about labeling of these foods. Next time you are in the supermarket, see if you can identify foods that are the result of biotechnology.

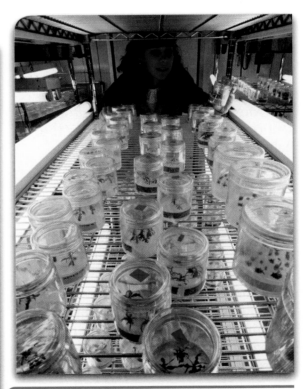

2-12 This USDA technician observes experimental peach and apple trees that are a product of food biotechnology.

Protection Agency (EPA) regulates the pest-resistant properties of biotech crops. These many checkpoints assure consumers and product developers of the safety of food biotechnology.

Improved food packaging is another way in which technology has affected the food supply. Researchers try to design packaging materials that will keep food safe without adding much to the cost of products. Plastic is one such material that is commonly used in food packaging. Plastics keep food fresh and protect food from contaminants in the air and on unclean surfaces. Another factor researchers must keep in mind when designing packaging is its impact on the environment. One option being studied is biodegradable packaging that will break down in landfills.

A packaging technology that preserves quality and extends shelf life of food is called **aseptic packaging.** This process involves packing sterile food into sterile containers. It is done in a sterile atmosphere. Bacteria cannot grow in aseptic packages. Therefore, food does not need to be refrigerated to remain wholesome. This means perishable foods can be kept in places where there is no refrigeration.

Food products can now be safely and quickly transported all over the world. Staple foods can be stored for extended periods and then used during times of food shortages. These foods can be shipped to areas where food production is low and people want to buy them.

The Economics of Food

Have you ever had to forego buying a candy bar because you were out of change? This is a minor example of the fact that it takes money to buy food. It also takes money to buy the seeds to grow food.

Economics has much to do with the availability of food. If a country cannot afford the agricultural supplies or other technological aids, such as tractors, food production is limited. If farmers cannot buy fertilizer, crop yields decrease. Poverty is a close relative of hunger.

Poor countries lack the resources to build food-processing plants and store food safely. This can result in up to 40 percent of crops being lost to spoilage and contamination. Poor countries also lack the dollars to import food from other more productive countries. The nutritional status of the entire population can suffer when a country's economy cannot afford to produce adequate food.

In wealthy countries, food prices and availability are also affected by global events and situations. For example, when corn is used for the production of ethanol gas, less corn is available for consumption or distribution. The price of corn in food stores goes up. When drought affects rice-growing countries and production decreases, the price of rice in the local supermarket goes up, too. As you follow news events, you can identify ways global events directly affect the availability and cost of food in your local stores.

The Politics of Food

The degree to which a country's economic resources are used to address food problems depends largely on politics. The people with political power make most of the decisions in some countries. Those who have political power may decide what lands will be used for food production. They might determine what crops will be grown. Sometimes the decision is made to raise crops that can be sold to other countries. Money from these crops often goes to the people in power rather than the farmers who grew the crops. While the politicians get rich, the farmers remain too poor to buy food. Land that could be used to raise nutritious food for hungry people is being used for the exported crops instead, **2-13**.

Some political decision makers invest a large percentage of a country's economic resources in military power. Sometimes leaders make these decisions to increase their personal power. Sometimes they feel compelled to channel resources to the military to protect their country from hostile neighbors. In any case, money spent on the military is not available to help develop a country's agricultural production. It cannot be used to buy food from other countries, either.

Political leaders may even decide how food will be distributed. Food needed by hungry people may be given to the military. People with higher status may receive more or better food than those who are poor.

Politics does not affect food only in other countries. The U.S. government sets many policies that relate to the food supply. Some policies concern food products that are imported from other countries. Some of these policies are intended to ensure the wholesomeness of foods. Other policies are designed to protect the market for products produced in the United States. Still other policies are made to keep trade relations friendly with other countries.

Many federal regulations mandate how food is to be produced and processed. The government requires that many foods, such as meat and poultry, be inspected to be sure they are wholesome. Guidelines state that manufacturers must pack foods in a sanitary setting. Laws require label information to be truthful. Federal acts designate what types of ingredients can be added to products, too. All these factors affect the foods that are available to you in the marketplace.

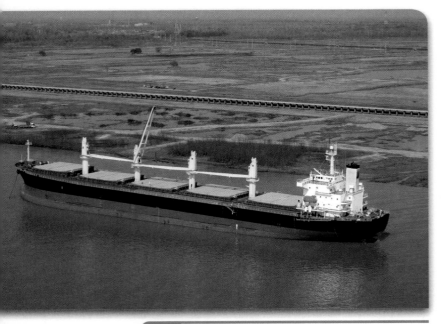

2-13 Many governments use land to raise crops for export rather than to produce food to feed people in their countries.

Nutrition Knowledge Affects Food Choices

This chapter has addressed a number of factors that affect your food choices. As you have read, factors ranging from your culture to government policies have an impact on the foods you select. One other factor that influences your food choices is how much you know about nutrition.

To illustrate this point, answer the following question: Should you avoid vegetable oil because it is high in cholesterol? If you said yes, you would be agreeing with 68 percent of respondents to a nationwide survey. Unfortunately, you would be wrong. Vegetable oil, like all other foods from plant sources, contains no cholesterol. Therefore, you would be avoiding a food based on misinformation. This example should help you see why correct information is so important. It can help you make knowledgeable food choices.

People have many beliefs about food and nutrition. The following are just a few examples reflecting a lack of knowledge that may lead people to make uninformed choices:

- *Certain foods have magical powers.* Eating fish will not make you a genius. Eating yogurt will not allow you to live to be over 100 years old. Eating an apple every day will not end your need for medical care. All nutritious foods have benefits for the body. However, you need to eat a variety of foods. No single food provides all the nutrients you need.

- *Taking vitamin and mineral pills eliminates the need to eat nutritious foods.* Some doctors suggest taking a multivitamin and mineral pill to help make up for lacks in the diet. However, no pill can replace the nutrients supplied by a nutritious diet. Depending on pills for good nutrition can interfere with a person's good dietary habits.

- *Foods grown without chemical pesticides have greater nutritional value than other foods.* Some people are concerned about the effects of chemicals used to control weeds and insects. They worry about the impact these chemicals may have on the environment and the food chain. However, farmers must use

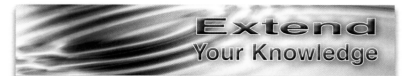

Extend Your Knowledge

The Power of Food

Research countries where there is strife and war. Find current reports in the media to understand the role food plays in these countries. How does the ability to safely grow or transport food to people impact the outcomes of the civil strife? Based on your findings, who do you think has the control to deny or permit the delivery of food to the hungry people? What are possible political solutions for reducing hunger?

chemicals within safety guidelines set by government agencies. According to tests, foods grown with and without chemical pesticides have similar nutritional value.

- *Certain foods can cure diseases.* Some people have heard a story about British sailors years ago. The story reports how the sailors stopped dying of scurvy when they started eating citrus fruits. Many people want to believe eating certain foods can similarly cure such diseases as arthritis and cancer. What these people may not understand is that scurvy is a nutrient-deficiency disease. The lack of vitamin C in the diet causes the disease. The vitamin C contained in the citrus fruit cured the sailors, not the fruit itself. Some foods have been shown to be useful in preventing and treating certain diseases not caused by nutrient deficiencies. For instance, research has shown that regularly eating onions and garlic may help prevent some types of cancer. However, diet is only one of several factors that play a role in disease prevention and treatment.

Where do you look for information about nutrition? Friends and relatives may offer advice, but they may lack knowledge. You can find an abundance of nutrition information through books, magazines, television, and the Internet, **2-14**. However, be aware that details from these sources can be incomplete or inaccurate. For reliable information, look for materials reviewed by registered dietitians. These professionals have expert knowledge of nutrition.

Knowledge about your health is also important for making the best food choices. Certain illnesses such as diabetes and hypertension require a modified diet. A qualified physician must correctly diagnose illnesses. Then a registered dietitian can help people with illnesses plan diets that will meet their special needs.

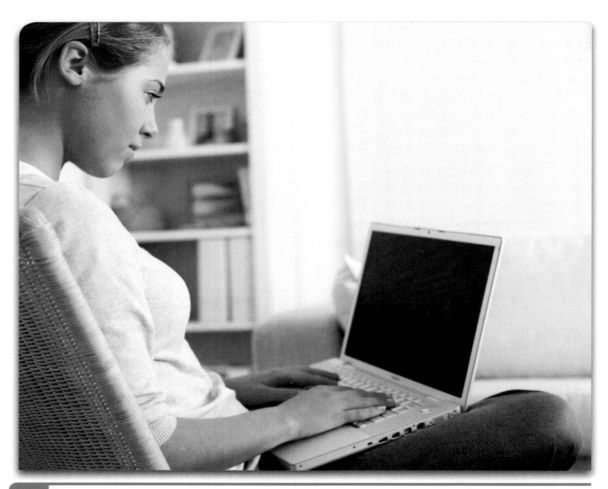

2-14 Choosing reliable reference materials will help you get accurate nutrition information.

Reading Summary

Choosing foods goes beyond satisfying hunger. Many factors influence people's food choices. Food choices often reflect a person's culture. Studying history can reveal how some foods became associated with a particular culture. Many foods have importance to certain ethnic groups. When people from an ethnic group settle together, their foods may become associated with a certain region. Religious beliefs about food are also an aspect of cultural cuisine.

People often choose food for social reasons. Family members influence the food choices children make. Friends can also influence food choices, especially for teens. The way people perceive the status of certain foods can affect people's interest in eating them. The media impact people's desire and willingness to eat certain foods, too.

Emotions are another factor that affects food choices. Some foods produce emotional responses in people. In the same way, some emotions cause people to desire certain foods. Some people use food to reward or punish themselves or others. Of course, personal preferences may be one of the biggest factors governing which foods people choose.

Agriculture, technology, economics, and politics affect what foods are sold in the grocery store. Foods that grow well in a region are likely to be widely available in that region. However, technological advances have made it easier for foods from all over the world to reach local supermarkets. Even when people need locally grown foods, the foods may be shipped to other countries for economic reasons. People with political power make decisions that affect the availability of food products among people in a country.

A final factor that affects food choices is nutrition knowledge. People are more likely to choose foods that are good for them when they understand their nutritional needs.

Review Learning

1. What three factors can help identify ethnic foods?
2. Why are certain foods more common in some regions of the United States than others?
3. What are four trends that have influenced family eating habits?
4. True or false. High-status foods have more nutritional value than other foods.
5. What are two ways in which the media influence people's food choices and eating habits?
6. When do people develop most of their emotional reactions toward foods?
7. True or false. People who have been rewarded with food as children may continue to reward themselves with food as adults.
8. What factors most affect individuals' food preferences?
9. What five resources are needed to grow plentiful crops?
10. Name three technological advances that have improved the food supply in modern history.
11. How can lack of food processing plants and food storage facilities affect food availability in an economically disadvantaged country?
12. List three examples of lack of nutrition knowledge that may lead people to make misinformed food choices.

Critical Thinking

13. **Analyze cause and effect.** In your opinion, what is the cause-and-effect relationship between food advertisements in the media and increasing obesity levels among all ages of Americans?

14. **Determine credibility.** When seeking knowledge about nutrition, how can you determine the credibility of a source?

15. **Draw conclusions.** Biotechnology has the potential to impact the world food supply in regard to feeding hungry people. Research current areas of study in biotechnology related to food. Draw conclusions about whether these research areas are likely to impact the world food supply.

Applying Your Knowledge

16. **Make a speech.** Identify and/or make one of your favorite meals. Prepare a brief speech explaining how the meal reflects you and your culture.

17. **Survey commercials.** Make a list of all the food commercials aired within a one-hour time segment. Note the techniques used to promote each product. Indicate which products on the list you have tried or would like to try.

18. **Analyze emotions and food.** List several emotions you commonly experience, such as anger, love, and fear. Then list a food you associate with each emotion. Compare your list with other students to decide if certain emotions make you think of the same foods.

19. **Food diary—new foods.** Try one new fruit, vegetable, or dairy product each week. Supermarkets, international food stores, and farmers' markets offer many choices. Keep a diary describing the taste and appearance of the food and also your personal reactions to the taste.

20. **Research misinformation.** Use media sources, the Internet, or personal interviews to discover a belief about nutrition or a particular food that is based on misinformation. Research the topic to disprove the belief. Share your findings with the class.

Technology Connections

21. **Chart food patterns.** Identify a country from another continent you wish to study. Use a minimum of two Web sites to learn about the country's geography, climate, and culture. Create a chart using spreadsheet or word processing software. In the first column, list the information you learned about the country's geography, climate, and culture. In the second column, describe how each factor in the first column affects food patterns in that country.

22. **Video presentation.** Using a camcorder, develop a three- to five-minute presentation of a family member preparing an ethnic food. Share information about how the food preparation techniques were learned and about any ingredients that may be unfamiliar to the class. Share with the class.

23. **Internet search.** Look up the Web site of your state's department of agriculture to learn which fruits and vegetables are grown locally and their growing seasons. Create a pamphlet that can be used as a reference for people interested in purchasing locally grown foods.

Academic Connections

24. **Social studies.** Research the dietary laws of an ethnic group in which you are interested. If possible, connect with a historian to learn where, why, and when the laws originated. Summarize your findings using presentation software.

25. **Math.** Examine the food section of a local newspaper, magazine, or Web site. Select articles and advertisements that might influence readers' food choices and eating habits. Identify the group that is being targeted, for example, children, teens, and so on. Calculate the percent of advertisements that is directed at each group.

26. **History.** Working in small groups, debate what aspect of food technology has had the greatest impact on food production in the last 50 years. Generate a list of five technologies on which the group can agree. Give reasons which support the position. Share the results with the rest of the class.

Workplace Applications

Analyze a Problem

The ability to gather and analyze information is an important skill in every workplace. Consider the following problem: As foodservice director for a multinational corporation, it has come to your attention that foods served in the company cafeterias are not meeting all cultural needs of employees. Most offices in the United States have many employees from Asian and Middle Eastern cultures. You need to make changes in some types of foods served, but need more information. Create a plan to gather and analyze needed information. List questions you need to ask and potential sources of reliable information.

Chapter 3
How Nutrients Become You

Reading for Meaning
Make a list of everything you already know about the topic of this chapter. As you read the chapter, check off the items that the chapter covers.

Concept Organizer
Use the flowchart diagram to identify the key parts of the digestive process. Identify concepts relevant to each part of the process.

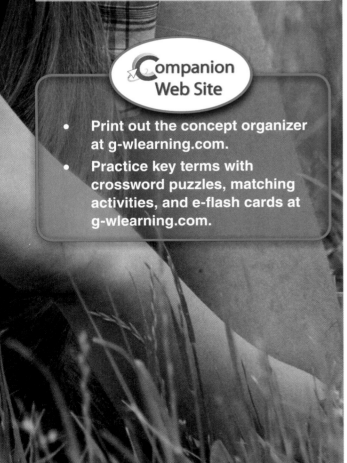

Terms to Know

kilocalorie
digestion
enzyme
gastrointestinal (GI) tract
mastication
peristalsis
gastric juices
chyme
bile
feces
absorption
villi
metabolism
ATP (adenosine triphosphate)
food allergy
food intolerance
diarrhea
constipation
indigestion
heartburn
ulcer
gallstones
diverticulosis

Companion Web Site

- **Print out the concept organizer at g-wlearning.com.**
- **Practice key terms with crossword puzzles, matching activities, and e-flash cards at g-wlearning.com.**

Objectives

After studying this chapter, you will be able to
- **identify** the six basic nutrient groups.
- **distinguish** the functions of the major parts of the digestive system.
- **summarize** the processes of absorption and metabolism.
- **analyze** how lifestyle behaviors and food patterns can affect digestion and absorption processes.
- **recognize** the characteristics associated with common digestive disorders.

Central Ideas

- Consuming foods from the six nutrient groups and good digestion are critical for physical wellness.
- Eating habits, emotions, food allergies and intolerances, and physical activity influence effective digestion.

The phrase "You are what you eat" is a true statement. Food is your body's fuel. When you eat, your body breaks down food and the nutrients it contains into simpler elements. Energy is released and nutrients are used to help build, repair, and maintain body cells. Then your body discards the by-products of this process as waste. This chapter will help you picture the process of how your body uses food from beginning to end.

Food, Nutrients, and Energy

Food plays more roles than simply satisfying hunger. The food you eat becomes part of you. Nutrients from food are your body's source of fuel and building materials.

The Six Nutrient Groups

There are six groups of nutrients your body needs. They are carbohydrates, fats, proteins, vitamins, minerals, and water. You must obtain these substances from the foods you eat. Each nutrient has specific jobs to perform in the body. Each of these nutrients, in recommended quantities, is vital to good health. Without adequate amounts of these nutrients over time, your risk of various health problems will increase.

Case Study: Chemistry of the Lunch Table

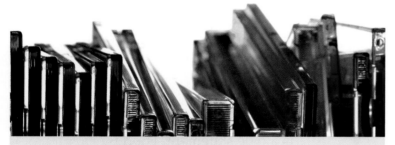

Josie and Linda were sitting in the school cafeteria. The girls brought their lunches from home today and are going to share food with each other.

Josie is taking both chemistry and nutrition this semester. She just learned that some of the elements in food are the same kind of elements she is studying in chemistry. Linda has not taken either chemistry or nutrition. When Linda saw Josie's lunch, she shouted, "What are you eating? The chemicals in your store-bought food are really bad for you. Eating fresh-grown foods and foods from health-food stores is much better for you. It is the only way to avoid all those chemicals they put in food." Josie disagrees and says, "Chemical elements are the foundation of all foods. Whether you eat food from your garden or from the store, you are still eating chemicals. In fact, you are made up mostly of chemical elements, too." Linda looks confused.

Case Review

1. Why do you think Linda believes only store-bought foods are composed of chemical elements?

2. With which girl do you agree? Why?

The Chemistry of Nutrition

Learning about health and nutrition requires some knowledge of chemistry. Your body and the foods you eat are composed of chemical elements. *Elements* are the simplest substances from which all matter is formed. *Matter* is anything that takes up space and has a measurable quantity. An *atom* is the smallest part of an element that can enter into a chemical reaction. A *molecule* is the smallest amount of a substance that has all the characteristics of the substance. Molecules are made up of two or more atoms that are bonded together. The atoms in a molecule may all be the same element, or they may be different elements. When atoms of different elements are bonded together, a *compound* is formed.

Hydrogen and oxygen are both elements. An atom of hydrogen can enter into a chemical reaction with another atom of hydrogen. These two atoms can be bonded together to form a hydrogen molecule. Two atoms of hydrogen can also bond to an atom of oxygen. The resulting substance would be a molecule of water. Because this molecule is made up of two different elements, water is a compound.

Five of the basic nutrient groups—carbohydrates, fats, proteins, vitamins, and water—are compounds. Minerals—the sixth basic nutrient group—are elements. There are at least 25 chemical elements involved in health and nutrition, including oxygen, hydrogen, carbon, nitrogen, sulfur, and cobalt.

It may be difficult to think of food as a list of chemicals. You do not need to carry out laboratory experiments to understand nutrition. However, having some chemistry background will help you grasp how nutrients interact in your body.

The Functions of Nutrients

Essential nutrients from food are used to

- build and repair body tissues
- regulate all body processes
- provide energy

When your body is performing all these functions in harmony, your potential for optimum wellness increases.

Build and Repair Body Tissues

Your body is made up of billions of cells. From before you are born until you die, cells divide. Each time a cell divides, it produces two new cells. These new cells account for your growth. New cells are also used to repair damaged body tissues and to replace old cells, **3-1**. All cells are formed with materials that come from food. Therefore, your body needs adequate amounts of nutrients to help make new cells.

Nutrient needs during periods of rapid growth are greater than at any other time. Such periods include the prenatal period, infancy, and adolescence. Lacking adequate nutrition during periods of growth may affect a person's physical size, strength, and health. His or her learning abilities and behavior patterns could be affected, too.

Every cell in your body contains genes. *Genes* carry hereditary information you received from your parents. Height, gender, skin color, and other details that are yours alone are on a genetic blueprint. However, good nutrition is necessary if you are to reach your full genetic potential. In other words, if your parents are tall, they may have passed along genes allowing you to become tall, too. However, your body needs nutrients to grow. If your diet does not provide these nutrients, you will not grow to your full height potential.

Regulate Body Processes

A second function of nutrients is to keep body processes running smoothly. For instance, the circulation of body fluids requires a balance of essential nutrients. Maintaining the correct

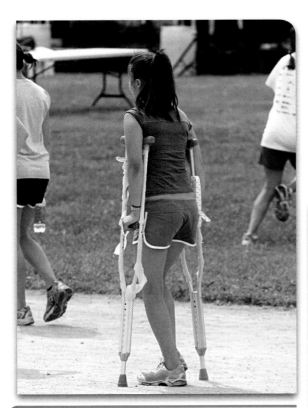

3-1 A key function of nutrients is to help the body repair damaged tissues.

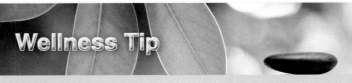

Wellness Tip

Chew on This!

What's the key to maintaining and losing weight? Chewing! Good digestion begins with chewing food well. As you chew, digestive enzymes begin their work releasing nutrients in your system. Chewing slowly not only releases nutrients, but it takes more time and can help you eat less which can help you to better manage your weight.

acid-base level in the blood is a function of nutrients. Digestion, absorption, and metabolism are also processes that rely on proper amounts of nutrients.

The chemical reactions that control body processes are complex. However, these reactions normally work well. You will not usually need to think about which foods cause which chemical reactions. Instead, you need only to focus on eating a nutritious diet, 3-2. This will ensure you are getting the nutrients you need to help your organs and tissues work properly.

Provide Energy

A third key function of nutrients is to provide energy. Food is to your body what gasoline is to a car. It is a source of energy for performance. The quality of the food you eat affects how well your body will run.

Energy is necessary for all life processes to occur. Your body needs energy to breathe, pump blood, move muscles, and provide heat. You need energy every minute of every day. If you go without food too long, your body will not have the energy needed to operate vital organs. The more active you are, the more energy you need to meet the physical demands placed on your body.

Chemical reactions that take place in your cells release energy from the nutrients you get from food. Carbohydrates and fats are the two main nutrients used for energy. Proteins may also be used, but the body prefers to save proteins for other vital functions. Vitamins, minerals, and water do not provide energy. However, the body needs these nutrients to help regulate the release of energy from carbohydrates, fats, and proteins. If just one nutrient is missing from the diet, energy release will be hampered.

The Energy Value of Food

The energy value of food is measured in units called **kilocalories**. A kilocalorie is the amount of heat needed to raise one kilogram of water one degree Celsius. Kilocalories may also be called *Calories*. In this book, the more common lowercase *calories* will be used. The prefix *kilo* means 1,000. A kilocalorie is 1,000 times larger than the calorie unit used in your chemistry or physics classes.

As mentioned earlier, only certain nutrients provide energy. Each gram of carbohydrate in a food product supplies the body with 4 calories of energy. Fats provide 9 calories per gram. Proteins yield 4 calories per gram. Water, vitamins, and minerals do not yield energy. Therefore, they have no calorie content. The more calories in a food, the more energy it will provide, 3-3.

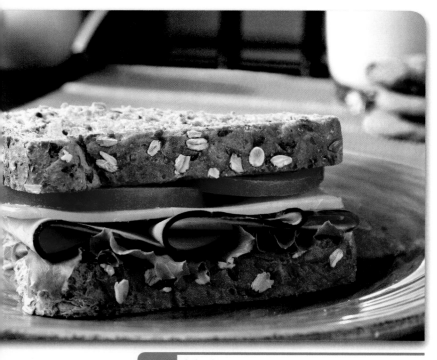

3-1 A balanced diet includes a variety of foods, which provide the nutrients needed to keep your body running right.

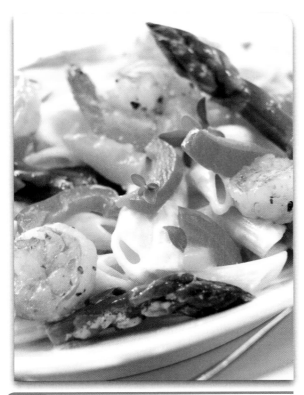

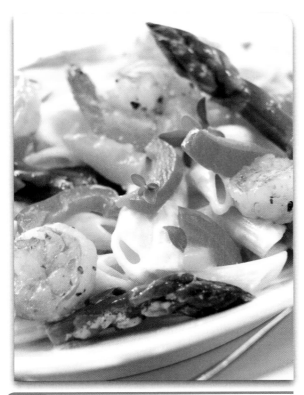

3-3 The calories in this dish come from carbohydrates in the pasta and vegetables, fat in the Alfredo sauce, and protein in the shrimp.

Alcohol provides 7 calories per gram consumed. However, alcohol is not considered a nutrient because it does not promote growth, maintain cells, or repair tissues. Alcohol is a drug. If consumed in excess, its harmful effects outweigh any positive energy contributions it might make to the diet.

The Process of Digestion

What happens to a piece of food after you put it in your mouth? A detailed answer to this question would describe the complex process of digestion. **Digestion** is the process by which your body breaks down food, and the nutrients in food, into simpler substances. The blood can then carry these simple substances to cells for use in growth, repair, and maintenance.

Digestion occurs through mechanical and chemical means throughout the digestive system. *Mechanical digestion* happens as food is crushed and churned. Chewing food is an observable form of mechanical digestion.

In *chemical digestion*, food is mixed with powerful acids and enzymes. **Enzymes** are a type of protein produced by cells that cause specific chemical reactions. For example, digestive enzymes cause food particles to break apart into simpler substances.

As food is digested, it passes through a muscular tube leading from the mouth to the anus. This tube is called the **gastrointestinal (GI) tract**. The GI tract is about 25 to 30 feet (7.6 to 9.1 m) in length. Each section performs important functions.

In the Mouth

Food enters the GI tract through the mouth. **Mastication**, or chewing, is the first step in the digestive process. The teeth and tongue work together

Math Link

Computing Snack Calories

Robert consumes a snack that contains 46 grams of carbohydrates, 9 grams of fat, and 2 grams of protein.
- Compute how many calories are in Robert's snack.

to move food and crush it into smaller pieces. This process prepares food for swallowing. Chewing your food well aids digestion because the body can break down small food particles faster than large particles.

There are about 10,000 taste buds that cover the surface of the tongue. These taste buds sense the flavors of food. This taste sensation, along with good food odors and the thought of food, trigger salivary glands in your mouth, 3-4. These glands produce and secrete a solution called *saliva*. Saliva is a mixture of about 99 percent water plus a few chemicals. One of these chemicals is an enzyme called *salivary amylase*. This enzyme, found only in the mouth, helps chemically break down (digest) the starches in foods.

Saliva plays other important roles in the digestive process besides the breakdown of starches. Without saliva, your mouth is dry and food seems to have little taste. Saliva moistens, softens, and dissolves food. It also helps cleanse the teeth and neutralize mouth acids.

In the Esophagus

As you chew, the muscles of your mouth and tongue form the food into a small ball. Your tongue moves this

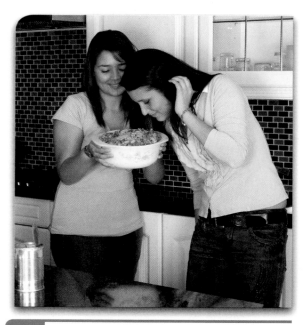

3-4 Appetizing smells, such as those from cooking food, trigger glands in the mouth to secrete saliva.

ball of food to the back of your mouth and you swallow it. As you swallow, food passes from the mouth to the stomach through the esophagus. The *esophagus* is a tube about 10 inches long. It connects the mouth to the stomach.

The esophagus is only one of two tubes in the throat. The other is the *trachea*, which is sometimes called the windpipe. When you swallow food, a flap of skin called the *epiglottis* closes to keep food from entering the trachea. Breathing automatically stops when you swallow food to help prevent choking.

A series of squeezing actions by the muscles in the esophagus, known as **peristalsis**, helps move food through the tube. Peristalsis is involuntary. It happens automatically when food is present. You cannot feel or control the muscles as they move the food toward the stomach. Peristaltic action occurs throughout the esophagus and intestine to help mechanically move and churn food.

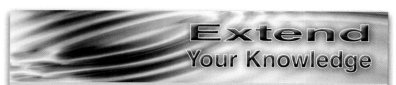

Extend Your Knowledge

What Affects the Sense of Taste?

Use print or Internet sources to learn more about factors that affect taste. If something smells good, do you think it tastes better? Why? How do certain medicines, illnesses, food colors, or serving utensils affect taste? How does the sense of taste develop? What flavors and tastes are recognized first as a child? How does age affect a person's sense of taste?

In the Stomach

When you eat, the stomach produces gastric juices to prepare for digesting the oncoming food. The term *gastric* means stomach. **Gastric juices** contain hydrochloric acid, digestive enzymes, and mucus. The mixture of gastric juices and chewed and swallowed food combine in the stomach. This mixture is called **chyme**.

The acid in the stomach is almost as strong as battery acid found in a car. The stomach wall has a thick lining, called the *mucosa*. The mucosa secretes mucus. *Mucus* is a thick fluid that helps soften and lubricate food. It also helps protect the stomach from its strong acidic juices.

Protein digestion begins in the stomach. The major gastric enzyme that begins to chemically break down protein is *pepsin*.

Most people can hold about one quart of food in their stomachs. Food generally remains in the stomach two to three hours, depending on the type of food. Liquids leave the stomach before solids. Carbohydrates and proteins digest faster than fats. Fatty foods stay in the stomach the longest, **3-5**. From the stomach, chyme moves to the small intestine.

In the Small Intestine

About 95 percent of digestion occurs in the small intestine. The small intestine is coiled in the abdomen in circular folds. It has three sections: the duodenum, the jejunum, and the ileum. The *duodenum* is the first section and is about 12 inches (30.5 cm) long. The *jejunum* is the middle section and is about 4 feet (1.2 m) long. The *ileum* is the last section and is 5 feet (10.5 m) in length. When stretched, the small intestine measures about 20 feet

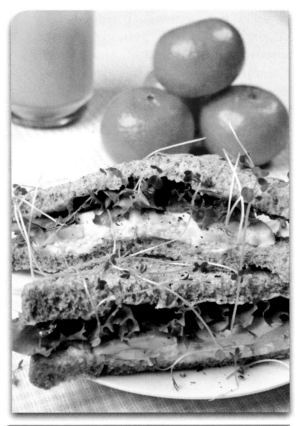

3-5 During digestion of this meal, liquids (orange juice) would leave the stomach first. They would be followed first by the carbohydrates (bread, fruit, lettuce), then by the protein (eggs), and finally by the fat (mayonnaise).

(6.1 m) in length and 1 inch (2.5 cm) in diameter.

It takes about 5 to 14 hours for food to travel from the mouth through the small intestine. During this time, strong muscular contractions constantly mix and churn food, aiding in mechanical digestion. Peristalsis moves food through the small intestine.

The small intestine needs a less acidic environment than the stomach to perform its work. The *pancreas*, an elongated gland behind the stomach, helps create the correct environment. The pancreas secretes *bicarbonate*, which neutralizes hydrochloric acid that has come from the stomach with the partially digested food.

The pancreas also produces digestive enzymes that aid in the chemical digestion that takes place in the small intestine. These enzymes break down proteins, fats, and carbohydrates into their most basic parts so your body can use them. *Amino acids* are the most basic parts of proteins. *Monosaccharides* are the most basic parts of carbohydrates. *Fatty acids, glycerol,* and *monoglycerides* are the most basic parts of fats. *Proteases* break down proteins into amino acids. *Lipases* are fat-digesting enzymes, which break down fats into fatty acids, glycerol, and monoglycerides. *Saccharidases* break carbohydrates into monosaccharides (simple sugars).

The liver is also involved in the chemical digestion that happens in the small intestine. The *liver* is a large gland that sits above the stomach. It produces a digestive juice called **bile**, which aids fat digestion. Bile helps disperse fat in the water-based digestive fluids. This gives enzymes in the fluids access to the fat so they can break it down. Bile is stored in a muscular sac called the *gallbladder* until it is needed for digestive purposes. It is secreted into the first part of the small intestine, **3-6**.

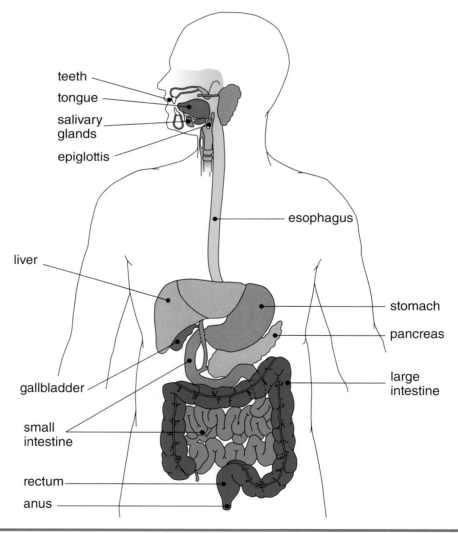

teeth
tongue
salivary glands
epiglottis
esophagus
liver
stomach
pancreas
gallbladder
large intestine
small intestine
rectum
anus

3-6 Each part of the digestive system performs important functions in breaking down food for use in the body.

In the Large Intestine

The small intestine is connected to the large intestine, which is sometimes called the *colon*. The large intestine measures about 3½ feet (1.1 m) in your body, or 5 to 6 feet (1.5 to 1.8 m) when stretched. Very little digestion occurs in the large intestine. The main job of the large intestine is to reabsorb water. (Chyme is very liquid when it enters the large intestine.)

Chyme usually stays in the colon for about one to three days before elimination. During this time, water is absorbed through the walls of the colon. Useful bacteria in the colon work on fiber. They also help manufacture small amounts of some vitamins.

Solid wastes that result from digestion are called **feces**. These wastes include mucus, bile pigments, fiber, sloughed off cells from the lining of the large intestine, and water. The end of the large intestine is called the *rectum*. Feces collect here until they are ready to pass from the body through the *anus*.

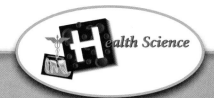

Health Science

Clinical Dietitian

Clinical dietitians provide nutritional services to patients in hospitals, nursing care facilities, and other institutions. They assess patients' nutritional needs, develop and implement nutrition programs, and evaluate and report the results. Clinical dietitians also confer with doctors and other health-care professionals to coordinate medical and nutritional needs. Some specialize in weight management or in the care of diabetic or critically ill patients. In addition, clinical dietitians may manage the food service department in nursing care facilities, small hospitals, or correctional facilities.

Education: Clinical dietitians need at least a bachelor's degree. Licensure, certification, or registration can vary by state.

Job Outlook: Average employment growth is projected. Applicants with specialized training, advanced degrees, or certifications beyond their particular state's minimum requirements should have the best job opportunities.

Absorption of Nutrients

After being digested in the small intestine, the nutrients in food are ready for absorption. **Absorption** is the passage of nutrients from the digestive tract into the circulatory or lymphatic system. Most nutrients pass through the walls of the small intestine. However, alcohol and a few other drugs can be absorbed in the stomach. Alcohol can be absorbed in the mouth, too.

The inside surface area of the small intestine is about 600 times larger than that of a smooth tube. This is because the wall of the small intestine is pleated with thousands of folds. The folds are covered with villi. **Villi** are tiny, fingerlike projections that give the lining of the small intestine a velvetlike texture. Each cell of every villus is covered with *microvilli*, which are like microscopic hairs that help catch nutrient particles.

Some nutrients can dissolve in water. They are called *water-soluble nutrients*. These nutrients include amino acids from proteins, monosaccharides from carbohydrates, minerals, most vitamins, and water. Tiny blood vessels in the villi, called *capillaries*, absorb water-soluble nutrients into the bloodstream. Then these nutrients are carried to the liver through the portal vein.

Some nutrients can dissolve in fat. They are called *fat-soluble nutrients*. These nutrients include a few vitamins as well as fatty acids, glycerol, and monoglycerides from fats. Lymph vessels in the villi, called *lacteals*, absorb fat-soluble nutrients into the lymphatic system. These nutrients then make their way to the bloodstream, **3-7**.

The large intestine finishes the job of absorption. Small amounts of water and some minerals are absorbed in the large intestine. Bacteria, plant fibers, and sloughed off cells from the lining of the large intestine make up the remaining waste material.

Metabolism

Once nutrients are digested and absorbed, the circulatory system takes over. The circulatory system carries nutrients and oxygen to individual cells. All the chemical changes that occur as cells produce energy and materials needed to sustain life are known as **metabolism**.

During metabolism, cells make some compounds. They use some of these compounds for energy and store others for later use. For example, cells can make new proteins to be used for growth. The body will slough off worn cells and replace them with new cells.

Through metabolism, cells convert some nutrients into energy. The body stores this energy as **ATP (adenosine triphosphate)**. ATP is the source of immediate energy found in muscle tissue. When the body needs energy, chemical reactions break down ATP to release energy. Every cell makes ATP to help meet all your energy needs.

The body must discard waste products that result from cell metabolism. Waste products leave the body through the kidneys, lungs, and skin. The *kidneys* are part of the urinary system. They act like a filter to remove wastes and excess water from the blood and form *urine*, a liquid waste material. The urine collects in the *bladder* until it is excreted. Drinking six to eight glasses of water daily helps keep waste products flushed out of your system.

Breath from your lungs and perspiration through your skin also excrete waste products from cell metabolism. The harder and faster you breathe, as when exercising, the more moisture and carbon dioxide you lose.

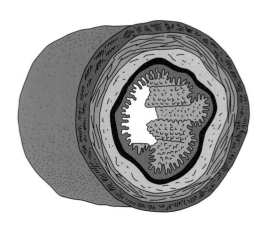

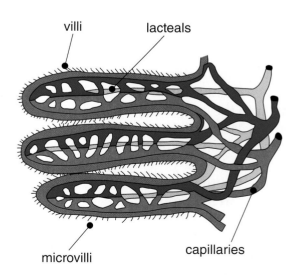

3-7 Villi lining the small intestine increase the surface area through which nutrients can be absorbed into the capillaries and lacteals.

Factors Affecting Digestion and Absorption

Have you ever been nervous or worried and felt food sitting in your stomach like a rock? The GI system usually works as it should. However, sometimes people have problems. Factors that affect this complex system include your eating habits and emotions, **3-8**. Food sensitivities and physical activity can affect digestion, too. Healthy lifestyle choices can help you avoid many GI problems.

Eating Habits

The foods you choose and how you eat them can affect digestion. If you eat too little food or your diet lacks variety, you may be missing important nutrients. The lack of a single nutrient can affect how your body will digest and absorb other nutrients. To ensure normal digestion, choose a nutritious diet that includes a wide range of foods.

Be sure to include fresh fruits and vegetables and whole-grain products in your varied diet. These plant foods are high in an indigestible material called *fiber*. Fiber helps strengthen intestinal muscles the way weight training helps strengthen arm and leg muscles. Fiber forms a mass in the digestive tract that creates resistance against which the muscles of the intestine can push.

Eating too much food too quickly places stress on the mechanical and chemical reactions needed for normal digestion. To avoid such stress, take time to enjoy your food instead of rushing through a meal. Also, be aware of the size of your portions. Eat moderate amounts of food rather than stuff yourself.

The makeup of a meal affects how long it will take your body to digest. Foods high in fat take longer to digest than foods high in carbohydrates or protein. In the stomach, fats separate from the watery part of the chyme and float to the top. They are the last food component to leave the stomach. A steak dinner, including baked potato with sour cream, oily salad dressing, and chocolate cream pie, is high in fat. This meal will take longer to digest than a high-carbohydrate meal, such as spaghetti, bread, and fruit salad. Because fats take longer to digest, you will feel full longer after eating the high-fat meal.

You should be aware of the wholesomeness of the foods you choose. Spoiled and contaminated foods are unsafe and can cause intestinal problems. Symptoms of these problems often include nausea, stomach cramps, and other intestinal disturbances. Illnesses caused by some contaminated foods can even lead to death.

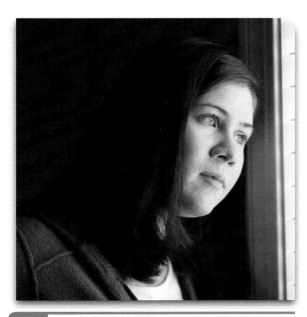

3-8 Emotions such as anxiety and depression can interfere with normal digestion.

Emotions

Emotions such as fear, anger, and tension can lead to digestive difficulties. You can avoid most of these problems by making a few lifestyle changes. Making a point of reducing stress and tension while eating will aid digestion. Try to enjoy food in a peaceful, quiet, cheerful atmosphere, **3-9**. Avoid arguments at mealtime. Also, chew foods slowly and thoroughly to ease swallowing. Taking these steps will help promote normal digestion.

Food Allergies and Intolerances

A **food allergy** is a reaction of your body's immune system to certain proteins found in foods. Allergic reactions to food occur in a small percent of the population. They occur more often during infancy and young adulthood. Reactions occur after a certain food is eaten and the immune system responds. The *immune system* is the body's defense system. The tonsils, thyroid, lymph glands, spleen, and white blood cells make up this system. The immune system protects the body against disease and foreign materials. It produces proteins called *antibodies*. Antibodies combat foreign materials that get into your bloodstream.

The protein that stimulates the immune system to produce antibodies is called an *allergen*. When an allergen enters the body, the release of antibodies leads to allergy symptoms. Vomiting, stomach pain, and intestinal distress are common symptoms of a food allergy. However, some people experience skin rashes, swelling, and breathing problems.

Experts cannot predict who will develop allergies or how allergies will affect people. Heredity seems to play a role in the development of some allergies. Very small amounts of an allergen may be a problem for one person. Another person may be able to tolerate much more of the same substance. Allergic reactions can change over a life span. As some children get older, their allergies go away. However, other people develop new allergies as adults.

Which foods can cause allergies? Most people are allergic to only one or two foods. The foods most often identified with allergic reactions are tree nuts, peanuts, eggs, milk, soybeans, wheat, fish, and shellfish. People who are allergic to such foods must eliminate or limit them. If milder reactions occur, after consuming a food, you may be sensitive to the food but not experience a full allergic reaction. People with food allergies must carefully read labels to be sure prepared foods do not contain allergens.

A **food intolerance** also causes an unpleasant reaction to food. Unlike a food allergy, a food intolerance does

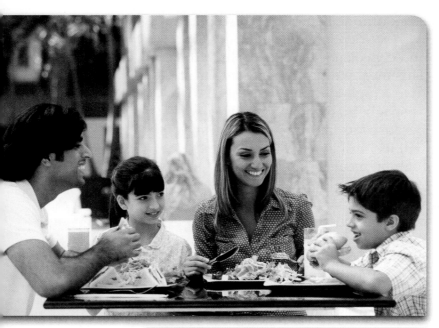

3-9 Dining in a relaxed atmosphere aids normal digestion.

not cause an immune system response. Usually, larger amounts of the food are consumed to experience intolerance problems. Allergic responses may occur with very little exposure to an allergen. Food intolerances are caused by deficiencies or reactions in the digestive tract. Intolerance can be experienced through a reaction to certain food colors, sulfates in food, or food contaminants from unhealthy bacteria. For example, some people lack the necessary enzyme in their digestive tract to digest milk properly. Some symptoms can be similar to an allergic response and may include elevated blood pressure, sweating, and headache. Treatment focuses on eliminating or reducing the amounts of the offending foods from the diet.

Physical Activity

Physical activity can improve health in many ways. It can aid digestion and metabolism. Physical activity stimulates a healthy appetite and strengthens the muscles of internal organs. It helps move food through the GI tract. It also helps reduce stress and adds to your total sense of well-being. For a healthy digestive system, include some physical activities in your lifestyle, **3-10**.

Digestive Disorders

Most people experience digestive disorders from time to time. Consumers spend many dollars on medications to relieve these problems. Most of these medications are not needed. The digestive system normally functions better without drugs. To help avoid problems, focus on eating a nutritious diet. Be sure to include a

Case Study: Adjusting to Food Intolerance

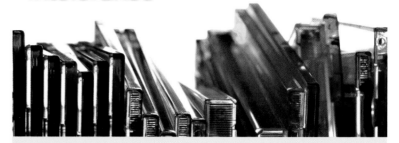

Tom, Sara, Katie, and Josh decided to go for burgers and drinks at a fast-food restaurant after school. They wanted to get a head start on their group science project. Tom watched as Josh pushed the hamburger bun from his plate and ate only the tomato, lettuce, pickle, and meat. Tom asked Josh, "Why don't you eat the bun? Are you on a diet or something?"

Josh said, "No, I am a celiac." Tom wondered if it was a contagious disease. Katie chimed in to ask, "What is that? It sounds weird!"

"I know what it is," said Sara, "He has an intolerance to the protein found in wheat and some other grains. My cousin has the same disease and she is on a gluten-free diet. It is not contagious!"

Case Review

1. How do you suppose Josh's life is impacted by having a food intolerance?

2. How could Josh's friends show their support and understanding the next time they go out to eat?

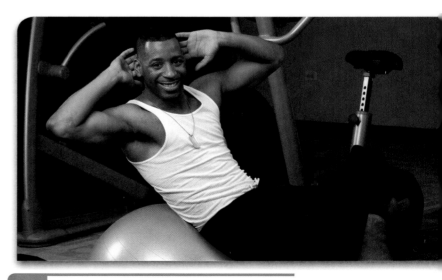

3-10 Physical activity stimulates a healthy appetite and helps the digestive system function properly.

variety of high-fiber fruits, vegetables, and whole-grain products.

Long-term illnesses, including ulcer and gallstones, can have more serious effects on digestion. They can alter the kinds and amounts of nutrients that reach the cells. Such illnesses require medical supervision.

Diarrhea

Diarrhea is frequent expulsion of watery feces. Food sensitivity, harmful bacteria, and stress are just a few of the factors that can cause diarrhea. Diarrhea causes food to move through the digestive system too quickly for nutrients to be fully absorbed. In addition, diarrhea can lead to a loss of body fluids. Drinking plenty of water will help restore fluid losses when diarrhea occurs. Prolonged diarrhea may be a sign of other health problems and indicates a need to see a doctor.

Constipation

Constipation occurs when chyme moves very slowly through the large intestine. When this happens, too much water is reabsorbed from the chyme. This causes the feces to become hard, making bowel movements painful. Straining during elimination can lead to the added problem of hemorrhoids. Hemorrhoids are swollen veins in the rectum.

Constipation can result from erratic eating habits, low fiber intake, and lack of physical activity. Drinking too little water and failing to respond to a bowel movement urge can also add to this problem.

Many people use laxatives when they are constipated. However, the body can start to depend on the use of laxatives. Therefore, laxatives can worsen constipation. A better approach

to treating and preventing constipation is to choose a diet high in fiber. Get regular physical activity and be sure to drink plenty of water, too, **3-11**.

Indigestion

Indigestion is a difficulty in digesting food. Indigestion may be caused by stress, eating too much or too fast, or eating particular foods. Symptoms of indigestion may include gas, stomach cramps, and nausea.

People often take antacids for indigestion. *Antacids* are medications that neutralize stomach acids. However, taking too many antacids can alter the acidity levels of the stomach and interfere with nutrient absorption rates. Frequent use of antacids can also cause constipation. Instead of taking antacids, try to modify your diet. Avoid eating too much of one food or too many calories at one meal. Avoid eating foods that seem to upset your stomach. Also, eat in a relaxed atmosphere to help reduce stress.

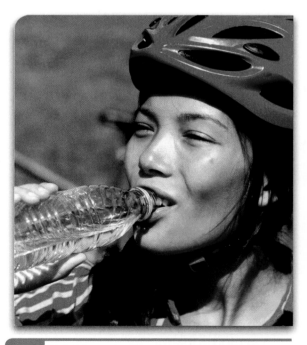

3-11 Drinking plenty of water can help prevent constipation.

Heartburn

Heartburn is a burning pain in the middle of the chest, but it has nothing to do with the heart. Stomach acid flowing back into the esophagus causes heartburn. This condition is known as *reflux*.

Many people have heartburn after a meal now and then. Antacids can help relieve occasional discomfort. However, you should see a doctor if you have ongoing or recurrent heartburn. This may be a sign of a more serious condition called *gastroesophageal reflux disease (GERD)*. This disease is common among older adults. If left untreated, it can cause damage to the esophagus and other complications.

Ulcer

An **ulcer** is an open sore in the lining of the stomach or small intestine. This disease is caused by a bacterium. The ulcerated area becomes inflamed, and the person who has the ulcer experiences a burning pain.

Some people get ulcers more quickly than others. People may have a hereditary tendency for the disease. Those who are under stress or use alcohol or aspirin excessively may also be at greater risk, **3-12**. You can avoid factors that contribute to ulcers by making healthful lifestyle choices.

Doctors generally prescribe antibiotic therapy for ulcer patients. Reducing the level of acid in your digestive system helps the healing process. Doctors also encourage ulcer patients to eat a nutritious diet. They recommend increasing physical activity and decreasing stress levels. They tell patients getting enough sleep is

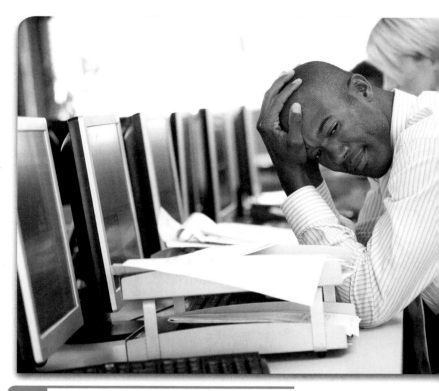

3-12 Individuals who have stressful jobs may be at increased risk for ulcers.

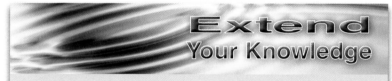

What Is Crohn's Disease?

Crohn's disease is a chronic inflammatory disease of the gastrointestinal tract that belongs to a group of illnesses called inflammatory bowel disease (IBD). Nutritional complications are common with this disease since it impacts the intestines. According to the National Institute of Allergy and Infectious Diseases, about one in 500 people suffer from IBD. Conduct research to learn about the occurrence, symptoms, and treatment of Crohn's disease. Is Crohn's disease hereditary? Is it more common in one gender than another? Which age groups are most affected? Which segments of the population are most affected? How is Crohn's disease treated? Is there a cure?

important. Avoid caffeine and alcohol in your diet. If you do have caffeine, combine it with a meal or snack. Eliminate foods that may cause added ulcer discomfort, such as chocolate, certain herbs, and spicy foods. Small meals throughout the day work better than one big meal. Tobacco is to be avoided.

Gallstones

Gallstones are small crystals that form from bile in the gallbladder. Bile, which is produced by the liver to help digest fat, is stored in the gallbladder. When food is present in the small intestine, the gallbladder contracts to release bile. When gallstones are blocking the duct between the gallbladder and the small intestine, this contraction causes severe pain. The presence of gallstones may slow fat digestion and cause fluids to pool and back up into the liver.

The treatment of gallstones often requires medical supervision. A physician may recommend a diet low in fats. In severe cases, the doctor may remove the gallbladder.

Diverticulosis

Diverticulosis is a disorder in which many abnormal pouches form in the intestinal wall. When these pouches become inflamed, the condition is called *diverticulitis*.

Diverticulosis can occur when intestinal muscles become weak, such as when the diet is too low in fiber. A high-fat diet and an inactive lifestyle can also increase the risk of getting this disease. The best prevention method is to eat a high-fiber diet, which will help keep intestinal muscles toned.

Reading Summary

Your body needs six types of nutrients—carbohydrates, fats, proteins, vitamins, minerals, and water. These nutrients, like your body, are made up of chemical elements. Your body uses them to build and repair tissues and control body processes. Carbohydrates, fats, and proteins are also used to provide energy. Energy is measured in units called Calories or kilocalories.

Your body breaks down the food you eat through a process called digestion. Digestion occurs in the gastrointestinal (GI) tract. The GI tract includes the mouth, esophagus, stomach, small intestine, and large intestine. Throughout the GI tract, crushing and churning help digest food mechanically. Enzymes and other fluids help digest food chemically.

After digestion, your bloodstream is able to absorb nutrients and carry them to your cells. Most absorption takes place in the small intestine. Once nutrients reach your cells, they undergo changes to produce energy and materials needed to sustain life. Together, these changes are known as metabolism.

Several factors can affect digestion and absorption. These include eating habits, emotions, food allergies and intolerances, and physical activity. Lifestyle behaviors that improve the digestive processes include eating a nutritious diet and reducing personal stress. Drinking six to eight glasses of water daily and getting regular physical activity can improve digestion, too.

The digestive system is complex. Normally all works well, but problems sometimes occur. Diarrhea, constipation, indigestion, ulcers, gallstones, and diverticulosis are among the digestive disorders that trouble some people. You can prevent most digestive problems by forming healthful lifestyle habits that aid digestion.

Review Learning

1. List the six nutrient groups and summarize the three main functions of nutrients in your body.
2. How is the energy value of food measured?
3. What is the difference between mechanical digestion and chemical digestion?
4. Why is saliva important in the digestive process?
5. How does the epiglottis help prevent you from choking on food while eating?
6. What is the function of mucus secreted in the stomach?
7. Describe the function of three digestive enzymes that help break down foods in the small intestine.
8. What is the main job of the large intestine?
9. What are the water-soluble and fat-soluble nutrients and how are they absorbed?
10. How does metabolism provide for the body's energy needs?
11. How can eating food too quickly or when you are stressed impact your digestion and absorption?
12. Describe the body's response when a food to which you are allergic is consumed.
13. Describe two digestive disorders and recommended treatment for each.
14. What is the difference between diverticulosis and diverticulitis?

Critical Thinking

15. **Analyze behaviors.** Analyze positive and negative behaviors that impact digestion. For each negative behavior, identify a change for improving digestion.
16. **Draw conclusions.** How can long-term use of acid-reducing medicines impact health? Make a list of your conclusions.

Applying Your Knowledge

17. **Lifestyle collage.** Prepare a collage illustrating healthful lifestyle choices that can help people avoid problems with digestion and absorption.
18. **Interview.** Peanut allergies are one of the most common types of food allergies for children. Interview a teacher of young children or the school foodservice manager to learn what the school does to promote a safe, allergen-free environment. What process is used by the school to learn if students have food allergies or intolerances? Share findings with the class.
19. **Identify treatment choices.** Visit the Web site of a store that sells medications for digestive disorders. List the various disorders and identify the names of drugs available to "treat" each one. Which disorder seems to offer the greatest variety of drug choices? Talk to the pharmacist to learn why so many choices are available. Report your findings in class.
20. **Article analysis.** Find a nutrition-related article, using an online newspaper service. Print out the article. Highlight three important facts you learned about how nutrients become you.

Technology Connections

21. **Electronic presentation.** Research the digestion and absorption process for alcohol. Prepare an electronic presentation on how alcohol is digested, absorbed, and metabolized in the body. Include in your report the effects of alcohol on the liver, kidneys, and other organs.
22. **Summarize credibility.** Evaluate the credibility of an Internet site reporting on causes, prevention, and treatment of a particular digestive disease. Write a summary of your findings.
23. **Online tour.** Take an online tour of the human body and its systems. Create a list the systems in the human body. Note an interesting fact that you learned about each system. Present your facts in class.

Academic Connections

24. **Biology.** Research how a cow's digestive system works. Compare the cow's digestive system to the human digestive system. How are they different? similar?
25. **History.** People have been studying human digestion throughout history. Understanding about digestion and the digestive organs has evolved over the centuries. Select a time period and learn about the accepted beliefs, myths, and traditions of that time regarding some aspect of human digestion. Share with the class.

26. **Science.** Use a reliable physiology resource to investigate how the various body systems relate to each other. Organize your findings in a chart.
27. **Speech.** In small groups, debate the topic "You are what you eat." Identify factors that support the expression referring to the facts of digestion. Identify factors that may interfere with the process of digestion.
28. **Science.** Research and write a paper on the changes that occur in the digestive system as people age. Compare the GI tract characteristics of a young person with that of a person in his or her later years.

Workplace Applications

Brainstorm Options

Presume you are the human resources director for a small manufacturing company. Recent research shows that employees who have good eating habits and total wellness have a positive impact on productivity. You are forming a workplace "Wellness Council." The members of your council are a group of creative-thinking employees who are dedicated to healthful living. Get together with your council members (two or more classmates) and brainstorm a list of several possible ideas for encouraging healthful eating among employees. Then narrow the list down to the three best options. How would you implement one of these options?

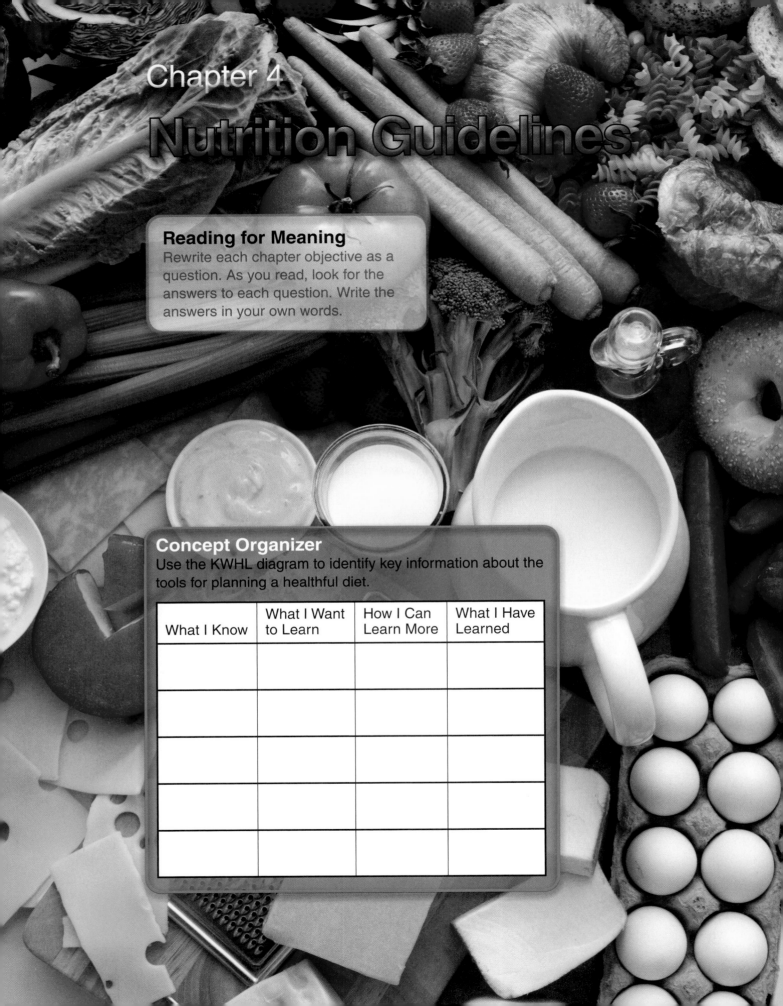

Chapter 4
Nutrition Guidelines

Reading for Meaning
Rewrite each chapter objective as a question. As you read, look for the answers to each question. Write the answers in your own words.

Concept Organizer
Use the KWHL diagram to identify key information about the tools for planning a healthful diet.

What I Know	What I Want to Learn	How I Can Learn More	What I Have Learned

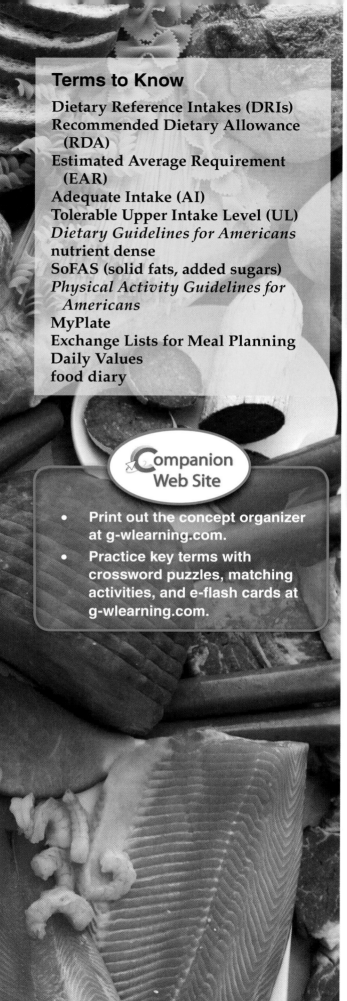

Terms to Know

Dietary Reference Intakes (DRIs)
Recommended Dietary Allowance (RDA)
Estimated Average Requirement (EAR)
Adequate Intake (AI)
Tolerable Upper Intake Level (UL)
Dietary Guidelines for Americans
nutrient dense
SoFAS (solid fats, added sugars)
Physical Activity Guidelines for Americans
MyPlate
Exchange Lists for Meal Planning
Daily Values
food diary

Companion Web Site

- **Print out the concept organizer at g-wlearning.com.**
- **Practice key terms with crossword puzzles, matching activities, and e-flash cards at g-wlearning.com.**

Objectives

After studying this chapter, you will be able to

- **differentiate** among the four types of Dietary Reference Intakes (DRIs).
- **summarize** the advice offered in the *Dietary Guidelines for Americans*.
- **apply** the MyPlate food guidance system to make healthy food choices.
- **use** percent Daily Values on food labels to evaluate a food's contributions to daily nutrient needs.
- **analyze** your current eating patterns using a variety of diet planning tools.

Central Ideas

- The tools for planning a healthful diet provide a road map for good nutrition and wellness.
- Utilizing food recommendations and guidelines for using them can help you eat a healthful diet and avoid health risks.

Many resources are available that are designed to promote wellness across the life span. This chapter introduces some common references and guidelines available to health professionals and consumers. You will read about guidelines for planning a healthful diet. You will then evaluate your eating pattern and practice applying the guidelines to your food choices.

Tools for Planning a Healthful Diet

Health experts are challenged to inform people about how to meet their nutritional needs. Many boards, councils, and committees work to develop tools to aid consumers in selecting a healthy diet. These tools continue to be revised as new information is discovered.

Dietary Reference Intakes

In the 1990s, the Food and Nutrition Board of the National Academy of Sciences and Health Canada began to work together to develop new dietary standards for both Americans and Canadians. In 2005, the final set of Dietary Reference Intakes (DRIs) was released. The **Dietary Reference Intakes (DRIs)** are reference values for nutrients and food components that can be used to plan and assess diets for healthy people, **4-1**. The purpose of the DRIs is to promote health, and prevent chronic disease and the effects of excessive or deficient nutrient intakes.

The DRIs include four types of nutrient reference standards—Estimated Average Requirement, Recommended Dietary Allowance, Adequate Intake, and Tolerable Upper Intake Level.

The **Estimated Average Requirement (EAR)** is a nutrient recommendation estimated to meet the needs of 50 percent of the people in a defined group. If a group of people consumes a nutrient at this level, half would be deficient. This standard is based on scientific evidence and is used for calculating the Recommended Dietary Allowance.

The **Recommended Dietary Allowance (RDA)** is the average daily intake of a nutrient required to meet the needs of most (97 to 98 percent) healthy individuals. RDAs are based on EARs. The RDA can be used as an aim for typical daily intake for an individual.

Adequate Intake (AI) is a reference value that is used when there is insufficient scientific evidence to determine an EAR. Since an EAR cannot be established for these nutrients, an RDA cannot be determined either. Instead, the intake recommendation is based on estimates and observations of people who appear to be healthy and well-nourished. As more research becomes available, AIs for some nutrients may be replaced by EARs and RDAs. AIs are used for all nutrients for infants.

The **Tolerable Upper Intake Level (UL)** is the maximum level of ongoing daily intake for a nutrient that is unlikely to cause harm to most people in the defined group. Daily intake above the UL for a nutrient could be harmful. ULs are not recommended levels of intake. Not enough information is available to set ULs for all nutrients.

DRIs are just one type of standard and should be used primarily by health professionals for planning and evaluating the diets of groups of people. To fully evaluate a diet, overall eating patterns and health conditions must be taken into consideration. Such factors as medications and illness can affect nutrient needs. A true nutrient lack or excess can be determined only through medical tests.

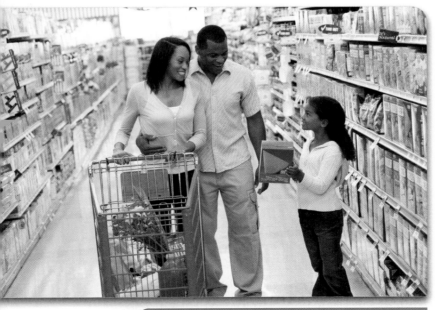

4-1   Many people want to know what foods they should choose to keep their bodies healthy.

For the most part, DRI values are used by scientists and nutritionists who work in research areas, such as sports medicine, or academic settings. Scientists analyze diets to determine the levels of nutrients being supplied. If the diet is not supplying enough of a nutrient, a disease state can result. Too much of some nutrients may be toxic.

DRIs can be used by nutritionists to develop menus that meet nutritional requirements for specific groups such as the elderly, a prison population, or the military. The DRIs also serve as a foundation for other nutrition-related guidance for Americans.

Dietary Guidelines for Americans

The *Dietary Guidelines for Americans* is published by the United States Departments of Health and Human Services and Agriculture. The **Dietary Guidelines for Americans** is a document that provides information and advice to promote health through improved nutrition and physical activity. Revised every five years, the *Guidelines* serve as

- authoritative advice for people two years and older about how proper dietary habits can promote health and reduce risk for major chronic diseases
- the basis of nutrition education programs, Federal nutrition assistance programs such as school meals and Meals on Wheel, and dietary advice provided by health professionals, **4-2**
- aid for policymakers in designing and implementing nutrition-related programs

Poor diet, physical inactivity, and overweight and obesity continue to be issues which undermine the health of Americans. These issues increase an individual's risk for a variety of chronic diseases. As a result, the population that the *2010 Dietary Guidelines* addresses

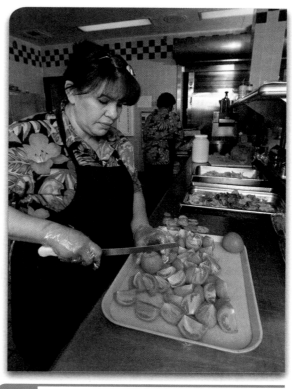

4-2   The *Dietary Guidelines for Americans* serve as a basis for school lunch menus. *(Photo by Ken Hammond, ARS/USDA)*

was revised for Americans two years and older, including those at increased risk of chronic disease.

The goal of the *Guidelines* is for Americans to meet the nutrient levels established in the DRIs by consuming a variety of foods. Two basic themes summarize the message of the *2010 Dietary Guidelines*.

- Maintain calorie balance over time to achieve and sustain a healthy weight.
- Focus on consuming nutrient-dense foods and beverages.

Maintain calorie balance over time to achieve and sustain a healthy weight. Reaching and maintaining a healthy body weight throughout life is important to good health and quality of life. Balancing calories taken in through eating with calories used by the body during physical activity is the key to healthy weight. Preventing unhealthy weight gain is much easier than losing weight.

Focus on consuming nutrient-dense foods and beverages. **Nutrient-dense** foods and beverages provide vitamins, minerals, and other substances that may have positive health effects, but supply relatively few calories. Foods that are high in calories from solid fats and/or added sugars, called **SoFAS**, should be limited or avoided. For example, whole-grain toast is a more nutrient-dense choice for breakfast than a doughnut, which is high in SoFAS. By decreasing the amount of SoFAS in the diet, intake of nutrient-dense foods can be increased without causing calorie imbalance and subsequent weight gain.

People sometimes use terms such as *junk food* or *health food* to describe a food's quality. As you begin to analyze foods, you will find there is no such thing as a perfect food. Likewise, there are few foods that supply absolutely no nutrients. Therefore, *junk food* and *health food* are less useful than the terms *low nutrient density* and *high nutrient density*. Every food has the potential to make a dietary contribution. For this to happen, you must make variety, moderation, balance, and adequacy a part of your daily food choices.

Physical activity is important not only for calorie balance, but also for prevention of many chronic diseases. The *2010 Dietary Guidelines* addresses the importance of physical activity in health. The *Dietary Guidelines* encourage Americans to meet the *2008 Physical Activity Guidelines for Americans*. The **Physical Activity Guidelines for Americans** specifies amounts and types of exercise that individuals at different stages of the life cycle should do to achieve health benefits.

MyPlate

In 2011, the United States Department of Agriculture (USDA) released a new food guidance system called **MyPlate** that is based on the *2010 Dietary Guidelines for Americans*. MyPlate replaced MyPyramid. MyPlate is a simple, visual message to help consumers build a healthy plate at mealtime. The Web site ChooseMyPlate.gov offers tools and resources to help consumers make changes in their eating habits that are consistent with the *Dietary Guidelines*, **4-3**.

MyPlate divides foods into five main food groups—fruits, grains, vegetables, protein foods, and dairy. Foods from each of these categories are required for a healthy diet. The plate is split into four sections representing fruits, grains, vegetables, and protein. The sections differ in size based on the recommended portion of your meal these foods should be. The circle next to the plate represents

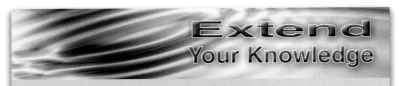

Extend Your Knowledge

Nutrition Evidence Library (NEL)

The first step in revising the *Dietary Guidelines* involves a committee reviewing and analyzing current scientific information on diet and health. The committee prepares a report summarizing its findings, which serves as a major resource for creating the *Guidelines*. The committee used the USDA's Nutrition Evidence Library (NEL) for its work on the *2010 Dietary Guidelines*. NEL is a government resource that evaluates, synthesizes, and grades food and nutrition-related research.

To facilitate its review of the scientific information, the committee submitted specific questions to NEL. The NEL process then found studies related to the question. The evidence from all the relevant studies was integrated. From this collection, a conclusion statement was formed and graded.

Locate the Nutrition Evidence Library online and learn what questions the committee submitted for its work on the *2010 Dietary Guidelines*. Select a question of particular interest to you. Find the summary of evidence for that question, the conclusion statement, and how it was graded.

the dairy group. The MyPlate image communicates the message that half of your meal plate should be fruits and vegetables. Oils are not a food group and are not included on the MyPlate image.

MyPlate Food Groups

The MyPlate food guidance system emphasizes eating a variety of foods from each of the food groups. It helps you identify what foods are in each group, what amounts you should eat, and how to make a healthy selection.

Fruits. This group is rich in nutrients and fiber. Examples of fruits include bananas, oranges, peaches, blueberries, and kiwifruit. Fruits may be fresh, frozen, puréed, or dried. Select whole fruit more often than fruit juice. Whole fruit contains fiber and is more nutrient dense than juice.

Grains. The grains group includes foods made from wheat, rice, oats, cornmeal, barley, and other grains. They can be either whole or refined grains. Guidelines from MyPlate recommend half of the grains you eat should be whole grains. Examples of whole grains include whole-wheat flour, bulgur, oatmeal, brown rice, and whole cornmeal. Refined grains include white bread, white rice, and other white flour products often used in pastas and crackers. Grains are a source of fiber, and some B vitamins and minerals.

Vegetables. Vegetables provide a variety of nutrients and fiber. MyPlate divides vegetables into the following five subgroups:
- *dark green vegetables,* such as broccoli, spinach, and kale
- *red and orange vegetables,* such as carrots, red peppers, tomatoes, and sweet potatoes
- *beans and peas,* such as kidney beans, soy beans, and lentils
- *starchy vegetables,* such as green peas, corn, and potatoes

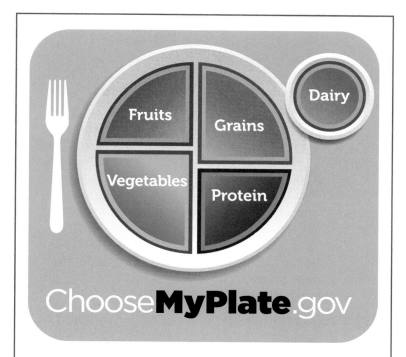

Balancing calories
- Enjoy your food, but eat less.
- Avoid oversized portions.

Foods to increase
- Make half your plate fruits and vegetables.
- Make at least half your grains whole grains.
- Switch to fat-free or low-fat (1%) milk.

Foods to reduce
- Compare sodium in foods like soup, bread, and frozen meals—and choose the foods with lower numbers.
- Drink water instead of sugary drinks.

4-3 MyPlate encourages consumers to focus on these key behaviors to create healthier eating plans. *Credit: USDA*

- *other vegetables,* such as celery, onions, and zucchini

Your plan recommends an amount from each group weekly. Foods from the vegetable group can be fresh, frozen, or canned.

Protein foods. This group supplies a variety of nutrients to the diet, including protein, essential fatty acids, B vitamins, iron, zinc, magnesium, and vitamin E. Meats, poultry, eggs, beans and peas,

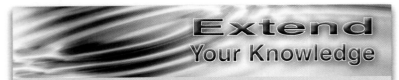

Choose Nutrient Dense

Individuals can consume only a limited number of calories if they want to avoid unhealthy weight gain. Therefore, you should choose foods that supply the nutrients you need for health, but add few additional calories from unnecessary solid fats and added sugars. In other words—choose nutrient-dense foods and beverages. Unfortunately, many Americans choose foods that are not nutrient dense. You do not have to give up your favorite foods, just choose the more nutrient-dense form of your favorite food.

Which food would you choose?

1 cup French fried potatoes (117 calories + 141 calories from frying fat)
or
✔ **baked potato** (117 calories)

1 cup sweetened applesauce (105 calories+ 68 calories from added sugar)
or
✔ **1 cup unsweetened applesauce** (105 calories)

✔ **3 ounces grilled chicken breast** (138 calories)
or
3 ounces fried chicken strips (138 calories + 108 calories from breading and frying fat)

nuts and seeds, and seafood are all found in this group. Choose lean meats and poultry to avoid saturated fats and cholesterol. Include at least eight ounces of cooked seafood per week. Beans and peas are also found in the vegetable group.

Dairy. The dairy group includes foods high in protein and calcium for bone health such as milk, cheese, milk-based desserts, and yogurt. It also includes calcium-fortified soymilk for people with lactose intolerance. Calcium fortified foods and beverages may provide calcium, but lack other nutrients supplied by foods in this group.

Oils. Oils are fats that are liquid at room temperature and are obtained from a variety of plants and fish. Oils are not a food group, but some are needed in the diet to provide essential nutrients. For this reason, there is an allowance for oils in your daily food plan. Only small amounts of oils are recommended because they are high in calories and can easily cause an imbalance between calories consumed and daily activity level. Foods that are rich in oils such as soft margarines, mayonnaise, and salad dressings are counted in this allowance for oils.

Fats that are solid at room temperature are *not* included in the allowance for oils. Common solid fats include butter, beef fat, chicken fat, pork fat, stick margarine, and shortening. The fat in milk is also considered solid fat because milk fat, or butterfat, is solid at room temperature. Solid fats are not necessary for good health and are considered *empty calories*. Empty calories such as those from foods high in solid fats and added sugars (SoFAS) provide few or no nutrients. Empty calories should be limited to avoid exceeding your recommended calorie intake.

A Daily Food Plan for You

The Web site at ChooseMyPlate.gov offers a number of interactive tools to help individuals plan and assess their daily food and activity choices. One of these tools is "Daily Food Plan" which helps you create a personalized food plan based on your age, sex, height, weight, and activity level. After you enter this data, the plan selects the food intake pattern that is right for you. Many teens require 2,000 calories daily, **4-4**.

The plan also aims to help people balance food intake and physical activity to promote healthy weight. Your level of physical activity influences the amount of food you consume.

My Daily Food Plan

Based on the information you provided, this is your daily recommended amount from each food group.

GRAINS 6 ounces	**Make half your grains whole** Aim for at least **3 ounces** of whole grains a day
VEGETABLES 2½ cups	**Vary your veggies** Aim for these amounts **each week**: **Dark green veggies** = 1½ cups **Red & orange veggies** = 5½ cups **Beans & peas** = 1½ cups **Starchy veggies** = 5 cups **Other veggies** = 4 cups
FRUITS 2 cups	**Focus on fruits** Eat a variety of fruit Choose whole or cut-up fruits more often than fruit juice
DAIRY 3 cups	**Get your calcium-rich foods** Drink fat-free or low-fat (1%) milk, for the same amount of calcium and other nutrients as whole milk, but less fat and calories Select fat-free or low-fat yogurt and cheese, or try calcium-fortified soy products
PROTEIN FOODS 5½ ounces	**Go lean with protein** Twice a week, make seafood the protein on your plate Vary your protein rountine—choose more fish, beans, peas, nuts, and seeds Keep meat and poultry portions small and lean

Find your balance between food and physical activity Be physically active for at least **60 minutes** each day.	**Know your limits on fats, sugars, and sodium** Your allowance for oils is **6 teaspoons** a day. Limit extras–solid fats and sugars–to **260 Calories** a day. Reduce sodium intake to less than **2300 mg** a day.

Your results are based on a 2000 calorie pattern. Name: _____

This calorie level is only an estimate of your needs. Monitor your body weight to see if you need to adjust your calorie intake.

4-4 Using the MyPlate system to plan daily food choices and exercise patterns can help you get the balance of nutrients and activity you need for good health. *Credit: USDA*

MyPlate also has tools for children, women who are pregnant or breast-feeding, and individuals who speak Spanish. You will want to access the other tools on ChooseMyPlate.gov as you read this textbook.

Measuring Food Amounts

You must know how to measure the various amounts of foods your Daily Food Plan recommends. People often have very different ideas about how big a serving size is. To avoid confusion,

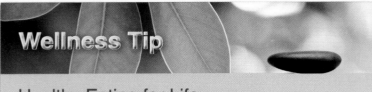

MyPlate uses volume and weight measures to tell you the amounts of food you should eat. The foods are often measured in cups, teaspoons, or ounces-equivalents.

Frequently eating more calories than you need to balance your activity level can cause you to gain weight. Therefore, it is important to be aware of the amounts your food plan recommends. Read the labels on food products to learn how many cups or ounce-equivalents are in packaged foods. The manufacturer does not determine serving sizes. Food labeling laws require that serving sizes be uniform and reflect the amounts people usually eat. They must be expressed on the label in common household and metric measures. However, you need to determine how the serving size on the label fits into your food plan.

Physical Activity

Physical activity is a key element in calorie balance and health. ChooseMyPlate.gov includes recommendations for how much physical activity is needed based on the *Physical Activity Guidelines for Americans*. The Web site has helpful resources such as a chart showing calorie use for various activities and tips for increasing physical activity. Staying active has many benefits such as
- reducing stress

- contributing to strong bones, muscles, and joints
- increasing endurance, muscle strength, and flexibility
- helping to achieve and maintain a healthy weight

Teens are encouraged to be physically active 60 minutes a day, most days of the week. Physical activity levels vary. Moderate physical activities include brisk walking, leisurely bicycling, light weight training, and dancing. More vigorous activities include aerobics, running or jogging at a faster pace, and swimming laps. To maintain good health, you must find your balance between food intake and physical activity.

Exchange Lists

Another tool that can be used to plan a healthy meal or follow a special diet is an exchange system. The **Exchange Lists for Meal Planning** system classifies foods into groups of similar nutrient and caloric content. In this system, one exchange of any food within a list has about the same amount of carbohydrate, protein, fat, and calories as other foods in that list. This makes estimating the nutrient content of any food or meal easier. The Exchange Lists were developed by the American Dietetic Association and the American Diabetes Association. The lists can be used to balance the amount of carbohydrate, protein, fat, and calories eaten each day. The system was originally used to help individuals with diabetes manage their food plan to help stabilize their blood sugar. The Exchange Lists can also be used successfully for weight management.

To use the Exchange Lists, you must first know which foods are included in each group. There are six basic lists used to organize foods.
- The *starch list* includes breads, cereals, grains, and starchy vegetables. One

food exchange from this group has 15 grams of carbohydrates, 3 grams of protein, 0 to 1 grams fat, and a total of 80 calories.

- The *fruits list* includes fruits in all forms, such as fresh, dried, canned, frozen, and juice. One fruit exchange has 15 grams of carbohydrates and 60 calories.

- The *milk list* includes milk and milk products that are further divided based on fat content—fat free, reduced fat, or whole fat. One fat-free milk exchange has 12 grams of carbohydrates, 8 grams of protein, 0 to 3 grams fat, and 90 calories.

- The *vegetable (nonstarchy) list* includes vegetables such as cooked green beans, salad greens, and vegetable juices. One vegetable exchange contains 5 grams of carbohydrates, 2 grams of protein, and 25 calories.

- The *meat and meat substitutes list* groups these exchanges based on fat content—very lean, lean, medium-fat, and high-fat. One very lean meat exchange has 7 grams of protein, 0 to 1 grams fat, and 35 calories per ounce. As the fat content of the meat exchange increases, the caloric content increases. Many of the meat substitute exchanges also contain carbohydrates.

- The *fats list* includes foods such as oil, butter, salad dressing, and mayonnaise. Most items in the fat exchange list contain 5 grams of fat and 45 calories.

Next, you must become familiar with the common exchange sizes for basic types of foods within each list. For example, breads are found in the starch list and their exchange size is typically one slice. Starchy vegetables such as corn and green peas are also found in the starch list. One exchange of starchy vegetables is usually one-half cup. Foods within an exchange list can

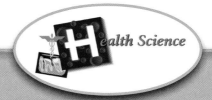

Dietetic Technician

Dietetic technicians assist dietitians in evaluating, organizing, and conducting nutrition services and programs for schools, hospitals, and industry. Under the supervision of dietitians, they gather and evaluate diet histories, assist in planning patient meals, conduct foodservice operations, and maintain records.

Education: Students wanting to become dietetic technicians should graduate from high school with a well-rounded program. High school business courses may prove helpful. Dietetic technicians must complete a two-year associate's degree program that is accepted by the American Dietetic Association. They must then meet other state requirements.

Job Outlook: Employment opportunities for dietetic technicians are expected to grow about as fast as the average. This is largely due to the emphasis that the medical community is placing on disease prevention through improved dietary habits. The growing aging population will also increase demand for dietetic technicians because they will need balanced meals and nutritional counseling.

be substituted for each other because the nutrient and caloric content of the foods on the list are about the same. When planning a meal that includes two starch exchanges, you could serve two slices of bread, one slice of bread and one-half cup of corn, or one cup of corn. You may substitute a small apple (one fruit exchange) for a small orange (one fruit exchange) because they are both about 60 calories with 15 grams of carbohydrates. However, you could not substitute a small banana (one fruit exchange) for a half-cup of green beans (one vegetable exchange) because these foods are in different groups.

To successfully use the Exchange Lists for Meal Planning, you must first know what your particular dietary requirements are and the number of calories you need each day. Often it is a doctor or dietitian who explains how many exchanges from each list are needed to meet daily requirements.

With practice, the exchange system can be used to plan a meal pattern that fits your individual dietary needs. The system gets more complicated as you begin to analyze the content of combination foods such as pizza or macaroni and cheese, but it is possible. Some foods are considered free foods and are found on a *free foods list*. Any food or drink that has less than 20 calories and 5 grams or less of carbohydrate per serving is a free food. Gum, water, plain coffee or tea, and diet soda are examples of free foods. Once an individual is familiar with the Exchange Lists, managing and balancing food intake becomes simple to master.

Food Labels and Daily Values

Reading food labels can help you plan and manage your diet. The law requires that most foods include nutrition information on the label. The Nutrition Facts panel on food labels is an easy-to-use tool when planning a healthful diet, **4-5**.

As you read the nutrition panel, you will see the term *Daily Value*. **Daily Values** are recommended nutrient intakes based on daily calorie needs. Daily Values based on 2,000- and 2,500-calorie diets for carbohydrate, fiber, fats, sodium, and sometimes protein are included on food labels when package size allows. (Protein must only be included if the food claims to be high in protein or is intended for infants and children under four years.) However, the *Percent (%) Daily Values* shown on Nutrition Facts panels are calculated using only the Daily Values for a 2,000-calorie diet. The % Daily Value shows the portion

Nutrition Facts		
Serving Size 1 cup (228g)		
Servings Per Container 2		

Amount Per Serving		
Calories 260 Calories from Fat 120		

		% Daily Value*
Total Fat 13g		**20%**
Saturated Fat 10g		**50%**
Trans Fat 1.5g		
Cholesterol 60mg		**20%**
Sodium 330mg		**14%**
Total Carbohydrate 31g		**10%**
Dietary Fiber 5g		**20%**
Sugars 10g		
Protein 5g		

Vitamin A 15%	Vitamin C 8%
Calcium 20%	Iron 2%

* Percent Daily Values are based on a 2,000 calorie diet. Your daily values may be higher or lower depending on your calorie needs:

	Calories	2,000	2,500
Total Fat	Less than	65g	80g
Sat Fat	Less than	20g	25g
Cholesterol	Less than	300mg	300mg
Sodium	Less than	2,400mg	2,400mg
Total Carbohydrate		300g	375g
Fiber		25g	30g

Calories per gram:
Fat 9   Carbohydrates 4   Protein 4

4-5   Nutrition Facts on a food label list the % Daily Value of various nutrients in each serving of the product.

of the daily requirement for a nutrient that is provided by one food serving. For example, if a cereal label states it supplies "20 percent Daily Value for dietary fiber," then one serving of the cereal supplies 20 percent of the fiber a person on a 2,000-calorie diet needs for one day.

Most food labels do not have enough room to list all nutrients for each age range and sex. Therefore, labels highlight only the nutrients most important to the health of today's consumer. Percent Daily Values are listed for fat, saturated fat, cholesterol, sodium, carbohydrate, fiber, vitamin A, vitamin C, calcium, and iron.

Learn to use the % Daily Values to see how foods contribute to your daily nutrient needs. Ask yourself what combination of foods you can eat throughout the day to get 100 percent of your Daily Values. You can also use the % Daily Values to compare the nutrient content of different brands and products. For instance, you might compare the fiber content of two brands of whole-grain bread. Then you might compare the fiber in whole-grain bread with the fiber in a bagel.

Math Link

Calculating % Daily Value

Jenna's food plan is 2,500 calories per day. Her goal is to select nutrient-dense foods as often as possible. One morning, she began reading the Nutrition Facts panel for the whole-grain bread she was toasting for breakfast. She discovered that each slice contained 3 grams of dietary fiber. She knows her Daily Value for dietary fiber is 30 grams.
- If Jenna has 2 slices of toast, what % Daily Value has she consumed?

Using Food Recommendations and Guidelines

You now know about a variety of diet planning tools. The next step is to learn how to use them to improve your diet.

Keep a Food Diary

Before you can determine whether you are getting enough nutrients, you need to know what foods you are eating. One way to be aware of what you eat is to keep a food diary. A **food diary** is a record of the kinds and amounts of foods and beverages consumed for a given time. Food diaries are sometimes called *food logs* or *journals*. The record includes snacks and foods eaten away from home. It also includes condiments, such as catsup, pickles, salad dressings, syrups, and jellies.

You need a complete diary if you want a true analysis of your diet. You will find it easy to forget what you ate if you wait too long to record information. Keeping a pad and pencil handy will help you remember to write down each food item you eat.

For your diet analysis to be valid, you need to accurately estimate food amounts

you are eating. Look at measuring utensils to help you become familiar with what amounts such as one tablespoon and one cup look like. Remember that 3 ounce-equivalents of meat or chicken is about the size of a deck of playing cards. Find out how many ounces your cups, bowls, and glasses hold. This will help you correctly list in your food diary the amounts of foods you consume.

You might want to record what you eat for several days. This will give you a more accurate picture of your eating habits than you will get from a one-day record. You will also get a better account if you record your diary on typical days. Avoid keeping a record on birthdays, holidays, and other days when you are likely to follow different eating patterns.

Analyze Your Diet

Use the information recorded in your food diary to see if you are meeting your daily nutrient needs. A number of software programs are available that can help you quickly analyze your diet with a computer. Most of these programs include a database of *food composition tables*. These tables are a reference guide listing the nutritive values of many foods in common serving sizes. You can enter data into the computer about the foods you ate. The program can then tell you such information as the calorie and nutrient values of those foods. You can make a detailed printout showing how your daily nutrient values compare to the RDAs and AIs. This comparison will show you which nutrient needs you have and have not met.

If you do not have access to diet analysis software, you can analyze your diet yourself. Make a chart with columns for the foods you ate, calories, and all the major nutrients. List the foods recorded in your food diary in the first column. Look up each food in a food composition table such as the USDA's Nutritive Value of Foods. Write the amounts of nutrients

supplied by each food in the appropriate columns of your chart.

After you have filled in all the information for each food, total the amounts in all the nutrient columns. Compare these totals to the RDAs and AIs.

As you complete your chart, remember to think about amounts. Compare the amount of each food you consumed to the amount listed in the table. If your amount differs, you will have to adjust the nutrient amounts you list in your chart. For instance, the amount listed in the table for milk is 1 cup. If you drank 1½ cups, you will have to multiply the quantity of each nutrient listed for milk by 1½.

You can also use the "Food Tracker" to help analyze your diet. Does your food diary show you are getting the recommended daily amounts from each food group? The different groups are good sources of different nutrients. Eating the recommended amounts from each group every day will help you get all the nutrients you need.

Case Study: Change for the Better

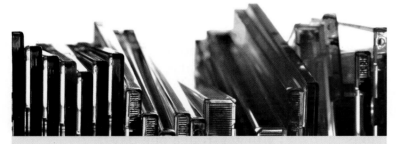

Kiara enrolled in a physical conditioning class for her physical education elective this semester. However, she is finding that she tires easily, is weaker than her peers, and has little stamina. One day, the class instructor was discussing the importance of nutrition for optimal health and performance. Kiara really isn't sure how good or bad her eating habits are, but she is pretty sure she could do better. Kiara is determined to improve her overall health—she just doesn't know where to start.

Case Review

1. What steps could Kiara take to achieve her goal of improving her overall health?

2. What resources might be helpful to Kiara during this process?

3. Do you think Kiara will succeed? Why?

Plan Menus Using Food Planner

Your diet analysis may show you are eating too much from some of the food groups and not enough of others. Planning a daily menu using the "Food Planner" at ChooseMyPlate.gov can help you correct such problems. Following this pattern will help you get the balance of nutrients you need. The plan guides you in selecting foods low in saturated fats, cholesterol, and added sugar, and rich in fiber and nutrients as needed for good health.

Eating right may be easier and tastier than you think. ChooseMyPlate.gov is flexible enough for anyone to use. It can suit different family lifestyles, ethnic backgrounds, and religious beliefs. It can accommodate all your favorite foods.

Reading Summary

Experts have developed a number of tools to help people evaluate their diets and make wise food choices. The Dietary Reference Intakes (DRIs) are reference values for nutrients and food components that can be used to plan and assess diets for healthy people. The *Dietary Guidelines for Americans* provides information and advice to promote health through improved nutrition and physical activity. MyPlate can be used for an individualized approach to planning and implementing a healthy diet.

The Exchange Lists for Meal Planning system classifies foods into groups of similar nutrient and caloric content. The Exchange Lists can be used to plan a healthy meal or follow a special diet. Daily Values on food labels show how servings of food products contribute to daily nutrient needs.

These tools can be used by health professionals and individuals to promote healthy food choices and physical activity. A food diary can be used to keep track of the kinds and amounts of foods and beverages consumed. This information can be analyzed to determine if an individual's daily nutrient needs are being met. Use the recommendations and tools from ChooseMyPlate.gov to plan balanced menus and track progress toward meeting nutrient needs.

Review Learning

1. True or false. Dietary Reference Intakes are used to plan and assess diets for individuals who have a chronic disease.
2. What are the two basic themes of the *2010 Dietary Guidelines for Americans*?
3. Why does the *2010 Dietary Guidelines* address physical activity?
4. What message is communicated by the MyPlate image?
5. How do you create a personalized food plan using MyPlate?
6. True or false. MyPlate uses volume and weight measures rather than number of servings to tell you the amounts of food you should eat.
7. How are foods in the same exchange list similar?
8. One fruit exchange from the fruit list has _____ grams of carbohydrates and _____ calories.
9. Percent Daily Values used as references on food labels are based on a _____-calorie diet.
10. Give two tips for keeping a food diary that will increase the validity of a diet analysis.
11. What is a food composition table?

Critical Thinking

12. **Make inferences.** Make four inferences supporting reasons why all Americans should fully utilize the nutrition guidelines available to them.
13. **Identify evidence.** What evidence can you give to support the theory that many people lack understanding about portion size? How can using the nutrition guidelines increase understanding and lead to healthful living?

Applying Your Knowledge

14. **Breakfast exchanges.** Use the Exchange Lists for Meal Planning to estimate the nutrient and calorie content of your breakfast.

15. **Guidelines survey.** Write a survey to assess people's adherence to the *Dietary Guidelines for Americans*. Also develop a rating scale respondents can use in answering the questions. Use your survey to interview three people in different age groups. Share your findings in class.

16. **Build MyPlate.** Dish up a meal on a plate using foods you typically eat at home. Use MyPlate to guide the amounts of each food you put on your plate. Take a photo of the plate and include it with a brief explanation how this compares with your typical meal.

17. **Implement recommendation.** Select one recommendation about healthy food choices or activity from this chapter. Write a plan to incorporate the recommendation in your daily life.

Technology Connections

18. **Consumer information.** Find consumer handouts on ChooseMyPlate.gov or from the *Dietary Guidelines for Americans* Web site. Obtain permission to create informative bulletin boards around the school using the handouts.

19. **Evaluate activities.** Complete interactive activities on ChooseMyPlate.gov and send feedback to the government committee planning future projects on your recommendations for site improvement.

20. **Track activity.** Track your physical activity on the President's Challenge Web site.

21. **Create PSA.** Find an audio or video podcast at ChooseMyPlate.gov and incorporate it in a brief public service announcement encouraging healthy eating.

Academic Connections

22. **History.** Research the history of the *Dietary Guidelines for Americans*. Discuss why they were developed, the intended audience, and how it has evolved. Write a brief summary of your findings.

23. **Social studies.** Research current legislation and regulations related to nutrition and wellness issues. Select one that interests you and write an opinion paper to publish in the school newspaper.

24. **Speech.** Create a one-minute media message promoting healthy food choices to broadcast over the school public announcement system. Formulate your message taking into consideration your audience. Practice delivering the nutrition message with enthusiasm.

25. **Language arts.** Research and create an informative pamphlet persuading students to make more nutrient-dense food choices. Include a list of foods that are popular with students and suggest more nutrient-dense options for each food.

Workplace Applications

Take Initiative

As a new employee, you are taking on the challenge of keeping your mind and body healthy. Part of this dedication includes taking initiative to maintain a healthy body weight. Use the "Food Planner" to plan healthful meals and the "Food Tracker" to keep track of your food and fitness activities. Continue using these tools found on ChooseMyPlate.gov for a month or more. After a couple of months, write a summary indicating how healthful eating and adequate physical activity have helped you maintain a healthy body weight. What would you tell other "employees" about the benefits of using these tools?

Part Two
The Health Effects of Energy Nutrients

Sautéing

Sautéing (saw tay ing) is a quick, healthy food preparation method. This method can be used to cook meat, poultry, fish, vegetables, and fruits. Precooked pasta and rice can be reheated by sautéing.

Sautéing is typically done using a shallow pan with sloped sides on the stove. This method cooks food over high heat using a small amount of fat—just enough to cover the bottom of the pan. To sauté properly, the pan and fat must be preheated before food is added. However, the fat must not be overheated. Some cooks heat the fat until it just begins to smoke and then quickly add the food to the pan. The amount of food added to the pan is important to the success of this method. If too much food is added, the pan cools down and food is not sautéed properly. For best results when sautéing meats, poultry, and fish, add no more than a single layer in the pan. When larger quantities are needed, cook a number of smaller batches. When sautéing vegetables, add vegetables that require a longer cooking time to the pan first. Add other vegetables later to ensure even cooking. For example, denser vegetables such as broccoli take longer to cook than less dense vegetables such as mushrooms. Cutting similar vegetables in uniform sizes also aids in proper cooking.

Sautéed Spinach (6 servings)

Ingredients

- 1½ pounds baby spinach leaves
- 2 tablespoons olive oil
- 6 cloves garlic, sliced
- ¼ teaspoon lemon juice
- salt and pepper to taste

Directions

1. Rinse spinach well and pat or spin dry.
2. Heat oil in a large pot over medium heat. Add garlic and sauté for about 1 minute, do not let garlic brown.
3. Add spinach, salt, and pepper to pot and stir about 1 to 2 minutes until wilted.
4. Place spinach in serving bowl and drizzle with lemon juice.

Chapter 5

Carbohydrates: The Preferred Body Fuel

Reading for Meaning

Read the review questions at the end of the chapter before you read the chapter. Keep the questions in mind as you read to help you determine which information is most important.

Concept Organizer

Use the spider diagram to identify the functions of carbohydrates. List several characteristics of each function.

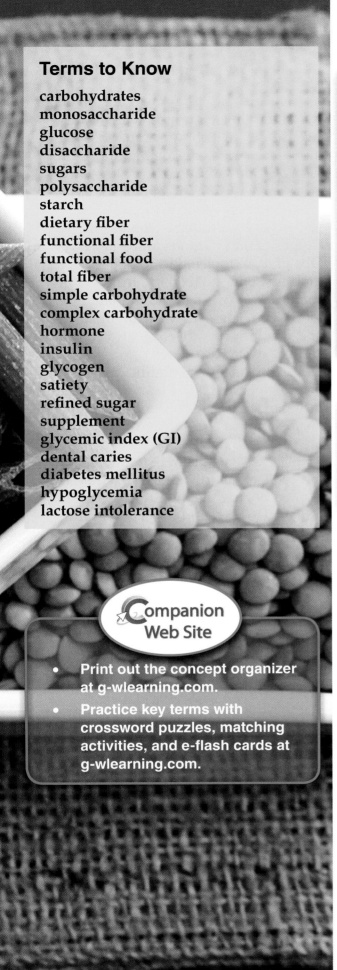

Terms to Know

carbohydrates
monosaccharide
glucose
disaccharide
sugars
polysaccharide
starch
dietary fiber
functional fiber
functional food
total fiber
simple carbohydrate
complex carbohydrate
hormone
insulin
glycogen
satiety
refined sugar
supplement
glycemic index (GI)
dental caries
diabetes mellitus
hypoglycemia
lactose intolerance

Companion Web Site

- Print out the concept organizer at g-wlearning.com.
- Practice key terms with crossword puzzles, matching activities, and e-flash cards at g-wlearning.com.

Objectives

After studying this chapter, you will be able to

- **summarize** the three types of carbohydrates and their food sources.
- **list** the major functions of carbohydrates.
- **interpret** how the body uses carbohydrates for energy production.
- **state** the relationship between adequate fiber in the diet and a healthy digestive system.
- **judge** the value and limitations of using the glycemic index.
- **evaluate** the role of carbohydrates in a variety of health issues.

Central Ideas

- Carbohydrates are the main energy source for the human body.
- To support their carbohydrate needs, people need to eat complex carbohydrates such as whole grains.

What comes to mind when you hear the word *carbohydrates*? If you are thinking potatoes, bread, rice, spaghetti, or fruits, you are correct. If your thoughts lead you to fattening foods, you might think differently after you read this chapter.

Carbohydrates are one of the six essential nutrients and are your body's main source of energy. They are the sugars, starches, and fibers in your diet. Except for the natural sugar in milk, nearly all carbohydrates come from plant sources. Carbohydrates should form the bulk of your diet.

Types of Carbohydrates

Carbohydrates are made of three common chemical elements—carbon, hydrogen, and oxygen. These elements are bonded together to form saccharides, or sugar units. The elements can be combined in several ways. The arrangement of the elements determines the type of sugar unit. Sugar units may be linked in various arrangements to form different types of carbohydrates, **5-1**.

Monosaccharides

Monosaccharides are carbohydrates composed of single sugar units. (The prefix *mono-* means one.) These are the smallest carbohydrate molecules. The three monosaccharides are glucose, fructose, and galactose. **Glucose** is sometimes called *blood sugar* because it circulates in the bloodstream. It is the body's source of energy. *Fructose* has the sweetest taste of all sugars. It occurs naturally in fruits and honey. *Galactose* does not occur alone as a monosaccharide in foods. Instead, it is found bonded to glucose. Together, these two monosaccharides form the sugar in milk.

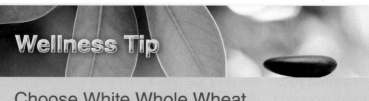

Wellness Tip

Choose White Whole Wheat

If you find the flavor and texture of whole-wheat bread unappealing, give white whole-wheat bread a try. Made from an albino variety of wheat, white whole wheat packs the same nutritional benefits and fiber as its red wheat counterpart.

Disaccharides

The **disaccharides** are made up of two sugar units. (The prefix *di-* means two.) The body splits disaccharides into monosaccharides during digestion. The disaccharides are sucrose, maltose, and lactose. All the mono- and disaccharides are collectively referred to as **sugars**.

Sucrose is the sugar you use in recipes or add to foods at the table. One glucose molecule and one fructose molecule bond together to form sucrose. Sucrose is found in many foods. Beet sugar, cane sugar, molasses, and maple syrup are concentrated sources of sucrose.

Lactose is found in milk. It is made of one glucose molecule and one galactose molecule that are bonded together. Lactose serves as a source of energy for breast-fed infants.

Maltose is made of two glucose molecules that are bonded together. It is formed during the digestion of starch. It may also be found in certain grains, such as malt.

Polysaccharides

Polysaccharides are carbohydrates that are made up of many sugar units. (The prefix *poly-* means many.) These units are linked in long, straight chains or branched chains. Like the disaccharides, the polysaccharides must be broken down during digestion. Starches and fibers are polysaccharides.

Starch is a polysaccharide that is the storage form of energy in plants. Starch is made of many glucose molecules that are bonded together. Grain products, such as breads and cereals, and starchy vegetables, such as corn, potatoes, and legumes, are high in starch.

Carbohydrate Structures

Monosaccharides

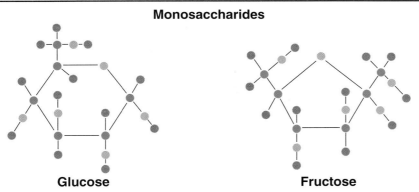

Glucose   **Fructose**

Both monosaccharide molecules contain 6 carbon atoms, 12 hydrogen atoms, and 6 oxygen atoms. However, the elements are arranged differently in each molecule.

Disaccharides

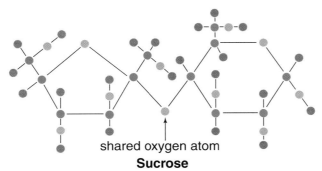

shared oxygen atom

Sucrose

A molecule of fructose bonded to a molecule of glucose forms the disaccharide sucrose. The two molecules share an oxygen atom. Notice that this disaccharide contains one fewer oxygen atom and two fewer hydrogen atoms than the two separate monosaccharide molecules. This is because a molecule of water (H_2O) was released when the bond was formed.

Polysaccharides

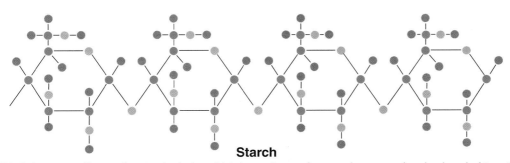

Starch

This is just a small part of a starch chain, which is made up of many glucose molecules bonded together.

Key
- carbon atom
- hydrogen atom
- oxygen atom

5-1   Carbohydrates are all made of different arrangements of carbon, hydrogen, and oxygen.

Three terms are used when discussing fiber—dietary fiber, functional fiber, and total fiber. **Dietary fibers** are the nondigestible carbohydrates and lignins that make up the tough, fibrous cell walls of plants, **5-2**. *Lignins* are not carbohydrates, but act as the binder in cell walls. Dietary fibers are found only in plant foods. **Functional fibers** are isolated, nondigestible carbohydrates that have beneficial effects in human health. Functional fiber is extracted from plants and prepared in a laboratory. For example, resistant starch is a functional fiber that is produced when cereals and grains are processed and baked. The resistant starch is then extracted from the original food source and added to other processed foods to enhance health benefits.

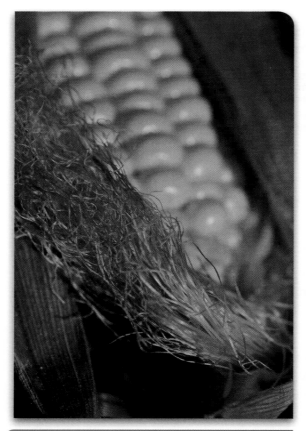

5-2   Corn plants store energy as starch in the kernels and are a good source of dietary fiber.

When food ingredients, such as fiber, are added to provide health benefits beyond basic nutrition, the foods are called **functional foods**. These foods are promoted in the media to improve health. This means the food is more than a source of nutrients. It also has the potential for preventing disease or promoting health.

Total fiber is the sum of dietary and functional fibers. Human digestive enzymes cannot digest fibers, but bacteria in the digestive tract can break down some fibers. Because most fibers pass through the digestive system unchanged, these carbohydrates provide almost no energy (calories). Look on food labels to find various terms for fiber such as *cellulose*, *gum*, β *glucan*, *psyllium*, and *pectin*. The AI for total fiber for 14- to 18-year-olds is 26 grams for females and 38 grams for males.

Because of their simple molecular structures, monosaccharides and disaccharides are considered **simple carbohydrates**. When people talk about eating simple carbohydrates, they are generally referring to foods that are high in simple sugars. Such foods include table sugar, candy, syrups, and soft drinks. Polysaccharides have a larger, more intricate molecular structure. Therefore, they are considered **complex carbohydrates**. When people talk about eating complex carbohydrates, they are referring to foods that are high in starch and fiber. Breads, cereals, rice, pasta, and vegetables are all sources of complex carbohydrates, **5-3**.

The distinction between simple and complex carbohydrates is important when making food choices. Choosing more food sources of complex carbohydrates and fewer sources of simple carbohydrates has health and nutrition benefits. You will read about these benefits later in the chapter.

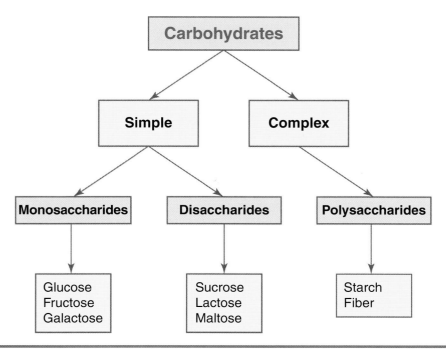

5-3   The arrangement of atoms and sugar units that make up carbohydrates determines their type and classification.

The Functions of Carbohydrates

Carbohydrates serve four key functions. They provide energy, spare proteins, assist in the breakdown of fats, and provide bulk in the diet.

Produce Energy

Meeting the energy needs of all your cells as they work to sustain life is your body's main goal. Carbohydrates provide 4 calories of energy per gram. Carbohydrates are the preferred source of energy because your body can use and store them so efficiently. Every time you are physically active you draw on the stores for energy. When the stored form of carbohydrates becomes depleted, you feel signs of fatigue. If you do not consume enough carbohydrates, your body begins to draw mainly on proteins for fuel needs. A small amount of fat can also be converted to energy during times of long physical activity.

Spare Proteins

If necessary, your body can use proteins as an energy source. Your body is less efficient in using proteins for energy than it is in using carbohydrates. More importantly, if you eat too little carbohydrate, your body is unable to use proteins to build and maintain cell structures. By eating adequate amounts of carbohydrates, you spare the proteins. That means you allow the proteins to be used for their more vital roles, **5-4**.

Break Down Fats

If the diet is too low in carbohydrates, the body cannot completely break down fats. When fats are not broken down completely, compounds called *ketone bodies* are formed. These compounds then collect in the bloodstream, causing the blood to become more acidic than normal. This acidity can damage cells and organs. This

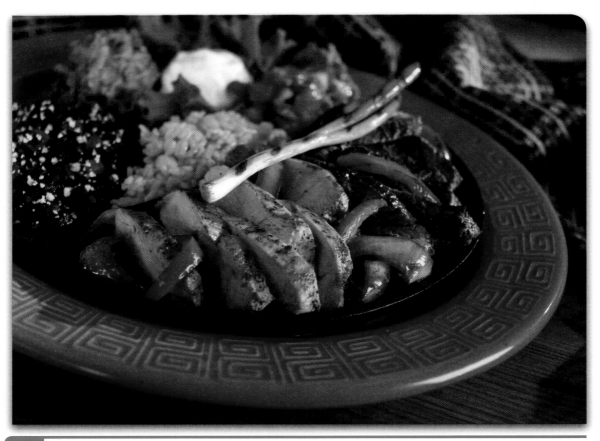

5-4   In this meal, the carbohydrates in the beans and rice supply energy, allowing the proteins in the meat to be used for other functions.

condition is called *ketosis*. The breath of a person in ketosis has the characteristic smell of nail polish remover. He or she also feels nauseous and weak. If the ketosis continues, the person can go into a coma and die.

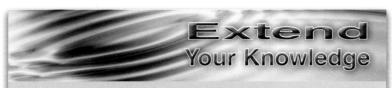

Carbohydrates and Sports Performance

Interview a sports nutritionist, registered dietitian, or certified athletic trainer about the role of carbohydrates in sports performance and physical endurance. Learn why carbohydrates are the energy fuel of choice for peak athletic performance.

Provide Bulk in the Diet

One other important function of carbohydrates is to add bulk to the diet. Fiber is the carbohydrate responsible for this task. It helps promote normal digestion and elimination of body wastes.

Like the muscles in your arms and legs, the muscles in your digestive tract need a healthy workout. Fiber is the solid material that provides this workout, helping intestinal muscles retain their tone.

Fiber acts like a sponge. It absorbs water, which softens stools and helps prevent constipation. Softer stools are easier to pass, reducing the likelihood of *hemorrhoids*, which are swollen veins in the rectum. Some fibers form gels that add bulk to stools. This helps relieve diarrhea.

Bulk in the diet has added benefits for people who are trying to lose weight. As fiber swells, the volume of food helps you feel full. Fiber also slows the rate at which the stomach empties. Fibrous food sources are usually lower in calories than foods high in fat, **5-5**.

Other Benefits of Fiber in the Diet

Fiber has been shown to have many benefits besides providing bulk in the diet. Current interest in fiber stems from observations made by British scientists around 1923. They noted African populations had lower rates of certain gastrointestinal (GI) tract diseases, such as colon cancer, than

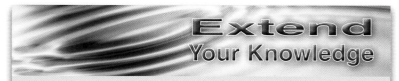

Where's the Fiber?

Review one week of your school lunch menu. Evaluate the menu for the use of whole-grain products, fruits, vegetables, legumes, and other high-fiber foods. Meet with the foodservice director to discuss the nutritional quality of school meals for meeting daily fiber needs. Inquire about the ratio of carbohydrates to fats and proteins in the meals served.

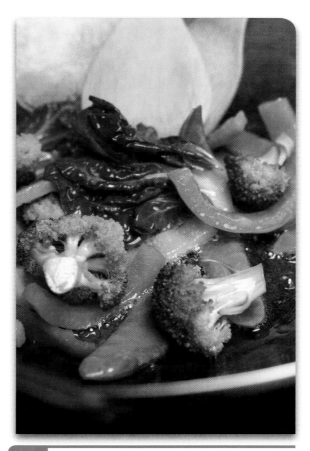

5-5 Vegetables are rich in fiber and low in calories.

Western industrialized populations. This led the scientists to study eating pattern differences. They found people in Western countries had rather low fiber intakes. In contrast, people in the African nations tended to have high fiber intakes. The scientists hypothesized the difference in the disease rate could be related to the difference in fiber consumption.

A variety of studies have been carried out to find out more about the role fiber plays in promoting wellness. Research results indicate including plenty of fiber in a low-fat diet appears to have many health benefits. For example, dietary fiber along with adequate fluids can help prevent *appendicitis*, which is an inflammation of the appendix. It may lower the risks of heart and artery disease. Dietary fiber may reduce the risk of colon cancer. It also helps control blood glucose levels.

Fibers vary in their composition and the jobs they perform in the GI tract. Eating a variety of fruits, vegetables, and whole grains gives you the full range of benefits from dietary fiber, **5-6**. These foods also provide health-promoting nutrients, including starch, protein, vitamins, minerals, and other important compounds.

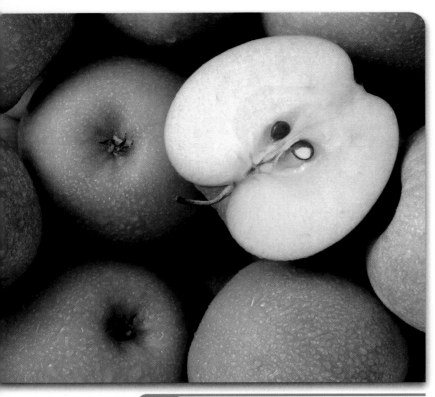

5-6   Apples are a source of dietary fiber called pectin.

How Your Body Uses Carbohydrates

Eating carbohydrates, regardless of their source, sets off a complex chain of events in your body. The way your body uses carbohydrates is explained here in simplified terms.

All carbohydrates must be in the form of glucose for your cells to use them as an energy source. To get them into this form, your digestive system first breaks down poly- and disaccharides from foods into monosaccharides. The monosaccharides are small enough to move across the intestinal wall into the blood. They travel via the blood to the liver. Any fructose and galactose in the blood is converted to glucose in the liver.

When the amount of glucose in the blood rises (this happens after you eat), a hormone called *insulin* is released from the pancreas. **Hormones** are chemicals produced in the body and released into the bloodstream to regulate specific body processes. **Insulin** helps the body lower blood glucose back to a normal level. It does this by triggering body cells to burn glucose for energy. It also causes muscles and the liver to store glucose. In healthy bodies, blood glucose is carefully managed. If carbohydrates are not broken down, then the body begins to break down protein and fats for energy. When blood glucose levels become too high, cells can be damaged. The disease related to insulin use and production is described in a later section.

If your cells do not have immediate energy needs, the excess glucose from the bloodstream is stored. The cells convert the glucose to glycogen. **Glycogen** is the body's storage form of glucose. Two-thirds of your body's glycogen is stored in your muscles for use as an energy source during muscular activity, **5-7**. Your liver stores the other one-third of the glycogen for use by the rest of your body.

Your liver can store only a limited amount of glycogen. You need to eat carbohydrates throughout the day to keep your glycogen stores replenished. However, suppose you eat more carbohydrates than your body can immediately use or store as glycogen. In this case, your liver converts the excess carbohydrates into fat. An unlimited amount of fat can be stored in the fatty tissues of your body. Unlike glycogen stores, fat stores cannot be converted back into glucose.

If a candy bar and a sandwich both end up as glucose, why does it matter which you eat? The candy bar provides

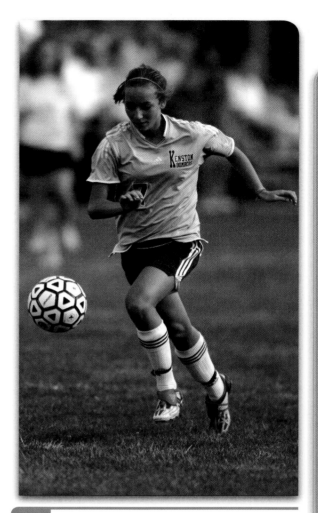

5-7 During physical activity, your body uses glycogen stored in the muscles for energy.

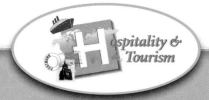

Bakers

Bakers mix and bake ingredients according to recipes to produce varying types and quantities of breads, pastries, and other baked goods. Bakers commonly are employed in commercial bakeries that distribute breads and pastries through established wholesale and retail outlets, mail order, or manufacturers' outlets. In these manufacturing facilities, bakers produce mostly standardized baked goods in large quantities, using high-volume mixing machines, ovens, and other equipment. Supermarkets and specialty shops produce smaller quantities of breads, pastries, and other baked goods for consumption on their premises or for sale as specialty baked goods.

Education: Bakers often start their careers as apprentices or trainees. Apprentice bakers usually start in craft bakeries, while trainees usually begin in store bakeries, such as those in supermarkets. Employment in both situations requires that bakers become skilled in baking, icing, and decorating. Many apprentice bakers participate in correspondence study and may work toward a certificate in baking through the Retail Bakers of America. Courses in nutrition are helpful for those selling baked goods or developing new recipes. If running a small business, bakers need to know how to operate a business. All bakers must follow government health and sanitation regulations.

Job Outlook: Highly skilled bakers should remain in demand because of growing interest specialty products and the time it takes to learn to make these products.

little more than simple sugars. The sandwich, on the other hand, supplies vitamins, minerals, and protein as well as complex carbohydrates.

In addition, complex carbohydrates take longer to digest than simple carbohydrates. This gives complex carbohydrates greater satiety value. **Satiety** is the feeling of fullness you have after eating food. The sandwich is higher in complex carbohydrates. Therefore, you are likely to feel full longer after eating the sandwich than after eating the candy bar.

Meeting Your Carbohydrate Needs

The RDA for carbohydrates for males and females is 130 grams. This represents only the sufficient amounts of carbohydrates needed to meet glucose needs for the brain and nervous system. More carbohydrates are needed to provide energy for daily activities. The *Dietary Guidelines* recommend 45 to 65 percent of total calories come from carbohydrates. Many popular foods, including whole-grain breads and cereals, pasta, nonfat milk, fruits, and vegetables, are rich sources of carbohydrates. Most foods that are high in carbohydrates are found in the grain group. MyPlate lists and describes a variety of carbohydrate foods to make up the foundation of a healthful diet. Grains are divided into two groups—whole grains and refined grains. At least half of your daily grain servings should be whole grains. Legumes, peas, beans, and nuts are also good sources of carbohydrates.

The typical diet in the United States fails to meet recommendations for carbohydrates. Even though most Americans eat more carbohydrates than recommended, too many are simple carbohydrates. Many diets fall short of recommended amounts of complex carbohydrates. How does your diet compare? Do you often choose foods such as milk shakes, candy, soft drinks, and pastries that are high in simple sugars? Do you choose complex carbohydrates such as brown rice, breads, vegetables, and legumes less often? What are your carbohydrate needs and how can you choose foods to meet them?

Sugars

You can divide sugars (simple carbohydrates) in foods into two categories. The first category includes sugars that occur naturally in foods. These sugars include lactose in milk and fructose in fruits. Naturally occurring sugars are generally accompanied by other nutrients in foods. Therefore, they do not cause great concern among nutrition experts.

The second category of sugars includes sugars added to foods at the table or during processing. These sugars are sometimes called *refined sugars*. **Refined sugars** are carbohydrate sweeteners that are separated from their natural sources for use as food additives. They come from such sources as sugar cane, sugar beets, and corn, **5-8**. Refined sugars function as more than sweetening agents. They may also be added to foods to increase bulk or aid in browning.

Soft drinks are the main source of sugar in teen diets. Many other foods high in sugar, such as candy, cakes, cookies, and donuts, are also high in fat. Eating too many of these foods can mean too many calories and not enough nutrients. This can lead to overweight and malnutrition.

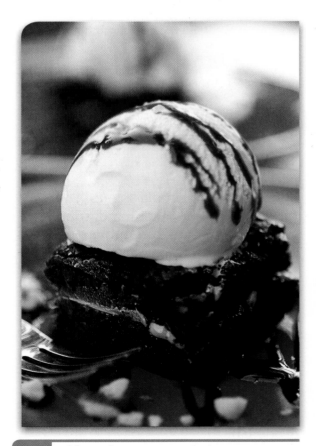

5-8   Most desserts get their sweet taste from refined sugars.

Many processed foods, such as catsup and cereals, are also high in added sugars. Although sugar is an excellent source of simple carbohydrates, it contributes no other nutrients to foods. In other words, sugars increase the calories a food provides without increasing the nutrients it provides. Added sugars reduce the nutrient density of processed foods.

High-fructose corn syrup (HFCS) is commonly used by food manufacturers to add sweetness to foods. HFCS is made by converting about half of the glucose found in cornstarch into fructose. The resulting product is sweeter than sucrose. HFCS is produced and sold to food manufacturers for its enhanced sweetening power. It is used in sports drinks, high-energy food bars, and other popular snack foods.

Reduced-fat and fat-free food products often contain much added sugar. Many consumers are aware that foods high in fat are also high in calories. To limit their calorie intake, consumers are buying products such as reduced-fat crackers and fat-free cookies. However, these products often have as many calories as regular crackers and cookies. Manufacturers often add sugar to products when they remove fat. Some consumers mistakenly think they can eat more when they choose reduced-fat snacks. These consumers may end up gaining weight rather than losing it. You can read food labels to determine the number of calories per serving to determine total calorie content.

Surveys show that added sugars make up about 16 percent of total calories in the American diet. Added sugars provide few or no essential nutrients and no fiber. The Dietary Guidelines suggest a healthy eating pattern would limit added sugars to roughly 6½ percent of total calories. A teaspoon of sugar

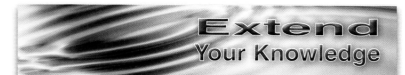

Extend Your Knowledge

Low-Calorie Sweeteners

Many people turn to low-calorie sweeteners to satisfy their sweet tooth while limiting calories. These low-calorie sweeteners contribute no or very few calories to foods and beverages, but provide more than 100 times the sweetening power of sugar. A number of low-calorie sweeteners have been approved for use in foods and drinks including

- Acesulfame potassium (known as acesulfame K or Ace-K)
- Aspartame
- Neotame
- Saccharin
- Rebaudioside A (Reb-A) stevia
- Sucralose

Saccharin, ace-K, sucralose, and Reb-A stevia can be substituted for sugar in baking. Refer to each product's package for directions on substitution amounts when replacing sugar in a recipe. Substitution equivalents vary depending on the product being used and its form (granular, liquid, or other). Neotame is stable when heated, but is not sold to consumers in packet or bulk form and does not include cooking instructions.

Another group of reduced-calorie sweeteners called polyols or sugar alcohols are most often used in desserts, candy, and chewing gum.

Search the Internet or study food labels at the supermarket to learn the brand names of the low-calorie sweeteners.

equals about 4 grams of carbohydrates. For a person following a 2,000-calorie diet, the daily limit would be about 32 grams of added sugars, or 8 teaspoons of sugar. This is the amount of added sugar in one can of most regular soft drinks, 5-9. The majority of added sugar consumed by teens comes from soda, energy drinks, and sports drinks.

The World Health Organization (WHO) recommends limiting the amounts of added sugars to no more than 10 percent of calorie intake. The

Added Sugar in Your Diet		
Food	**Added Sugar**	
	Grams	**Teaspoons**
12-ounce carbonated soft drink	40	10
¾ cup ready-to-eat cereal, chocolate-flavored puffs	12	3
8-ounce fruit yogurt	14	3½
1.7-ounce candy bar, milk chocolate	31	7¾
granola bar	12	3
cake with frosting	36	9
1 Tbsp. catsup	3	¾

5-9   You may be surprised how quickly the teaspoons of added sugar can total up in your diet.

American Heart Association suggests limiting added sugars to approximately 7 percent of calorie intake. For most men and women, this means less than 35 grams of added sugar per day.

Starches

Starches are the preferred source of fuel for your diet. Your body can burn them efficiently for energy, and they have greater satiety value than simple sugars. Many starchy foods are also excellent sources of vitamins, minerals, and fiber.

Nutrition experts agree that your carbohydrate intake should primarily consist of fruits, vegetables, whole-grain breads and cereals, and beans. Following MyPlate helps you achieve this goal. The grain group is an excellent source of foods high in starch. Foods in the vegetable group and legumes from the protein foods group are also high in starch.

Fiber

The DRI for fiber is 38 grams per day for males ages 14 through 50. The DRI is 26 grams per day for 14- to 18-year-old females. For women ages 19 through 50, the DRI decreases to 25 grams daily. These recommendations are based on intakes that have been shown to help protect against heart disease. Most people must at least double their current fiber intakes to meet these recommendations.

You can begin increasing your fiber intake by choosing whole-grain products in place of refined-grain products whenever possible. Whole-grain products contain all three edible parts of the grain kernel—bran, germ, and endosperm, **5-10**.

- *Bran* is the outer layer of the grain, which is a good source of fiber.
- *Germ* is the nutrient-rich part of the kernel.
- *Endosperm* is the largest part of the kernel and contains mostly starch.

Processing removes the bran, germ, and most of the fiber to produce refined-grain products. White flour and white rice are examples of refined-grain products.

Some people use fiber supplements to add fiber to their diets. A **supplement** is a concentrated source of a nutrient, usually in pill, liquid, or powder form. Supplements do not offer the range of nutritional benefits provided by food sources of nutrients.

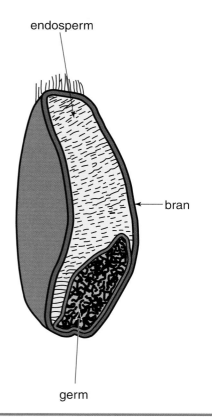

5-10 The germ and the fiber-rich bran layer are removed when grains are refined. Choose whole-grain bread and cereal products for the nutrients contained in all three parts of the kernel.

For most people, fiber supplements are unnecessary. Meeting your fiber needs is fairly easy if you eat the recommended amounts from MyPlate. An average serving of most whole-grain breads and cereals, vegetables, or fruits provides three grams of fiber. Dry beans provide up to eight grams per serving. Other high-fiber foods include foods such as cooked lentils, peas, and nuts.

As you change your eating habits, increase your intake of dietary fiber slowly. This helps your body adjust. A sudden large increase of dietary fiber may cause digestive discomfort. Be sure to drink plenty of water as you increase your fiber intake.

Using Food Labels to Meet Your Carbohydrate Needs

Reading food labels can help you meet your carbohydrate needs. The amount of total carbohydrate provided by a food is listed in grams on the Nutrition Facts panel. Total carbohydrate includes starches, fiber, and sugars present in the food product. Underneath the total carbohydrate, the numbers of grams of dietary fiber and sugars per serving are given. The amount listed for sugars includes both naturally occurring sugars—as found in milk or fruit—as well as any added sugars.

Find out how much added sugar the product contains by reading the ingredient list. Ingredients must be listed in descending order by weight. The ingredients present in the largest amounts will appear near the beginning of the list. Check to see if an added sugar, such as corn syrup or fruit juice concentrate, appears near the beginning of the list. In addition, check to see if more than one type of sugar is listed, **5-11**. These are both indications a product is high in refined sugars.

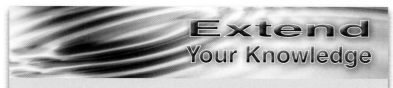

Extend Your Knowledge

A Better Recipe

Ask a registered dietitian or use Internet resources to learn how to add fiber to a recipe and reduce the amount of refined sugars. Find out how recipes, such as baked goods, soups, sauces, and other prepared foods, can be nutritionally modified to improve nutrient density. Try applying what you learn to one of your favorite recipes and prepare it.

Identifying Added Sugars on the Label

- Brown sugar
- Cane juice
- Cane syrup
- Corn sweetener
- Corn syrup
- Dextrose
- Fructose
- Fruit juice concentrate
- Glucose
- High-fructose corn syrup
- Honey
- Invert sugar
- Lactose
- Maltose
- Malt syrup
- Molasses
- Raw sugar
- Sucrose
- Syrup

5-11   Look for other names used for added sugars when reading the ingredient lists on food labels.

Math Link

Converting to Grams

Every morning, Tonya starts her day with a serving of cereal and half-cup of milk. According to their Nutrition Facts panels, these foods contain the following Total Carbohydrates:

cereal—24 g
milk—6 g

Tonya follows an 1,800-calorie food plan. Her goal is to obtain 60% of her calories from carbohydrates.

- How many more grams does Tonya need to meet her daily goal?

Reading the ingredient list can also help you increase your intake of whole grains. When selecting carbohydrate foods, look for the word "whole" in the first ingredient listed. For example, choose breads that list whole-wheat flour as the first ingredient rather than simply wheat flour or enriched flour. Other whole-grain ingredients include whole-grain cornmeal, brown rice, wheat berries, whole-grain rye, oats, and buckwheat.

The Glycemic Index (GI)

The term *glycemic index* is frequently used when making carbohydrate choices for people on special diets or trying to lose weight. The **glycemic index (GI)** is a measure of the speed at which various carbohydrates are digested into glucose, absorbed, and enter the bloodstream. Pure glucose raises blood glucose levels more quickly than any other carbohydrate. Foods with a high GI produce a quick, steep increase in blood glucose often followed by a fast drop in levels. Foods with lower GI result in slower, less dramatic increases in blood glucose levels. Glycemic index may be a helpful tool for individuals trying to prevent or manage chronic illnesses such as heart disease and diabetes.

A food is assigned a GI based on how it compares to an equal amount of pure glucose (GI=100). GI scores can be affected by how the food is prepared, food combinations, and differences in individuals' metabolisms. A person can have different GI scores for the same food eaten at different times of the day. Carbohydrates consumed with fat, protein, or fiber are digested and absorbed more slowly. Therefore, a plain slice of white bread has a much higher GI than a slice of white bread with peanut butter, **5-12**.

The gylcemic index is designed to help people who must regulate their blood glucose levels to maintain good health. If the research is accurate, less glucose builds up in the blood when foods with lower GI values are consumed. Data from research has mixed results. Usefulness of predicting blood glucose levels remains in question. Using the glycemic index can be a valuable strategy when combined with other tools that help you select healthful whole-grain foods, legumes, and nuts along with a varied selection of

Glycemic Indexes of Common Foods		
Glycemic Index		**Food Item**
High	100	pure glucose
	85	baked potato
	81	cornflakes
	80	jelly beans
	73	white bread
	72	popcorn
	68	chocolate ice cream
	64	spaghetti
	51	banana
	48	orange
	40	apple
Low	13	peanuts

Source: Data from Kaye Foster-Powell, Susanna HA Holt and Janette C. Brand-Miller, "International table of glycemic index and glycemic load values: 2002," American Journal of Clinical Nutrition, Vol. 76, No. 1, 5-56, 2002.

5-12   These glycemic index values are measured using glucose as a reference.

other fruits and vegetables. These foods are absorbed slowly and provide more stable levels of blood glucose levels.

Remember, complex carbohydrates take longer to digest than simple carbohydrates. This gives complex carbohydrates greater satiety value. Since it is higher in complex carbohydrates, oatmeal might be a better choice than a doughnut for breakfast. Also, you are likely to feel full longer after eating a whole-grain cereal than after eating a donut. Eating more complex carbohydrates helps people who are trying to reduce their calorie intake. These carbohydrates often contain other beneficial nutrients as well.

Health Questions Related to Carbohydrates

As you read about the importance of carbohydrates in your diet, you may find yourself thinking of specific questions. Many teens and their parents want to know the answers to these frequently asked questions.

Are Starchy Foods Fattening?

Some people believe eating foods high in starch causes weight gain. Starchy foods are rich in carbohydrates. Gram per gram, carbohydrates have the same amount of calories (4) as protein. They have less than half the calories (9) of fat.

One reason some people think starchy foods are fattening may be related to the way these foods are served. Pasta is often served with cream sauce, rice with gravy, and baked potatoes with sour cream. Such high-fat toppings can send the total calories in carbohydrate dishes soaring. Consider the example of a slice of bread, which has about 12 grams of carbohydrate and 65 calories. Spreading the bread with a teaspoon of butter would add 4 grams of fat and 36 more calories. If you are trying to cut calories out of your diet, try limiting the fatty toppings, not the carbohydrates.

Is Sugar a Hazard to Your Teeth?

There is a clear connection between sweets and **dental caries** (tooth decay). People who eat much sugar are likely to have a higher incidence of tooth decay than people who eat less sugar. However, sugar is not the only culprit. Starches can promote tooth decay, too.

Bacteria that live in the mouth feed on the carbohydrates in food particles. The bacteria form a sticky substance called *plaque* that clings to teeth. As the bacteria grow, they produce acid that eats away the protective tooth enamel, forming pits in the teeth. In time, these pits can deepen into cavities.

The risk of dental caries depends on two main factors—the type of food and when you eat it. Sticky, carbohydrate foods, such as raisins, cookies, crackers, and caramels, tend to cling to teeth. They are more harmful than foods that are quickly swallowed and removed from contact with the teeth. Likewise, sugars and starches eaten between meals tend to be more harmful to tooth enamel than carbohydrates consumed at meals. Food particles from between-meal snacks tend to remain in the mouth—and in contact with teeth—for longer periods.

Carbohydrates eaten during meals are removed from the mouth by beverages and other foods eaten with them.

Avoiding sticky carbohydrate-rich foods between meals is good advice for keeping teeth healthy. If you do eat sticky foods, drink plenty of water to wash the teeth. If brushing and flossing your teeth are possible, this is even better, **5-13**.

People who care for young children should know tooth damage can begin in early infancy. Regularly allowing a baby to sleep with a bottle in his or her mouth can destroy the baby's teeth. The acids formed by constant contact of bacteria with sugars in the milk will

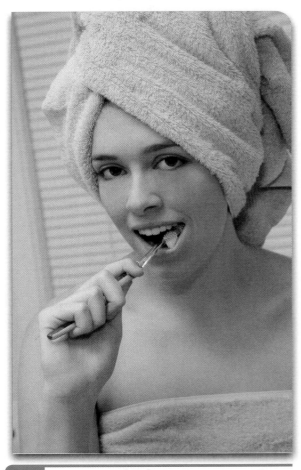

5-13   Brushing teeth after eating will help prevent a buildup of plaque that can lead to tooth decay.

erode the baby's tooth enamel. After feeding, caregivers should gently clean babies' gums and teeth by wiping them with a soft, clean cloth.

Does Sugar Cause Hyperactivity?

Hyperactivity is a condition in which a person seems to be in constant motion and is easily distracted. Children with this condition may disrupt their classmates and have trouble concentrating on their schoolwork. Many teachers and parents observe that children are more active after parties and other events at which sweets are served. This has led some people to believe sugar causes hyperactivity.

Although researchers have conducted many studies, they have found no proof that consuming sugars causes behavior changes in most people. It is true eating sugars gives children energy needed to fuel activity. However, children at a party may exhibit rowdy behavior simply because they are excited. After all, eating and playing with friends are fun social activities. Caregivers may find leading children in less-active games at the end of a party helps reduce post-party excitement, **5-14**.

Caregivers should also keep in mind that children who eat large amounts of sweets may be missing some important nutrients. If you know a child who has trouble concentrating, look at his or her total diet. Eating a well-balanced diet that includes fewer sweets and more nutritious snacks can help improve performance.

Is Sugar Addictive?

Some people seem to crave sweets all the time. There are those who

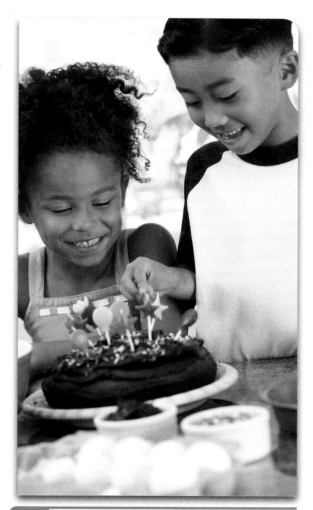

5-14 Unruly behavior following a children's party is more likely to be caused by excitement than sugar consumption.

believe this type of craving qualifies as an *addiction*, or a habitual need.

Experiments have shown that if animals do not have a nutritious diet, they will eat excessive amounts of sugar. When the animals are allowed to eat a variety of foods, they seem to be less dependent on sugar. This indicates the animals did not truly need the sugar. Therefore, *addiction* is not the best word to use to explain the animals' excessive use of sugar.

Research has shown people are born with a preference for sweet-tasting foods.

Case Study: Too Much Sugar?

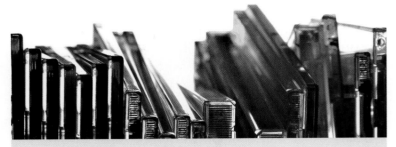

Mary was told she is addicted to sugar. She usually has a soft drink for breakfast, has a candy bar for mid-morning snack, and brings cupcakes for lunch at school. In the evening her parents always have ice cream or cookies for dessert. She often has soft drinks and more sweet snacks during the evening while studying.

Case Review

1. Is Mary addicted to sugar?

2. What advice would you give to improve Mary's eating behaviors?

However, people may not respond to sugar in the same way as test animals. Researchers now seem to think the need for sugar is more psychological than physiological. In other words, people seem to eat sweets because they enjoy them, not because they are addicted to them.

Will Too Much Sugar Cause Diabetes?

Diabetes mellitus is a lack of or an inability to use the hormone insulin. Sugars and starches in the foods you eat are converted to glucose, which then enters the bloodstream. Insulin regulates the blood glucose level by stimulating cells to pull glucose from the bloodstream. When the body does not make enough insulin, or fails to use insulin correctly, glucose builds up in the bloodstream.

There are two main types of diabetes. In type 1 diabetes, the pancreas is not able to make insulin. This type of diabetes occurs most often in children and young adults. People with type 1 diabetes must take daily injections of insulin to maintain normal blood glucose levels. This type represents 5 to 10 percent of all diagnosed cases.

In type 2 diabetes, body cells do not respond well to the insulin the pancreas makes. This type of diabetes is much more common and represents about 90 to 95 percent of all diagnosed cases. Sometimes called *adult onset diabetes*, this type usually occurs in adults over age 40. However, as overweight problems increase for a growing number of young people, so does the incidence of type 2 diabetes. People who are overweight and eat diets high in refined carbohydrates and low in fiber are at greater risk of developing this type of diabetes. People in the later stages of this disease may require insulin injections. In the earlier stages, however, type 2 diabetes can often be controlled with diet and physical activity, **5-15**.

Both types of diabetes tend to run in families. Symptoms of both types include excessive hunger and thirst accompanied by weakness, irritability, and nausea. Changes in eyesight; slow healing of cuts; drowsiness; and numbness in legs, feet, or fingers are symptoms, too.

In both types of diabetes, the blood glucose level rises too high. Although eating sugar increases the blood glucose level, it does not cause diabetes to develop. However, diabetics need to

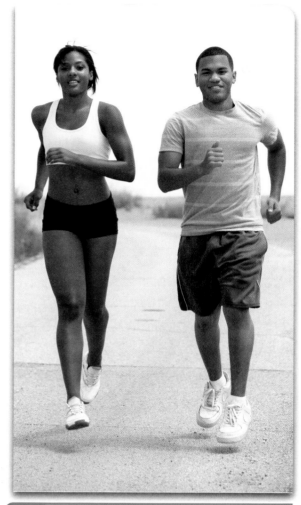

5-15   Regular physical exercise plays an important role in controlling type 2 diabetes.

regulate their sugar intake by following a diet plan prescribed by a physician or registered dietitian.

What Is Hypoglycemia?

Hypoglycemia refers to a low blood glucose level. An overproduction of insulin causes blood sugar to drop sharply two to four hours after eating a meal. The central nervous system depends on a constant supply of glucose from the blood. Low blood sugar causes physical symptoms of sweating, shaking, headaches, hunger, and anxiety.

A medical test is required to diagnose true hypoglycemia. This condition is rare and may point to a more severe health problem. Many people who believe they have hypoglycemia may just be reacting to stress.

The dietary advice for people with hypoglycemia is sensible for all people. That is, avoid eating large amounts of sugar all at once. Also, eat nutritious meals at regular intervals.

What Is Lactose Intolerance?

Lactose intolerance is an inability to digest lactose, the main carbohydrate in milk. This condition is caused by a lack of the digestive enzyme lactase, which is needed to break down lactose. People who are lactose intolerant may experience gas, cramping, nausea, and diarrhea when they consume dairy products.

Lactose intolerance is common throughout the world. It occurs more often among nonwhite populations and tends to develop as people age.

Milk and other dairy products are the chief sources of calcium and vitamin D in the diet. These nutrients help build strong bones and teeth. They are especially important for children and pregnant women. People who do not consume dairy products must use care to eat and drink adequate sources of calcium and vitamin D.

People who are unable to drink milk must meet their calcium needs from other sources. Some people can tolerate small amounts of milk if they consume it with a meal. They may also be able to consume milk alternates such as yogurt, cheese, and butter-milk, **5-16**. Lactose in these products is changed to lactic acid or broken down into glucose and galactose during the culturing process. Another option is to take lactase pills or add lactase drops to dairy foods.

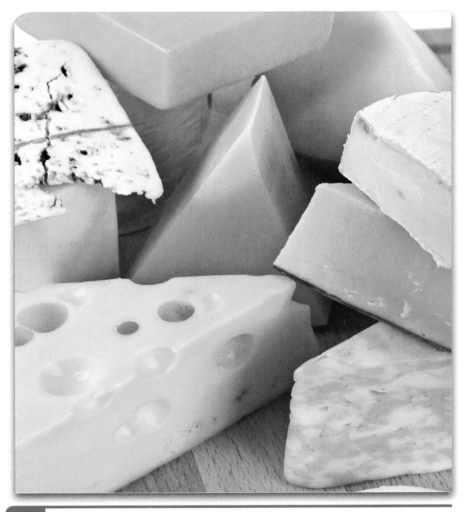

5-16   Someone who is lactose intolerant may be able to digest cheese more easily than milk.

Reading Summary

Carbohydrates are sugars, starches, and fibers in the diet. Simple carbohydrates are called sugars. They include the mono- and disaccharides. Complex carbohydrates include starches and fibers. They are also called polysaccharides. Breads, pasta, rice, vegetables, fruits, milk, yogurt, legumes, and sweets are all sources of carbohydrates.

Carbohydrates supply four calories per gram and are the body's most important energy source. They spare proteins in the diet for other important functions. Carbohydrates also help with fat metabolism and provide bulk in the diet as fiber. In addition, fiber may help people manage weight and lower risks of heart disease, cancer, and intestinal disorders.

During digestion, carbohydrates are broken down and converted into glucose with the help of the liver. The bloodstream delivers glucose to cells where it is used for energy or converted to glycogen for storage. Insulin from the pancreas helps regulate this process. Excess carbohydrates are converted into fat.

Carbohydrates should make up a large portion of your diet. About 45-65 percent of your daily calories should come from carbohydrates. However, the American Heart Association recommends limiting your intake of refined sugars to no more than 7 percent of daily calories. They also suggest most people increase their intake of dietary fiber. Reading food labels can help you meet these dietary goals. The glycemic index (GI) is sometimes used as a tool to indicate which foods are quickly digested to form blood glucose and which are slower in this process.

Sugars and starches that remain in contact with the teeth promote dental caries, but good dental hygiene can reduce problems. Also, sugar has not been proven to cause hyperactivity, nor has it been shown to be addictive.

Diabetes type 1 and type 2 affect how the body responds to carbohydrates. Sugar does not cause diabetes; diabetes is an insulin related problem. Hypoglycemia, which is a low blood glucose level, can often be controlled by regularly consuming meals high in complex carbohydrates. Lactose intolerance, which is an inability to digest milk sugar, may be controlled through careful use of dairy products.

Review Learning

1. Identify the monosaccharide units that make up each of the three disaccharides.
2. How do simple carbohydrates differ from complex carbohydrates?
3. If the diet does not provide enough carbohydrates, how does the body meet its needs for energy?
4. What are two benefits of fiber in the diet for people who are trying to lose weight?
5. True or false. A person is likely to feel full longer after eating popcorn than after eating cotton candy.
6. Where is the body's glycogen stored and how is it used?

7. Why do refined sugars in the diet cause greater concern among nutrition experts than naturally occurring sugars?

8. If a person eats 3,000 calories per day, about how many of those calories are recommended come from carbohydrates? What is the preferred type of the carbohydrates?

9. List three good food sources of dietary fiber.

10. What two factors affect the risk of dental caries?

11. Describe the difference between type 1 diabetes and type 2 diabetes?

12. What causes lactose intolerance?

Critical Thinking

13. **Draw conclusions.** What conclusions can you draw about the "misinformation" people have about carbohydrate foods?

14. **Analyze behavior.** What reasons can you identify for people choosing simple carbohydrates over complex carbohydrates? What factors may impact this behavior?

Applying Your Knowledge

15. **Create a list.** Make a list of snacks that are high in refined sugars. Then make a list of snack alternatives that are high in naturally occurring sugars and/or complex carbohydrates. Make sure half of your alternative snacks are whole grain. Share your lists with the class.

16. **Product chart.** Analyze five cereal product labels. Make a chart and record the amount of total carbohydrate, dietary fiber, and sugars in each product. Also list all the types of refined sugars included in each product. Rank the cereals based on their nutritional value. Present your rankings to the class.

17. **Bulletin board.** Prepare a bulletin board or showcase showing how to use information about carbohydrates found on food labels. Highlight the differences between simple and complex carbohydrates.

18. **Dentist interview.** To find out more about the relationship between nutrition and dental health, interview a dentist. Implement strategies you learn to keep your teeth healthy.

Technology Connections

19. **Research additives.** Review the ingredient lists on three canned or frozen meals to identify the carbohydrate additives. Use the Internet to research the major functions of each additive listed. Share your findings in class.

20. **Electronic presentation.** Use the American Diabetic Association Web site and other useful sites to prepare an electronic presentation on healthful eating plans for a person who is diabetic. Include a discussion of why and how carbohydrates are counted. Give your presentation to the class.

21. **Write a PSA.** Write and video record an entertaining and informative public service announcement (PSA) for television that encourages people to increase their fiber intake.

22. **Create a puzzle.** Use a puzzle-maker program found on the Internet to prepare a word search or crossword puzzle. Use the list of vocabulary words from this chapter.

Academic Connections

23. **Math.** Select four bread products. Be sure to include a variety such as whole-grain bread, plain bagel, rye bread, and so on. Using the information provided from their Nutrition Facts panels, create a histogram comparing the grams of fiber found in each product.
24. **Writing.** Research a grain that you have never eaten. Write a brief paper summarizing your findings.
25. **Social studies.** Prepare a global map showing where crops are grown to produce sweeteners, such as sugar cane, beets, and corn. Compare the climates and topographies of the growing areas.
26. **Science.** Use Internet or print resources to research the prevalence of lactose intolerance in various populations and age groups. Briefly summarize the theories explaining these differences and formulate your own conclusion. Share your conclusion with the class.

Workplace Applications

Teaching Others

The ability to teach skills to others is a transferrable skill that employers desire. Presume your new employer has noticed you have this ability. A group of employees has decided to form a team of runners to train for a fundraising marathon next spring. Because you are a dedicated marathon runner and have knowledge about healthful eating, your employer has asked you to lead a lunchtime discussion group once a week. This week's topic is the importance of eating the right carbohydrates, especially when training for a marathon. What questions would you ask your coworkers about their carbohydrate intake? What information would you want to teach them about carbohydrate choices?

Chapter 6

Fats: A Concentrated Energy Source

Reading for Meaning

Before reading, skim the chapter and examine how it is organized. Look at the bold or italic words, headings of different colors and sizes, bulleted lists or numbered lists, tables, charts, captions, and features.

Concept Organizer

Use the T-chart diagram to identify key chapter concepts. In the left column, write the main ideas. In the right column, write details about subtopics.

Main Ideas About Fats	Supporting Details

Terms to Know

lipid
triglycerides
fatty acid
saturated fatty acid
unsaturated fatty acid
monounsaturated fatty acid
polyunsaturated fatty acid
hydrogenation
trans fatty acid
rancid
phospholipids
lecithin
emulsifier
sterols
cholesterol
essential fatty acid
adipose tissue
chylomicron
lipoprotein
very low-density lipoprotein (VLDL)
low-density lipoprotein (LDL)
high-density lipoprotein (HDL)
coronary heart disease (CHD)
plaque
atherosclerosis
heart attack
stroke
hypertension
blood lipid profile
omega-3 fatty acids
cancer
fat replacer

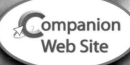

Companion Web Site

- **Print out the concept organizer at g-wlearning.com.**
- **Practice key terms with crossword puzzles, matching activities, and e-flash cards at g-wlearning.com.**

Objectives

After studying this chapter, you will be able to
- **contrast** the characteristic differences between saturated and unsaturated fatty acids.
- **list** five functions of lipids in the body.
- **summarize** how the body digests, absorbs, and transports lipids.
- **explain** the role fats play in heart health.
- **identify** 11 heart-health risk factors.
- **evaluate** food choices within the different food groups for their types and amounts of fat content.
- **select** foods that follow recommended limits for dietary fats and cholesterol.

Central Ideas
- Lipids are vital for many body functions.
- Choosing the right types of fats is important to good health.

Fat seems to be a common topic when discussing health and nutrition these days. "Americans are eating too much fat." "How many grams of fat are in that food?" "Have you tried the latest low-fat diet?" You might hear comments like these through the media, at the grocery store, and even in the halls at school.

There are some good reasons to be concerned about fat. Too much fat in the diet is linked to a variety of health problems. However, fats are not all bad. In fact, fats perform many important functions in the body. You need to eat foods containing some fat every day. The goal is to choose foods with the recommended amounts and types of fat for a healthful diet, **6-1**.

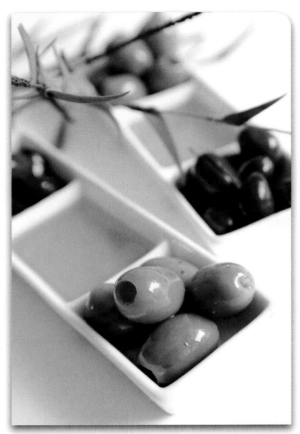

6-1   The type of fat found in olives and olive oil is a good choice for a healthful diet.

What Are Lipids?

You are familiar with the word *fat*, but the word *lipid* may be new to you. **Lipid** is a broader term for a group of compounds that includes fats, oils, lecithin, and cholesterol. Lipids can be grouped into three main classes—triglycerides, phospholipids, and sterols.

What Are Triglycerides?

Triglycerides are the major type of fat found in foods and in the body. Triglycerides are sometimes called *blood fat*. In excess, triglycerides are stored in the fat cells and in the liver. Triglycerides consist of three fatty acids attached to a glycerol molecule. *Glycerol* is an alcohol that has three carbon atoms. It is the backbone of the triglyceride molecule. **Fatty acids** are organic compounds made up of a chain of carbon atoms to which hydrogen atoms are attached. The last carbon atom at one end of the chain forms an *acid group* with two oxygen atoms and a hydrogen atom. Fatty acid chains vary in length. The most common fatty acids in food have 16 to 18 carbon atoms.

Saturated and Unsaturated Fatty Acids

Fatty acids can be saturated or unsaturated. **Saturated fatty acids** have no double bonds in their chemical structure. They have a full load of hydrogen atoms. An **unsaturated fatty acid** has at least one double bond between two carbon atoms in each molecule. If a double bond is broken, two hydrogen atoms can be added to the molecule. The number of double bonds and hydrogen atoms in the fatty acid chain determine the degree of saturation. A **monounsaturated fatty acid** has only one double bond between carbon atoms. A **polyunsaturated fatty acid** has two or more double bonds, **6-2**.

Nearly all fats and oils contain a mixture of the three types of fatty acids. For instance, corn oil is 13 percent saturated, 25 percent monounsaturated, and 62 percent polyunsaturated. The fats in meat and dairy products, including beef fat, lard, and butterfat, tend to be high in saturated fatty acids. Fats from plants are usually higher in unsaturated fatty acids. Olive and peanut oils are high in monounsaturated fatty acids. Corn, safflower, and soybean oils are high in polyunsaturated fatty acids. The tropical oils, such as coconut and palm oils, are an exception to the rule about fats from plants. These oils are high in saturated fatty acids.

Types of Fatty Acids

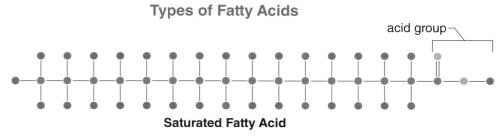

Saturated Fatty Acid

The carbon atoms in the chain are all linked with single bonds. The chain is saturated with as many hydrogen atoms as the carbon atoms can hold.

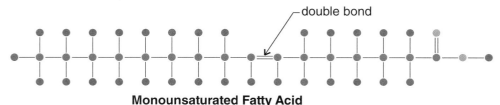

Monounsaturated Fatty Acid

The chain of carbon atoms contains one double bond. The two carbon atoms linked by the double bond could each hold another hydrogen atom.

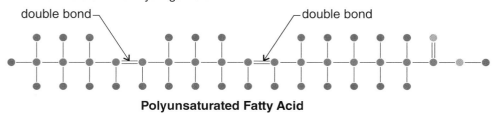

Polyunsaturated Fatty Acid

The chain of carbon atoms contains more than one double bond. Each of the carbon atoms linked by double bonds could hold another hydrogen atom.

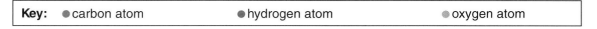

| **Key:** | ●carbon atom | ●hydrogen atom | ●oxygen atom |

6-2   The number of double bonds and hydrogen atoms determine whether a fatty acid is saturated, monounsaturated, or polyunsaturated.

The prevalent type of fatty acid determines whether a lipid is liquid or solid at room temperature. Lipids that are high in saturated fatty acids tend to be solid at room temperature. Lipids that are high in unsaturated fatty acids tend to be liquid at room temperature. Unsaturated fats have a lower melting point than more highly saturated fats. This is why chicken fat melts at a lower temperature than butterfat, which is more highly saturated.

Trans Fatty Acids

Unsaturated fatty acids can be hydrogenated. **Hydrogenation** is the process of breaking the double carbon bonds in unsaturated fatty acids and adding hydrogen. These fatty acids are known as ***trans* fatty acids**, also called *trans* fats or partially hydrogenated vegetable oils. This process converts liquid oils into solid fats. For instance, hydrogen is added to some of the double bonds in unsaturated liquid vegetable oil to make solid margarine.

Besides changing the texture, the main reason for hydrogenating oils is to improve their keeping quality. Oils turn rancid if they are exposed to air or stored for a long time. **Rancid** describes a food oil in which the fatty acid molecules have combined with oxygen. This causes them to break down, and the oil spoils. Rancid oils have an unpleasant smell and taste. Food manufacturers often prefer to use hydrogenated fats over unsaturated oils. The longer shelf life of the hydrogenated fats saves the manufacturers money and improves consumer satisfaction.

Research shows *trans* fat acts much like saturated fat in the body. Saturated fat is known to contribute to heart disease, as do *trans* fat and dietary cholesterol. *Trans* fats have been found to increase levels of fatty deposits on the walls of the arteries, which increases the chance for heart disease. *Trans* fats in the diet are also linked to high blood cholesterol levels. Reducing saturated and *trans* fats in your diet helps reduce heart health risks. This is important because heart disease is a leading cause of illness and death worldwide.

Processed foods made with partially hydrogenated vegetable oils provide about 80 percent of the *trans* fats in the diet. They are often found in vegetable shortenings, solid margarines, crackers, candies, cookies, chips, French fries, baked goods, and other favorite snack foods, **6-3**. However, *trans* fats are inherent in some foods such as beef, lamb, and butterfat. It is not understood whether these naturally occurring *trans* fats have the same effect as manufactured ones.

The American Heart Association (AHA) recommends no more than one percent of your total daily calories be *trans* fat. If you consume 2,000 calories per day, no more than 20 calories (about 2 grams) should come from *trans* fats. Less is preferred. To limit your intake of *trans* fats, read the Nutrition Facts label to determine the amount that food

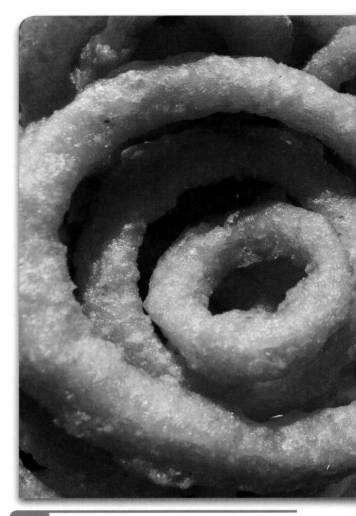

6-3   Fried snack foods may be a source of *trans* fats.

supplies. The amount listed includes both naturally occurring and added *trans* fats.

Since manufacturers can list *trans* fat content as 0 grams if a food contains less than 0.5 grams, you should also read the ingredient list. Avoid foods that list partially hydrogenated oil as an ingredient. Look for fast-food chains and restaurants that have switched from *trans* fat oils to healthier soybean, corn, or sunflower oils. Several states have laws that forbid restaurants from using *trans* fats in their cooking. For heart health, choose grilled or baked food products.

Phospholipids

Phospholipids are lipids that have a phosphorus-containing compound in their chemical structure. **Lecithin** is a phospholipid. Lecithin is made by the liver, so it is not essential to the diet. However, lecithin is found in many foods, including egg yolks. You will see *lecithin* on the ingredient lists of some food products. Soy lecithin is added to chocolate candy and commercially baked products.

Lecithin, like other phospholipids, is an emulsifier. An **emulsifier** is a substance that can mix with both water and fat. For example, egg yolk acts as an emulsifier in mayonnaise to prevent the oil and vinegar from separating. The lecithin in the egg yolk keeps the oil particles suspended in the watery vinegar.

In the body, lecithin is part of cell membranes. Some health food stores claim lecithin is a magical nutrient, but it is not. Lecithin supplements have no known benefits to your health. Lecithin is broken down during digestion. Therefore, the body no longer recognizes it as lecithin when it is absorbed.

Sterols

Another class of lipids is called **sterols**. Sterols have a complex molecular structure. They include some hormones, vitamin D, and cholesterol. Sterols are not to be confused with steroids, which is a manufactured chemical substance and is a drug. Sterols are often associated with heart health.

Cholesterol, a type of sterol, is a white, waxy lipid. This fat-like substance performs essential functions in the body. Cholesterol provides structure for all cell membranes. Cholesterol is made by the body and found

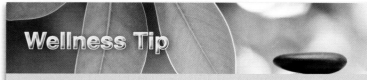

Wellness Tip

Check the Fat

To maintain a healthy weight, monitoring how much fat you eat can be a help. Start with the Nutrition Facts panel to identify the types and amount of fat in your favorite foods. Then look at the label ingredient list and note which items are listed first. If a type of fat is one of the first ingredients listed, you may want to look for a lower-fat alternative.

in every cell. For example, your body uses cholesterol to make sex hormones and bile acids. Because cholesterol is manufactured in your body, it is not essential in the diet.

Cholesterol is found only in animal tissues. It is never present in plants. Therefore plant foods, such as peanut butter and corn oil margarine, contain

Math Link

Calculating Grams of *Trans* Fat

The American Heart Association (AHA) says that calories from *trans* fats account for about 2 percent of the diet for most Americans. This is twice the amount the AHA recommends. The AHA recommends limiting your *trans* fat intake to no more than 1 percent of your daily calories.

- Calculate the maximum number of grams of *trans* fat the AHA recommends for an individual requiring 3,000 calories per day.

no cholesterol. All animal foods, including milk, cheese, hamburgers, eggs, and butter, contain cholesterol. It is abundant in egg yolks, organ meats (liver and kidney), crab, and lobster.

Phytosterols are compounds from plants that are similar in structure to cholesterol. Phytosterols include plant sterols and stanols. Although plant sterols and stanols are different from animal cholesterol, they carry out similar cellular functions in plants. Stanols and sterols are essential components of plant membranes. Both stanols and sterols can only be obtained through dietary sources. They are present naturally in small quantities in many fruits, vegetables, nuts, seeds, cereals, legumes, vegetable oils, and other plant sources. Foods containing phytosterols may have beneficial effects for health. Including plant sterols and stanols in the diet may help lower LDL cholesterol levels and the risk for heart disease.

Functions of Lipids

Lipids serve many important functions in the body. You need a number of fatty acids for normal growth and development. Your body can make most of these. However, two polyunsaturated fatty acids, *linoleic acid* and *linolenic acid*, are called **essential fatty acids**. Your body cannot make them. You must get them from your diet. If your diet is missing these nutrients, the skin, reproductive system, liver, and kidneys may all be affected. Most people include plenty of fats and oils in their diets, so lacks of the essential fatty acids are rare.

Lipids provide a concentrated source of energy. All lipids, whether butter, margarine, corn oil, or some other type of fat or oil, provide 9 calories per gram. In comparison, proteins and carbohydrates provide only 4 calories per gram. Your body can conveniently store fat calories for future energy needs.

The body stores a large share of lipids in **adipose tissue**. About half of this tissue is just under your skin. It serves as an internal blanket that holds in body heat, **6-4**. The fat cells in adipose tissue can expand to hold an almost unlimited amount of fat. Overweight people have excess stores of fat in their adipose tissue.

Body fat surrounds organs such as the heart and liver. This fat acts like a shock absorber. It helps protect the organs from the bumps and bruises of body movement.

Vitamins A, D, E, and K dissolve in fat. They are carried into your body along with the fat in foods. Lipids also help move these vitamins around inside your body.

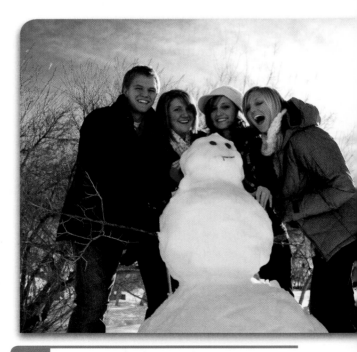

6-4   A layer of adipose tissue under the skin helps insulate the body in cold weather.

Lipids are part of the structure of every cell. You need lipids for the formation of healthy cell membranes. They are also used to make some hormones, vitamins, and other secretions.

Fats play roles in foods as well as in your body. Both naturally occurring and added fats affect the tastes, textures, and aromas of foods. Fats make meat moist and flavorful. They make biscuits tender and pie crusts flaky. Fats help fried foods become brown and crisp. They disperse the compounds that allow you to smell bacon cooking, too.

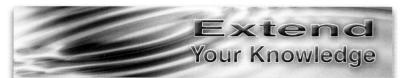

Extend Your Knowledge

What's on Your Bread?

Compare several types of margarine, such as stick margarine, soft spreads, and reduced-calorie margarine. Compare their costs, tastes, and textures with traditional butter. Examine the Nutrition Facts panels on the label for grams of saturated fat, as well as polyunsaturated and monounsaturated fats if listed. Compare amounts of *trans* fats in each type of product. Decide for whom and when you might use the various products. Which brands do you think would be most heart healthy? Why?

Lipids in the Body

You probably include sources of fat in your diet throughout the day. You may have an egg for breakfast, a cheese sandwich for lunch, and a pork chop for dinner. How does your body use the fats in foods to perform vital functions?

Lipid Digestion and Absorption

Remember that most of the fats in foods are triglycerides. After chewing and swallowing, fat reaches the stomach along with carbohydrates, proteins, and other food elements. The fat separates from the watery contents of the stomach and floats in a layer on top.

When fats reach the small intestine, they are mixed with bile, which acts as an emulsifier. Bile helps break fats into tiny droplets and keeps them suspended in watery digestive fluid. Breaking fat into tiny droplets increases its surface area. This makes it easier for pancreatic enzymes to break triglycerides down into glycerol, fatty acids,

and monoglycerides. (A monoglyceride is one fatty acid attached to a glycerol molecule.) Bile's emulsifying effect improves the absorption of the fat by the cells lining the intestine.

Lipid Transport in the Body

Lipids travel in the bloodstream to tissues throughout the body. Glycerol and short-chain fatty acids resulting from fat digestion pass through the intestinal lining directly into the bloodstream. In the intestinal cells, monoglycerides and long-chain fatty acids are converted back into triglycerides and clustered together. These clusters of triglycerides are thinly coated with cholesterol, phospholipids, and proteins to form **chylomicrons**. The chylomicrons are then absorbed into the lymphatic system and eventually move into the bloodstream.

Keep in mind that blood is made up mostly of water, which does not mix well with fats. The protein and phospholipid coat on chylomicrons allows fats to remain dispersed in

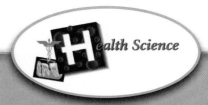

Research Dietitian

Research dietitians implement, collect, and enter food records. They also develop nutrition education materials. Research dietitians primarily work with dietary-related research in the clinical aspect of nutrition in disease and foodservice aspects in issues involving food. Many research dietitians work with the biochemical aspects of nutrient interaction in the body. They normally work in a hospital or university research facilities. Quality improvement in dietetics services is also an area of research.

Education: Research dietitians often have a master's degree. They must have a strong background in health science including anatomy, chemistry, biochemistry, biology, physiology, and nutrition.

Job Outlook: Employment in the dietetics field will grow about as fast as the average for all occupations. Factors that underlie the steady expansion of the health services industry include population growth and aging, and emphasis on health education.

water-based blood. Once chylomicrons enter the bloodstream, they are again broken down to fatty acids and glycerol. This process helps fats from your diet move efficiently through your blood vessels to the tissues where fatty acids can be absorbed for fuel or stored.

Chylomicrons are one type of lipoprotein. **Lipoproteins** are a combination of fats and proteins that help transport fats in the body. **Very low-density lipoproteins (VLDL)** are a second type. They carry triglycerides and cholesterol made by the liver to body cells. Once in the bloodstream, some of the triglycerides in VLDL are broken down into glycerol and fatty acids and released. Losing triglycerides causes VLDL to become more dense and contain a larger percentage of

cholesterol. At this point, VLDL become **low-density lipoproteins (LDL)**. LDL carry cholesterol through the bloodstream to body cells. A fourth type of lipoprotein is the **high-density lipoproteins (HDL)**. HDL pick up cholesterol from around the body and transfer it to other lipoproteins for transport back to the liver. The liver processes this returned cholesterol as a waste product for removal from the body. You will read more about LDL and HDL later in this chapter.

Lipid Use for Energy

Fats are an important source of energy. The enzymes on the lining of blood vessels break down the triglycerides in chylomicrons and VLDL into glycerol and fatty acids. Body cells can take up fatty acids from the bloodstream. Cells can break fatty acids down further to release energy for immediate needs. If the cells do not have immediate energy needs, they can rebuild the fatty acids into triglycerides. The cells store these triglycerides for future energy needs.

Most cells can store only limited amounts of triglycerides. However, fat cells can hold an almost limitless supply. When needed, fat cells can break down stored triglycerides. They send fatty acids through the bloodstream to other body cells that use lipids for fuel.

Fats and Heart Health

Fats, especially the wrong kind of fats in the diet and in the body, play a major role in the health of your heart. **Coronary heart disease (CHD)** refers to disease of the heart and blood vessels. CHD is the leading cause of death in the United States.

Arteries are the blood vessels that carry oxygen and nutrients to body tissues. Fatty compounds made up largely of cholesterol can attach to the inside walls of arteries, forming a buildup called **plaque**. Plaque begins to form early in life in everyone's blood vessels, 6-5. A number of factors affect the rate at which plaque buildups form.

As plaque increases, it hardens and narrows the arteries. This condition is called **atherosclerosis**, the most common form of heart disease. The heart has to work harder to pump blood through narrowed arteries. This strains the heart and causes blood pressure to rise.

Blood clots are more likely to form at the sites of plaque buildups. Blood clots can become lodged in narrowed arteries and cut off the blood supply to tissues fed by the arteries. A buildup of plaque in the arteries feeding the heart muscle can lead to a **heart attack**. A buildup of plaque in the arteries leading to the brain may result in a **stroke**. These conditions can be life threatening. In both cases, cells are destroyed because the blocked arteries cannot supply enough nutrients or oxygen to the tissue.

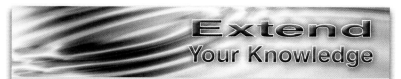

Women and Heart Health

More recently, medical research has identified special health concerns for women and heart health. This information is coming to light as more research is focused on women's health issues. Historically, heart health research focused on the male gender. Visit the National Heart, Lung, and Blood Institute to read "The Healthy Heart Handbook for Women" to learn about heart disease symptoms, the risks of heart attack, and treatment for women.

Scientists have identified a number of risk factors that contribute to CHD. The chances of developing CHD increase rapidly as more factors begin to apply to you. You can reduce the risks of factors beyond your control by carefully managing the factors within your control.

The Uncontrollable Heart-Health Risk Factors

Unfortunately, you cannot control some factors that greatly affect your

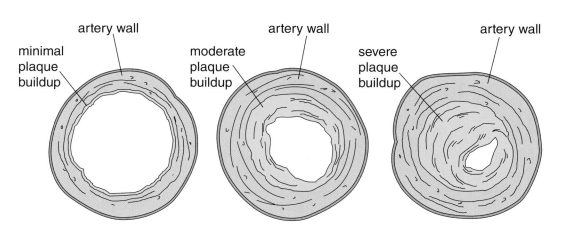

artery wall   artery wall   artery wall

minimal plaque buildup   moderate plaque buildup   severe plaque buildup

6-5   A heavy buildup of plaque in the arteries is the most common cause of coronary heart disease.

state of health. Risks for CHD are associated with certain age, gender, and race groups. Certain inherited traits present risks, too. If any of these risks applies to you, getting regular medical checkups can help detect potential problems.

Age

The risk of heart attack increases with age. Most heart attacks occur after the age of 65. Following healthy lifestyle behaviors when you are young can help prevent heart disease later in life.

Gender

If you are male, you are at a greater risk of coronary heart disease than females, **6-6**. Female hormones tend

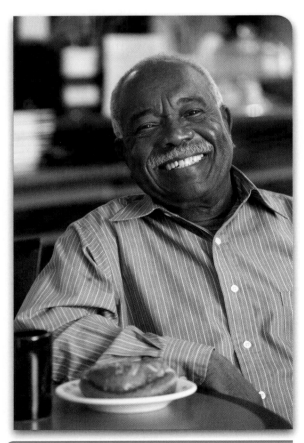

6-6 Advanced age and male gender are both factors that increase the risk of heart disease.

to protect against CHD. Hormonal changes that occur during menopause reduce this protective factor in older women. Therefore, if other factors are equal, women over age 50 have a risk for CHD equal to men.

Ethnic Group

Some ethnic groups are at greater risk of heart disease than others. For instance, African Americans are twice as likely to have heart attacks as members of some other races. African Americans also have a higher incidence of high blood pressure. The reasons for this are unclear. However, members of these groups should make an extra effort to manage controllable risk factors.

Family History

If one or more of your blood relatives have had heart disease or stroke, your risk increases. Blood relatives include parents, grandparents, aunts, uncles, brothers, and sisters.

The Controllable Heart-Health Risk Factors

Is it possible to do something to prevent heart attacks? People who have survived heart attacks are the first to tell you that you can change lifestyle behaviors. Many heart attack victims are motivated to make some drastic changes. They quit smoking. They start exercising more. They learn how to manage stress. They also lose weight and eat diets low in saturated fats and *trans* fatty acids.

The biggest risk factors for CHD are smoking, high blood pressure, and high blood cholesterol. Diabetes mellitus, inactivity, stress, and overweight are risk factors, too. Through your lifestyle choices, you have some control over all these risk factors. Changing lifestyle behaviors to control these factors could reduce CHD risk for up to 95 percent of the population.

Smoking

Heart attacks before age 55 can often be traced to cigarette smoking. Smokers have two to four times more risk of dying from a heart attack than nonsmokers. Smoking constricts blood vessels which might be narrowed with plaque. Therefore, a smoker's heart must work harder to get needed blood and oxygen to body cells. When the heart has to work harder, the risk of CHD increases.

By quitting, people can undo most of the damage caused by smoking. The best advice for a healthy heart is to never begin smoking, **6-7**.

High Blood Pressure

Abnormally high blood pressure, or **hypertension**, is a heart-health risk factor. It involves an excess force on the walls of the arteries as blood is pumped from the heart. A normal blood pressure reading is less than 120/80 mm of mercury. The first number in this reading measures *systolic pressure*. This is the pressure on the arteries when the heart muscle contracts. The second number in a blood pressure reading measures *diastolic pressure*. This is the pressure on the arteries when the heart is between beats.

Hypertension affects 20 to 25 percent of the adult population in the United States. People with hypertension have a systolic value at or above 140. A diastolic reading at or above 90 also defines high blood pressure. High blood pressure is a strong indicator of coronary disease.

High blood pressure places added stress on the heart. It contributes to

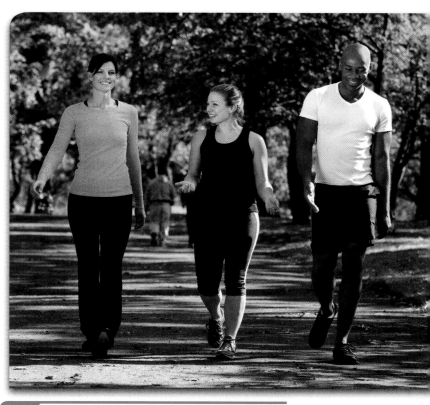

6-7   An active lifestyle is important for heart health.

CHD by damaging the walls of the arteries. The walls then accumulate plaque more easily.

Doctors cannot cure high blood pressure. However, some people can control it through diet, exercise, and stress management. Doctors often prescribe medication for people who have trouble controlling their blood pressure.

High Blood Cholesterol

Blood serum refers to the watery portion of blood in which blood cells and other materials are suspended. One of these materials is cholesterol. This cholesterol is known as *serum cholesterol*. Do not confuse serum cholesterol with *dietary cholesterol*, which is the cholesterol found in food.

Artery-clogging plaques are made up largely of cholesterol. Therefore, a large amount of serum cholesterol is a risk factor for CHD.

You should know your blood cholesterol level. If you have a family history of high cholesterol or high blood pressure, you should have your cholesterol level checked, **6-8**. A **blood lipid profile** is a medical test that measures cholesterol, HDL, LDL, and triglycerides in the blood. Test results identify the number of milligrams of each of these components found in a deciliter (0.1 liter) of blood.

The HDL and LDL measurements in a blood lipid profile are heart-health indicators. HDL are sometimes called "good cholesterol" because these lipoproteins carry excess cholesterol to the liver to be discarded. Therefore, a high level of HDL in the blood indicates a low risk of CHD. On the other hand, LDL are sometimes called "bad cholesterol." They carry cholesterol that is deposited in body tissues. A high level of LDL in the blood indicates a high risk of CHD.

The American Heart Association (AHA) recommends calculating your cholesterol ratio by dividing your HDL cholesterol into your total cholesterol. The goal is to keep your total cholesterol/HDL ratio at or below 4 to 1. A higher ratio indicates a higher risk of heart disease; a lower ratio indicates a lower risk.

People who have other risk factors for CHD should also be aware of their blood triglyceride levels, **6-9**. High levels of blood triglycerides are usually associated with high levels of serum cholesterol and may increase the risk of CHD for people with other risk factors.

Diabetes Mellitus

Diabetes mellitus causes blood vessels to become damaged or blocked with fat. This reduces blood circulation beyond the effects of normal plaque buildups. Therefore, people with diabetes mellitus are at a higher risk of CHD.

People with type 1 diabetes cannot view their disease as a controllable heart-health risk factor. They must take insulin injections to manage their condition. They cannot control it through lifestyle behaviors. However, about 80 percent of people who have diabetes mellitus have type 2. These people do have some control over this risk factor. Type 2 diabetes can often be managed with diet and physical activity.

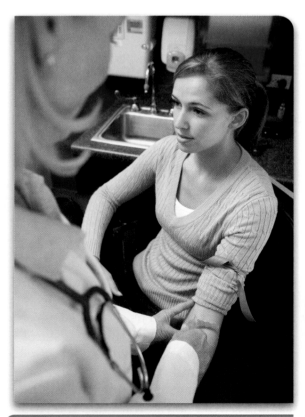

6-8   A blood lipid profile will reveal your blood cholesterol level.

Desirable Blood Lipid Levels

Total Cholesterol—less than 200 mg/dL
HDL Cholesterol—60 mg/dL and above
LDL Cholesterol—less than 100 mg/dL
Triglycerides—less than 150 mg/dL

6-9   Desirable blood lipid levels lower an individual's risk for heart disease.

Excess Weight

Because fats are such a concentrated source of energy, calories from fat mount up surprisingly fast. For example, a tablespoon of peanut butter adds 72 fat calories to a slice of bread. The body can easily convert excess calories from fat into adipose tissue. Excess calories from carbohydrates and proteins are stored as body fat, too.

Every pound of stored body fat is equal to 3,500 calories of energy. One way your body can get energy needed between meals is to break down these fat stores. However, many people regularly consume more calories than they need. Many teens exercise too little. Therefore, their fat stores continue to build rather than being burned for energy. This causes these people to become overweight.

As fat stores in the body increase, the number of blood vessels must increase to nourish the added tissue. This creates more work for the heart, which increases blood pressure. High blood pressure causes blood vessels to become stretched and injured. Points of injury attract cholesterol, adding to plaque buildups. If blood pressure remains high, blood vessels begin to lose their elasticity. This makes it harder to control blood pressure.

Overweight people, statistically, have a shorter life span. Being overweight increases a person's risk of diabetes mellitus and high blood cholesterol as well as high blood pressure. Each of these factors is also a risk factor for CHD. Therefore, an overweight person is more likely to have a combination of heart-health risk factors. Multiple risk factors place a person's heart health in greater danger than a single factor.

If you are like most people, you are concerned about how you feel. You want to keep your weight at a healthy level. Eating a nutritious diet and getting plenty of exercise will help you maintain a healthy weight. Reducing fat in your diet and increasing activity are two key steps for preventing excess weight gain.

Dieting to lose excess weight is not recommended for most teens. A calorie reduced diet for a teen can result in failure to get enough essential nutrients. Normal growth can be impaired. Be sure to check with your health care provider or a registered dietitian before starting any weight loss program.

Inactivity

A lack of physical activity contributes to many people's excess weight problems. In addition, inactive people fail to give their heart the kind of regular workout it needs to remain healthy. People who spend much time sitting need to make a point of getting some exercise nearly every day, **6-10**.

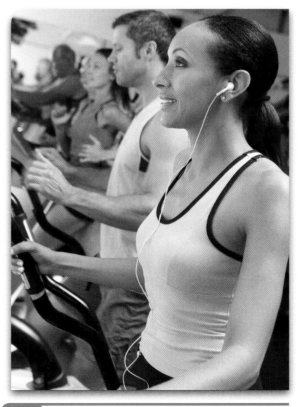

6-10   Exercising regularly may help you avoid becoming overweight.

Exercise helps people manage weight, reduce stress, control cholesterol, and strengthen the heart muscle. Exercise improves the flexibility of your arteries. Muscles receive their blood supply more efficiently. All of these benefits have a positive impact on heart health.

Strength training and lifting weights is important. When you contract your muscles, you begin to improve the ability to use glucose and respond with insulin more effectively. Keeping muscles, strong protects against high blood pressure and can lower blood sugar.

Stress

Research has linked stress and personality to a person's potential for developing heart disease. People who overreact to life's demands on a continuous level may suffer negative heart health. Those who are competitive, impatient, irritable, and easily angered may also be at greater risk.

People can learn ways to reduce stress and work toward emotional balance. They can acquire skills that will help them adapt to the stresses in life, too. For instance, eating right and getting enough rest and exercise can give people the strength they need to handle stress. Finding enjoyable hobbies can help them get their minds

off stressful conditions. Setting priorities and using time effectively can keep some stressful situations from arising. Using these and other techniques can help people manage this heart-health risk factor.

Recommended Limits

Experts have linked too much cholesterol and fat—especially saturated and *trans* fats—in the diet with heart and blood vessel diseases. The National Cholesterol Education Program recommends a maximum intake of 300 mg of cholesterol per day. Many people in the United States include more cholesterol than this in their daily diets. Studies show that too much dietary cholesterol raises serum cholesterol for some people, increasing their risk of CHD. These people must strictly limit their intake of such high-cholesterol foods as egg yolks and organ meats.

People who have high serum cholesterol may also want to increase their intake of plant foods. In fact, all people can benefit from a diet high in plant foods. Plant foods provide fiber and other heart-protective substances—such as plant sterols and stanols—that can help lower blood cholesterol.

For most people, dietary cholesterol does not affect serum cholesterol as much as total dietary fat, especially saturated and *trans* fats. The *Dietary Guidelines* recommends no more than 20 to 35 percent of the total calories in your diet come from fats. Less than 10 percent of your total daily calories should come from saturated fats. Keep *trans* fats to less than one percent of daily calories. A heart-healthy diet is one that reduces total fat calories from all food groups.

Active teenage boys should eat no more than 123 grams of fat per day. No

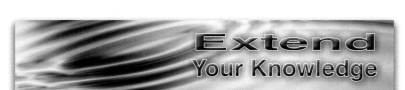

Hearts Around the World

Using world health statistics, research the incidence of coronary heart disease in three different countries including the United States. Investigate typical diet patterns in each country. As you compare the countries' health statistics and diets, do you find a link between diet and CHD?

more than 35 grams should be from saturated fats. Active teenage girls should eat no more than 92 grams of fat daily. Teen girls should limit saturated fats to 26 grams per day. However, many teens go beyond these recommendations.

Suppose a teen chooses a quarter-pound cheeseburger, French fries, and a milk shake for lunch. How much fat do you think would be in this meal? The answer is about 43 grams, 17 of which are saturated—nearly the fat equivalent of half a stick of butter! Now suppose the teen chooses a sausage and egg biscuit for breakfast. Dinner includes fried chicken, coleslaw, and ice cream. Throw in a bag of chips and a handful of cookies for snacks. The total for the day would be 147 grams of fat, with over 54 of those grams being saturated. Clearly, this is beyond the daily recommended limits. Keep in mind that these examples did not include all side dishes. Hash browns with the breakfast biscuit would add 8 more grams of fat.

By choosing other meals and snacks with care, however, a teen could include hamburgers and fries in a nutritious diet, **6-11**. For instance, the teen could select a bowl of cereal and fresh strawberries for breakfast. Roasted, skinless chicken and a tossed salad with low-fat dressing could be chosen for dinner. Popcorn and an apple would be lower in fat than the other snack choices. Now the day's meals would supply 54 grams of total fat, with only 20 grams of saturated fat.

Fish Oils and Heart Health

A number of years ago, the health community focused much attention on the effects of fish oils on heart health. The attention arose from the observation that the incidence of coronary

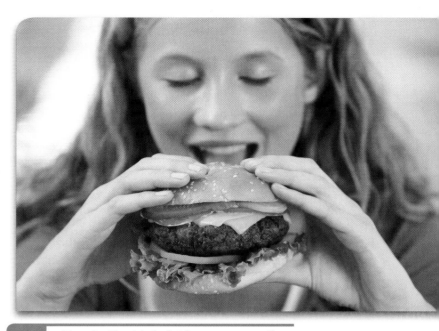

6-11   Foods like high-fat burgers can fit into a balanced diet if you use care when making other food choices.

heart disease was low among native Alaskans. When analyzing the diet of this culture, researchers found that the Alaskans ate high-fat, high-cholesterol fish. This led the researchers to question why the high-fat diet did not cause the Alaskans to have clogged arteries.

The researchers discovered that fish oils contain a certain type of polyunsaturated fatty acids called **omega-3 fatty acids**. Researchers found that omega-3 fatty acids lowered the risk of heart disease. This finding led people to ask if taking fish oil in pill form would improve their health.

The American Heart Association has found no conclusive evidence that fish oil pills lessen the risks of heart disease. In fact, including large amounts of fish oil supplements in the diet can cause health problems. Large amounts of fish oil have been found to thin the blood and may prevent clotting of the blood. Some fish oil, such as cod liver oil, contains dangerously high amounts of vitamins A and D.

Case Study: Change of Heart

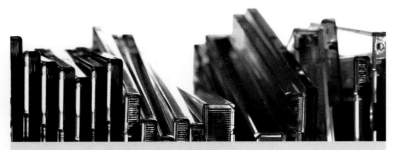

George is 14 years old. He is 5 feet 4 inches (162.6 cm) tall and weighs 210 pounds (95.3 kg). He knows he is overweight, but had not given the problem much thought until recently. His 43-year-old uncle suffered a heart attack this year.

George frequently enjoys his favorite foods, which include fried chicken, mashed potatoes with gravy, and French fries. Most mornings he buys a breakfast sandwich and hash browns at the fast-food restaurant on his way to school. He has never been an active person. He never learned to ride a bike, swim, or play sports. George spends his free time playing video games or on the computer. He usually snacks on a bag of potato chips and a cola while watching TV.

Case Review

George worries that he might suffer an early heart attack like his uncle. He wants to make changes to improve his health, but does not know how to begin.

1. Do you think George has risk factors that are within his control?

2. What lifestyle changes can George make to reduce his risk of future heart disease problems?

Fish contain high quality protein and a variety of vitamins and minerals as well as omega-3 fatty acids. You cannot get this range of nutrients from fish oil pills or foods fortified with omega-3 fatty acids, alone. Including fish in your diet at least once a week offers more benefits than taking fish oil supplements. *Dietary Guidelines* recommends eating eight ounces or more per week from a variety of fish and seafood.

Fats and Cancer

Cancer is a general term that refers to a number of diseases in which abnormal cells grow out of control. This is in sharp contrast to normal cell growth, which is highly regulated. Cancers can spread throughout the body. As a group, they are the second largest cause of death in the United States.

Scientists have spent years researching the causes and prevention of cancer. Much remains to be learned. However, researchers have determined that many factors increase your chances of developing cancer. Diet is among these factors. Up to half of all cancer cases appear to be related to diet.

The American Institute for Cancer Research (AIRC) reports that lifestyle choices have a great impact on cancer development. Lifestyle choices can be grouped as cancer promoting or cancer protective. For example, the AIRC suggests you should be choosy about the types and amounts of fat you eat. A diet that includes foods high in saturated fats may promote the development of colon, prostate, breast, and some other types of cancer. However, choosing a diet that includes monounsaturated fats and foods high in omega-3 fatty acids may protect against cancer. The amount of dietary fat may contribute to risk as much as the type of fat. Eating large amounts of fatty foods results in weight gain, and excess weight increases cancer risk.

Adding a variety of fruits, vegetables, and grains to your daily eating plan is a cancer-protective lifestyle choice. These foods are often low in fat, and contain fiber and certain chemicals that have anticancer effects. Maintaining a healthy weight and being physically active daily are cancer-protective factors as well. This lifestyle helps to prevent a high percentage of body fat, which increases the risks of some types of cancer.

Limiting Fats and Cholesterol in Your Diet

Selecting foods low in total fat, as well as cholesterol and saturated and *trans* fats, is important for most Americans over the age of two. By adolescence, most people already have some buildup of fat deposits in their arteries. To keep dietary fat at a recommended level, you need to know where fats are in foods. Then you need to be willing to select a diet that contains no more than 35 percent fat.

Be a Fat Detector

If you are going to limit fat and cholesterol in your diet, you need to be a fat detector. If you know where the fat is in foods, you can learn how to limit or avoid it.

Lipids can be deceiving to the eyes. Sometimes they are easy to see, but sometimes they are not. The *visible fats* are those that you can clearly see. Butter, fat on meats, and salad oil are visible fats. You know you need to limit your intake of these foods because you can see the fat.

Many times you cannot see the fat, but it is there. The *invisible fats* are those that are hidden in foods. Baked goods, snack foods, and luncheon meats are often sources of invisible fat. For instance, one hot dog has about 145 calories, and 117 of them come from fat. You may be more likely to consume excess fat and calories when you cannot see the fat in foods.

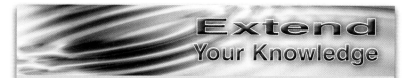

Extend Your Knowledge

What Is the Mediterranean Style of Eating?
Some evidence suggests there are benefits to eating as they do in the Mediterranean region of the world. Claims are made that this diet is protective against heart disease and cancer. Locate countries that are near the Mediterranean Sea. What popular foods are grown in the area? What are the key elements of the Mediterranean food plan? Compare the Mediterranean food plan with the MyPlate food guidance system. How are they different? similar?

Foods that are high in added fats and sugars are found in all the food groups. Foods such as biscuits and muffins with invisible fat are found in the MyPlate grains group. These types of foods should be used sparingly because they add more fat and possibly cholesterol to your diet. A better choice would be nutrient-dense selections from the grains group, such as oatmeal or whole-wheat bread.

The other food groups can also contribute fat to your diet. Vegetables served with butter and fruits topped with cream are sources of fat. Whole milk and yogurts are high in fat. A gradual change from whole-fat to low-fat and finally to fat-free dairy products will help reduce solid fat intake. Drinks such as cappuccinos and lattes contain fat. To reduce the fat content, ask for them to be made with fat-free dairy products. Eggs, nuts, and many meat cuts can be fat sources from the protein foods group. For products with a Nutrition Facts label, select those with less fat and saturated fat. You need to carefully choose the recommended daily amounts from each food group.

When you buy prepared food, read the Nutrition Facts panel on the product label, **6-12**. The label states how many calories per serving come from

Nutrition Facts

Serving Size 6 crackers (28g)
Servings Per Container About 13

Amount Per Serving

Calories 120	Calories from Fat 40

	% Daily Value*
Total Fat 4.5g	7%
Saturated Fat 1g	5%
Trans Fat 0g	
Polyunsaturated Fat 2.5g	
Monounsaturated Fat 1g	
Cholesterol 0mg	0%
Sodium 180mg	8%
Potassium 110mg	3%
Total Carbohydrate 19g	6%
Dietary Fiber 3g	12%
Sugars 0g	
Protein 5g	

Vitamin A 0%	•	Vitamin C 0%
Calcium 0%	•	Iron 4%
Phosphorus 10%		

* Percent Daily Values are based on a 2,000 calorie diet. Your daily values may be higher or lower depending on your calorie needs:

	Calories:	2,000	2,500
Total Fat	Less than	65g	80g
Sat Fat	Less than	20g	25g
Cholesterol	Less than	300mg	300mg
Sodium	Less than	2,400mg	2,400mg
Potassium		2,400mg	2,400mg
Total Carbohydrate		300g	375g
Dietary Fiber		25g	30g

INGREDIENTS: WHOLE WHEAT, SOYBEAN AND/OR PALM OIL, SALT.

CONTAINS: WHEAT.

6-12   Information about fats and cholesterol on the Nutrition Facts panel can help you determine how foods fit into your total diet plan.

fat. Remember the recommendation is that no more than 35 percent of your total daily calories should come from fat. The label also tells you the percent Daily Value for fat, saturated fat, and cholesterol provided by a product. A product is considered low in any nutrient for which it provides five percent or less of the Daily Value. A low DV percent is good for nutrients that you want to limit such as total fat, cholesterol, saturated and *trans* fats, and sodium.

Making Diet Changes

Old eating habits are not easy to change. As a teen, your habits are not so old. You are young and your body is strong. You are in a good position to make a fresh start. Forming a program of good nutrition will help you feel your physical and mental best.

Most people in the United States need to reduce their consumption of saturated fats, *trans* fats, and cholesterol to meet current recommendations. When making diet changes, where do you start? First, decide how you are doing right now. You need to keep a food diary for a few days, writing down everything you eat and drink. Use the information in your food diary to find out about the fats in your diet. Diet analysis software or a food composition table can help you.

Your analysis should help you determine which foods in your diet contribute most to elevated blood lipids. Learn how many grams of fat you are consuming each day. You should be able to calculate the number and percentage of calories in your diet that are coming from fat. What percentage of your fat intake is coming from saturated, monounsaturated, and polyunsaturated fats? Your analysis should show you your daily cholesterol intake, too.

Decide what is good about your current diet. Then identify changes you can make to help reduce blood triglycerides and cholesterol. Set realistic goals for yourself to make these changes gradually. Then make choices that support your goals. For instance, you might decide to eat French fries no more than once a week. Sticking with this decision might mean ordering a salad with low-fat dressing instead of fries at your next meal.

Support from your family can affect your ability to reach your dietary goals. Talk to family members about your desire to make changes in your diet. See if they might be willing to make changes as well. If not, ask for their respect and encouragement as you work to change your eating habits, **6-13**.

Using Fat Replacers

Have you tasted the new foods with fat replacers in them? **Fat replacers** are used as ingredients in food products. They are designed to replace some or all the fat typically found in those products. There are three categories of fat replacers—carbohydrate-, protein-, or fat-based. They are developed to have a flavor and texture similar to fats and oils, but contain less fat and fewer calories. For example, a tablespoon of regular mayonnaise provides 11 grams of fat and 100 calories. A tablespoon of fat-free mayonnaise made with a fat replacer, provides no fat and only 10 calories. Some of the fat replacers can be used only in foods that are not cooked for a long time. You may find them in foods such as salad dressings, cheese, and ice cream.

Scientific research on animals and human beings shows fat replacers are safe. However, some of them have drawbacks. For instance, some products containing fat replacers have an after-taste. One type of fat replacer may cause digestive problems and inhibit absorption of some nutrients.

Fat replacers may allow you to more easily enjoy some traditionally high-fat foods as part of a nutritious diet. However, you need to be aware that some foods containing fat replacers have added sugar. Therefore, they may not be much lower in calories than their high-fat counterparts. Read labels carefully when buying products to compare fat, calories, and sugars.

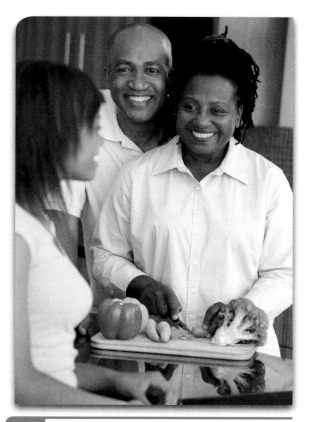

6-13 Support from family members and friends can improve success in making dietary changes.

You have many choices available to help reduce fat in your diet. Foods containing fat replacers are not a simple answer to poor food habits. They are not a quick-fix substitute for lifestyle changes, either. You should check out all your options before deciding how often you will include foods that contain fat replacers.

Guidelines for Food Choices

The American Heart Association (AHA) recommends eating more fruits, vegetables, whole-grain products, and low- or fat-free dairy products. They also recommend eating no more than 6 ounces (170 g) of cooked fish, skinless poultry, or lean meat a day. Go easy on fried foods, such as potato chips and fried chicken, **6-14**. Limit visible

Choices for a Healthier Heart

- Limit your intake of foods high in saturated and *trans* fats such as shortening, cakes, cookies, butter, and snack foods
- Select low-fat or fat-free milks, yogurts, and cheeses
- Watch your intake of foods high in cholesterol such as eggs, organ meats, and shellfish
- Use more vegetable oils, such as corn, soy, safflower, cottonseed, and sunflower
- Include more monounsaturated fats such as olive, canola, and peanut oils
- Choose foods high in omega-3 fatty acids such as cold-water fish (salmon, mackerel), avocados, walnuts, and flaxseeds

6-14 Making healthy food choices can protect your heart over your lifetime.

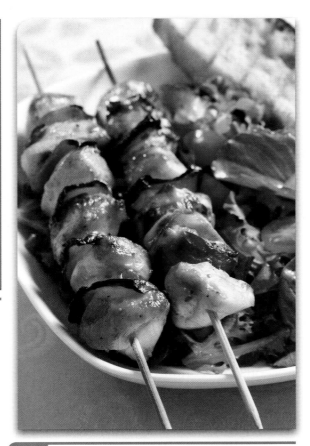

6-15 Choosing lean cuts, using low-fat cooking methods, and limiting portion sizes allow meats to fit easily into a healthy diet.

fats, such as butter, cream, and salad dressing, too.

Some people do not enjoy drinking fat-free milk because they miss the thick, rich flavor of whole milk. These people may find it easier to switch to reduced-fat milk for a while before trying fat-free milk. Manufacturers continue to look for new ways to make fat-free milk taste better.

A good percentage of the fat in many people's diets comes from meat products. You can reduce the amount of fat you get from meats by choosing lean cuts. Trim all visible fat before cooking. Use low-fat cooking methods, such as roasting, broiling, and grilling, **6-15**. Limit portion size to 3 ounces (85 g) of cooked meat, which is about the size of a deck of playing cards.

People who make changes to reduce dietary fat generally see an improvement in their blood lipid profile within six months.

Eating for good health does not just happen. You have to be informed about what will make your body strong and healthy for a full, productive life. Following through on your knowledge requires a commitment to a healthy lifestyle. Deciding to improve your diet is not just a goal for yourself. It will affect those around you, too. The better you feel, the more you are free to interact positively with others.

Reading Summary

Lipids, which include all fats and oils, are made up of different types of fatty acids. Saturated fatty acids contain the maximum number of hydrogen atoms. Monounsaturated fatty acids have a double bond between just one pair of carbon atoms. Polyunsaturated fatty acids have double bonds between two or more pairs of carbon atoms. A high percentage of saturated fatty acids tends to make lipids solid at room temperature. A high percentage of unsaturated fatty acids tends to make lipids liquid at room temperature. When oils are hydrogenated, they become more solid at room temperature.

Most of the lipids in foods and in the body are triglycerides. Other classes of lipids are phospholipids and sterols.

Lipids are important to the diet for several reasons. They provide essential fatty acids. They provide a concentrated source of energy. Lipids carry the fat-soluble vitamins A, D, E, and K. They are needed to form cell membranes and various secretions in the body. They provide an internal blanket to hold in body heat. Lipids also cushion body organs.

The body must digest and absorb fats before using them as an energy source. Most fat digestion takes place in the small intestine where bile keeps fats emulsified while pancreatic enzymes break down triglycerides. Chylomicrons carry fats from foods into the bloodstream following digestion. Other types of lipoproteins help transport fats made in the body away from and back to the liver.

Fats in the body can form deposits in the arteries, which can lead to coronary heart disease. A number of factors contribute to a person's risk of CHD. Some of these factors, such as age, gender, race, and heredity, are beyond a person's control. However, people can control a number of lifestyle factors to help reduce their risk of CHD. Controllable heart-health risk factors include smoking, inactivity, stress and personality type, overweight, diabetes, high blood pressure, and high blood cholesterol.

Learn to identify sources of visible and invisible fats in your diet. Limit fat intake to 20 to 35 percent of your total calories, with less than 7 percent coming from saturated fats. Avoid too much cholesterol.

Review Learning

1. What are the three main classes of lipids?
2. Give two food sources that are high in each of the three types of fatty acids.
3. By what process is corn oil made into margarine?
4. How do saturated and *trans* fats contribute to heart disease?
5. What are three major food sources of cholesterol?
6. What are five major functions of lipids in the body?
7. How do lipoproteins play a role in moving lipids in the body?
8. What is the difference between a heart attack and a stroke?
9. What age and gender groups are at increased risk for CHD?
10. True or false. Changing lifestyle behaviors could reduce coronary heart disease risk for up to 95 percent of the population.
11. What does a blood lipid profile measure?
12. What is the recommended limit for cholesterol in the diet?

13. What is a food source of omega-3 fatty acids?
14. What effect does diet have on cancer development?
15. When should most people begin limiting saturated fats, *trans* fats, and cholesterol in their diets?
16. Give five guidelines for making food choices to reduce fats, saturated fats, *trans* fat, and cholesterol.

Critical Thinking

17. **Analyze behavior.** Why should teens be concerned about heart health? What behavior changes can teens make for healthful living throughout the life span?
18. **Draw conclusions.** Identify conclusions you can make about choosing heart-healthy fats in your diet. What other lifestyle changes can you make to maintain or improve heart health?

Applying Your Knowledge

19. **Food display.** Prepare a display showing examples of foods high in saturated, monounsaturated, or polyunsaturated lipids.
20. **Evaluate information.** The American Heart Association instituted a check mark system to quickly and easily spot heart-healthy foods in the supermarket. Find examples of three different foods with the AHA check mark on it. Evaluate if you think this is an effective way to inform consumers of healthy eating practices. Write a summary of your evaluation.
21. **Create a poster.** Design a poster illustrating the major functions of lipids in the body. Share your poster in class.
22. **Survey awareness.** Write a survey to assess people's awareness of risk factors for coronary heart disease. Use your survey to interview three people in different age groups. Share your findings in class.
23. **Menu planning.** Develop a "heart-healthy" menu for a breakfast, lunch, or dinner meal. Using diet analysis software, determine how many grams of fat and saturated fat are in the meal. Also notice how many milligrams of cholesterol the meal provides. Share your meal plan and analysis results with others in your class.

Technology Connections

24. **Calculate fat.** Use the American Heart Association's fat calculator to determine your recommended daily fat intake. Determine your daily calorie needs for maintaining or achieving a healthy weight.
25. **Create a brochure.** Using desktop publishing software, prepare a brochure suggesting ways to improve heart health. Distribute it at a school health fair.
26. **Electronic presentation.** Research current recommendations provided by the National Institutes of Health or the U.S. National Library of Medicine on heart health and disease prevention. Prepare an electronic presentation describing three recommended preventive strategies for maintaining heart health over the lifecycle. Explain similarities and differences between heart disease prevention and stroke prevention.

27. **Podcast quiz.** Listen to free podcasts from the National Heart, Lung, and Blood Institute on such topics as chronic heart disease, heart attack, heart disease risk factors, physical activity and your heart, or other heart-health topics. After listening to one of the podcasts, use word-processing software to prepare a short 10 item quiz on the topic. Have the class listen to the podcast and take the quiz. Share the correct answers.

Academic Connections

28. **Math.** Find the nutrient analysis information from three different fast-food restaurant menus on the Internet or at the restaurant. Prepare a histogram to compare the amounts of cholesterol, and saturated, *trans*, and unsaturated fats in each restaurant's leading menu item.

29. **Language arts.** Interview a medical professional to learn the recommendations for lowering cholesterol. Questions should focus on both lifestyle behaviors and the pros and cons of prescription medicines. Share your findings in class.

30. **Speech/writing.** Prepare a 15-minute presentation for a parent education or child development class on raising children in a heart-smart lifestyle. Practice the use of effective presentation skills. Include discussion of the rising rate of childhood obesity, high cholesterol, and hypertension. Outline what parents can do to help prevent childhood health and heart problems.

31. **History.** Research the history of the Framingham Heart Study. Write a brief summary of your findings. Discuss societal changes that occurred as a result of this study. Note the risk factors for heart health presented in the study. Compare their findings to those presented in this chapter.

32. **Writing.** Use the Internet and print resources to research the connection between cancer risk and high-fat diets. Write a three-page research paper summarizing the outcomes of recent (year 2005 or later) studies and your own conclusions.

Workplace Applications

Communicate Information

Effective writing ability is an important workplace skill. As newsletter editor for your company, it is your responsibility to write the *Health & Wellness* column in the monthly employee e-newsletter. This month's topic is on limiting and choosing healthful dietary fats. As you gather information for your article, remember to address *who, what, when, where, why,* and *how.* Keep your target audience in mind as you write the article.

Chapter 7

Proteins: The Body's Building Blocks

Reading for Meaning
Read the chapter title and write a paragraph describing what you know about the topic. After reading the chapter, summarize what you have learned.

Concept Organizer
Use a T-chart diagram to show the functions of protein in the body. For each function, list specific examples.

Functions of Protein	Details About Functions

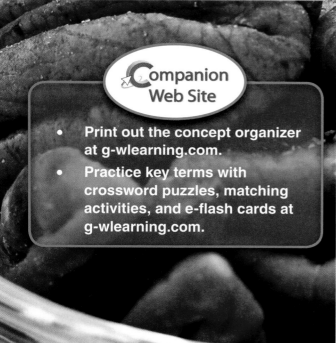

Terms to Know

protein
amino acid
denaturation
dispensable amino acid
indispensable amino acid
antibody
acid-base balance
buffer
legume
vegetarianism
complete protein
incomplete protein
complementary proteins
nitrogen balance
deficiency disease
protein-energy malnutrition (PEM)
kwashiorkor
marasmus

Companion Web Site

- **Print out the concept organizer at g-wlearning.com.**
- **Practice key terms with crossword puzzles, matching activities, and e-flash cards at g-wlearning.com.**

Objectives

After studying this chapter, you will be able to

- **compare** the structure and functions of protein with the other energy nutrients.
- **explain** the difference between indispensable and dispensable amino acids.
- **identify** animal and plant food sources of protein.
- **calculate** your daily protein needs.
- **differentiate** between protein needs of an athlete and a nonathlete.
- **summarize** problems associated with protein deficiencies and excesses.

Central Ideas

- Protein is a complex nutrient essential to many important functions in the body.
- Protein needs can be met by eating a variety of food sources.

Mothers often tell children, "You have to eat your meat and drink your milk to get your protein." These mothers are right about meat and milk being good protein sources. However, they may not fully understand what protein does in the body and where protein can be found. They may not realize how much protein children really need, either. Although protein is an important nutrient, people often misunderstand it. Myths about how much you need and the power it has to build strong bodies abound.

Proteins make important contributions to your diet. You need to be sure to eat recommended amounts of protein each day. This chapter will help you determine your protein needs. It will also help you understand the effects of too little and too much protein in the diet.

What Is Protein?

Protein is an energy-yielding nutrient composed of carbon, hydrogen, oxygen, and nitrogen. The presence of nitrogen in the molecular structure makes this nutrient different from carbohydrates and fats.

Amino acids are the building blocks of protein molecules. Most proteins are made up of different patterns and combinations of about 20 amino acids, which are linked in strands. (Although additional amino acids have been discovered, they rarely appear in proteins.) Part of the amino acid structure is the side chain. The side chains give identity and a unique chemical makeup to each amino acid. Most amino acids have the following basic chemical structure:

$$NH_2 \leftarrow \text{amino group}$$
$$\text{side chain} - C - COOH \leftarrow \text{acidic carboxyl group}$$
$$| $$
$$H$$

The body probably has at least 30,000 types of protein. Each type performs a specific job. The number of amino acids and the order in which they are linked determine the type of protein. Think of amino acids as letters in the alphabet. You can combine the different letters to make words. The words can contain any letter in any sequence. There is no limit to the number of letters in a word. That is why it is possible to have so many different words. In a similar way, amino acids are combined in different sequences to form different proteins. The amino acids can be arranged one after the other in a straight line. However, they may be stacked up and branched like a tree. Each protein structure serves a specialized function.

DNA *(deoxyribonucleic acid)* is found in the nucleus of every cell. It provides the instructions for how the amino acids will be linked to form the proteins in your body.

Protein molecules can change their shape and take on new characteristics. This is called **denaturation**. Heat, acids, bases, and alcohol are among the factors that can denature proteins. You can see the effects of denaturation when you cook an egg or marinate a roast—both high-protein foods. Applying heat to an egg changes it from a runny fluid to a solid mass, **7-1**. Soaking a roast in an acidic marinade makes the meat more tender. The shapes of the protein molecules in these foods have changed. Once proteins are denatured, they can never return to their original state. For example, a hard-boiled egg can never become liquid again.

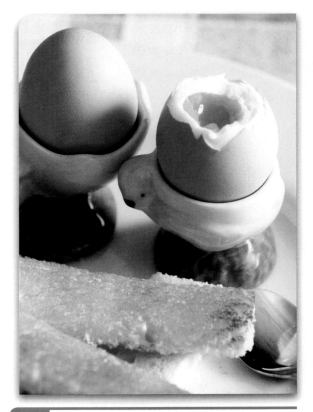

7-1   Heat denatures the proteins in eggs. This is why eggs become firm when they are cooked.

Types of Amino Acids

You need all the amino acids to make the proteins your body needs for good health. Your body can synthesize 11 of the amino acids from the other amino acids. (*Synthesize* means your body can use one or more compounds to make a new and different compound.) The amino acids your body can make for itself are called **dispensable amino acids** (also called nonessential amino acids). However, your body is not able to make the remaining 9 amino acids. These are called **indispensable amino acids** (also called essential amino acids). You must get indispensable amino acids from the foods you eat since your body cannot make them.

Certain health conditions interfere with the body's ability to make a dispensable amino acid from an indispensable amino acid. When this happens, a dispensable amino acid becomes a *conditionally indispensable amino acid* (sometimes called conditionally essential amino acid). Since the body is no longer able to create the amino acid, it must be obtained through a dietary source.

Protein in the Body

When you eat a protein food, stomach acids denature the proteins. This makes it easier for enzymes in the stomach to begin breaking down large protein molecules into smaller pieces. As these protein pieces move into the small intestine, other enzymes break them down into single amino acids. The amino acids are absorbed into the bloodstream. The blood then carries amino acids to body cells that need them.

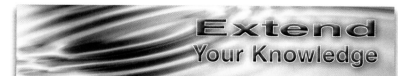

22 Amino Acids?

The study of nutrition and food science is ongoing and evolving. In recent years, two new amino acids were discovered making a total of 22 identified amino acids. Research print and Internet resources to learn the names of these amino acids. How common are they in nature? Who discovered them?

Functions of Protein

Your cells can use amino acids from food proteins to build new proteins. Cells can also convert amino acids to other compounds, including other amino acids.

The proteins built by cells are custom designed to perform a wide variety of functions in the body. The roles proteins play depend on where they are located and how your body needs them. The following sections describe several key functions of proteins.

Build and Maintain Tissues

Protein is a necessary part of every cell. You need protein to form the structure of muscles, organs, skin, blood,

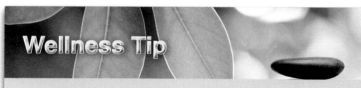

Consider Quinoa

Quinoa (KEEN-wah) is a grain that has been a staple for the people of the Andes Mountains for 5,000 years. Quinoa is considered a high quality protein because it supplies the indispensable amino acids. It is gluten free and a good source of iron and magnesium.

hair, nails, and every other body part. As your body grows, it uses protein to help make new tissues. This is why it is important for people to get enough protein during the growth years. Otherwise, they will not grow as tall and strong as they should.

Protein makes up about 18 to 20 percent of your body. Skeletal muscle accounts for more than half of body protein, **7-2**. About three percent of this protein is broken down each day. Besides building new tissues, therefore, you need protein to maintain existing tissues. Each cell has a limited life span. Your body constantly makes new cells to replace those that have died.

When you eat a nutritious diet and exercise regularly, your body uses proteins to build lean muscle mass. Before you can build muscles, however, you must meet your protein needs for normal growth and repair of tissues.

Where Body Protein Can Be Found

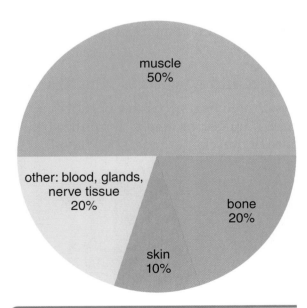

muscle
50%

other: blood, glands,
nerve tissue
20%

bone
20%

skin
10%

7-2   The largest amount of body protein is stored in muscle tissue. Protein is also located in bone, skin, blood, and all other cell tissue.

Growth and repair are possible only when your diet provides the necessary mix of amino acids.

Make Important Compounds

Your body uses proteins to make a number of important compounds. These compounds include enzymes, which cause specific chemical reactions in the body. For instance, digestive enzymes cause a chemical breakdown of carbohydrates, fats, and proteins from foods. Proteins are also used to make some hormones. Hormones are chemicals released into the bloodstream to control specific body processes. For example, the hormone insulin helps regulate the level of glucose in the blood. Your body's immune system uses proteins to make antibodies. **Antibodies** are proteins that defend the body against infection and disease, **7-3**.

Regulate Mineral and Fluid Balance

Proteins help carry the minerals sodium and potassium from one side of cell walls to the other. These minerals and other proteins control the flow of water through cell membranes. A balance of fluid inside and outside the cells is crucial. This balance is needed for normal functioning of the heart, lungs, brain, and every other cell.

Maintain Acid-Base Balance

Proteins help maintain the acid-base balance of the blood. **Acid-base balance** refers to the maintenance of the correct level of acidity of a body fluid. A life-threatening condition can result if the blood becomes too acidic. Proteins in the blood act as chemical buffers. A **buffer** is a compound that can counteract an excess of acid or base in a fluid.

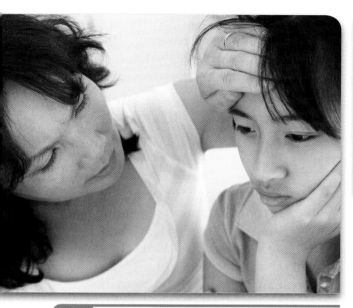

7-3   The body's immune system uses proteins to defend itself against infection and disease by making antibodies.

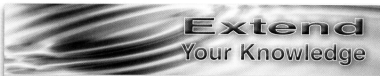

Follow the Proteins

Choose one of the listed functions of proteins. Research how the body uses proteins to perform that specific function. Create a diagram to illustrate how the process works.

Carry Vital Substances

Proteins linked with fats form *lipoproteins*, the compounds used to carry fats in the bloodstream. A protein is also used to transport iron and other nutrients. Oxygen transport in the blood depends on the presence of a protein, too. Each cell in the body has proteins that act as "cargo carriers." Protein is the carrier of chromosomes and other bundles of protein to other parts of cells. Health suffers if proteins are not available to carry these vital substances to needed points throughout the body.

Provide Energy

Only protein can perform the critical functions of cell growth and repair. However, the body's number one priority is to provide the cells with the energy they need to exist. Therefore, if carbohydrates and fats are lacking in the diet, the body uses proteins as an energy source. Protein can also be converted to glucose, which can be used as fuel. Proteins yield 4 calories of energy per gram. When proteins are used to provide energy, they cannot be used for other purposes, such as building cells.

A shortage of dietary carbohydrates and fats is not the only condition that causes the body to burn proteins for energy. The body also uses proteins as an energy source when there is an excess of protein in the diet.

Food Sources of Protein

Most people meet their protein needs by eating both animal and plant food sources. Many factors influence which protein foods people choose. Availability, cost, health concerns, food preferences, religious beliefs, and environmental factors all affect people's food choices.

Animal Sources of Protein

Animal flesh is by far the largest source of protein in a meat-eating culture, such as the United States. Animal foods include beef, veal, pork, lamb, poultry, and fish, **7-4**. Other animal sources of protein include eggs, milk, yogurt, and cheese.

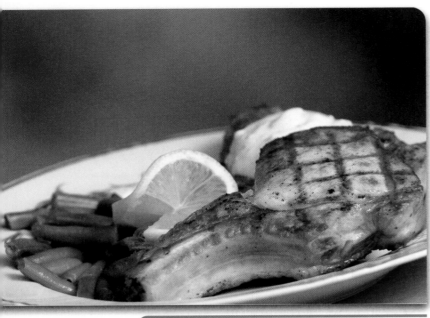

7-4 Pork is a popular source of animal protein.

The USDA reports that U.S. citizens eat an average of 200 pounds (90.7 kg) of meat, poultry, and seafood annually. Over the last 100 years, meat consumption has increased dramatically. The fast-food chains, serving hamburgers, chicken, and fish sandwiches, provide much of the protein in teen diets.

Although meat is an excellent source of protein, some meat products are quite high in fat. The same is true of some dairy products. For instance, 57 percent of the calories in regular ground beef come from fat. Of the calories in whole milk, 48 percent come from fat. Much of the fat in foods from animal sources is saturated. These foods provide no dietary fiber, either.

The cost of protein from animal sources is high. For example, one ounce (28 g) of a pork loin roast would provide about 8 grams of protein. One ounce (28 g) of sliced Swiss cheese would provide about 7 grams of protein. The cost of the pork roast is about 31 cents and the cost of the cheese is about 46 cents. In contrast, a ½-cup serving of baked beans provides about 6 grams of protein and costs only about 9 cents. High costs often limit the amount of animal protein low-income families can buy.

Plant Sources of Protein

A plentiful supply of protein is available from plant foods. Protein is found in grains, nuts, seeds, and legumes. **Legumes** are plants that have a special ability to capture nitrogen from the air and transfer it to their protein-rich seeds. Examples include peanuts, black-eyed peas, kidney beans, black beans, lentils, chickpeas, and lima beans.

Soybeans are an especially rich source of plant protein. These legumes can be processed and modified to form a variety of food products. For example, tofu is a curd product made from soybeans. It is used as a meat alternative in some dishes. Other pastes and meatlike products can also be made from soybeans.

Vegetarianism

Vegetarianism is the practice of eating a diet consisting entirely or largely of plant foods. Fruits, vegetables, grains, nuts, and seeds are the mainstays of a vegetarian diet. Some vegetarians also eat dairy products and eggs.

Forms of vegetarianism have existed since history began. Today, as in the past, many people choose to avoid eating foods from animal sources. Interest in vegetarianism, especially among young people, seems to be growing. This may explain the increasing popularity of vegetarian cookbooks and restaurants. The eating patterns of people who call themselves vegetarians vary greatly, **7-5**.

Types of Vegetarians
Vegans, or strict vegetarians, eat no foods from animal sources. Their diet is limited to foods from plant sources.
Fruitarians eat vegan diets based on fruits, nuts, and seeds. Vegetables, grains, beans, and animal products are excluded.
Lacto-vegetarians eat animal protein in the form of milk, cheese, and other dairy products. They do not eat meat, fish, poultry, or eggs.
Ovo-vegetarians do not eat meat or dairy products, but do eat eggs. The prefix "ovo" comes from the Latin word for egg. Many people are ovo-vegetarians because they are lactose-intolerant.
Lacto-ovo vegetarians eat animal protein in the form of dairy products and eggs. However, they do not eat meats, fish, or poultry.
Pescetarians eat any combination of vegetables, fruits, nuts, beans, and fish or seafood, but reject animal or poultry food products.
Semivegetarians, or partial vegetarians, eat dairy products, eggs, poultry, and seafood. They eat little or no red meat—beef, veal, pork, and lamb.

7-5   Vegetarians are identified by the degree to which they refrain from eating animal foods.

In recent years, health benefits of vegetarianism have received much attention. Most of the fats in plant protein foods are polyunsaturated. Plant foods contain no cholesterol, and the foods are generally high in fiber and low in saturated fat. These are positive factors in terms of heart health and cancer risk reduction.

Plant-based protein is not as easily digested as meat-based protein. Despite the decreased digestibility, the RDAs for protein are no different for vegetarians. Most people can easily meet their protein needs by eating a variety of whole grains, legumes, nuts, seeds, and vegetables in adequate amounts on a daily basis. Ask a vegetarian why he or she prefers not to eat foods from animal origin. The answer may simply be the person grew up in a vegetarian household. Other reasons may include the following:

- *Religious reasons* for vegetarianism are cited by followers of many Eastern religions, such as Buddhists and Hindus. Seventh-Day Adventists and Trappist monks from the Roman Catholic Church also choose a vegetarian diet.

- *Health reasons* are mentioned by people who want to avoid the fat and cholesterol in meat. They may also want to avoid certain hormones and chemicals used in raising livestock. Some people are concerned about illnesses that can be transmitted by animal foods, too. These people may claim some animal foods give them digestive problems. They say they feel better when they eat primarily fruits, vegetables, and cereals.

- *Socioeconomic reasons* are given by people who believe eating animals is wasteful. About 90 percent of the soybeans, corn, oats, and barley grown in the United States is fed to livestock. These crops would feed many more people directly than can be fed by the animals that eat the crops, **7-6**.

- *Environmental reasons* are given by people who say animal grazing is hard on land. These people may also mention that meat processing uses a tremendous amount of water and energy.

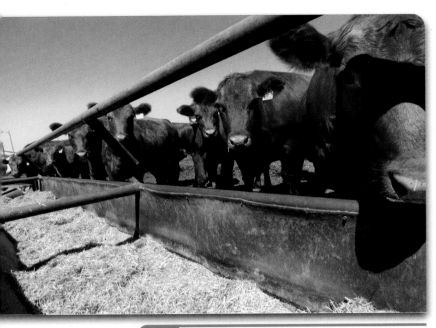

7-6 Large quantities of grain are fed to cattle to prepare them for market.

- *Humanitarian reasons* are stated by people who believe sacrificing the life of an animal for food is wrong. Some oppose the conditions in which animals are raised and prepared for slaughter.

Protein Quality

Proteins in various food sources differ in their quality. The quality of the protein in meat, poultry, and fish is very high. Animal foods are sources of **complete proteins**. This means all the indispensable amino acids humans need are present in the proteins. Eggs, milk, cheese, and yogurt are excellent sources of high-quality protein, too.

The protein provided by plant sources is of lower quality than that provided by animal sources. Plants furnish **incomplete proteins**. These proteins are missing or short in one or more of the indispensable amino acids.

Your body needs the right balance of amino acids to build tissues and other compounds. If one or more indispensable amino acids are missing, your cells will not be able to make needed proteins. To understand this concept better, think about a group of students working on an election campaign. They want to make 10 large sets of signs of the individual letters in the word *vote*. One student volunteers to make the *V*s, *T*s, and *E*s. Another student volunteers to make the *O*s. However, through lack of communication, the second student makes only eight *O*s. Instead of having 10 good signs, 2 signs are incomplete and unusable. Now suppose each letter represents a different indispensable amino acid. You can see how not having enough of all the indispensable amino acids leaves some proteins incomplete and unusable.

Complementary Proteins

You can get the amino acids missing from one incomplete protein source by combining it with another incomplete source. When eaten within the same day, these two incomplete protein foods become a source of complete protein. Two or more incomplete proteins that can be combined to provide all the indispensable amino acids are called **complementary proteins**.

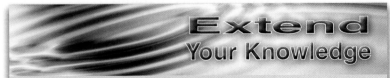

Meat Substitutes

Find out how textured-vegetable protein is used to make meat substitutes. Research the comparative costs and nutritional value of these meat substitutes with the foods they are intended to replace. Sample a product made from textured-vegetable protein and evaluate its taste. Report your findings in class.

How do you know which plant foods complement each other? A general guideline is to combine grains, nuts, or seeds with legumes. For example, peanuts (legumes) and wheat (grain) are complementary proteins. They are both incomplete sources of protein. When peanut butter is combined with wheat bread, however, the sandwich becomes a source of complete protein, **7-7**.

People from all over the world combine complementary proteins. For example, Mexicans often serve corn tortillas with refried beans (grain plus legumes). People in the Middle East combine sesame seeds and chickpeas (seeds plus legumes) to make a dip called *hummus*. How many combination foods and meals can you think of that contain complementary protein food sources?

Another way to extend the quality of incomplete protein foods is to combine them with complete protein foods. For instance, you might add a small amount of pork (complete protein) to a large amount of rice (incomplete protein). This extends the protein value of the rice.

Strict vegetarians must think carefully about using complementary proteins. High-quality protein is essential if normal growth and development are to occur. Diets that focus on only one source of incomplete protein, such as rice, are harmful to long-term good health.

How Much Protein Do You Need?

Your body does not store protein. Therefore, you need protein every day. The amount of protein you need is related to age, gender, and body size. It

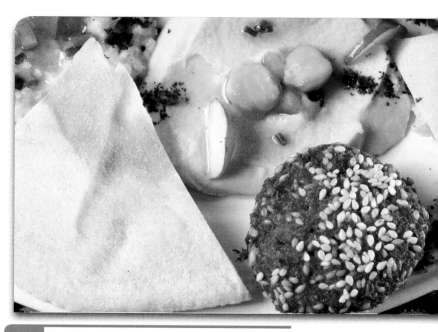

7-7 Falafel, a popular Middle Eastern dish made from garbanzo beans, is often served with a sesame seed paste called *tahini*. This dish is an example of complementary proteins.

also depends on your state of health. If you are like most people in the United States, you need less protein than you are consuming.

As children and teens grow, their bodies are building new tissue as well as maintaining existing tissue. Therefore, children and teens have a higher proportional need for protein than people who are no longer growing. In other words, they need more protein per pound of body weight. Similarly, women who are pregnant need extra protein to support the growth of their babies. Women who are breast-feeding need extra protein, too. They need protein to produce milk.

Protein needs vary between males and females. The body needs protein to replace lean tissue that wears out and is lost on a daily basis. Men generally have a higher percentage of lean tissue than women. Therefore, teen and adult males usually require more protein than females of similar age and body size, **7-8**.

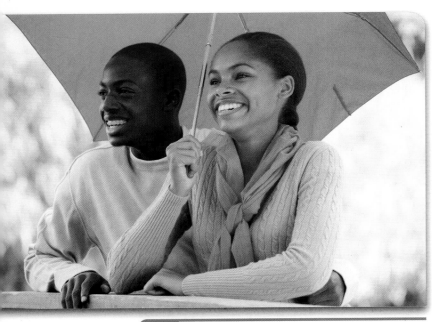

7-8 Because they have a larger proportion of lean muscle tissue, men typically need more protein than women.

Math Link

Converting Pounds to Kilograms

In the United States, an individual's weight is typically stated in units of pounds. The scientific field commonly uses the metric system of measurement. The metric system measures weight in units called kilograms (kg). One kilogram is equivalent to 2.2 pounds. To convert pounds to kilograms, divide the number of pounds by 2.2. To convert kilograms to pounds, multiply the number of kilograms by 2.2.

1. Convert 135 pounds to kilograms. (round to one decimal place)
2. Convert 48 kilograms to pounds. (round to one decimal place)

The more lean tissue a person has, the more protein is needed to maintain it. Therefore, a large, tall person has a slightly greater protein need than a small, short person.

Illness and injury increase the need for protein. When someone is sick, his or her immune system needs extra protein to build antibodies. When someone is injured, extra protein is needed to rebuild damaged tissue.

Protein Intake Recommendations

The RDA for protein is 52 grams per day for 14- to 18-year-old males. The RDA is 46 grams of protein daily for females in the same age range. RDAs for this age range are calculated based on 0.85 grams of protein per kilogram of body weight per day. After age 19, most individuals meet their protein needs with 0.8 grams of protein per kilogram of body weight per day. These are generous allowances that include a margin of safety. RDAs are designed for healthy individuals who eat adequate amounts of carbohydrates and fats. They are also based on the assumption that people are choosing high-quality sources of protein.

For ages 4 to 18 years, the DRI for protein is 10 to 30 percent of calories. For individuals 19 years and older, the range is 10 to no more than 35 percent. This means a physically active 18-year-old woman who needs 2,400 calories a day, should include around 240 calories from protein. Other health organizations recommend lower limits of 10 and upper limits of 15 percent of total calories from protein. Protein intake depends on a person's size. One of the clearest ways to compute protein needs is to calculate the DRI for most people as 0.8 grams for each kilogram (2.2 pounds) of healthy body weight. This amount will help you cover your need to replace the lost protein in tissue and worn out cells each day.

By reading the Nutrition Facts panel on food products, you can estimate how much protein you consume each day. A daily food diary will also help you analyze what percentage of calories in your diet is from protein. How does your daily intake of protein compare with your calculated RDA? Are you eating more or less than the RDA for protein?

Do Athletes Need More Protein?

Some athletes associate eating a solid piece of meat with building greater masses of body muscle. Serious athletes may wonder if they need more protein in their daily diet than others who are less active. Many athletes—competitive and casual—are able to meet their needs by consuming their RDA for protein, **7-9**. Following the MyPlate plan allows for adequate protein to meet the daily needs of most athletes.

Exercise involves a big increase in energy expenditure when compared to the resting state. The availability of energy from carbohydrates during exercise impacts the body's protein needs. For this reason, an athlete needs to consume adequate carbohydrate and fat in his or her diet so protein can be used to build and repair muscle rather than for energy. Other factors impact the body's protein needs during exercise. Such factors include the intensity, duration, and type of exercise, as well as, the gender and age of the athlete.

The athlete's gender and age may influence his or her protein needs. Some studies report that during distance running events, female athletes may use less protein as an energy source than males. Due to their age, teens may need more protein since they are still growing. The additional protein is needed for both development and energy needs.

Most research studying the impact of exercise intensity on protein needs focuses on sports involving strength, or resistance, training. Due to the high intensity of these activities, the athlete's protein needs are greater than athletes participating in low intensity sports. For example, weight lifting requires high muscular intensity with few repetitions (low endurance) to build muscle. To support this muscle growth, weight lifters require sufficient amounts of amino acids from protein. Heavy resistance training along with adequate protein intake improves muscle mass.

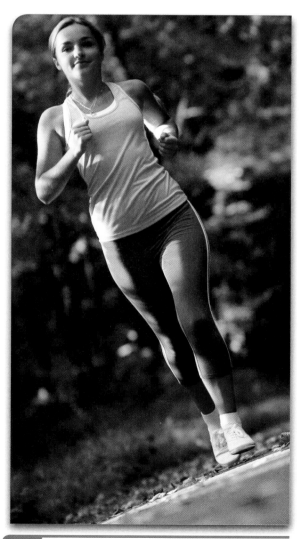

7-9 A runner who trains every day needs extra protein to build muscle and provide energy.

Protein Requirements for Different Activity Levels					
If the Individual Is a(n)	**Body Weight**		**Protein Needs**		**Total Protein**
Sedentary adult	68 kg	x	0.8 g/kg	=	54 g
Growing teen athlete	68 kg	x	1.5–2.0 g/kg	=	102–136 g
Adult in strength/resistance training	68 kg	x	1.5–1.7 g/kg	=	102–116 g
Adult in endurance training	68 kg	x	1.2–1.7 g/kg	=	82–116 g
Note: These figures represent commonly recommended findings from the American College of Sports Medicine, American Dietetic Association, and the Dietitians of Canada.					

7-10   Protein requirements may vary based on a number of factors.

When researchers study how duration of an activity impacts protein needs, endurance sports such as long distance cycling, marathons, or triathlons are the focus. Distance runners are involved in high endurance activity of low intensity and may require protein in excess of the RDA. However, since increasing muscle mass is not the goal of these endurance athletes, their protein needs are typically less than those of strength (high intensity) athletes, **7-10**.

Most athletes can meet additional protein needs by including a few more protein foods in their meal plans. Protein and amino acid supplements or large servings of red meat are usually not necessary. Supplements may actually create greater health problems and interfere with performance gains. Most athletes perform at their peak by consuming natural foods. Good sources of protein in foods include dairy, meat, fish, cheese, eggs, and beans, **7-11**.

The evidence that athletes perform better with dietary protein in excess of RDAs is not scientifically consistent or clear. In general, active individuals and competitive athletes should aim for 60 to 65 percent of total calories from carbohydrates. (It is important to remember the primary need is for energy.) Athletes should stay at the low end of the range for fats—20 to 25 percent of total calories. If the remaining 10 to 20 percent of calories comes from protein, an athlete's nutritional needs will be adequately met.

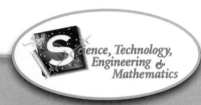

Science, Technology, Engineering & Mathematics

Food Scientist

Food scientists work to create food products that are healthy, safe, tasty, and easy to use. They find better ways to preserve, process, package, store, and deliver foods. Some food scientists discover new foods and analyze foods to see how much fat, sugar, or protein is in them. Others search for better food additives. Some food scientists work in the food processing industry, while others work in universities and government agencies.

Education: Most jobs require a bachelor's degree, but a master's or doctoral degree is usually required for research positions at universities. Students preparing to be food scientists take courses, such as food chemistry, food analysis, food microbiology, food engineering, and food processing operations.

Job Outlook: Job growth in food science should be faster than the average for all occupations. This growth will stem primarily from efforts to increase the quantity and quality of food produced for a growing population.

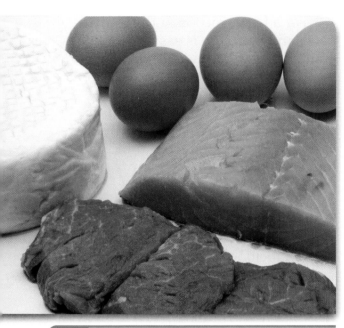

7-11 Most athletes can meet their protein requirements by consuming foods that are good sources of protein.

Drinking fluids before, during, and after exercise is important. Sweating and heat can easily result in dehydration.

Meeting the Protein RDA

One of the simplest ways to meet protein needs is to follow the recommendations of MyPlate. The protein foods and dairy groups are your primary food sources of protein.

Two to three cups or the equivalent are recommended from the dairy group every day. One cup of yogurt, one and one-half ounces of cheese, or two ounces of processed cheese are equivalent to one cup of milk.

For most teens, five to six ounce-equivalents from the protein foods group are recommended daily. One ounce of meat, fish, or poultry, one-fourth cup of cooked dry beans or peas, one egg, or one tablespoon of peanut butter counts as one ounce-equivalent.

When choosing protein sources, avoid the health risks of a diet high in saturated fats. Choose low-fat protein foods often. Fat-free milk, low-fat cheese, most fish, and dry beans and peas are low-fat protein sources. Trim visible fat from meats and remove skin from poultry. Use low-fat cooking methods such as grilling, baking, or poaching. Avoid adding high-fat cooking oils, sauces, and gravies to protein foods.

The Risks of Too Little or Too Much Protein

As with all nutrients, you need to consume enough protein, but you should avoid getting too much. A lack of protein and a surplus of protein can both cause health problems.

Nitrogen balance is a comparison of the nitrogen a person consumes with the nitrogen he or she excretes. Protein is the only energy nutrient that provides nitrogen. Therefore, nitrogen balance is used to evaluate a person's protein status. Most healthy adults are in *nitrogen equilibrium*. This means they excrete the same amount of nitrogen they take in each day. A person who is building new tissue takes in more protein than he or she excretes. This person is said to be in *positive nitrogen balance*. A pregnant woman or a growing child would be in positive nitrogen balance. Someone whose tissues are deteriorating would be losing more nitrogen than he or she consumes. This person is said to be in *negative nitrogen balance*. A person whose body is wasting due to starvation would be in negative nitrogen balance, **7-12**.

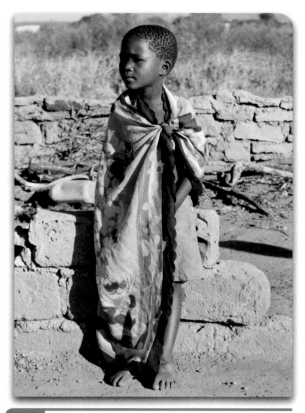

7-12 Protein deficiencies are common among the people in some African nations where high-quality sources of protein are scarce.

Protein Deficiency

A deficiency is a shortage. In nutrition, deficiency refers to an amount of a nutrient less than the body needs for optimum health. A **deficiency disease** is a sickness caused by a lack of an essential nutrient.

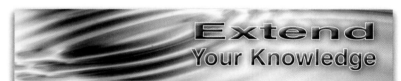

Where Does Hunger Exist?

Using the Internet or print resources, learn where hunger is occurring in the world. Select one country and learn the causes for the hunger problem. Give an oral report describing the country, the reasons for the food insecurity, the population that is most impacted, and their typical diet.

For a large portion of the U.S. population, protein is easy to get in amounts that exceed daily recommendations. Among people who are fighting poverty, however, protein deficiency is not uncommon. This is especially true in countries where there is simply not enough food. If the only foods eaten are low in protein, a protein deficiency is likely to occur.

Protein-energy malnutrition (PEM) is a condition caused by a lack of calories and proteins in the diet. Symptoms of PEM include diarrhea and various nutrient deficiencies.

A form of PEM is **kwashiorkor**, which is a protein deficiency disease. This disease most frequently strikes a child when the next sibling is born. The disease is common in poor countries where mothers stop breast-feeding an older child to begin breast-feeding a newborn. The weaned older child is no longer receiving protein-rich breast milk. He or she begins eating a diet that is much lower in protein.

A child suffering from kwashiorkor does not reach his or her full growth potential. The child develops a bloated abdomen and has skinny arms and legs. Lack of protein also affects the body's fluid balance and immune system. Many children die of such simple illnesses as a fever or the common measles.

Another PEM disease is marasmus. **Marasmus** is a wasting disease caused by a lack of calories and protein. It most often affects infants. The muscles and tissues of these children begin to waste away. The children become thin, weak, and susceptible to infection and disease. In short, they are suffering from starvation.

Excess Proteins in the Diet

If you are like most people in the United States, you consume more than the RDA for protein. On the average, women in the United States eat almost one and one-half times the RDA for protein. Men eat nearly twice the RDA for protein.

Some people take protein or amino acid supplements, believing these products offer health benefits, **7-13**. Others simply enjoy eating diets rich in high-protein foods. These people should consider the problems associated with high-protein diets. Several health issues and serious complications have been identified.

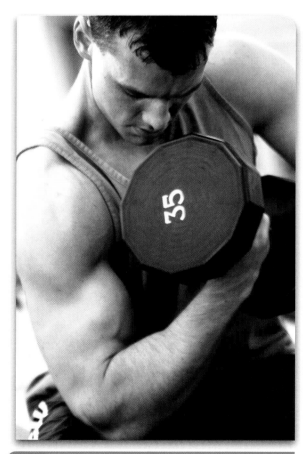

7-13 Bodybuilders should be aware of the health risks of taking amino acid supplements and eating a high-protein diet.

Case Study: Building Muscle

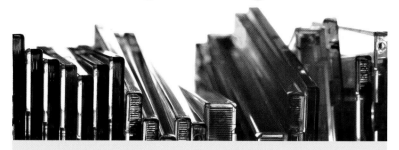

Spence is 15 years old and wants to build up his muscles. He does not enjoy much physical activity, but he would like to change the way his body looks. All the guys his age seem to be taller and stronger. Spence decided he would add more protein to his diet in order to build his muscles. His friends told him about protein drinks he could buy and other protein food supplements that might help him out. Spence added the following to his usual daily food plan: 2 whey protein shakes, 3 hard-boiled eggs, and 1 protein snack bar.

Case Review

1. What results do you think Spence will have with his new food plan?

2. What advice would you give Spence?

Liver and Kidney Problems

A high-protein diet produces an overabundance of nitrogen waste. The body must excrete this waste before it builds up to toxic levels. The liver turns nitrogen waste into urea. The kidneys are responsible for excreting urea in urine. Therefore, excess protein creates extra work for the liver and kidneys. Stress on these organs can be a problem and may cause them to age prematurely. Extra work for the kidneys is a special problem for diabetics, who may already have problems with kidney disease.

Calcium Loss

Several studies have shown diets high in protein from animal sources may contribute to calcium losses in the bones. A loss of calcium weakens the bones, which leads to a number of other health problems. This occurs through increased urinary calcium losses. Other health problems may follow. A person whose diet is low in calcium is particularly at risk.

Excess Body Fat

Many common high-protein foods, such as whole milk, beef, and cheese, are also high-fat foods. Extra calories from fat can contribute to weight problems. Foods high in fat are also associated with heart-health and cancer risks, **7-14**.

The body cannot store excess amino acids as a protein source. However, it can store them as an energy source by converting them to body fat. Whether fat accompanies the protein in food or is manufactured from excess amino acids, the consequences are the same. Excess body fat is associated with a number of health problems.

Comparing Protein Sources	
Extra Lean Ground Beef Patty	**White Beans**
4 ounces	1/2 cup
290 calories	116 calories
112 mg cholesterol	0 mg cholesterol
high in saturated fat	low in saturated fat
0 g fiber	7 g fiber

7-14   Compare protein sources to determine which foods contribute more total nutrition.

Reading Summary

Protein is an energy-providing nutrient. Proteins in the diet are made of 20 amino acids. Nine of the amino acids are indispensable and cannot be manufactured by your body.

Proteins serve multiple functions. They provide for growth and maintenance of body tissues. Proteins are used to make important compounds, such as enzymes, hormones, and antibodies. They regulate fluid and acid-base balance. They carry vital substances, and they provide energy under special conditions.

Proteins come from animal food sources, including meat, fish, poultry, milk, and eggs. They also come from plant sources, such as cereals, legumes, seeds, and nuts. Animal sources of protein are complete; plant sources are incomplete. Complete proteins provide all the indispensable amino acids; incomplete proteins do not. Incomplete sources of protein can be combined to make a complete protein. This is important information for vegetarians, who eat little or no animal protein.

Protein needs depend on age, gender, body build, and state of health. Growing children need proportionally more protein than adults. Pregnant women need additional protein for building new tissue, and breast-feeding mothers need it to produce milk. Men tend to need more protein than women because they have a higher percentage of lean tissue. Individuals who are sick or injured need proteins to build body tissues. Athletes may have slightly higher protein needs than less active people. However, athletes can easily meet these needs by eating a nutritious diet.

RDA for protein can be met by following your MyPlate recommendations for food amounts from the dairy and protein foods groups. Most people in the United States consume more than the recommended amount of protein. Kwashiorkor and marasmus are two types of protein-energy malnutrition that are common in developing countries. These diseases especially affect young children, who then become susceptible to other life-threatening diseases and infections.

Review Learning

1. Compare the chemical structure of protein with that of carbohydrates and fats.
2. What is the difference between an indispensable and a dispensable amino acid?
3. What role do stomach acids play in protein digestion?
4. How does protein affect growth during the teen years?
5. How do carbohydrates and fats impact the body's use of protein?
6. Name three specific animal sources and three specific plant sources of protein.
7. Describe two reasons vegetarians might give for eating little or no food from animal sources.
8. How can vegans meet their needs for complete sources of protein?
9. About what percentage of daily calories should come from protein?

10. Give three dietary tips for limiting fat intake while meeting protein needs.
11. Compare the nitrogen balance status of a healthy teen with one who is undernourished.
12. A disease brought on by a protein deficiency is called _____.
13. What factors might impact an athlete's requirements for protein in his or her food plan?
14. What are three problems associated with high-protein diets?

Critical Thinking

15. **Draw conclusions.** Research vegan diets and lifestyles using print and Internet resources. Interview two people who are vegans. Based on your findings, write a persuasive paper arguing for or against the merits of a vegan diet.
16. **Analyze options.** Use the Internet to research three possible solutions to the problem of protein-energy malnutrition in developing countries. Write an opinion paper or give an oral report on the solution you think is most viable. Give reasons for your choice.

Applying Your Knowledge

17. **Assess your intake.** Keep a daily food diary for three days. Use diet analysis software to compare your actual daily protein consumption with the RDA.
18. **Food preferences.** Survey three teens and two adults to find out their favorite sources of protein. Compile your findings with those of your classmates. Work together to make a poster listing the calorie, fat, and protein content of the top 10 favorites.
19. **Vegetarian menu.** A friend who is visiting with you is a vegetarian. The person eats no meat, fish, or poultry but does enjoy dairy products and eggs. Write a one-day vegetarian menu that accommodates your friend's dietary restriction. Be sure to include the use of complementary proteins. Draw arrows to show where protein complements occur.
20. **Community service.** Contact a local food bank to learn what foods are in greatest need. Identify nonperishable protein food items that could be donated. Organize a nonperishable food donation drive at your school.

Technology Connections

21. **Internet research.** Use the Internet to find the various nutritional supplies the World Food Programme distributes to people during emergencies or in refugee situations. Use spreadsheet software to prepare a bar chart comparing the calories and protein content of the various products to the RDA.
22. **Nutrient analysis.** Collect food diaries from a vegetarian and a nonvegetarian friend. Complete a diet analysis to determine if protein needs are met in both cases. Using the ChooseMyPlate.gov website, select the Interactive Tools and click on the "Food Tracker" to assess food intake.

Academic Connections

23. **Science.** Interview the biology teacher to learn how muscle develops. How does resistance training make muscle stronger? What other factors are important for muscle builders to consider?

24. **Science.** Construct a model of a protein molecule using materials such as toothpicks, marshmallows, and other materials available in the classroom or at home.

25. **Research.** Investigate the foundation for a manufacturer's claims about their amino acid supplements. Determine whether the claims are valid. Compare the cost and nutritional value of these supplements to whole food protein sources. Consider any dangers the use of these products might pose. Videotape yourself role-playing an investigative reporter presenting the findings.

Workplace Applications

Solving a Protein Problem

Presume you are a department manager at a local social service agency. Your department works with people who have limited resources for food, especially families with young children and older adults. For most clients, obtaining adequate daily protein is a financial problem. In order to better serve your clients, you have decided to put together a fact sheet on available local protein sources and their typical costs. Locate protein foods from both plant and animal sources. Identify the cost per ounce. Then prepare the fact sheet to help your clients more accurately calculate and budget costs for protein foods.

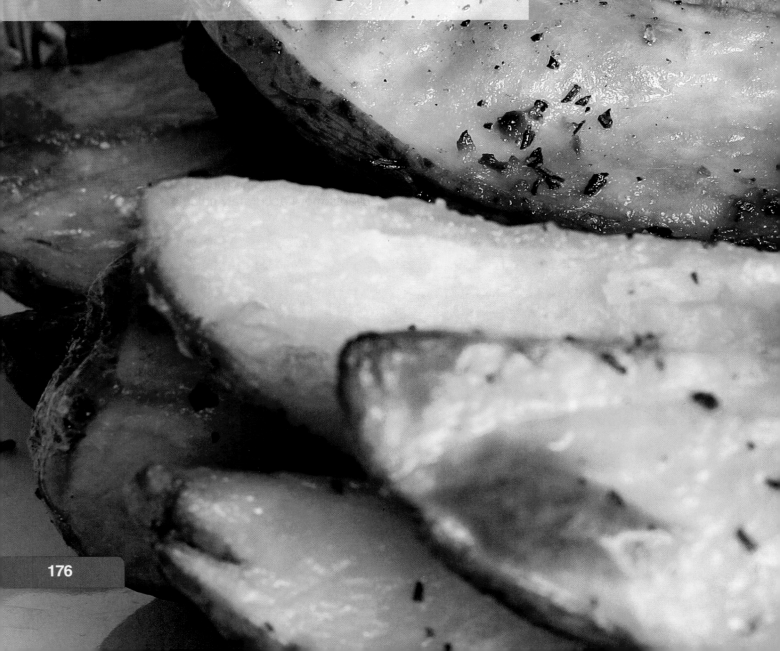

Part Three
The Work of Noncaloric Nutrients

Roasting

Roasting is a preparation method that cooks food by surrounding it with dry heat. Meats and poultry are often placed on a rack for roasting. This allows fats to drip away and air to circulate evenly around the food. Vegetables and fruits can also be roasted. Roasting creates a tasty, browned finish that enhances the flavor of foods. Additional herbs, spices, and other seasonings can be added to further develop the flavor of roasted foods.

When no additional fat is added during cooking, roasting is a healthy food preparation option. Procedures for roasting poultry often recommend periodic ladling of butter, drippings, or other fat over the food during cooking. This process is called basting and is intended to keep the food moist. Rather than using a fat, food can be basted with a low-sodium broth or other flavorful low-fat liquid.

Oven Roasted Potato Wedges (6 Servings)

Ingredients

- 1¼ pounds Russet potatoes
- 1 tablespoon canola oil
- ¼ teaspoon garlic powder
- ¼ teaspoon paprika
- ¼ teaspoon pepper
- ¼ teaspoon salt

Directions

1. Mix oil and seasonings in large bowl.
2. Wash and dry potatoes. Cut potatoes in half lengthwise. Cut each half into 4 wedges.
3. Add potatoes wedges to oil and seasonings and toss to coat.
4. Spray sheet pan with cooking spray and place potatoes on pan in a single layer.
5. Roast potatoes in a 375°F oven for 45 to 60 minutes. Turn potatoes over halfway through cooking.

Chapter 8

Vitamins: Drivers of Cell Processes

Reading for Meaning

As you read the chapter, record any questions that come to mind. Indicate where the answers to the questions can be found: within the text, by asking your teacher, in another book, on the Internet, or by reflecting on your own experiences. Pursue the answers to your questions.

Concept Organizer

Use the modified star diagram to identify the fat-soluble and water-soluble vitamins.

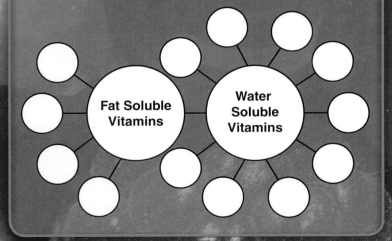

Terms to Know

vitamin
provitamin
fat-soluble vitamin
water-soluble vitamin
toxicity
epithelial cells
night blindness
fortified food
rickets
osteomalacia
antioxidant
free radical
erythrocyte hemolysis
coagulation
coenzyme
enriched food
beriberi
pellagra
pernicious anemia
scurvy
collagen
phytochemicals
probiotics
prebiotics
placebo effect

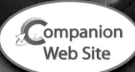

Companion Web Site

- **Print out the concept organizer at g-wlearning.com.**
- **Practice key terms with crossword puzzles, matching activities, and e-flash cards at g-wlearning.com.**

Objectives

After studying this chapter, you will be able to

- **recall** the major roles of vitamins in the diet.
- **classify** vitamins as fat-soluble or water-soluble.
- **summarize** functions and sources of specific vitamins.
- **recall** symptoms of various vitamin deficiencies and excesses.
- **evaluate** the use of vitamin supplements.
- **compare** ways to select, cook, and store foods to maximize vitamin content.

Central Ideas

- Vitamins are essential nutrients that regulate body processes.
- You can obtain the vitamins your body needs by eating a variety of healthful foods.

Although nutrition research began in the nineteenth century, vitamins were not identified until the beginning of the twentieth century. Today, vitamins continue to be in the news. Scientists have learned much about vitamins. However, many questions concerning the roles of vitamins in the diet remain.

Will taking extra vitamin C prevent a cold? Should you take vitamin pills rather than trying to get vitamins from food? Do fresh, raw vegetables supply more vitamins than canned or cooked vegetables? These are among the questions for which researchers have already found answers. You will learn about these and other topics related to vitamins as you study this chapter.

What Are Vitamins?

A **vitamin** is an essential nutrient needed in tiny amounts to regulate body processes. Vitamins have no calorie value because they yield no energy. However, the body needs vitamins for the chemical reactions involved in releasing energy from other nutrients, **8-1**.

Vitamins in the diet are vital to health and wellness. Each vitamin has specific functions. As a nutrient group, vitamins assist with the following functions:

- nutrient metabolism
- energy production and release
- tissue maintenance
- normal digestion
- infection resistance

Vitamin Names

In 1912, Casimir Funk, a food science professor in Poland, coined the word *vitamine. Vita* means life; *amine* refers to a certain chemical structure that contains nitrogen. After years of research, it was discovered few vitamins had the amine structure in their chemical compounds. Therefore, the final *e* was dropped to avoid confusion with the amine groups found in the chemical structure of proteins.

Vitamins were named as they were discovered. The first vitamin discovered was named vitamin A. Logically, the next vitamin discovered was named vitamin B. However, it was later discovered that vitamin B was really several different vitamins. Also, some compounds originally thought to be vitamins turned out not to be. Therefore, the pattern to the naming of the vitamins became harder to recognize.

You may wonder how researchers prove whether a compound is a vitamin. Vitamins are essential for life for a specific species. A compound that is essential for humans may not be essential for earthworms. However, the compound is essential for all humans. This means removing the compound from the human diet will eventually cause all humans to develop deficiency symptoms. Conversely, if removing the compound does not result in deficiency symptoms, the compound is not a vitamin.

Today, there are 13 known vitamins. Some are most often referred to by a letter, such as vitamins A, C, D, E, and K. Most of the B vitamins

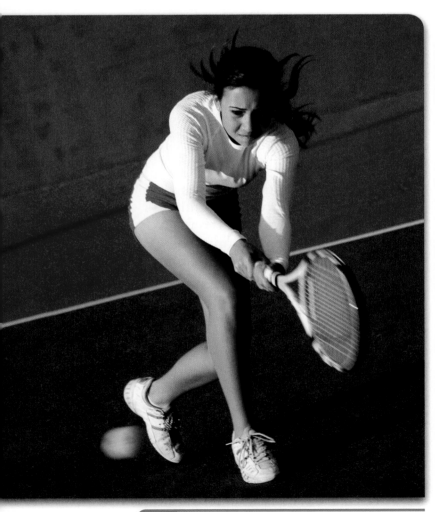

8-1   Vitamins help the body release energy needed for physical activity.

are better known by a name, such as riboflavin, thiamin, and niacin.

Most vitamins have several *active forms*, or types that perform in the body. All the active forms have similar molecular structures. However, they may not all be able to do every function associated with the vitamin. The different active forms are like different car models. Some models have navigation systems and some do not, but they can all provide transportation. There are different names for each form of the same vitamin. For example, *pyridoxine*, *pyridoxal*, and *pyridoxamine* are all forms of vitamin B_6. You may have noticed some of these complex names on the ingredient lists of food labels, **8-2**.

INGREDIENTS: WHOLE OAT FLOUR, WHEAT, BARLEY, BROWN SUGAR, CORN, RICE, SALT, MALT FLAVORING, RICE BRAN. VITAMINS AND MINERALS: IRON (FERRIC PHOSPHATE), VITAMIN E (ALPHA TOCOPHEROL ACETATE), NIACINAMIDE, ZINC (OXIDE), CALCIUM PANTOTHENATE, VITAMIN B_6 (PYRIDOXINE HYDROCHLORIDE), VITAMIN B_2 (RIBOFLAVIN), VITAMIN A (PALMITATE), VITAMIN B_1 (THIAMIN HYDROCHLORIDE), FOLIC ACID, BIOTIN, VITAMIN B_{12} AND VITAMIN D.

Morning Crunch

Whole Grain Cereal

Nutrition Facts

Serving Size	1 cup (56 g)
Servings Per Container	9

Amount Per Serving	
Calories	90
Calories from Fat	10

	% Daily Value
Total Fat 1g	2%
Saturated Fat 0g	0%
Trans Fat 0g	
Cholesterol 0mg	0%
Sodium 180mg	8%
Total Carb. 15g	5%
Fiber 2g	
Sugars 1g	
Protein 2g	

Vitamin A 15%		Vitamin C 15%	
Calcium 2%		Iron 25%	

Percent Daily Values are based on a 2,000 calorie diet. Your daily values may be higher or lower depending on your calorie needs:

	Calories:	2,000	2,500
Total Fat	Less than	65g	80g
Sat Fat	Less than	20g	25g
Cholesterol	Less than	300mg	300mg
Sodium	Less than	2,400mg	2,400mg
Total Carbohydrate		300mg	375g
Dietary Fiber		25g	30g

Calories per gram:
Fat 9   Carbohydrate 4   Protein 4

INGREDIENTS: WHOLE OAT FLOUR, WHEAT, BARLEY, BROWN SUGAR, CORN, RICE, SALT, MALT FLAVORING, RICE BRAN. VITAMINS AND MINERALS: IRON (FERRIC PHOSPHATE), VITAMIN E (ALPHA TOCOPHEROL ACETATE), NIACINAMIDE, ZINC (OXIDE), CALCIUM PANTOTHENATE, VITAMIN B_6 (PYRIDOXINE HYDROCHLORIDE), VITAMIN B_2 (RIBOFLAVIN), VITAMIN A (PALMITATE), VITAMIN B_1 (THIAMIN HYDROCHLORIDE), FOLIC ACID, BIOTIN, VITAMIN B_{12} AND VITAMIN D.

8-2   Ingredient lists on food labels often include the complex chemical names of added vitamins.

The Chemistry of Vitamins

Unlike carbohydrates, fats, and proteins, the different vitamins do not share a typical molecular structure. Each vitamin is unique. All vitamins are *organic compounds*, which means they contain carbon. They also contain hydrogen and oxygen. Some contain nitrogen, sulfur, or cobalt in their structures, too.

Several vitamins have provitamin forms. **Provitamins** are compounds that are not vitamins, but the body can convert them into the active form of a vitamin. For example, *beta-carotene* is a provitamin for vitamin A. Beta-carotene is a deep-yellow compound found in dark green and deep yellow fruits and vegetables, including carrots. When you eat this compound, your body can change the beta-carotene into vitamin A.

How Much of the Vitamins Are Needed?

Long ago, doctors wondered why just small amounts of specific foods improved health problems such as scurvy and night blindness. They learned the answer with the discovery of vitamins. They found the amounts of vitamins you need for growth, maintenance, and reproduction were tiny. In fact, you need only about one ounce of vitamins for every 150 pounds (2,400 ounces) of food you eat. All the vitamins you need in one day add up to only one-eighth of a teaspoon.

Nutrition experts make recommendations stating how much of various vitamins people need each day for good health. Eating a nutritious diet that meets the Adequate Intakes (AIs) or Recommended Dietary Allowances (RDAs) is an important daily

goal. However, if your intake of some vitamins is short now and then, there is no serious harm. The first symptoms of a vitamin deficiency take a month or so to appear in most people.

There are two main causes of vitamin deficiency diseases. The first cause is an insufficient amount of a vitamin in the diet. In cases of poverty, people may lack the variety of foods that would provide all the vitamins they need. Even with a bounty of different foods, however, some people simply fail to choose rich sources of some vitamins.

Getting enough vitamins in the daily food plan can be more of a challenge for people who have increased vitamin needs. Pregnant women need larger amounts of many nutrients, including most vitamins. Infants and adolescents need extra nutrients to aid in the growth of body tissues, **8-3**. People who are sick or recovering from injuries have greater needs, too. Lifestyle behaviors can also increase needs for certain vitamins. For instance, cigarette smokers need more vitamin C in their diets than nonsmokers.

The second cause of a vitamin deficiency disease is a failure of the body to absorb a vitamin. For instance, changes in the body that occur with age can affect a person's ability to absorb vitamin B_{12}. When food moves through the intestinal tract too quickly, vitamins do not have a chance to be absorbed adequately. Diarrhea or a very high-fiber diet may affect absorption in this way. Malabsorption of some nutrients can also be due to a lack of other nutrients.

Vitamin Classifications

All vitamins are grouped in two categories—fat-soluble or water-soluble. *Soluble* refers to a substance's

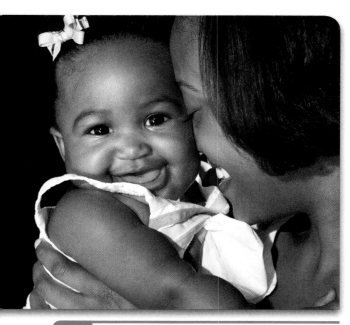

8-3 Infants need relatively large amounts of vitamins to support their rapid growth.

ability to dissolve. Some vitamins dissolve in fats. The four **fat-soluble vitamins** are vitamins A, D, E, and K. Other vitamins dissolve in water. The nine **water-soluble vitamins** are the B-complex vitamins and vitamin C.

Your body stores excess fat-soluble vitamins when you take in more than you can use. An advantage of this is it is not crucial to consume the fat-soluble vitamins every day. A disadvantage is toxicity can result if amounts of these vitamins that are stored become too large. **Toxicity** is a poisonous condition. Vitamins A and D are especially toxic if consumed in large amounts over long periods. Toxicity does not occur from eating vitamin-rich foods. It occurs when people take large amounts of vitamin supplements.

Your body does not store water-soluble vitamins to any great extent. Excesses are normally excreted in the urine. With excess vitamins, your urine may change color, sometimes becoming more yellow. Therefore, water-soluble vitamins do not readily build up to

toxic levels in the body. Without large stores of these vitamins, however, deficiency symptoms may not take long to develop. Therefore, you need to be sure to consume enough of the water-soluble vitamins every day.

The Fat-Soluble Vitamins at Work

The fat-soluble vitamins, A, D, E, and K, are present in a wide range of foods in the diet. They are absorbed through the intestinal walls with fats from foods. Your body can draw on stored reserves of these vitamins when your intake is low.

Vitamin A

Vitamin A deficiency is the leading cause of preventable blindness in children living in Africa, Asia, and South America. Up to 500,000 children go blind each year because their diets lack this vitamin.

Functions of Vitamin A

Vitamin A is necessary for the formation of healthy epithelial tissue. The **epithelial cells** are the surface cells that line the outside of the body. Epithelial tissue also covers the eyes and lines the passages of the lungs, intestines, and reproductive organs. Because of this function, vitamin A plays a role in keeping skin and hair healthy. Adequate amounts of vitamin A help keep the eyes free from dryness and infections, **8-4**. Vitamin A also helps the linings of the lungs and intestines stay moist and resistant to disease.

Maintaining healthy eyesight is another main function of vitamin A. Without sufficient vitamin A, the cells in the eyes cannot make the

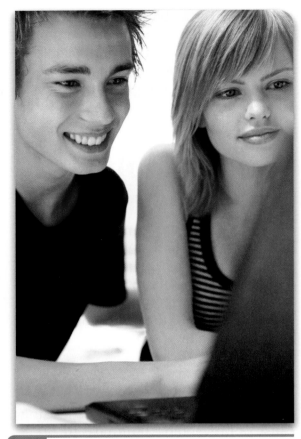

8-4 Vitamin A helps keep skin, hair, and eyes healthy.

compounds needed by the eyes to see well in dim light. That means the eyes adapt slowly to darkness and night vision becomes poor. This condition is called **night blindness**.

Vitamin A is also crucial for the development of bone tissue. If bone formation is hampered, normal growth will not occur.

Meeting Vitamin A Needs

The RDA for vitamin A is 900 micrograms for males ages 14 and older. The RDA is 700 micrograms for females over age 14. (Males need more of many nutrients to support their higher percentage of lean body tissue.)

Another unit of measure for vitamin A is the *retinol activity equivalent (RAE)*. This unit is used to measure how strong various vitamin A

compounds are and how easy they are for the body to use.

Vitamin A in foods exists in two basic forms—one from animal sources and the other from plant sources. Animal foods usually provide vitamin A as a *preformed* vitamin. This is an active form the body can use. Plant foods provide vitamin A as provitamin *carotenes*, including alpha- and beta-carotene. The body can convert these compounds into the more usable form of vitamin A. However, they are not in an active form your body can use when you consume them. Therefore, they have a lower RAE value than preformed vitamin A.

Liver, fish oils, egg yolks, and whole-fat dairy products are good sources of preformed vitamin A. Removing the fat from dairy products removes the fat-soluble vitamin A, too. Therefore, reduced-fat dairy products are fortified with vitamin A. **Fortified foods** are those that have one or more nutrients added during processing. Good sources of provitamin A carotenes include winter squash, carrots, broccoli, cantaloupe, and apricots, **8-5**.

Eating a nutritious diet is the best way to meet vitamin A needs. Try to select rich sources each day.

Effects of Vitamin A Deficiencies and Excesses

People who drink little milk or eat few vegetables may show signs of vitamin A deficiency. Symptoms of the deficiency may include night blindness; dry, scaly skin; and fatigue.

Vitamin A deficiency is one of the major causes of blindness in the world. It is a serious problem in under-developed nations. Without adequate vitamin A, the membrane covering the eyes becomes dry and hard. Infection and blindness can develop. If detected

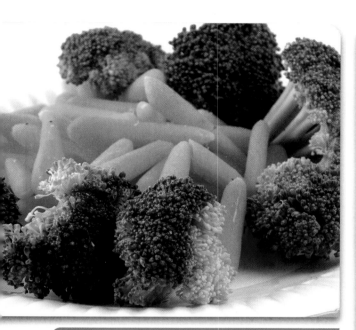

8-5   Dark green and deep orange fruits and vegetables, including broccoli and carrots, are good sources of beta-carotene. The body can convert beta-carotene into vitamin A.

early enough, vision problems caused by deficiency can be reversed with large doses of vitamin A.

Getting enough vitamin A is important. However, getting too much can cause health problems. The Tolerable Upper Intake Level (UL) for 14- to 18-year-olds is 2,800 micrograms. The body can store vitamin A to toxic levels. Symptoms of vitamin A toxicity include severe headaches, bone pain, dry skin, hair loss, vomiting, and liver damage. Toxicity poses a greater risk for children. Very high vitamin A intakes are especially dangerous during pregnancy. Such intakes can cause babies to be born with disabilities.

Vitamin D

Vitamin D is a unique fat-soluble vitamin. With direct exposure to sunlight, your body can make all the vitamin D it needs, **8-6**. Of course, you can also obtain vitamin D from your daily diet.

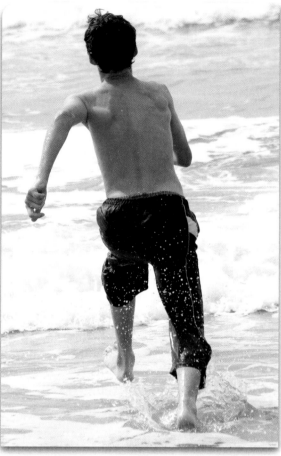

8-6   The body can make vitamin D with exposure to sunlight.

Functions of Vitamin D

An important function of vitamin D is to help regulate the levels of calcium in the bloodstream. Normal amounts of calcium in the blood are needed for healthy nerve function, bone growth and maintenance, and other functions. Vitamin D performs this function by triggering the release of calcium from the bones. Vitamin D also controls blood calcium levels by enhancing the absorption of calcium from the intestines. When blood calcium levels are low, vitamin D also reduces the amount of calcium the kidneys excrete.

Vitamin D plays a major role in bone health. Bone tissue is the chief user of blood calcium. This mineral makes bones rigid and strong.

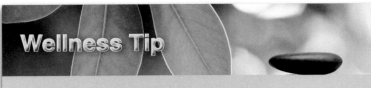

Wellness Tip

Hold That Supplement

Buying supplements is a costly way to get nutrients. In addition, vitamin tablets provide no fiber, energy, or taste. You cannot enjoy supplements as you do foods. Most nutritionists agree people benefit more from spending their money on a nutritious diet than on vitamin supplements.

However, nerve, muscle, and other cells also require calcium drawn from the bloodstream to function properly. Therefore, vitamin D plays a role in maintaining all body tissues. More recently, vitamin D has been discovered to play a major role in regulating the cell cycle. It affects the growth and differentiation of many types of cells.

Meeting Vitamin D Needs

A growing body of research indicates that both calcium and vitamin D deficiency is widespread throughout the world as well as in the United States, particularly in adults 70 and older. The RDA for vitamin D is 15 micrograms per day for all people through age 70. The RDA is higher for older adults. This is to help older adults avoid developing porous, fragile bones—a condition that is more common in later life.

Vitamin D occurs in 10 different forms. The two forms important to humans are the provitamins D_2 (ergocalciferol) and D_3 (cholecalciferol). The provitamin D_2 is found in plant foods. D_3 is found in animal foods, but is also made by the human body in the skin when exposed to sunlight. When sunlight shines on skin, a cholesterol-like compound in the skin forms the D_3 provitamin. The liver and kidneys then change the provitamin into the form of vitamin D best used by the body.

Spending too much time in the sun without protecting the skin increases the risk of skin cancer. Fortunately, the skin does not need prolonged sun exposure to make vitamin D. A light-skinned person can make enough vitamin D to meet the body's needs in 15 minutes of sun exposure. Dark-skinned people require a somewhat longer time to produce the same amount of vitamin D. Anything that filters sunlight, including clouds, smog, window glass, sunscreen, and heavy clothing, inhibits vitamin D production. People living in the Northern hemisphere can experience many days with little or no sunshine. Anyone who does not receive enough sunshine must get vitamin D from food sources.

Vitamin D occurs in a limited number of foods. Fatty fish and fish oils, eggs, butter, and vitamin D fortified milk and margarine are the best food sources, **8-7**.

Effects of Vitamin D Deficiencies and Excesses

Rickets was once a common childhood disease. **Rickets** is a deficiency disease in children caused by lack of vitamin D. Without adequate vitamin D, not enough calcium is deposited in the bones. This causes the bones to be soft and misshapen. The leg bones may bow in or out. The chest bones may bulge outward. The disease is now rare in the United States. It may occur where infants do not receive vitamin D supplements with breast milk or formula. Children who receive little exposure to sunlight, or who live in smog-filled urban areas, are at greater risk for vitamin D deficiency.

A similar vitamin D deficiency disease in adults is called **osteomalacia.** It can cause the leg and spine bones to soften and bend. Osteomalacia is different from *osteoporosis*, which is a bone condition due to a calcium deficiency that affects older adults.

Too much vitamin D can be poisonous and toxicity occurs most quickly in children. Too much sun exposure does not cause vitamin D toxicity. Getting an excessive amount of vitamin D from food would be difficult. Therefore, toxic intakes are usually the result of consuming supplements in amounts greater than the UL. The UL for vitamin D is 100 micrograms per day for anyone over eight years old.

Excessive amounts of vitamin D cause too much calcium to be absorbed into the bloodstream. This surplus calcium is then deposited in the kidneys and other soft organs. This causes the organs to become hard and unable to perform their vital functions.

Vitamin E

Vitamin E may be the most advertised vitamin. Salespeople boost its popularity by making dramatic claims about its benefits. They have promoted vitamin E as an aid for enhancing athletic performance and reducing the signs of aging. However, research does not support such claims.

Functions of Vitamin E

Vitamin E helps maintain healthy immune and nervous systems. However, the main function of vitamin E in your body is as an antioxidant. **Antioxidants** are substances that react with oxygen to protect other substances from harmful effects of oxygen exposure. Vitamin C

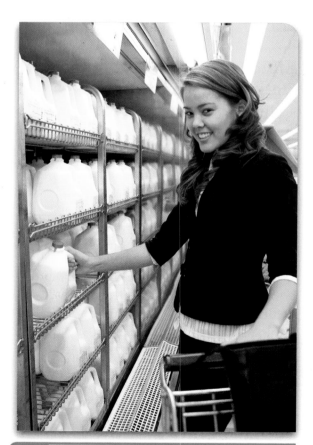

8-7 Fortified milk is an excellent source of vitamin D.

Math Link

Subtracting Micrograms from Grams

When weighing small amounts using the metric system, weights are expressed in units called grams (g). Prefixes are used to identify units less than one gram. For example, the prefix micro (μ) means millionth. Therefore, one microgram is equal to one millionth of a gram. Other prefixes include
  milli (m)—one thousandth
  centi (c)—one hundredth
  deci (d)—one tenth
* Subtract 900 micrograms from 7 grams.

and provitamin A are also antioxidants. As an antioxidant, vitamin E ties up oxygen that could damage the membranes of white and red blood cells. It also protects the cells of the lungs.

Oxygen usually occurs as two oxygen molecules bonded together. When bound together, they are stable. However, when a single oxygen molecule is present, it is highly reactive. This molecule wants to react with other compounds as quickly as possible. Such a highly reactive, unstable single oxygen molecule is called a **free radical**. Free radicals regularly form in the body due to ordinary cell processes and environmental conditions. These single oxygen molecules can generate a harmful chain reaction that can damage tissue.

Vitamin E and other antioxidants help deactivate or transform free radicals. If vitamin E does not step in, tissue damage can lead to disease.

Meeting Vitamin E Needs

The RDA for vitamin E is 15 milligrams per day for males and females over the age of 14. Research provides no strong support for consuming large amounts of vitamin E. There is also no support for taking vitamin E supplements instead of getting it from food sources.

A varied diet includes many sources of vitamin E. The best sources are vegetable oils, some fruits and vegetables, and margarine. Wheat germ, multigrain cereals, and nuts are also good sources, **8-8**.

High temperatures destroy vitamin E. Therefore, foods that are prepared or processed with high heat lose their vitamin E value.

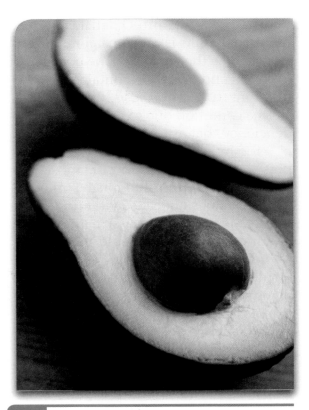

8-8   Avocados are rich sources of vitamin E.

Effects of Vitamin E Deficiencies and Excesses

Because sources of vitamin E are widespread in the diet, deficiencies are not common. However, deficiencies have been seen in premature babies. This is because babies store vitamin E during the last few weeks of their mothers' pregnancies. If babies are born prematurely, they do not have vitamin E stores. These deficiencies cause red blood cells to break, a condition called **erythrocyte hemolysis**, which makes the babies weak and listless. Premature babies almost always receive a vitamin E supplement when they are born to prevent these problems. Vitamin E deficiency in adults negatively affects speech, vision, and muscle coordination.

Vitamin E is less toxic than other fat-soluble vitamins. However, large doses have caused digestive problems and nausea. Excessive amounts of vitamin E may interfere with blood clotting. The UL for 14- to 18-year-olds is 800 milligrams per day.

Vitamin K

Facing surgery is difficult for many people. Bleeding injuries, such as those caused by cuts and wounds, can also become serious. However, if you must face these difficult situations, you will be glad for the action of vitamin K.

Functions of Vitamin K

The main function of vitamin K is to make proteins needed in the coagulation of blood. **Coagulation** means clotting. This is the process that stops bleeding. Vitamin K is also needed to make a protein that helps bones collect the minerals they need for strength.

Meeting Vitamin K Needs

The need for vitamin K increases throughout childhood, the teen years, and young adulthood. For 14- to 18-year-old males and females, the AI for vitamin K is 75 micrograms per day.

Bacteria in the intestinal tract help meet a significant part of your vitamin K needs. These bacteria can synthesize vitamin K.

A varied diet will help you meet the rest of your vitamin K needs. Good food sources of vitamin K include green leafy vegetables and liver. Fruits, milk, meat, eggs, and grain products also supply small amounts of this vitamin.

Effects of Vitamin K Deficiencies and Excesses

There are few cases of vitamin K deficiency. However, a deficiency can occur among people who take antibiotics that kill intestinal bacteria. Newborns can also be at risk for vitamin K deficiency. This is because they do not yet have enough bacteria in their intestines to synthesize the vitamin. Newborns almost always receive a vitamin K supplement, **8-9**. This helps meet their needs until bacteria in their intestines can begin producing enough vitamin K.

Although vitamin K can be toxic, toxicity is rare. A symptom of toxicity is *jaundice*, which is a yellow coloring of the skin. Vitamin K toxicity can cause brain damage. There is no UL established for vitamin K at this time.

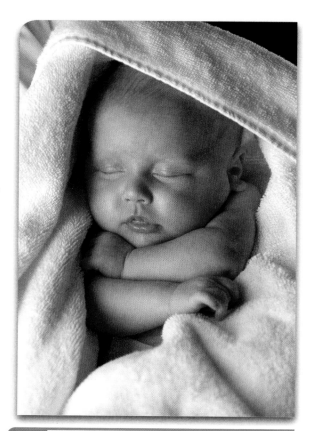

8-9   Newborns may lack vitamin K because they have not yet developed the intestinal bacteria that make it.

The Water-Soluble Vitamins at Work

The water-soluble vitamins include all the B vitamins and vitamin C. Lean tissues may store surpluses of these vitamins for short periods. However, excesses are generally excreted in the urine. Therefore, the accepted recommendation is that you include them in your diet every day.

The Teamwork of B Vitamins

The B vitamins are thiamin, riboflavin, niacin, pantothenic acid, biotin, B_6, folate, and B_{12}. These vitamins work as a team. They are all parts of coenzymes.

A **coenzyme** is a nonprotein compound that combines with an inactive enzyme to form an active enzyme system. Think of an inactive enzyme as a car without wheels. The vitamin coenzyme is like the wheels. When you put the wheels on the car, the car can move. Just as a car does not work without wheels, an inactive enzyme does not work without the vitamin coenzyme.

The metabolism of energy nutrients is one critical area requiring the joint action of enzymes and coenzymes. Without coenzymes, the enzymes that release energy from carbohydrates, fats, and proteins could not do their jobs. As parts of the coenzymes, the B vitamins help provide the energy needed by every cell in the body.

The B vitamins are found in many of the same food sources. Therefore, deficiency symptoms are often due to a shortage of several vitamins rather than a single vitamin. Deficiencies of B vitamins can cause a broad range of symptoms. These symptoms include nausea and loss of weight and appetite. Severe exhaustion, irritability, depression, and forgetfulness may also occur. The heart, skin, and immune system may be affected, too.

Besides their roles as a group, each of the B vitamins has individual functions. These will be discussed in the following sections.

Thiamin

Thiamin was named for its molecular structure. *Thi-* means "sulfur," which is one of the elements in a thiamin molecule.

Functions of Thiamin

Thiamin plays a vital role in energy metabolism. It is also required for normal functioning of the nerves and the muscles they control.

Meeting Thiamin Needs

The more calories you burn, the more thiamin you need. Teens who are 14- to 18-years-old have fairly high daily calorie needs. The thiamin RDA that corresponds with these needs is 1.2 milligrams per day for males. The RDA for females is 1.0 milligrams per day.

Whole-grain breads and cereals are sources of thiamin as well as several other B vitamins, **8-10**. Refined-grain products are commonly enriched with these vitamins and iron. **Enriched foods** have had vitamins and minerals added back that were lost in the refining process. Enriched foods can be important sources of nutrients.

Other foods that are good sources of thiamin include pork products, dried beans, nuts, seeds, and liver. Because the body does not store much thiamin, you need to consume thiamin-rich foods daily.

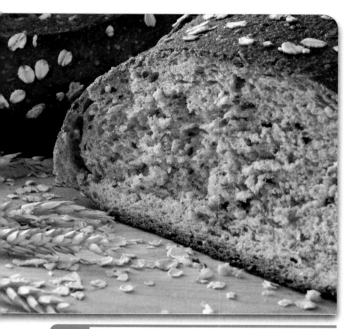

8-10 Enriched and whole-grain breads and cereals are good sources of several B vitamins.

Effects of Thiamin Deficiencies and Excesses

Beriberi is the thiamin deficiency disease. *Beriberi* means "I can't, I can't." Without enough thiamin, the body cannot perform the tasks required for everyday living. Symptoms include weakness, loss of appetite, and irritability. Poor arm and leg coordination and a nervous tingling throughout the body are also symptoms of thiamin deficiency. Some people develop edema and heart failure. Edema is an excess accumulation of fluid.

The disease of alcoholism increases the risk of thiamin deficiency because alcohol diminishes the body's ability to absorb and use thiamin. A diet in which a large percentage of calories comes from alcohol also lacks calories from nutritious food sources.

Symptoms of thiamin toxicity have not been identified. However, nutrition experts state there is no health benefit in consuming thiamin at levels higher than the RDA. The UL for thiamin has not been established.

Riboflavin

The word riboflavin comes from the yellow color of this vitamin compound. *Flavus* means "yellow" in Latin.

Functions of Riboflavin

Riboflavin helps the body release energy from carbohydrates, fats, and proteins. You also need it for healthy skin and normal eyesight.

Meeting Riboflavin Needs

Daily riboflavin needs for males 14 years and older is 1.3 milligrams per day. The RDA for 14- to 18-year-old females is 1.0 milligrams per day, but increases to 1.1 milligrams per day for 19 years and older. Milk and milk products are excellent food sources for meeting these needs, **8-11**. Enriched and whole-grain cereals, meats, poultry, and fish are also good sources of riboflavin.

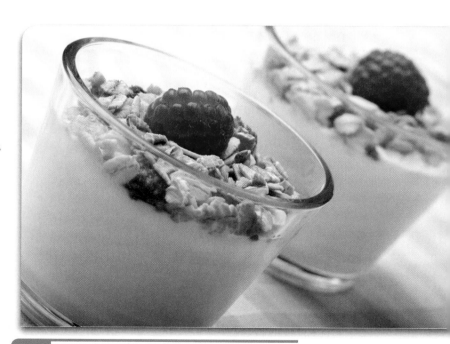

8-11 Yogurt, like other dairy products, is a source of riboflavin.

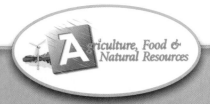

Biochemist

Biochemists study the chemical composition of living things. They analyze the complex chemical combinations and reactions involved in metabolism, reproduction, and growth. Many conduct further research to understand the effects of foods, drugs, serums, hormones, and other substances on tissues and vital processes of living organisms.

Education: Most biochemists need a Ph.D. (doctorate) in biology to work in independent research or development positions. Other positions are available to those with a master's or bachelor's degree in the field.

Job Outlook: Employment for biochemists is expected to increase much faster than the average for all occupations, although there will continue to be competition for some basic research positions.

Healthy people who eat a nutritious diet generally get enough riboflavin. People who do not drink milk or eat milk products may be at risk for developing a deficiency.

Effects of Riboflavin Deficiencies and Excesses

Many symptoms are associated with riboflavin deficiency. They include an inflamed tongue and cracked skin around the corners of the mouth. Various eye disorders and mental confusion are symptoms, too.

Toxicity symptoms have not been reported. Established ULs have not been set. Extra riboflavin is excreted in the urine.

Niacin

There are several types of niacin. These include *nicotinic acid* and *nicotinamide*. All types of niacin are water-soluble.

Functions of Niacin

Like the other B vitamins, niacin is involved in energy metabolism. It also helps keep the skin and nervous system healthy. It promotes normal digestion, too.

Meeting Niacin Needs

Niacin in foods is available as a preformed vitamin. It is also available in a provitamin form—tryptophan, which is one of the amino acids in many protein foods.

The RDA for niacin is stated in terms of *niacin equivalents (NE)*. This unit accounts for both the provitamin and preformed forms of niacin. Males in the 14- to 18-year age range need the equivalent of 16 milligrams of niacin daily. Females in this age range need the equivalent of 14 milligrams.

Whole-grain and enriched breads and cereals, meat, poultry, and nuts are popular sources of niacin, **8-12**. Tryptophan is found in protein foods, such as meats and dairy products.

Effects of Niacin Deficiencies and Excesses

Pellagra is the niacin deficiency disease. The symptoms of pellagra are often known as the *four Ds*. These symptoms are diarrhea, dermatitis (dry, flaky skin), dementia (insanity), and death. Early disease symptoms include poor appetite, weight loss, and weakness.

Niacin can be toxic when too much is consumed through supplements. Toxicity is characterized by dilated blood vessels near the surface of the skin. The resulting painful rash is sometimes called *niacin flush*. Nausea, dizziness, and low blood pressure are also symptoms of too much niacin. Tolerable Upper Intake Level for 14- to 18-year-olds is 30 milligrams daily.

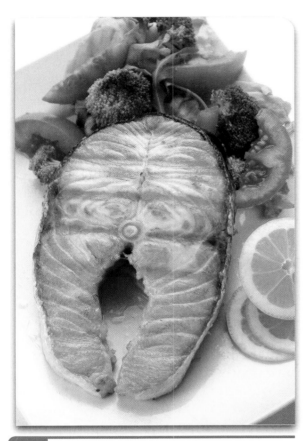

8-12   Salmon is an excellent source of niacin.

Pantothenic Acid

Pantothenic acid is another B-complex vitamin. It gets its name from the Greek word *pantothen*, which means "from all sides." This name seems appropriate because pantothenic acid is found in all living tissues.

Functions of Pantothenic Acid

Pantothenic acid promotes growth. It is part of a coenzyme that is critical to the metabolism of the energy nutrients. It is also involved in synthesizing a number of vital substances in the body.

Meeting Pantothenic Acid Needs

Studies on pantothenic acid have not produced enough conclusive data to set an RDA. Therefore, an AI has been established as a guide for intake. For people ages 14 years and older, the AI for pantothenic acid is 5 milligrams per day.

Effects of Pantothenic Acid Deficiencies and Excesses

Pantothenic acid is found in many food sources. Therefore, deficiency symptoms are rarely a problem. Toxicity is also rare and no UL has been established for this vitamin.

Biotin

Biotin gets its name from the Greek word for "sustenance," which means something that helps support life.

Functions of Biotin

Biotin helps activate several enzymes involved in the release of energy from carbohydrates, fats, and proteins. Biotin also helps the body make fats and glycogen.

Meeting Biotin Needs

Like pantothenic acid, there is no RDA for biotin. The AI for males and females ages 14- to 18-years-old is 25 micrograms per day.

Biotin is widespread in foods. Egg yolks, yeast, beans, nuts, cheese, and liver are especially good sources, **8-13**.

Effects of Biotin Deficiencies and Excesses

Because biotin is widely available in foods, deficiencies among people who eat nutritious diets are uncommon. A biotin deficiency produces similar symptoms of the circulatory and muscular systems as a thiamin deficiency. These symptoms include abnormal heart rhythms, pain, weakness, fatigue, and depression. Nausea; loss of appetite; dry, scaly skin; and hair loss are other symptoms.

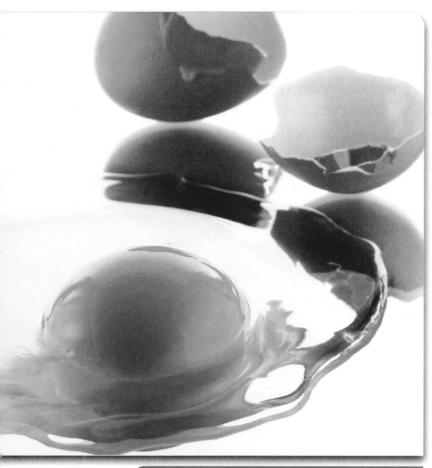

8-13   Egg yolks are a good source of biotin.

Nutrition researchers have found no evidence of biotin toxicity. Although there may be no health risk, there are no advantages to biotin intakes above the recommended range.

Vitamin B₆

The diet must supply only 9 of the 20 amino acids that make up proteins. This is because the body can make sufficient amounts of the other 11 amino acids. However, the body could not do this without the help of vitamin B_6.

Functions of Vitamin B₆

Vitamin B_6 plays a key role in synthesizing dispensable amino acids. It is needed to convert the amino acid tryptophan to niacin. Vitamin B_6 helps make the protein that allows red blood cells to carry oxygen. It also affects the health of the immune and nervous systems.

Meeting Vitamin B₆ Needs

The RDA for vitamin B_6 for males ages 14 through 50 is 1.3 milligrams per day. Females ages 14 to 18 need 1.2 milligrams per day. Needs increase to 1.3 milligrams daily for adult females through age 50. Vitamin B_6 needs increase for people of both sexes after age 50.

Vitamin B_6 is found in meats, fish, and poultry. Dairy products and some fruits and vegetables, such as bananas, cantaloupe, broccoli, and spinach, are also good sources.

Effects of Vitamin B₆ Deficiencies and Excesses

Vitamin B_6 deficiencies are rare. Symptoms of vitamin B_6 deficiencies are related to poor amino acid and protein metabolism. Symptoms include skin disorders, fatigue, irritability, and convulsions.

People who have taken large doses of vitamin B_6 have reported symptoms of toxicity. The UL is set at 80 milligrams per day for 14- to 18-year-olds. These symptoms include walking difficulties and numbness in the hands and feet. Irreversible nerve damage can also result from excessive intakes of this vitamin.

Folate

Folate, which was also called *folacin* in the past, is another B vitamin. The term *folate* is derived from the Latin word *folium*, which means "leaf." This is a logical name because leafy green vegetables are good sources of folate. *Folic acid* is a synthetic form of this vitamin found in nutrient supplements and fortified foods.

Functions of Folate

The main function of folate is to help synthesize DNA, the genetic material in every cell. Without folate, cells cannot divide to form new cells.

Another function of folate is especially important to any woman of childbearing age. Women who have inadequate folate intakes are more likely to give birth to babies with *neural tube damage*. Such damage affects the brain and spinal cord and can cause mental retardation, paralysis, and premature death.

Meeting Folate Needs

The RDA for folate is 400 micrograms per day for everyone age 14 and over. Pregnancy increases folate needs. Pregnant women need 600 micrograms of folate daily.

Dark green, leafy vegetables are excellent sources of folate. Liver, legumes, oranges, cantaloupe, and broccoli are also good sources. In addition, most enriched breads, flours, and other grain products are fortified with folic acid.

Meeting daily folate recommendations is especially important for women of childbearing age. This is because neural tube damage occurs during the first weeks of pregnancy, before many women realize they are pregnant. Fully meeting folate requirements before becoming pregnant reduces a woman's risk of having a baby with neural tube damage.

Research confirms that folic acid from fortified foods and supplements reduces the risk of neural tube damage. Researchers do not know if the folate that occurs naturally in foods has the same preventive effect. Therefore, health care providers recommend all

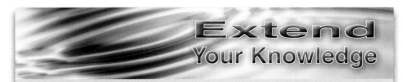

Alcohol's Effect on Vitamins

How does excessive use of alcohol affect nutrient absorption? When people consume large amounts of alcohol—especially in the case of alcoholics—appetite suppression often occurs. Poor eating habits and greater alcohol consumption tend to go hand-in-hand. In addition to taking in fewer nutrients, alcohol can interfere with the way the body absorbs nutrients, especially vitamins. For example, alcohol interferes with the way the body metabolizes and absorbs folacin, vitamin A, and vitamin B_{12}.

women of childbearing age consume 400 micrograms of folic acid daily from supplements or fortified foods. Eating a nutritious diet will provide additional folate from foods, **8-14**.

Effects of Folate Deficiencies and Excesses

You have already read about the increased risks of neural tube damage due to folate deficiency in pregnant women. Additional complications during pregnancy may include spontaneous miscarriage or the placenta separating from the uterus before delivery. Other population groups can also be affected by folate deficiencies.

Folate deficiencies are not uncommon. They usually result from low intakes of folate. Several medications, such as aspirin and oral contraceptives, can interfere with the body's ability to use folate.

The first signs of a folate deficiency appear in the red blood cells. Without sufficient folate, the red blood cells are fragile and cannot mature and carry oxygen. With a reduced number of mature red blood cells, a person feels tired and weak. Other symptoms of a

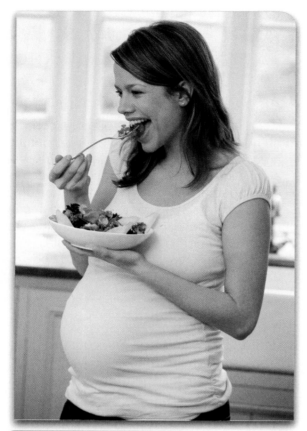

8-14   Women should be sure to meet their folate needs before and during pregnancy to help prevent neural tube damage in their babies.

folate deficiency include diarrhea and increased risk of infection.

Little information is available about folate toxicity. However, large intakes of folate can conceal symptoms of a vitamin B_{12} deficiency. This reduces the likelihood the vitamin B_{12} deficiency would be diagnosed and treated. Irreparable nerve damage could result. The UL for 14- to 18-year-olds is 800 micrograms of folate per day.

Vitamin B_{12}

Vitamin B_{12} is a chemical compound that contains cobalt. That is why the vitamin is sometimes called *cyanocobalamin.*

Functions of Vitamin B_{12}

Vitamin B_{12} helps folate function. It is needed for growth, maintenance of healthy nerve tissue, and formation of normal red blood cells. It also is needed for the release of energy from fat.

Meeting Vitamin B_{12} Needs

The RDA for vitamin B_{12} for males and females ages 14 and over is 2.4 micrograms per day. People who eat foods from animal sources easily meet these needs. Meat, poultry, fish, eggs, and dairy products are all good sources. Vitamin B_{12} does not naturally occur in foods from plant sources, **8-15**.

Effects of Vitamin B_{12} Deficiencies and Excesses

Pernicious anemia, the deficiency disease associated with vitamin B_{12}, is actually caused by an inability to absorb the vitamin. Impaired absorption is due to the lack of a compound made in the stomach. An injury or a rare genetic disorder can cause the stomach to stop producing this important compound. As people grow older,

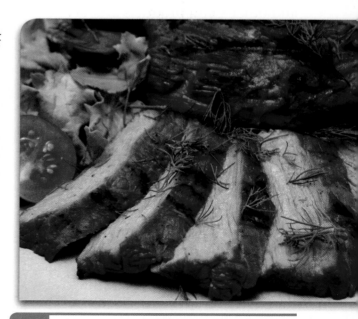

8-15   Meat and other animal foods are good sources of vitamin B_{12}.

they may lose their ability to make this compound. Pernicious anemia prevents red blood cells from maturing and dividing properly. This causes a person to feel tired and weak.

Symptoms of pernicious anemia also include a red, painful tongue and a tingling or burning in the skin. Nerve damage can eventually lead to walking difficulties and paralysis. Nerve damage can cause memory loss and mental slowness, too.

Fortunately, pernicious anemia can be treated. Injections of vitamin B_{12} periodically, perhaps throughout life, will allow red blood cells to mature normally. (The vitamin must be injected due to the body's inability to absorb a supplement taken by mouth.) With vitamin B_{12} present, the insulation remaining around nerve cells will be maintained. However, nerve damage that occurred before the deficiency was diagnosed usually cannot be reversed.

People who eat animal foods and can absorb vitamin B_{12} are unlikely to develop deficiencies. Strict vegetarians, who eat no animal products, must include alternative sources of vitamin B_{12} in their diets. Such sources might be vitamin supplements and fortified soy milk. Older adults are also at risk for developing pernicious anemia. Regular blood tests can help identify those people who need vitamin B_{12} injections.

The body can maintain long-term stores of vitamin B_{12}. However, no toxicity symptoms are known. There is no reported Tolerable Upper Intake Level.

Vitamin C

Vitamin C is often referred to as *ascorbic acid*. Long before this vitamin was identified, sailors who went on lengthy voyages often developed the deadly disease scurvy. In a search for

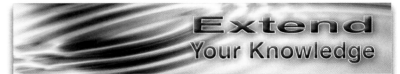

Marketing Vitamin Supplements

Claims made about vitamin pills can be confusing. Some advertisements claim the product is "all-natural." Others target certain groups such as chewable, grape-flavored vitamin supplements for children; performance vitamins for athletes; or vitamin supplements "designed just for women."

Compare the amounts of each vitamin listed on the labels to the DRIs for the various consumer groups being targeted. Include the same information for a generic multivitamin supplement. Note the price for each vitamin supplement. Organize your findings in a chart. Write a paragraph explaining your opinion whether the vitamin supplements with special claims are worth any difference in price.

a cure, a British doctor, James Lind, carried out the first nutrition experiment using human subjects. He added different substances to the diets of each of several groups of sailors with scurvy. Lind found those sailors who ate citrus fruits were cured.

Nutritionists now know it was the vitamin C in the citrus fruits that helped cure the disease. **Scurvy** has been correctly identified as a disease caused by vitamin C deficiency.

Functions of Vitamin C

Vitamin C performs a number of important functions in the body. It assists in the formation of collagen. **Collagen** is a protein substance in the connective tissue that holds cells together. Collagen is needed for healthy bones, cartilage, muscles, and blood vessels. Collagen helps wounds heal quickly. It also helps maintain capillaries and gums.

Vitamin C increases iron and calcium absorption. It plays a role in synthesizing thyroxine, the hormone that controls basal metabolic rate. Vitamin C is also vital to the body's immune system.

Vitamin C is an antioxidant. It works with vitamin E to protect body cells from free radicals. Some experts believe this may allow vitamin C to help prevent some cell damage. This may include the cell damage that leads to the development of some cancers, cataracts, and heart disease.

Meeting Vitamin C Needs

The RDA for vitamin C for males ages 14 to 18 is 75 milligrams per day. After age 19, it increases to 90 milligrams per day. For females ages 14 to 18, the RDA is 65 milligrams per day. After age 19, it increases to 75 milligrams per day. The body does not store vitamin C, so a daily intake is necessary.

People exposed to tobacco smoke need extra vitamin C. The exposure to smoke results in increased free radicals in the body. More vitamin C is needed to function as an antioxidant and protect cells from the free radicals. Smokers and anyone exposed to smoke should include an extra 35 milligrams of vitamin C in their daily diets.

Vitamin C is found in many fruits and vegetables. Fruits rich in vitamin C include citrus fruits, cantaloupe, and strawberries, **8-16**. Good vegetable sources include sweet peppers, broccoli, cabbage, and potatoes.

Effects of Vitamin C Deficiencies and Excesses

Most people in the United States meet their daily needs for vitamin C through diet. However, low intakes of vitamin C are not unusual among older adults. As a group, they tend to eat diets that contain fewer fruits and vegetables.

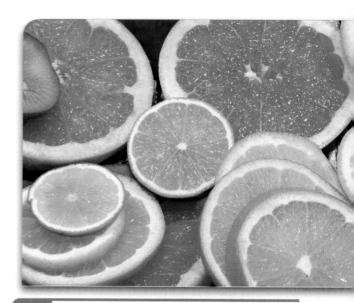

8-16   Citrus fruits and juices are excellent sources of vitamin C.

What happens if there is inadequate vitamin C in the diet? Scurvy is the most severe form of vitamin C deficiency. It rarely occurs in developed countries because the causes and cure of the disease are known. In poorer countries where diets are inadequate, however, scurvy is not uncommon.

The symptoms of scurvy are many. They include tiredness, weakness, shortness of breath, aching bones and muscles, swollen and bleeding gums, and lack of appetite. Wounds heal slowly. The skin can become rough and covered with tiny red spots. The marks are small patches of bleeding just under the skin that appear as capillaries break.

The UL for Vitamin C is set at 1800 milligrams per day for 14- to 18-year-olds. Some extra vitamin C may not be harmful. Most excess vitamin C is excreted. However, large doses of one to three grams (1,000 to 3,000 milligrams) have had reported side effects. People taking large doses have complained of nausea, diarrhea, and stomach cramps. Large doses may also reduce the ability of vitamin B_{12} to function.

Many people believe that taking extra vitamin C can prevent or cure the common cold. Current research does not support this claim. However, adequate amounts of vitamin C do help protect the body against infections.

Nonvitamins and Other Nonnutrients

A number of substances have been discovered to have vitaminlike qualities. Examples include *choline* and *inositol,* which play roles in energy metabolism similar to B vitamins. These compounds are active in the body. However, research has not shown them to be vital for human life. Therefore, they are not currently regarded as vitamins. Future studies may lead researchers to add some of these substances to the list of essential nutrients.

Other compounds sometimes labeled as vitamins include *laetrile* (sometimes called vitamin B_{17}) and *pangamic acid* (sometimes called vitamin B_{15}). These substances have no vitamin value for humans. Some people use these compounds to treat diseases for which the compounds have not been proven effective. This may keep these people from seeking reliable medical care.

Health food fans promote the benefits of dietary supplements such as melatonin and ephedrine. Like the nonvitamins just described, many of these substances are active in the body. However, they are not essential to human nutrition. Therefore, they may be viewed as nonnutrients. Although these nonnutrients may be advertised and sold, claims made for many of them are unproven. Some of them have caused harmful reactions.

Case Study: A Pill to Cure Janet's Cold?

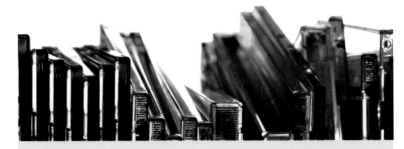

Janet and LaTisha were at the mall shopping. Janet had just spent the last of her money in the food court on French fries and a soft drink. Janet has been feeling like she is coming down with a cold. She asks LaTisha if she could borrow some money to buy some vitamin C supplements and cough drops containing vitamin C at the nutrition store in the mall. Janet believes the extra vitamin C will help her avoid a cold.

Case Review

1. If you were LaTisha, would you loan Janet the money to purchase the vitamin C supplement? Why?

2. Why do you think people buy and use vitamin supplements?

Phytochemicals

Although some nonnutrient substances seem to be of little value, scientific studies document the benefits of others. Among the helpful nonnutrients are some **phytochemicals**. These are health-enhancing compounds in plant foods that are active in the body's cells. Plants make hundreds of phytochemicals to protect themselves against such factors as ultraviolet light, oxidation, and insects. Scientists have just begun to learn about the useful roles some of these compounds play in the human body.

One major group of phytochemicals is *flavonoids*, also known as *polyphenols*. The flavonoids contribute a strong antioxidant effect. Green tea, extra virgin olive oil, and pomegranates are good sources of flavonoids.

Research has shown flavonoids and other phytochemicals may help prevent heart disease and some forms of cancer. They achieve this preventive effect through various chemical reactions in the body. Prompting the body to make enzymes, binding harmful substances, and acting as antioxidants are among the ways phytochemicals work.

Currently there are no recommendations for intake of phytochemicals. More research is needed. Studies citing the value of certain phytochemicals have led many nutrition faddists to buy phytochemical supplements. Research has not proven these supplements to be safe and effective. The combinations of phytochemicals and nutrients found in foods cannot be duplicated in a supplement. Therefore, supplements cannot perform the same way foods can.

Eating a variety of plant foods in a rainbow of colors is the best way to include phytochemicals in your diet. Include a variety of fruits, vegetables, herbs, spices, legumes, and whole grains to maximize phytochemicals in your diet, **8-17**.

Phytochemicals	
Classes	**Major Food Sources***
Carotenoids	Pumpkin (canned), carrot juice (canned), spinach (cooked), sweet potato (baked), pumpkin (cooked), papaya, tomato paste, watermelon, spinach (frozen, cooked), kale (frozen, cooked)
Chlorophyll Chlorophyllin	Spinach (raw), parsley (raw)
Curcumin	Tumeric
Fiber	Legumes, cereals, grains, fruits, vegetables, nuts, seeds
Flavonoids	Red, blue, and purple berries; red and purple grapes; teas; chocolate; citrus fruits; yellow onions; kale; broccoli; apples; parsley; thyme; hot peppers; soybeans; legumes
Garlic (Organosulfur compounds)	Garlic, onions
Indole-3-Carbinol	Broccoli, Brussels sprouts, cabbage, cauliflower
Isothiocyanates	Broccoli, Brussels sprouts, cabbage, horseradish, mustard, radish
Lignans	Flaxseeds, sesame seeds
Phytosterols	Wheat germ, sesame oil, corn oil
Resveratrol	Red grape juice, peanuts
Soy Isoflavones	Soybeans, tofu
*Lists are not all inclusive.	

8-17 Food rich in phytochemicals can improve health and decrease risks for certain diseases.

Probiotics and Prebiotics

Probiotics are known as the "good" microorganisms found in foods that offer health benefits when eaten in sufficient amounts. These good microorganisms help to counterbalance the "bad" microorganisms in your intestinal tract. The evidence is not clear for all people. For some people, there is evidence that probiotics help boost the immune system. For others, bowel regularity may be helped. Evidence must be gathered to support other health claims, such as the possibility of lowering cholesterol. Yogurt is promoted as containing probiotics. Probiotics found in food are considered safe for healthy people.

Prebiotics are the nondigestible food ingredients that stimulate the growth of good microorganisms in the colon. Prebiotics can be found in foods such as whole grains, onions, bananas, garlic, honey, leeks, and artichokes.

Both probiotics and prebiotics are present naturally in some foods and beverages. They can also be added through fortifying foods and beverages or as dietary supplements. The health benefits result from the improved environment that results in the gastrointestinal tract (GI). If you think of the probiotic as a sunflower seed, the prebiotic is the water and plant food that is needed for the seed to flourish and become a flower. Foods high in probiotics and prebiotics are considered functional foods because they are promoted as having added beneficial health effects.

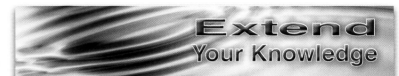

Tracking Down Probiotics

Visit a supermarket and find as many foods as you can that contain probiotics. Note the name of the food, any health claims are listed on the label, and its price per serving. Compare the cost per serving with a similar food that does not contain a probiotic. Report results of your survey.

Are Vitamin Supplements Needed?

In the United States, people spend billions of dollars on vitamin supplements each year. Why? Is it necessary? Many people worry their diets are lacking in vitamins. Their schedules are busy and they may not take time to eat nutritiously. Others are convinced they have more energy when they take a vitamin pill. However, these people may feel stronger or more energetic due to the placebo effect. The **placebo effect** is a change in a person's condition that is not a result of treatment given, but of the individual's belief that the treatment is working. The individual's expectation and belief cause the change in condition rather than the pill.

Those who sell vitamin supplements have profited from consumer concerns about health and nutrition. They promote numerous benefits of taking vitamin supplements to persuade people to spend more money. Contrary to some advertisements, vitamins are not "miracle cures" for everything from acne to AIDS. Vitamins cannot pep you up when you are feeling tired and run-down. They do not make you strong, attractive, or more popular. Supplements do not make up for poor eating habits, either. The only symptoms a vitamin supplement relieves are those caused by a lack of that vitamin. For example, a thiamin supplement relieves the symptoms of beriberi.

Some groups of people may need supplements to augment the vitamins provided by their diets. Doctors may advise pregnant and breast-feeding women to take supplements, 8-18. Doctors may recommend supplements for infants, older adults, and patients who are ill or recovering from surgery. Doctors also occasionally prescribe large doses of vitamins for pharmaceutical purposes. For instance, large doses of vitamin A are sometimes prescribed for their drug effects in treating a particular eye disease. Few

people outside these groups need vitamin supplements. A diet including the recommended servings from all the food groups supplies most people with the vitamins they need.

People who decide to use supplements have a number of choices available. They may choose products in pill, liquid, or powder form. They may also choose between natural and synthetic vitamins. *Natural vitamins* are extracted from foods. *Synthetic vitamins* are made in a laboratory. Advertisers may claim natural vitamins are superior. Chemically speaking, there is no advantage of a natural vitamin over a synthetic vitamin. The body uses both types of vitamins the same way. However, synthetic vitamins are less expensive and are usually purer than natural vitamins.

People who choose to use supplements should also be aware that some supplements provide large doses of vitamins. Amounts may be many times higher than the recommended daily levels. You know vitamins have specific functions and only very small amounts are needed for good health.

The Food and Drug Administration (FDA) regulates the sale of vitamin supplements. They require scientific research to back up health claims made on product labels or in advertising. However, the FDA has little authority to regulate the amounts of vitamins supplements contain.

Taking more vitamin supplements than needed can cause health problems. The body can store toxic levels of fat-soluble vitamins. Excess water-soluble vitamins are normally excreted in the urine. However, large doses of some water-soluble vitamins produce negative effects for some people. For instance, too much vitamin C in the diet can irritate the gastrointestinal system. Also, an excess of one nutrient may affect how the body uses other nutrients.

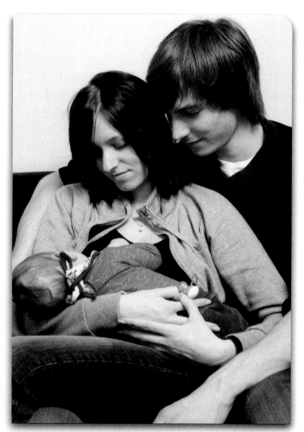

8-18   Doctors often recommend vitamin supplements for breast-feeding women to help meet the extra needs caused by producing milk.

Preserving Vitamins in Foods

Eating vitamin-rich foods should ensure you are meeting your body's need for vitamins. Right? Wrong! Many vitamins are unstable. Careless food storage can destroy some vitamins. Cooking techniques can affect vitamin retention, too. In this section, you will learn how to select foods high in vitamins. You will also learn how to preserve the vitamins that are present in foods.

Selecting Foods High in Vitamins

Modern processing methods minimize nutrient losses. Therefore, canned, frozen, and dried foods are comparable to fresh in terms of vitamin content. Choose the form that is most convenient for you. However, be aware of products that contain large amounts of added fat, sugar, and sodium. Read Nutrition Facts panels to help you choose foods that are rich in nutrients.

Knowing signs of quality can help you avoid foods that may have suffered excessive vitamin losses. When buying fresh fruits and vegetables, choose items that have bright colors and firm textures, **8-19**. Avoid pieces with wilted leaves, mold growth, or bruised spots. When selecting canned products, do not buy cans that are dented or bulging. These signs may indicate a broken seal and possible contamination of the food. Choose foods from the freezer case that are firmly frozen. Avoid frozen foods that have a layer of ice on the package. This indicates the food may not have been stored at a constant low temperature. Partial thawing can result in

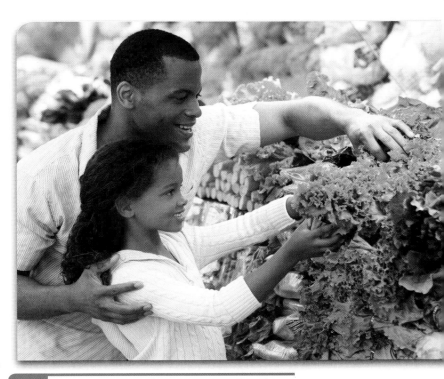

8-19   Buying fresh foods and eating them soon after they are purchased will help you get maximum vitamin value.

nutrient losses and a general decrease in quality. When buying dried foods, look for packages that are securely sealed.

Storing Foods for Vitamin Retention

The way you handle food can affect its nutritional value. Exposing foods to air, light, and heat during transportation and storage causes vitamin losses. If fresh foods are not properly stored, they may have fewer vitamins than frozen or canned foods.

The following suggestions help to minimize nutrient losses during handling and storing of food:

- Keep freezer temperatures at zero degrees or lower to retain vitamin content of frozen foods. Try to use frozen foods within several months. Avoid thawing and refreezing foods, which causes some vitamin losses.

- Store canned foods in a cool, dry storage area. The liquid in which foods are canned contains nutrients. Serve the canning liquid with the food or use it in cooking.
- Store milk in opaque containers to protect its riboflavin content. Riboflavin is destroyed by light.
- Ripen fresh fruits and vegetables at room temperature away from direct sunlight.
- Store fresh vegetables promptly in a vegetable crisper in the refrigerator. The low temperature and high humidity of the crisper help preserve the vitamins in the vegetables.
- When storing cut foods, be sure to wrap them tightly. This prevents vitamins from being destroyed by oxidation. Storing foods promptly in the refrigerator reduces the action of enzymes that can break down vitamins.

Preparing Foods to Preserve Vitamins

Water, heat, acids, and alkalis used in cooking can all destroy vitamins. Knowing how vitamins respond to different cooking methods can help you preserve vitamins when preparing foods. The following guidelines may be helpful:

- To preserve water-soluble vitamins, do not soak fruits or vegetables in water. Instead, rinse fresh foods with water before cutting and serving. If foods are to be peeled, wash the food before peeling.
- Many vitamins are located just under the skin of fresh produce. Therefore, avoid paring and peeling fruits and vegetables, if possible.
- Keep foods in large pieces to avoid exposing large amounts of surface area to light, air, and water.

- Cut up fruits and vegetables just before you are ready to cook or eat them, **8-20**. This reduces air and light exposure, which can damage vitamins.
- Choose steaming over boiling to help retain water-soluble vitamins. If you do boil vegetables, do not add them to cooking water until the water begins to boil. Use only a small amount of water and cook the vegetables just until tender. Avoid adding baking soda, which is an alkali, to vegetables. It can destroy some vitamins. Use cooking water in soups, gravies, or sauces.
- Use a pressure cooker or microwave oven to help preserve nutrients by reducing cooking times.

In general, keep cooking times short and use little water. Overcooking destroys heat-sensitive vitamins. Water-soluble vitamins leach into cooking water.

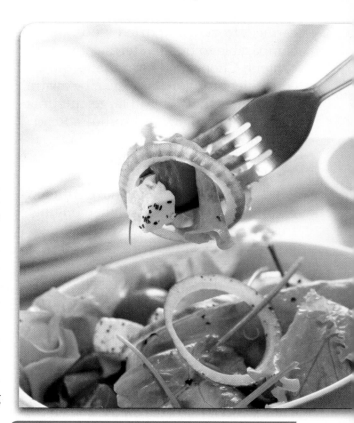

8-20   Prepare salads as close to serving time as possible to avoid exposing vitamins to air and light for long periods.

Reading Summary

Vitamins are essential nutrients. No one food supplies all the vitamins needed. Choosing a variety of foods is likely to supply all the vitamins most people need.

Vitamins perform a number of major roles in the body. They are needed to release energy from carbohydrates, fats, and proteins. They help maintain healthy body tissues. They are required for the normal operation of all body processes. They also help the body's immune system resist infection.

The fat-soluble vitamins are vitamins A, D, E, and K. They dissolve in fats and are found in foods containing fats. Fat-soluble vitamins can be stored in body tissues to toxic levels.

The water-soluble vitamins include the B vitamins (thiamin, riboflavin, niacin, pantothenic acid, biotin, vitamin B_6, folate, and vitamin B_{12}) and vitamin C. Excess water-soluble vitamins are generally lost through the urine. However, large doses of some water-soluble vitamin supplements, especially niacin and vitamins B_6 and C, can produce toxic symptoms.

Substances have been discovered that have vitaminlike qualities, but have not been proven to be vital to human life. Groups of phytochemicals found in foods are active beneficially at the cellular level and work to help prevent disease. Probiotics and prebiotics work together and yield health benefits when eaten in sufficient amounts.

Doctors may advise extra vitamin supplements for some people with special health or dietary needs. However, most people who use vitamin supplements should choose those that provide no more than the RDA or AI for each vitamin. Most nutritionists agree foods are the preferred source of vitamins.

Storing and preparing foods carefully helps preserve vitamins. Avoid exposing foods to excess heat, light, water, and alkalis, all of which can destroy vitamins. Cooking with low temperatures for short periods using a small amount of water also saves vitamins.

Review Learning

1. List five basic functions vitamins assist within the body.
2. True or false. Most vitamins have several active forms, which have similar molecular structures.
3. What are two main causes of vitamin deficiency diseases?
4. List three differences between fat-soluble vitamins and water-soluble vitamins.
5. What form of vitamin A is provided by plant foods?
6. Why do some people not need vitamin D in their diets?
7. What is the main function of vitamin E in the body?
8. What is the main function of vitamin K in the body?
9. Name three deficiency symptoms shared by all the B-complex vitamins.
10. What is the name of the thiamin deficiency disease?
11. List three food sources of riboflavin.
12. True or false. Because niacin is water-soluble, it cannot build up to toxic levels in the body.
13. What is the RDA for pantothenic acid?
14. Why is adequate folate intake especially important to women of childbearing age?

15. What group of people has an increased need for vitamin C and why?
16. List two ways phytochemicals help prevent heart disease and some cancers.
17. Name three groups of people for whom doctors might recommend vitamin supplements.
18. What is the difference between the sources of natural vitamins and the sources of synthetic vitamins?
19. Give three tips for selecting foods high in vitamins.
20. List five ways to prevent vitamin losses when storing and preparing foods.

Critical Thinking

21. **Draw conclusions.** Continuing research has identified additional functions of Vitamin D. Draw conclusions about why you think many people are deficient in this vitamin. What might be some long-term effects of this deficiency?
22. **Determine credibility.** When you hear an advertisement about supplements, how can you tell if the information is credible? What sources can you use to verify data?

Applying Your Knowledge

23. **Vitamin poster.** Create a poster or bulletin board showing foods that are good sources for each of the vitamins. Organize the foods under headings for fat-soluble and water-soluble vitamins. Incorporate the message that eating a variety of foods is the best way to obtain all the vitamins you need each day.
24. **Food diary.** Examine how well your diet meets vitamin needs. Complete a food diary listing all the foods you eat for a three-day period. Find diet analysis software online and use it to analyze your vitamin intake for each day. Which vitamin needs have you met and which are low? Identify foods you could add to your diet to increase intakes of needed vitamins.
25. **Vitamin research.** Visit a health food store to find a "vitamin" supplement that was not discussed in the chapter such as vitamin P or coenzyme Q10. Write to the manufacturer requesting evidence to support claims made on the product label or in advertising. Share your findings in class.
26. **Antioxidant poster.** Prepare a poster showing pictures of foods high in antioxidants. Include a summary of the roles antioxidants play in maintaining good health. Display the poster in your school cafeteria.

Technology Connections

27. **Internet research.** Use the Internet to research the relationship of vitamin K to successful surgery outcomes. Prepare a summary of current medical thinking on how to prepare for surgery to avoid excessive bleeding during and after surgery.
28. **Vitamin bingo.** Find a printable bingo card game Web page to prepare a "Know Your Vitamins" bingo game. Include words on the card that are listed on the key terms at the beginning of the chapter. Add others as you find them in the chapter (carotene, dietary supplement). Use legume seeds as markers.

29. **Vitamin spreadsheet.** Use spreadsheet software to prepare a chart of vitamins. Headings on the chart should include Vitamin Name, Functions, Deficiency Symptoms, Toxicity Symptoms, RDA/AI, UL, and Common Food Sources.

30. **Electronic brochure.** Use desktop publishing software to prepare a brochure about foods commonly served on the school lunch menu that are good sources of phytochemicals. Explain the benefits of phytochemicals in the diet. Obtain permission to distribute the brochure in your school cafeteria.

31. **Electronic puzzle.** Using an Internet to locate the *Discovery Education* Web site. Use the "puzzlemaker" to create a fruits and vegetable word search. Include as many different kinds of fruits and vegetables that you have tasted or would like to taste. Exchange word searches with classmates to find solutions.

Academic Connections

32. **Science.** Draw a flowchart of pictures describing how healthy human cells change to cancerous cells. Include a description of how the oxidation plays a role.

33. **Speech.** In small groups, debate the following topic: "Use the rainbow as a guide for choosing a healthy food plan." Support or refute the position that choosing colorful foods are enough for guiding the selection of a nutritious food plan.

34. **Science.** Research how free radicals form in the body and how antioxidants may prevent free radical damage. Identify common sources of free radicals and antioxidants. Use presentation software to prepare an electronic presentation. Be sure to include diagrams and sketches to explain the damage that can occur as a result of free radical activity. Share your findings with the class.

35. **History.** Research the history of food fortification practices. Write a paper summarizing when each practice began, which foods are commonly fortified with vitamins and phytochemicals, and the pros and cons of this practice. Include your opinion about food fortification.

Workplace Applications

Interpreting Information

The ability to read and interpret information in context is an important workplace skill. Presume you work for a food manufacturer who typically fortifies its products with vitamins B and C. The company is considering adding vitamin D to some products, but wants you to evaluate and interpret some research on the additional need for vitamin D in the body. You will need to locate at least three reliable sources of information. Read and interpret the information on vitamin D. Then write a report summarizing your findings.

Chapter 9

Minerals: Regulators of Body Functions

Reading for Meaning

Before you read the chapter, read all of the chart and photo captions. What do you know about the material covered in this chapter just from reading the captions?

Concept Organizer

Use the fishbone diagram to identify the macrominerals. Identify details about functions, sources, and effects of deficiencies and excesses.

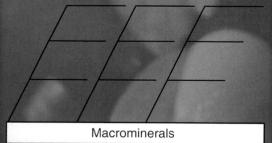

Macrominerals

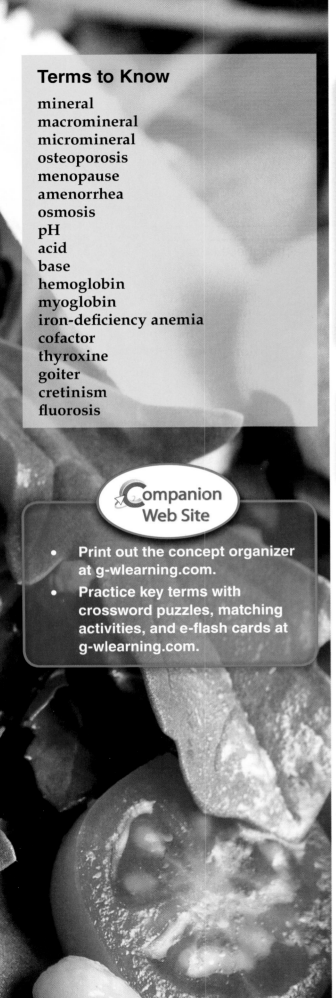

Terms to Know

mineral
macromineral
micromineral
osteoporosis
menopause
amenorrhea
osmosis
pH
acid
base
hemoglobin
myoglobin
iron-deficiency anemia
cofactor
thyroxine
goiter
cretinism
fluorosis

Companion Web Site

- **Print out the concept organizer at g-wlearning.com.**
- **Practice key terms with crossword puzzles, matching activities, and e-flash cards at g-wlearning.com.**

Objectives

After studying this chapter, you will be able to

- **recall** the major roles of minerals in the diet.
- **identify** functions and sources of specific macrominerals and microminerals.
- **recall** symptoms of various mineral deficiencies and excesses.
- **explain** the relationship between calcium intake and bone health.
- **outline** guidelines for maximizing mineral absorption and availability in the body.

Central Ideas

- Minerals are essential for regulating body processes.
- Whole foods are likely better sources of minerals than highly processed foods.

Like vitamins, **minerals** are nutrients needed in small amounts to perform various functions in the body. Also like vitamins, minerals provide no calories. Vitamins are organic compounds. This means they are made of different elements bonded together, and one of the elements is carbon. In contrast, minerals are *inorganic elements*. This means they are not compounds, and they do not contain carbon.

Minerals in nutrition are the same as those listed on the periodic table of elements found in most chemistry classrooms. Nutritionists know a number of minerals, including calcium, phosphorus, zinc, and iron, are vital to good health. However, they are still studying the roles and functions of other minerals, such as tin, lead, and lithium. This chapter will discuss the minerals most researchers believe to be essential in the diet, **9-1**.

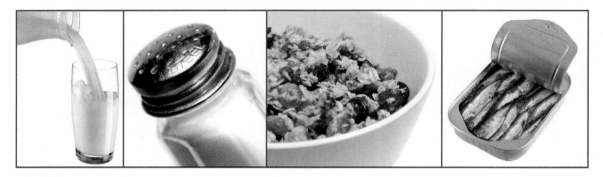

9-1 Can you identify the minerals that are in each of these foods?

How Minerals Are Classified

At least 21 mineral elements are currently known to be essential to good health. Dietary Reference Intakes have been established for 15 of the minerals. These minerals can be classified into two major groups. The first group is **macrominerals**, which are also called *major minerals*. These are minerals required in the diet in amounts of 100 or more milligrams per day. The second group is **microminerals**, or *trace minerals*. These are minerals required in amounts of less than 100 milligrams per day. Microminerals are just as important for health as macrominerals. The biological function of the *ultratrace minerals* in humans remains unclear. More research may show their increased importance for maintaining good health, **9-2**.

All the minerals in your body combined make up only about four percent of your body mass. Although your mineral needs are small, meeting those needs is critical to good health. Minerals serve a variety of complex functions which include
- helping enzymes complete chemical reactions
- becoming part of body components
- aiding normal nerve functioning and muscle contraction

Classification of Minerals		
Macrominerals (Major Minerals)	**Microminerals (Trace Minerals)**	**Other Microminerals (Ultratrace)**
Calcium	Iron	Arsenic
Phosphorus	Zinc	Boron
Magnesium	Iodine	Nickel
Sulfur	Fluoride	Silicon
Sodium	Selenium	Vanadium
Potassium	Copper	
Chloride	Chromium	
	Manganese	
	Molybdenum	

9-2 Minerals are classified as macrominerals or microminerals based on the amount that is recommended every day for good health.

- promoting growth
- regulating acid-base balance in the body
- maintaining body fluid balance

Studying key minerals will help you understand their specific, individual functions.

The Macrominerals at Work

The macrominerals include calcium, phosphorus, magnesium, sulfur, sodium, potassium, and chloride. Each of these minerals serves specific functions in the body. Learning about food sources and daily needs will help you plan diets rich in minerals.

Calcium

The macromineral found in the largest amount in the body is calcium. Calcium represents about two percent of body weight. This means the body of a 150-pound person contains about 3 pounds of calcium.

You may have heard a parent say to a child, "Drink your milk." There is good reason for parents to be concerned about their children's dairy intake. Milk, cheese, and other dairy products are great sources of calcium for people of all ages, **9-3**. Informed parents know how important calcium is for normal growth.

Functions of Calcium

Nearly all the calcium in your body is stored in your bones. Calcium from your diet is absorbed from your small intestine into your bloodstream. The blood then carries the calcium to your bones. Bones are always being rebuilt. Calcium in the blood is added to and removed from bones as needed

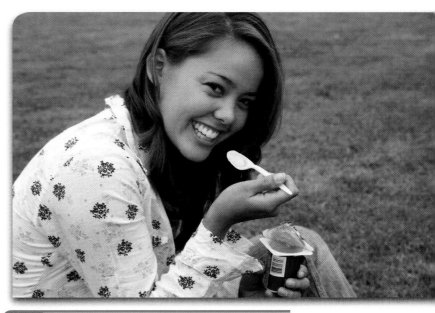

9-3   Yogurt, like milk and other dairy products, is a good source of calcium.

throughout life. The calcium that is in the bloodstream must be maintained within a very narrow range. This balance is essential so that calcium is available for the many important jobs it performs in the body.

Calcium from your food intake is deposited in your bones to build and strengthen them. This process builds bone mass. Bone mass refers to the extent to which the bone tissue is filled up with minerals. Bone tissue at the ends of long bones looks something

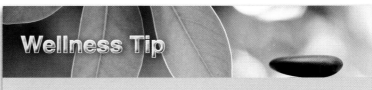

Wellness Tip

Support Bone Health—Limit Soft Drinks

Recent research shows that teens today consume more carbonated soft drinks than milk. Daily consumption of these beverages (high in phosphoric acid) can put teens at greater risk of bone fracture, especially teen females. To protect your bone health, limit soft drinks to special occasions and consume milk and other calcium-rich foods to support bone health.

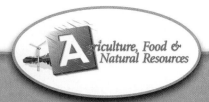

Soil Scientist

Soil scientists study how soils help plants grow. They also study the responses of various soil types to fertilizers, tillage practices, and crop rotation. Many soil scientists conduct soil surveys, classifying and mapping soils. They provide information and recommendations to farmers and other landowners about the best use of land and plants to avoid or correct problems, such as erosion. They work to ensure environmental quality and effective land use.

Education: Most jobs in soil science require a bachelor's degree, but a master's or Ph.D. (doctoral) degree is usually required for university research positions. Soil scientists take courses including plant pathology, soil chemistry, entomology, plant physiology, and biochemistry.

Job Outlook: Job growth among soil scientists should be faster than average for all occupations. They also will be needed to balance increased agricultural output with protection and preservation of soil, water, and ecosystems.

like a sponge covered by a shell layer. Healthy bone tissue is dense. The cells of the sponge are small, and the walls of the cells are thick. The shell layer is hard. When sufficient calcium is available for bone building, you are more likely to achieve your full growth potential. Peak bone mass occurs in the late 20s or early 30s when bone development ends. In a similar way, calcium is used to build strong teeth.

Many people associate calcium with bones and teeth. They often overlook the fact that a tiny amount of calcium is found in every cell of the body. This calcium plays many vital roles. It helps muscles contract and relax, and assists in blood-clotting processes. Calcium also helps transmit nerve impulses. These roles are so important that if there is insufficient calcium in the diet, the body takes the calcium from the bone to ensure these functions continue.

Amount of Calcium Needed

The Recommended Dietary Allowance (RDA) for calcium for males and females ages 14 through 18 is 1,300 milligrams per day. After age 19, the recommended amount decreases to 1,000 milligrams per day. The RDA increases again for women over age 50 and men over age 70.

Adequate calcium intake coupled with physical activity is particularly important during the preteen, teen, and early adult years. During this stage, your body requires more calcium to build bones to keep up with your body as it grows. Weight-bearing exercise helps build strong, dense bones.

Many teens and young adults fail to recognize the importance of eating good sources of calcium. Including adequate amounts of calcium in your diet at this stage protects your bone health in the future. One study reported only 15 percent of 12- to 16-year-old females met their daily need for calcium. Males in this age group fared better with 53 percent meeting their need for calcium.

Teenage males may get more calcium than teenage females simply because the males eat more food. Many teen women limit their food intake to lose weight. Some consume less than 300 milligrams of calcium per day. Individuals who are restricting calories should remember there are foods that are low in calories and rich in calcium.

Sources of Calcium

Foods found in MyPlate's dairy group are your primary source of calcium. Consuming the recommended daily amounts will help you meet your calcium needs.

Relying on the dairy group may be difficult for people who are lactose intolerant. However, they still have a number of options for meeting their calcium needs. They can add the enzyme lactase to fluid milk to aid digestion. Some people experience digestive problems with milk, but may tolerate cheese and yogurt as calcium sources. These products often contain much less lactose than milk. They can also choose calcium-rich foods from other food groups.

People on low-calorie food plans sometimes avoid dairy products thinking they are too high in fat and calories. If you are restricting calories, consider choosing fat-free milk and yogurt, reduced-fat cheese, and other low-fat or nonfat dairy products. These foods are good sources of calcium and low in fat and calories.

A variety of nondairy foods supply calcium. Leafy green vegetables, legumes, and sardines eaten with the bones all provide calcium. Some foods are processed with added calcium. For instance, orange juice is sometimes fortified with calcium, making it a good mineral source. Read food labels to identify calcium-fortified products, **9-4**.

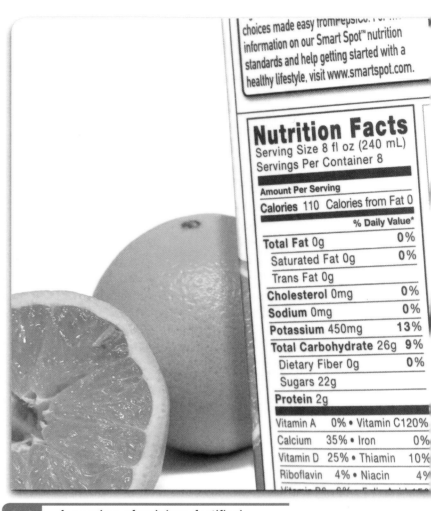

9-4   A serving of calcium-fortified orange juice may provide as much calcium as a serving of milk.

Effects of Calcium Deficiencies and Excesses

Cells get the calcium they need from a supply found in the blood. Your life depends on the maintenance of normal blood calcium levels at all times. If your diet is calcium deficient, your blood pulls calcium from your bones. When bones lose calcium, they become less dense. The cells of the tissue become larger and the walls of the cells become thinner. The outer layer of the bone becomes brittle.

Calcium deficiencies are more likely to occur when the body's need for calcium is high. People have greater demands for calcium during certain stages of the lifecycle. For example, infants and adolescents are in peak growth periods. Their calcium needs are high because their bones and teeth are developing. If their calcium needs are not met, their bones and teeth may not develop normally. Pregnant and breast-feeding women need calcium to meet their babies' needs in addition to their own. If these women do not consume enough calcium, the calcium stored in their bones is used.

People who fail to eat a calcium-rich diet through their young adult years do not reach maximum bone mass. This increases their risk of problems due to bone loss later in life. Conversely, people who achieve a higher bone density in their youth are less likely to experience problems as they age. To illustrate this point, think about a bone that lacks mass as a toothpick. Think about a bone that has reached maximum mass as a 2-inch by 4-inch board. Suppose both "bones" lose the same amount of calcium. The one that started out as a toothpick is much more likely to break. By age 40, many people begin to gradually lose bone density if they are inactive and consume too little calcium. Smoking and alcohol in excess can contribute to decreased bone mass and should be avoided at any age.

A gradual loss of bone mass that continues for many years may lead to **osteoporosis**. Osteoporosis is a condition that results when bones become porous and fragile due to a loss of calcium. The signs of this bone loss usually appear only after many years as the bones become fragile and lose their strength.

With the older adult, breaks of wrist and hip bones are frequently the result of osteoporosis. A loss of mineral density and mass causes the bones to be less strong. Tooth loss may occur due to weakening of the jaw bone. Bones in the spinal area can compress, causing height to decrease by several inches, **9-5**.

Osteoporosis affects more than half the female population age 60 and older. Although osteoporosis occurs

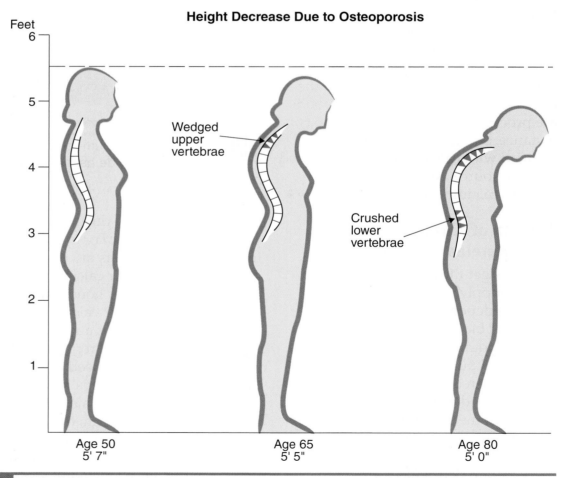

Height Decrease Due to Osteoporosis

Feet

Wedged upper vertebrae

Crushed lower vertebrae

Age 50
5' 7"

Age 65
5' 5"

Age 80
5' 0"

9-5   Compression of bones in the spinal column due to osteoporosis results in a decrease in height.

most often in women, it can occur in men as well. Women are at greater risk for osteoporosis for several reasons. First, their bones are smaller and loss of mass makes the bones more fragile at an earlier age. Pregnancy and breast-feeding place extra demands on the calcium stored in their bones. Women also have a longer life expectancy than men and, therefore, have more time to experience bone mass losses.

Hormonal changes are another factor that places women at greater risk of osteoporosis than men. At around age 50, women go through menopause. **Menopause** is the time of life when menstruation ends due to a decrease in production of the hormone estrogen. Among other functions, estrogen plays a role in maintaining bone tissue. Therefore, bone density loss occurs more rapidly in women after menopause due to the drop in estrogen levels.

Middle-aged women are not the only ones at risk of bone losses due to hormonal changes. A number of teenage and young adult women develop **amenorrhea**. This means they stop having menstrual periods. This condition is fairly common among females who have eating disorders. It also occurs among female athletes who exercise excessively. The hormonal changes caused by amenorrhea are just like those that occur during menopause. They have the same effect on bone tissue, causing a loss of bone mass that can lead to osteoporosis.

Genetics and body frame size also play a role in bone health. Some people have greater bone density than others. These individuals may have built more bone density when they were young or inherited a family trait for greater bone density.

You should note that a loss of bone mass is not necessarily age related. It is largely related to diet and exercise.

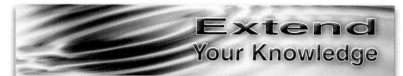

Boning Up on Bones

The number of people with osteoporosis is increasing in the United States primarily due to an aging population. The main goal of treating people with this disease is preventing fractures. Along with a diet containing foods rich in calcium and vitamin D, some doctors prescribe medications. These medications are designed to reduce bone loss and increase bone density especially in the hip and spine. Many of these drugs belong to a group of drugs called *bisphosphonates*. People who take such drugs should ask their doctors about the side effects and the risk of a rare type of fracture in the thigh bone associated with some drugs. What other treatments are available for osteoporosis? Research such reliable Web sites as the National Institutes of Health and the Centers for Disease Control for more information.

People who eat calcium-rich diets and engage in weight-bearing exercise do not lose much bone mass as they age. On the other hand, even teens can lose bone mass if they follow extreme diet and exercise practices. Excess sweating that occurs with athletes, can lead to calcium losses. Low calcium intakes compound these problems.

The good news is that people who have lost bone mass can restore it—at least partly. Calcium supplementation and exercise can help to replace lost bone mass.

Although low calcium intakes are fairly common, calcium excesses from dietary sources are relatively rare. Excesses are generally the result of taking too many supplements. Possible problems from excess calcium intake include kidney stones, constipation, and gas.

Eating an energy-balanced diet that is rich in calcium can protect bones and teeth. Moderate exercise that places weight on the bones can also help keep bones dense and strong over a lifetime. Lifestyle choices of physical activity to reduce bone loss include walking, dancing, and jogging, **9-6**. The effects of bone loss will depend partly on the amount of calcium you store in your bones now.

Calcium Supplements

One out of two women will face osteoporosis at some point in their lives. With the common problem of poor calcium intake and the effects of inactivity, you may wonder about the value of calcium supplements. Calcium

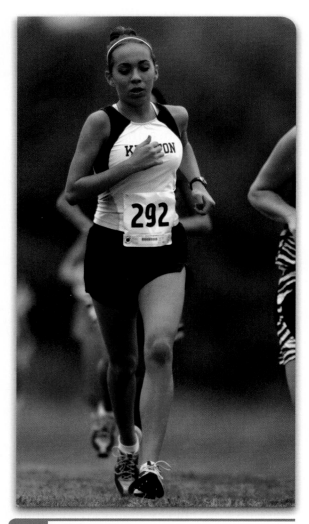

9-6   Weight-bearing exercise, such as running, helps increase bone density.

supplements can benefit some people, especially those who cannot consume dairy products.

A number of types of calcium supplements are available. The body can absorb some types better than others. For instance, compounds of concentrated calcium, such as calcium carbonate, calcium phosphate, and calcium citrate are the best choices. Supplements made from powdered calcium-containing materials, such as bones and oyster shells, are not recommended. They may contain contaminants, such as lead or other impurities. People (usually older adults) who produce little stomach acid, should take supplements with meals. This is so any acid produced during digestion can aid calcium absorption.

Calcium supplements help reduce the risk of osteoporosis. Along with this advantage, taking calcium supplements can have some disadvantages. Calcium supplements can also hinder the absorption of some other nutrients, such as iron and zinc. Most nutritionists agree getting calcium from food sources is preferred to using supplements.

Phosphorus

Phosphorus is the mineral found in the second largest amount in the body. It makes up one to one and one-half percent of your body weight. Phosphorus and calcium together represent more than half of all the mineral weight in your body.

Functions of Phosphorus

Phosphorus works with calcium to help form strong bones and teeth. It helps maintain an acid-base balance in the blood. It is part of ATP (adenosine triphosphate), which is the source of immediate energy found in muscle tissue. Phosphorus is also in cell membranes and is part of some enzymes. Like calcium, it is part of every cell.

Meeting Phosphorus Needs

The Recommended Dietary Allowance (RDA) for phosphorus for males and females ages 14 through 18 is 1,250 milligrams daily. Phosphorus is easily found in the diet and is absorbed efficiently. Therefore, typical U.S. diets supply adequate amounts of phosphorus.

Phosphorus is found in protein-rich foods including milk, cheese, meats, legumes, and eggs. Peas, potatoes, raisins, and avocados are good sources, too. Baked products, chocolate, and carbonated soft drinks are also sources of phosphorus.

Effects of Phosphorus Deficiencies and Excesses

Phosphorus deficiencies are virtually unknown. However, too much phosphorus in the diet can hinder the absorption of other minerals. For example, excess phosphorus can reduce calcium absorption and utilization, and contribute to bone loss.

The typical diet of a U.S. teen contains roughly two to four times more phosphorus than calcium. A high protein diet combined with additives found in baked goods and other processed foods increases the chances of calcium-phosphorous imbalance. Carbonated soft drinks with phosphoric acid are a high source of phosphorous, **9-7**. Teens who replace milk with soft drinks may have insufficient intakes of calcium and vitamin D. Such a diet greatly increases the risk of less than optimal bone density. Researches have noted that the imbalance can cause calcium to be drawn from the bone into the blood to neutralize the acidic effect of

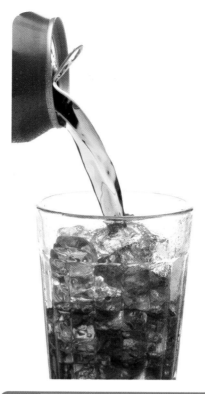

9-7   An excess of carbonated soft drinks may contribute to decreased bone density.

phosphorus. Too much phosphorous with insufficient calcium and vitamin D are contributing factors for osteoporosis, and gum and teeth problems.

Magnesium

Like calcium and phosphorus, most of the magnesium in the body is in the bones. Additional magnesium is found in muscle tissue. However, the amount of magnesium is much smaller than the amounts of the other two minerals. The magnesium content in the body of an adult is less than two ounces.

Functions of Magnesium

Magnesium is involved in over 300 enzymatic reactions in the body. Magnesium makes the enzymes active and lets them work more efficiently. Magnesium also activates the ATP in your body so it can release energy.

Case Study: Fast-Food Choices

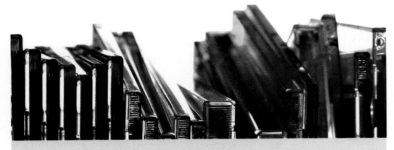

Jerry, a 16-year-old male, is at a fast-food restaurant with his friends. He has just read the chapter in his textbook about the need for calcium for strong bones and good health. Last week, he read about the importance of protein for muscle growth. He learned that milk is a source of both calcium and protein. Jerry thinks this is perfect because he loves milk shakes and ice-cream sundaes!

However, Jerry is on the wrestling team and the coach has reminded him he must make his weight category. Strong muscles and bones are important in wrestling. Jerry realizes he must pay more attention to his food choices. He wants to meet his calcium needs, but is concerned about too many calories from saturated fats. He has learned saturated fats can negatively impact weight and health. He looks at the menu to see his choices.

Case Review

1. What are several food choices commonly found on fast-food restaurant menus that will help Jerry meet his calcium and protein needs, and are also low in saturated fats?

2. Do you think Jerry should rely on fast-food restaurants to meet his daily calcium needs? Why?

It helps the lungs, nerves, and heart function properly. Magnesium is also tied to your body's use of calcium and phosphorus and therefore important for bone health.

Meeting Magnesium Needs

The RDA for magnesium is 360 milligrams per day for women ages 14 through 18 years. For men in the same age group, the RDA is 410 milligrams per day. Many people in the United States consume less than the RDA for magnesium.

Good sources of magnesium include leafy green vegetables, potatoes, legumes, seafood, nuts, dairy foods, and whole-grain products, **9-8**. Hard water, which has a high concentration of minerals, is also a source of magnesium.

Effects of Magnesium Deficiencies and Excesses

Few Americans are deficient in magnesium. The body can store magnesium, so deficiency symptoms develop slowly in most people. Magnesium deficiencies are often the result of other health problems. For instance, starvation or extended periods of vomiting or diarrhea can cause low magnesium levels. Alcohol increases magnesium excretion. Therefore, alcoholics are at an increased risk of magnesium deficiency. Deficiency symptoms include weakness, heart irregularities, disorientation, and seizures.

Too much magnesium in the blood occurs mainly when the kidneys are not working properly. Excess magnesium from food sources is not considered a health concern. However, daily intakes of over 350 milligrams of magnesium from supplements may produce toxicity symptoms in teens and adults. Lower intakes from supplements may produce toxicity symptoms in children. Magnesium toxicity can cause weakness and nausea.

Sulfur

Sulfur is present in every cell in your body. Sulfur is in high concentrations in your hair, nails, and skin. If you have ever burned your hair, you may have recognized the sulfur smell.

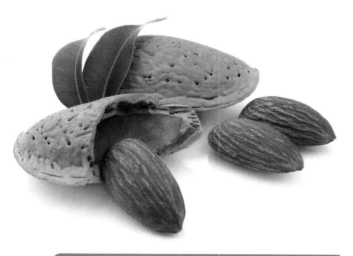

9-8 Almonds are a good source of magnesium.

Functions of Sulfur

Sulfur is part of the protein in your tissues. It is also part of the vitamins thiamin and biotin. It helps maintain a normal acid-base balance in the body. It also helps the liver change toxins into harmless substances.

Meeting Sulfur Needs

There is no RDA for sulfur. You can easily meet your sulfur needs through diet. You get sulfur from protein foods and sources of thiamin and biotin.

Effects of Sulfur Deficiencies and Excesses

Sulfur presents no known deficiency symptoms. There is no danger of toxicity associated with sulfur from food sources.

Sodium, Potassium, and Chloride

Sodium, potassium, and chloride are grouped together because they work as a team to perform similar functions. (Chloride is the form of the mineral chlorine that is found in the body.)

Functions of Sodium, Potassium, and Chloride

Water makes up a large percentage of your body weight. There is water inside every type of cell, from muscle to bone. There is also water in the spaces surrounding the cells. Most sodium is found in fluids outside the cells. Most potassium is found within the cells. Chloride is found both inside and outside cells.

If all body compartments do not contain the right amount and type of fluid, they cannot function properly. If a continuous fluid imbalance occurs, it can cause a serious medical condition and may lead to heart failure. Sodium, potassium, and chloride help regulate the fluid balance in cells and body compartments.

The membrane that encloses each cell in your body is *semipermeable*. This means water can flow freely through the membrane but particles, such as minerals, cannot.

When the mineral concentrations on each side of the membrane are different, water is drawn across the membrane. Water moves from the side with fewer particles to the side with more particles. This helps equalize the concentrations of mineral particles on each side of the membrane. This movement of water across cell membranes is known as **osmosis**, 9-9.

Pumping mechanisms help draw potassium into body cells and sodium out of body cells. This controls the flow of water in and out of cells as the water moves to balance mineral concentrations.

Controlling osmosis is not the only function of sodium, potassium, and chloride. They also play an important role in maintaining the acid-base balance in the body. The term **pH** is used to express the measure of a substance's acidity or alkalinity.

The Process of Osmosis

Side A   Side B

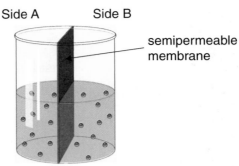

semipermeable membrane

A container is divided with a semipermeable membrane. Side A and side B contain equal amounts of an equally concentrated solution. The volume of water and the concentration of mineral particles is equal on both sides of the membrane.

Side A   Side B

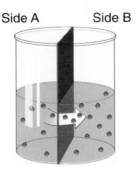

Particles are pumped across the membrane from side A to side B. The concentration of mineral particles becomes unequal.

Side A   Side B

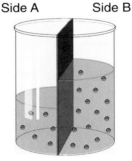

Water follows the particles across the semipermeable membrane from side A to side B to dilute the concentrated solution. The volume of water on either side of the membrane becomes unequal as the concentration of mineral particles becomes equal.

9-9   Osmosis helps balance the concentration of fluids that are inside and outside body cells.

This measure is expressed on a scale from 0 to 14. Water and other neutral substances have a pH of 7. Compounds that have a pH lower than 7 are acidic and are called **acids**. Compounds that have a pH greater than 7 are *alkaline* and are called *alkalis* or **bases**. The more acidic a solution is, the lower its pH will be. Conversely, the more basic a solution is, the higher its pH will be, **9-10**.

All body fluids must remain within a narrow pH range for essential life processes to occur. For instance, blood must maintain a near-neutral pH of 7.4. Gastric juice is a strong acid with a pH of about 1.5. Pancreatic juice, with a pH of 8,

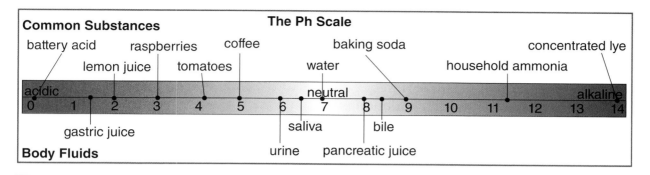

9-10   The pH of a substance represents its acidity or alkalinity. On the pH scale, an extreme acid is pH 0 and an extreme alkali is pH 14. The neutral point is 7.

is a weak base. Sodium and potassium combine with other elements to form alkaline compounds. This helps maintain the proper pH levels of body fluids by neutralizing acid-forming elements in your body. Chloride combines with other elements to form acids.

Sodium, potassium, and chloride play other important roles in the body. They aid in the transmission of nerve impulses. Potassium helps maintain a normal heartbeat. Chloride is a component of the hydrochloric acid in your stomach.

Meeting Sodium, Potassium, and Chloride Needs

The Adequate Intake (AI) of sodium for adolescents and adults is 1,500 milligrams a day. The AI for chloride for these age groups is 2,300 milligrams. For people over 50 years old, the AI is reduced to 1,300 milligrams sodium and 2,000 milligrams chloride to reduce adverse effects related to hypertension.

Sodium occurs naturally in many foods. However, the primary dietary source of both of these minerals is table salt, which is chemically known as *sodium chloride*. One teaspoon of salt equals roughly 5,000 milligrams: 2,000 milligrams of sodium and 3,000 milligrams of chloride.

Much salt in the typical U.S. diet is added to food during cooking and at the table. However, you may not realize the majority of salt in the diet comes from processed foods. Some experts estimate as much as 75 percent of sodium in the diet comes from processed foods. Salt is often added during processing to enhance flavors and preserve foods. Pickles, cured meats, canned soups, frozen dinners, and snack items are among the foods that are often high in sodium, **9-11**. Because salt contains chloride as well as sodium, foods containing added salt are also sources of chloride.

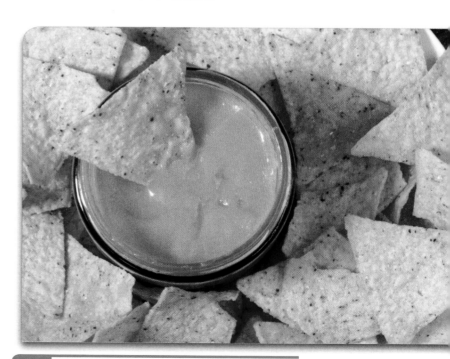

9-11   Many snack foods and condiment sauces are high in sodium.

Many people in the United States consume well over 3,000 milligrams of sodium per day. For this reason, the *Dietary Guidelines* recommend reducing daily sodium intake to less than 2,300 milligrams. The recommendation is further reduced to 1,500 milligrams for individuals who are over 51 years and those of any age who are African American or have hypertension, diabetes, or chronic kidney disease.

The Nutrition Facts panel on food labels can you identify sources of sodium in your diet. Foods are considered low in sodium if they contain less than 140 milligrams of sodium per serving.

The AI for potassium for adolescents and adults is 4,700 milligrams per day. Fresh fruits and vegetables are rich sources of potassium. Milk and many kinds of fish are also good sources.

Effects of Sodium, Potassium, and Chloride Deficiencies and Excesses

Deficiencies are rarely the result of too little sodium in the diet. More often, fluid losses, such as vomiting or diarrhea, cause a drop in the body's sodium level. The kidneys respond to these losses by increasing retention of sodium and water. A typical diet soon makes up for these sodium losses. Increased fluid intake is needed to replace missing water. Sodium deficiency can cause muscle cramps, nausea, vomiting, and perhaps even death. If a person is on a very low-calorie diet and loses body fluids through sweat, symptoms will occur.

Sodium losses through perspiration during normal exercise are usually negligible. If you lose more than three percent of body weight through perspiration, however, you may need to replace sodium. Adding salt to your food can restore your sodium needs. Some sports drinks and nutritional energy bars may contain extra sodium. There is no need to take salt tablets—you may be consuming more sodium than you lost in sweat. The additional sodium could cause stomach cramps.

The average person in the United States consumes several times the AI for sodium each day. In most healthy people, the kidneys filter excess sodium from the blood and excrete it in the urine. However, about 10 to 15 percent of the population is *sodium sensitive*. In these people, the kidneys have trouble getting rid of extra sodium.

Too much sodium in the blood can provoke hypertension in sodium-sensitive people. Someone who has hypertension has excess force on the walls of his or her arteries. Sodium draws water into blood vessels, causing the volume of blood to expand. Arteries are elastic. They stretch as blood volume expands. However, an excess of sodium causes blood volume to expand too much. This puts increased pressure on the arteries. If arteries are overstretched too much, they weaken, lose their elasticity, and may become damaged. If left untreated, hypertension can lead to heart attack or stroke.

Factors other than eating habits, including heredity, overweight, smoking, inactivity, and stress, affect the development of hypertension. You cannot prevent high blood pressure by

Math Links

Calculating Percentage

The label on a can of tomatoes states the entire contents of the can contains 525 mg sodium. The can contains 3½ servings of tomatoes.

- What percent of the AI for sodium does one serving of tomatoes contain?

reducing sodium in your diet. However, sodium-sensitive people can reduce their blood pressure by decreasing their salt intake, **9-12**. Also, the chance of becoming sodium sensitive increases with age. Therefore, experts recommend all people in the United States choose and prepare foods with less salt. Experts recommend people have their blood pressure checked yearly, too.

Potassium needs must be kept in balance for a healthy heart. Too little potassium can cause the heart to malfunction. Other symptoms of potassium deficiency include muscle cramps, loss of appetite, constipation, and confusion. Like sodium, potassium can be lost with body fluids during bouts of vomiting and diarrhea. Fluid losses that happen with the use of some high blood pressure medications can also lead to potassium deficiencies.

Due to the quantity of chloride provided by salt in the typical diet, chloride deficiencies are rare. Deficiency symptoms are similar to those for sodium and are likely to appear under the same circumstances. Excess chloride in the diet does not normally produce toxicity symptoms.

The Microminerals at Work

There are at least nine microminerals needed by the body. These include iron, zinc, iodine, fluorine, selenium, copper, chromium, manganese, and molybdenum. Several other trace minerals may also play a role in human nutrition. They include arsenic, boron, nickel, silicon, and vanadium, which currently do not have established

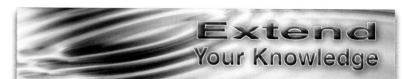

When Is DASHing Good?

DASH is the acronym for the Dietary Approaches to Stop Hypertension eating plan from the U.S. Department of Health and Human Services. To learn about the DASH eating plan, search such reliable Web sites as the National Institutes of Health or the USDA Dietary Guidelines for Americans sites. Explain the DASH guidelines and identify who would benefit from the DASH diet plan. Then plan a sample one-day menu of your own making.

Ways to Reduce Sodium in Your Diet

- Taste foods before adding salt to them during cooking or at the table.
- Use pepper, lemon juice, and herbs and spices instead of salt to flavor foods.
- Choose fresh fruits, vegetables, meats, fish, and poultry often. They generally contain less sodium than processed products.
- Check the Nutrition Facts panel on processed foods, frozen foods, and canned foods. Choose those products that provide the least amount of sodium per serving.
- Use cured and processed meats, such as hot dogs, sausage, and luncheon meats, sparingly.
- Use condiments, such as soy sauce, catsup, mustard, chili sauce, pickles, and olives, sparingly.
- Choose low- or reduced-sodium versions of foods when they are available.
- Limit use of salty snack foods.

9-12   Following these tips can help you reduce the amount of sodium in your diet.

known human needs. Trace minerals present a high risk for toxicity. A pile containing all the microminerals from your body would fit in the palm of your hand. However, these tiny amounts perform a variety of important functions.

Trace mineral research is one of the newest areas in the science of nutrition. Much of what nutritionists know about trace minerals has been identified in just the last 30 years. Many questions about trace minerals still remain. Could the average diet be low in some essential, yet unidentified mineral? Are trace minerals that occur naturally in foods removed when foods are refined and processed? Can trace mineral supplements serve as a safety net for people who fail to eat nutritious diets? Researchers will continue to seek the answers to these and other questions about how microminerals can affect wellness, **9-13**.

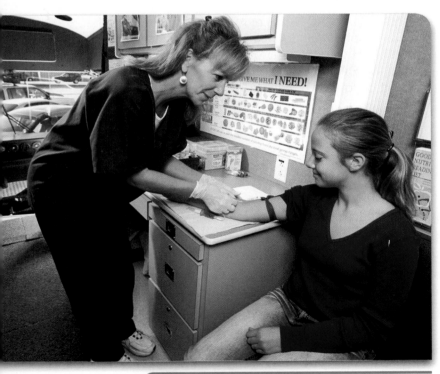

9-13   Nutrition researchers conduct studies to learn more about the roles microminerals play in the diet. *(Photo by Stephen Ausmus, ARS/USDA)*

Iron

The total amount of iron in your body is about one teaspoon. This may seem to be a trivial amount. However, iron plays a critical role in maintaining your health.

Functions of Iron

Most of the iron in your body is found in your blood. It is part of **hemoglobin**. This is a protein that helps red blood cells carry oxygen from the lungs to cells throughout the body. It is what makes blood red. Hemoglobin also carries carbon dioxide from body tissues back to the lungs for excretion.

Another iron-containing protein is **myoglobin**. This protein carries oxygen and carbon dioxide in muscle tissue.

Bone marrow stores some iron in the body, which is used to build red blood cells. The liver releases new red blood cells into the bloodstream. Red blood cells perform their oxygen delivery and carbon dioxide removal duties for three to four months before they die. Then the liver and spleen harvest the iron from the dead red blood cells. They send the iron back to the bone marrow for storage until it is recycled into new hemoglobin molecules.

Besides carrying oxygen, iron helps the body release energy from macronutrients. It is also needed to help make new cells and several compounds in the body.

Meeting Iron Needs

The RDA for iron for 14- through 18-year-old males is 11 milligrams per day. During these growth years, males have a significant increase in muscle mass. Extra iron is needed as myoglobin carries more oxygen and carbon dioxide in growing muscles. After age 19, the body is no longer growing, so the iron RDA for males drops to 8 milligrams daily. Maintaining muscle does not require as much iron as building new muscle.

Because iron is part of red blood cells, whenever blood is lost, iron is lost. Females lose blood every month through menstruation. Therefore, the RDA for iron for females ages 14 through 18 is 15 milligrams per day. Iron needs increase to 18 milligrams per day for females ages 19 to 50. Iron needs drop to 8 milligrams daily for women over 50, who are assumed postmenopausal.

Iron in foods is found in two forms—*heme* and *nonheme*. Heme iron is found in the hemoglobin and myoglobin of animal foods. Nonheme iron is found in plant and animal foods. The body can absorb heme iron more easily than nonheme iron. Vegetarians must pay attention to having adequate iron levels.

Red meat, fish and shellfish (clams, oysters), poultry, and organ meats (liver) are excellent sources of iron. Legumes, dark-green leafy vegetables, and whole grains are good iron sources, too. Many bread and cereal products are enriched with iron. Acidic foods, such as tomatoes, also become good sources when they are cooked in iron pans. The acid helps liberate some of the iron from the cookware. This liberated iron remains in the food, **9-14**. Consuming good sources of vitamin C along with iron-rich foods will increase iron absorption. This is because vitamin C helps the body absorb iron.

Milk is a very poor source of iron. This is why infant formulas and cereals are fortified with iron. The addition of iron has helped reduce the number of iron deficiencies among young children.

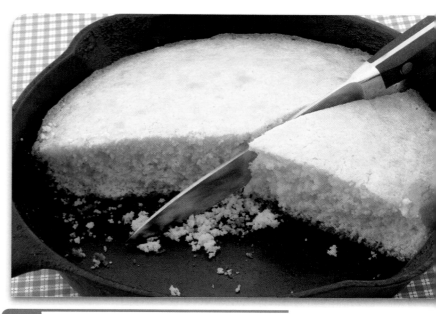

9-14   Cooking some foods in iron cookware can help increase their iron content.

Effects of Iron Deficiencies and Excesses

As the body's iron stores become depleted over time, and the food intake does not provide enough iron, an iron deficiency occurs. The body makes fewer red blood cells, and each cell contains less hemoglobin. The smaller number of red blood cells means the blood has a decreased ability to carry oxygen to body tissues. Symptoms of this condition include pale skin, fatigue, loss of appetite, and a tendency to feel cold. A person who has this condition has **iron-deficiency anemia**. This is the most common type of anemia found worldwide.

Iron-deficiency anemia is common during the teen years, especially among females. One reason for this is iron needs increase during the teenage growth spurt. In addition, females are beginning their menstrual cycles and losing iron supplies that must be replaced. Females also tend to eat less than males and, therefore, have trouble getting enough iron in their diets.

The problem of low iron stores persists into adulthood for many women. In times of illness or pregnancy, the likelihood of an iron shortage increases. Doctors advise some women to take an iron supplement to help meet their daily needs.

Some people have an inherited disorder that causes them to absorb too much iron. This results in a condition called *iron overload*. The consequent buildup of iron is toxic and can damage the liver. Iron toxicity can also result from overdoses of iron supplements. This is a leading cause of accidental poisoning among children in the United States. Besides liver damage, iron toxicity can cause infections and bloody stools.

Case Study: The Missing Nutrient

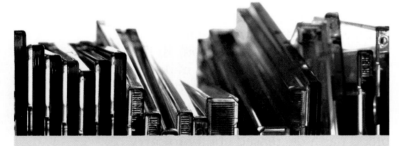

Melinda wants to lose ten pounds. She is a fast growing 15-year-old girl. Her favorite sport is basketball because she has a height advantage. One day she hopes to be a fashion model. She has decided to cut her food eating patterns in half. She avoids meats and poultry and barely eats vegetables and fruits. Eating beans and peas makes her feel fat. For several weeks she has been trying to keep up with her new eating behaviors. But today, she really feels tired, looks pale, and is irritable with her friends.

Case Review

1. What do you think might be the cause of how Melinda feels?

2. What could be going on in her body?

3. How would you convince a peer that drastic diet restrictions can have health consequences?

Zinc

Zinc is an amazing trace mineral that plays many important roles in the body. It is involved in most every physiological human function.

Functions of Zinc

Zinc serves a wide variety of functions. It aids in body growth and sexual development, **9-15**. It serves as a cofactor for many enzymes. A **cofactor** is a substance that acts with enzymes to increase enzyme activity. Zinc is also necessary for the successful healing of wounds and acid-base balance. It affects the body's storage and use of insulin. Zinc helps with the metabolism of protein and alcohol. Zinc performs an important role in the body's resistance to infections, too.

Meeting Zinc Needs

Zinc is particularly important during periods of rapid growth and sexual development. The RDA for zinc is 9 milligrams per day for females ages 14 through 18. The RDA is 8 milligrams per day for all females over age 19. The RDA for zinc for all males over age 14 is 11 milligrams per day.

A protein-rich diet, including seafood and red meats, is rich in zinc. Good plant sources include whole grains, legumes, and nuts.

Effects of Zinc Deficiencies and Excesses

A zinc deficiency will hinder a child's growth and sexual development. A number of other deficiency symptoms may appear. These include loss of appetite, reduced resistance to infections, and a decreased sense of taste and smell.

People are unlikely to get too much zinc from a nutritious diet. Excess

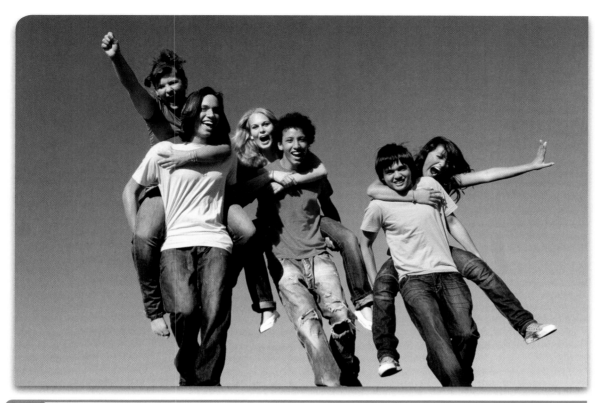

9-15 Zinc is especially important during the teen years and other periods of rapid growth.

zinc, resulting in toxicity, is most often due to the use of supplements. Zinc supplements are often used to reduce the symptoms of the common cold. There is no clear data to show they are effective. The danger is associated with excess zinc reducing the body's ability to absorb iron and copper. Large doses of zinc may impair the immune system and reduce good cholesterol (HDL) levels. Toxicity symptoms include diarrhea, nausea, vomiting, and impaired functioning of the immune system.

Iodine

The percentage of children with mental retardation and lagging growth is greater in countries where malnutrition is widespread. This is because women in these countries are often unable to obtain adequate sources of an essential mineral during pregnancy. This mineral is iodine.

Function of Iodine

Most of the iodine in your body is concentrated in one area, the thyroid gland. The thyroid produces a hormone called **thyroxine**. This hormone helps control your body's metabolism. As part of thyroxine, iodine plays a role in metabolic functions.

Meeting Iodine Needs

How much iodine do you need in your diet? The RDA is 150 micrograms per day for most people over age 14. However, many people in the United States consume more than this amount.

Iodine is present in food as the compound iodide. Lobster, shrimp, oysters, and other types of seafood are rich sources of iodide, **9-16**.

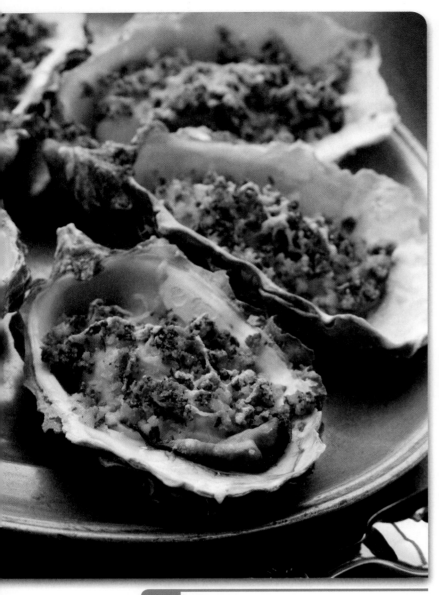

9-16   Oysters, like most seafood, are a good source of iodine.

In addition, *iodized* salt is a common source. Milk and bakery products also contain iodide, which is a result of processing.

Effects of Iodine Deficiencies and Excesses

Iodine must be available for the thyroid gland to make thyroxine. When iodine levels are low, the thyroid gland works harder to produce the hormone. This causes an enlargement of the thyroid gland called a **goiter**. Other symptoms of iodine deficiency include weight gain and slowed mental and physical response.

Fortunately, iodine deficiency is less of a problem worldwide. Iodine is more commonly added to the salt people use. If a woman's diet is iodine-deficient during pregnancy, the development of the fetus may be impaired. The child may have severe mental retardation and dwarfed physical features. This condition is called **cretinism**.

A goiter is not only a symptom of iodine deficiency; it is also a symptom of iodine excess. Iodine is toxic in large amounts.

Fluoride

Fluoride is important for strong, healthy bones and teeth. Some scientists suggest it may help prevent the onset or decrease the severity of osteoporosis. Fluoride also helps prevent tooth decay. Children who drink fluoridated water have a much lower incidence of dental caries.

The AI for fluoride is 3 milligrams per day for all females over age 14. For males ages 14 to 18, the daily recommendation for fluoride is 3 milligrams. Adult males should consume 4 milligrams per day.

Tea, seaweed, and seafood are the only significant food sources of fluoride. Fluoride occurs naturally in some water. In the United States, most people get fluoride from fluoridated water. Many communities add fluoride to their drinking water, **9-17**.

There is no evidence fluoridating water is harmful. A very high fluoride intake can cause teeth to develop a spotty discoloration called **fluorosis**.

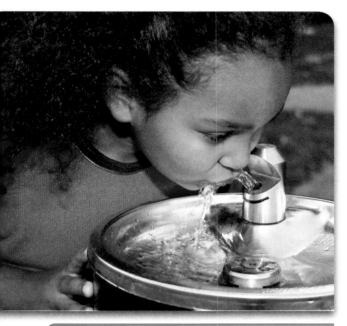

9-17 Fluoridated drinking water is a primary source of fluoride for many people in the United States.

Selenium

Selenium works with vitamin E in an antioxidant capacity. It assists an enzyme that helps reduce damage to cell membranes due to exposure to oxygen. Antioxidants have been shown to play a role in the prevention of certain cancers. However, there is no clear evidence selenium will reduce the production of cancer cells.

The RDA for selenium is 55 micrograms daily for all males and females 14 years and older. Most teens in the United States have little trouble getting this amount.

Selenium is found in meats, eggs, fish, and shellfish. Grains and vegetables grown in selenium-rich soil are also good sources of the mineral.

A deficiency of selenium causes heart disease. Too much selenium is toxic, producing such symptoms as nausea, hair loss, and nerve damage.

Other Microminerals

Several other minerals have been identified as having important roles in the body. Each has varying and specific functions. Without them, health suffers. Many of the minerals are connected to energy metabolism and the body's ability to recover after expending great amounts of energy.

The two values used for daily micromineral recommendations are based on scientific knowledge that is available at this time. When research is inconclusive, daily recommendations are given as AIs. RDAs are given when research is more conclusive.

Copper helps the body make hemoglobin and collagen. It also helps many enzymes work. The RDA for copper is 890 micrograms daily for all teens ages 14 to 18. Rich sources are organ meats, seafood, seeds, nuts, and beans, **9-18.** Deficiencies are uncommon but can result in anemia. Excesses can cause liver damage.

Chromium works with insulin in glucose metabolism. The AI for chromium is 35 micrograms daily for 14- to 18-year-old males. The AI is 24 micrograms daily for females in this age group. Chromium is found in meat, poultry, fish, and some cereals. Deficiencies lead to impaired glucose metabolism. Excesses can cause kidney failure.

Manganese helps many enzymes work. It plays a role in carbohydrate metabolism and in normal skeletal development. The AI for manganese is 2.2 milligrams for 14- to 18-year-old males and 1.6 milligrams for 14- to 18-year-old females. Excesses of this mineral can be toxic.

Molybdenum is an essential part of several enzymes. The RDA for males and females ages 14 through 18 years is 43 micrograms daily. Beans, whole

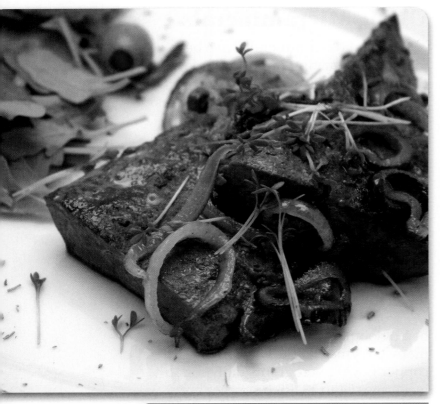

9-18   Organ meats such as liver are a rich source of copper.

grains, and nuts are good food sources. Excess molybdenum in the diet may affect the reproductive system.

Do not attempt to self-diagnose mineral deficiencies. If you have symptoms you suspect are due to a mineral deficiency, discuss them with a doctor. If he or she diagnoses a deficiency, a registered dietitian can help you evaluate your diet for good mineral sources.

Minerals and Healthful Food Choices

Information from this chapter can help you make healthful decisions about foods. You can put the facts you have read about minerals and their functions into practice at a personal level.

Mineral Values of Foods

The mineral content of plant foods depends on the soil, water, and fertilizers used to grow them, **9-19**. Thus, it is difficult to determine exactly how much of a mineral a given plant food will provide. Because animals eat plants, the mineral content of foods from animal sources is also hard to determine.

Most minerals in grains are located in the outer layers of the grain kernel. Most minerals in fruits and vegetables are located near the skin. Therefore, for maximum mineral value, choose whole grains and avoid peeling fruits and vegetables.

Generally, the most concentrated food sources of minerals are meat, fish, and poultry. Plant foods are rich in minerals, however, they provide a less concentrated source of minerals. People who eat no animal foods may be low in some minerals. They need to carefully plan their diets to include mineral-rich foods of plant origin.

Processing tends to decrease the mineral value of many foods. You are likely to find more minerals in whole foods than in processed foods. Fresh fruits and vegetables, whole grains, meat, poultry, and dairy products are rich sources of minerals. Fats, sugars, and refined flour are low in essential minerals.

Mineral Absorption and Availability

You take in minerals when you consume food and beverages. These minerals are absorbed into the bloodstream mostly through the small intestine. Your body does not absorb all the minerals you consume. In fact,

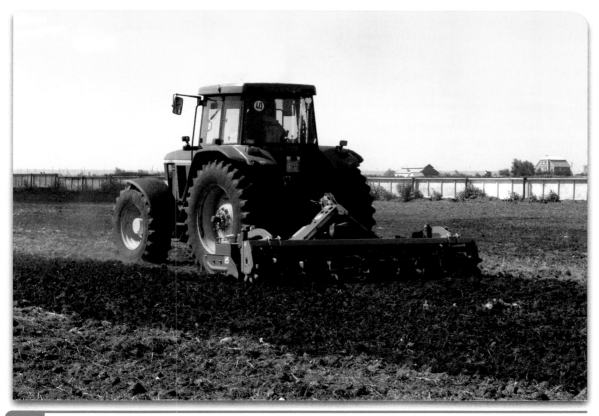

9-19   The mineral content of soil will affect the mineral content of foods grown in it.

most adults absorb less than half of the minerals they consume through food. Only the amounts of minerals your body absorbs are available to perform important functions. Unabsorbed minerals will be excreted with other body wastes.

What can you do to maximize absorption of minerals needed for growth and regulation of body processes? You should learn what dietary factors decrease and increase the availability of minerals for absorption.

Aside from being toxic, an excess of some minerals can interfere with the absorption of others. For instance, excess zinc can hinder the absorption of iron and copper. Absorption problems usually occur only when people take supplements. Therefore, avoid taking mineral supplements unless a doctor or registered dietitian advises you to do so.

High-fiber diets can decrease absorption of some minerals, including iron, zinc, and magnesium. Fiber binds these minerals and the minerals are excreted with body wastes. Although getting adequate fiber in the diet is important, exceeding daily recommendations is not advisable.

Drugs and caffeine can affect the availability of minerals in many complex ways. If you are taking prescription drugs, ask your doctor about any effects they may have on mineral absorption. Caffeine is a diuretic, which increases urine output. It thereby increases the loss of certain minerals excreted in urine. Avoid unneeded medications and excess caffeine.

The presence of certain vitamins can promote the absorption of some minerals. For example, the presence of vitamin D improves calcium and phosphorus absorption. Also, foods high in vitamin C increase iron absorption.

Your body's ability to absorb many minerals increases with your need for those minerals. This is a lifesaving defense in times of starvation or illness. It also helps the body meet increased mineral demands, such as those that occur during growth spurts and pregnancy, **9-20**.

Conserving Minerals in Food During Cooking

Minerals are not as fragile as vitamins. Minerals are not affected by heat or enzyme activity. However, minerals can be lost when foods are washed or cooked in liquid. Therefore, to preserve mineral content, avoid soaking foods when cleaning them. Also, cook foods using the smallest amount of water possible. Retain the minerals that have leached into cooking liquid by using it to make sauces, soups, and gravies.

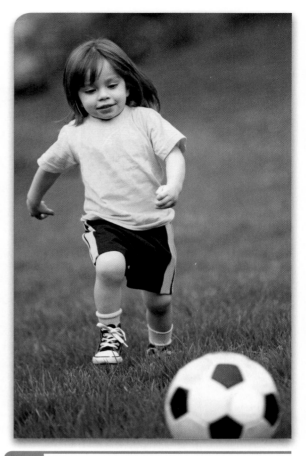

9-20   The body absorbs many nutrients very efficiently during the childhood years when growth is occurring rapidly.

Reading Summary

Minerals are inorganic elements that can be divided into two classes. The macrominerals, or major minerals, include calcium, phosphorus, magnesium, sulfur, sodium, potassium, and chloride. The microminerals, or trace minerals, include iron, zinc, iodine, fluoride, selenium, copper, chromium, manganese, and molybdenum.

Although you need only small quantities of minerals, getting the right amounts is a key to good health. Without adequate intakes, deficiency symptoms can occur. At the same time, you need to avoid mineral excesses, which can be toxic.

Each mineral plays specific roles in the body. The vital functions of minerals include becoming part of body tissues. Many minerals help enzymes do their jobs. Some minerals help nerves work and muscles contract. Minerals also promote growth and control acid-base balance in the body. They help maintain fluid balance, too.

Minerals are widely found throughout the food supply. Selecting fresh and wholesome foods is preferred over the use of supplements. A health problem, such as osteoporosis, may require the use of a supplement. Choose a variety of plant and animal foods. Limit your use of highly processed foods. Eat the recommended daily amounts from each group in MyPlate. Following this basic nutrition advice should provide you with most of your mineral needs.

Review Learning

1. True or false. Because they are needed in larger amounts, macrominerals are more important for health than microminerals.
2. Where is nearly all the calcium in the body stored?
3. Which group from MyPlate is the primary source of calcium?
4. Give two reasons women are at greater risk than men for developing osteoporosis.
5. What is the relationship of meeting adequate phosphorus needs to good health?
6. What are five dietary sources of magnesium?
7. Where are high concentrations of sulfur found in the body?
8. What process helps equalize the fluid balance inside and outside of body cells?
9. What is the pH of a neutral substance, such as water?
10. What minerals are contributed by salt, and what is the primary source of salt in the diet?
11. What organ is affected by potassium deficiencies and excesses?
12. What mineral is part of a protein that helps red blood cells carry oxygen?
13. Give two reasons why iron-deficiency anemia is common among teenage females.
14. What is the most common source of excess zinc resulting in toxicity?
15. Where is most of the iodine in the body concentrated?
16. What is the importance of fluoride in the body?
17. What is the main function of selenium?

18. Name two microminerals other than iron, zinc, iodine, fluoride, and selenium and give a function of each.
19. What are three factors that affect the mineral content of plant foods?
20. True or false. An excess of some minerals can interfere with the absorption of others.

Critical Thinking

21. **Identify evidence.** What evidence can you give about whether it is better to eat whole, fresh foods or take supplements for minerals that may be lacking in the diet?
22. **Analyze behavior.** What human behaviors are detrimental to absorption of essential minerals?

Applying Your Knowledge

23. **Menu plan.** Write a one-day menu that meets the RDA for calcium for a friend who refuses to drink milk. Your friend is not lactose-intolerant and likes cheese and other dairy products.
24. **Showcase display.** Create a showcase display titled "Tracking the Sodium in Your Diet." Mount labels illustrating the high sodium content of popular snack foods and convenience products. Beside each label, identify the sodium content of a low-sodium alternative. Include information on how to read the Nutrition Facts panel to determine foods that are low in sodium.
25. **Mineral brochure.** Prepare a brochure describing factors that increase and decrease mineral absorption and availability. Share your brochures at school.
26. **Food technique.** Select one of the techniques for choosing, preparing, and/or storing foods carefully to maximize the mineral content of your diet. Implement the technique in your personal life. Share the change you have made with the class.

Technology Connections

27. **Prepare a PSA.** Select one of the minerals discussed in this chapter. Research the health benefits associated with consumption of that mineral. Using the information from your research, write and video-record a public service announcement (PSA) promoting the benefits and sources of the mineral you selected.
28. **Sodium quiz.** Sodium intake is a controllable risk factor for high blood pressure. Take *The Scoop on Sodium* quiz on the American Heart Association Web site to test your knowledge about sodium and your health.
29. **Electronic presentation.** Research recommendations for teens on the use and selection of mineral supplements on the National Institutes for Health Web site. Prepare an electronic presentation to communicate what you learn with others.

30. **Calcium quiz.** Take the *Calcium Quiz* on the Dairy Council of California Web site to assess your calcium intake. Complete the section on goals for increasing or maintaining calcium in your diet and print them off as a reminder.

Academic Connections

31. **Science.** With the help of the science department, use litmus paper to identify the pH of 10 food items and record your findings in a chart. Then investigate why eating foods that are acidic does not drastically affect the pH of your digestive tract. Share what you learn in a brief oral report.
32. **Speech.** Working in pairs, role-play a discussion between two people—one loves fruits and vegetables and the other does not. The fruit and vegetable lover must convince the other person to try new foods rich in minerals and vitamins.
33. **Math.** Keep a one-day food diary of all the food and beverages you consume. Include amounts of any salt added to your food at the table. Use food labels, appendix C, or Internet nutrient analysis to determine the total milligrams of sodium consumed. The *Dietary Guidelines* recommendation is not to exceed 2,300 milligrams of sodium in one day. Calculate your intake as a percent of the recommended maximum intake of 2,300 milligrams.
34. **History.** Learn about the history of iodine. Who discovered it? Was that person searching for an essential mineral when he or she discovered iodine? Write a brief paper summarizing your findings.
35. **Science.** Use a reliable anatomy and physiology resource to investigate the urinary system's role in regulating fluid-electrolyte balance in humans. Write a brief summary describing the role of the various system organs.

Workplace Applications

Interpersonal Skills

Presume you are a dietitian. Your interpersonal skills—your ability to listen, speak, and empathize—are a great asset in working with clients. Lilly is your latest client. She was recently diagnosed with osteoporosis. In addition to the medicine her doctor prescribed, Lilly was instructed to seek nutrition counseling about ways to increase the calcium in her diet. What calcium-rich foods would you recommend to Lilly? How much should she have daily?

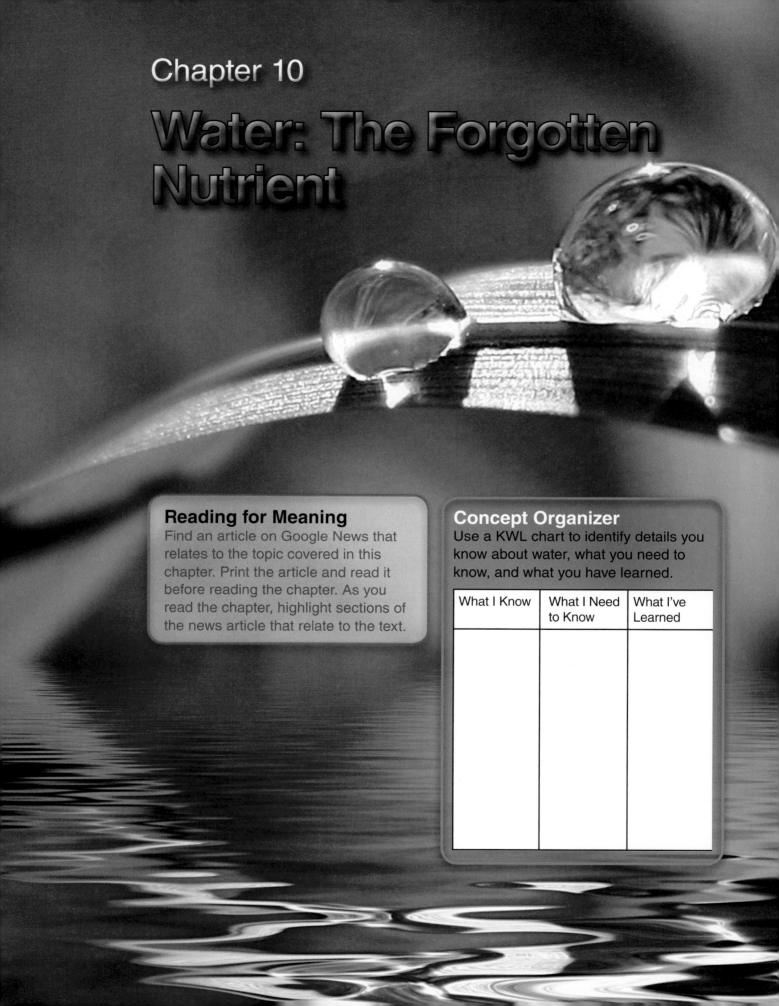

Chapter 10

Water: The Forgotten Nutrient

Reading for Meaning

Find an article on Google News that relates to the topic covered in this chapter. Print the article and read it before reading the chapter. As you read the chapter, highlight sections of the news article that relate to the text.

Concept Organizer

Use a KWL chart to identify details you know about water, what you need to know, and what you have learned.

What I Know	What I Need to Know	What I've Learned

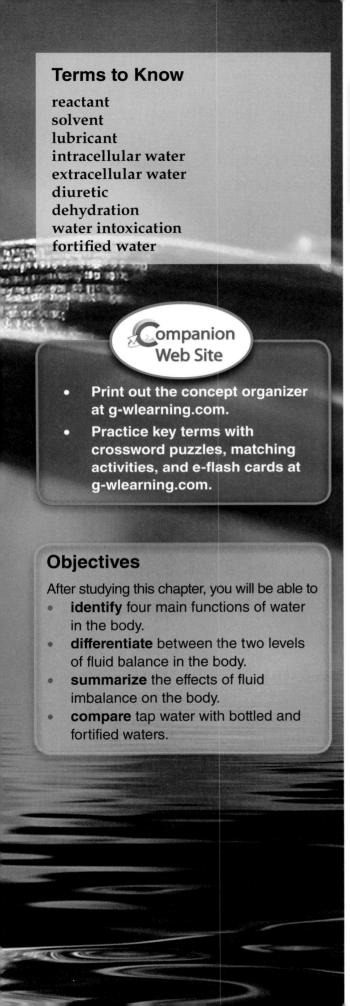

Terms to Know

reactant
solvent
lubricant
intracellular water
extracellular water
diuretic
dehydration
water intoxication
fortified water

Companion Web Site

- **Print out the concept organizer at g-wlearning.com.**
- **Practice key terms with crossword puzzles, matching activities, and e-flash cards at g-wlearning.com.**

Objectives

After studying this chapter, you will be able to
- **identify** four main functions of water in the body.
- **differentiate** between the two levels of fluid balance in the body.
- **summarize** the effects of fluid imbalance on the body.
- **compare** tap water with bottled and fortified waters.

Central Ideas
- Because water is part of every body cell, it is essential to consume water daily.
- Foods, as well as water and healthful beverages, help meet the body's need for water.

Carbohydrates, fats, proteins, vitamins, minerals, and water are the six major nutrients you need for survival. Of these, water is the one that is most often overlooked. This seems odd considering you could make a good argument for viewing water as the most critical nutrient.

Water is an essential nutrient that must be replaced every day. Depending on your state of health, you may be able to survive 8 to 10 weeks without food. Without water, however, you can survive only a few days. This chapter will highlight the vital role water plays in promoting health and wellness.

The Vital Functions of Water

Water is in every body cell. In fact, the presence of water determines the shape, size, and firmness of cells, **10-1.**

For most adults, body weight is about 50 to 75 percent water. That equals roughly 10 to 12 gallons (38 to 46 L). Fat tissue is about 20 to 35 percent water whereas muscle tissue is about 75 percent water. Therefore, the total percentage of body weight from water depends on the ratio of fat to lean body tissue. This ratio varies from person to person. People who have a higher percentage of lean tissue

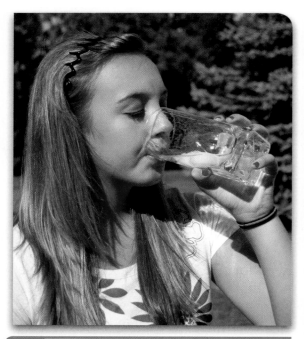

10-1 Much more than a thirst quencher—water is a vital nutrient.

have a higher percentage of water weight. Men typically have a higher percentage of lean tissue and, thereby, more water weight than women. Young people usually have a higher percentage of lean tissue and water weight than older people.

Body fluids include saliva, blood, lymph, digestive juices, urine, and perspiration. Water is the main component in each of these fluids. Your diet must include adequate amounts of water to allow your body to form enough fluids. Otherwise, body fluids will not be able to perform their functions normally. For example, without enough water intake you will not be able to produce enough sweat to cool your body. A buildup of heat in the body can cause such symptoms as headache, nausea, dizziness, and loss of consciousness. If body temperature is not lowered, death can result.

Water performs a number of functions in the body. It helps chemical reactions take place. It carries nutrients to and waste products from cells throughout the body. Water is the substance that reduces friction between surfaces. It also controls body temperature.

Facilitates Chemical Reactions

Most chemical reactions in the body need water to take place. This includes the reactions involved in breaking down carbohydrates, fats, and proteins for energy. It also includes reactions that result in the formation of new compounds, such as the making of dispensable amino acids. Water seems to help some enzymes perform their functions. It dilutes concentrated substances in the body, too.

Water is a reactant in many chemical reactions in the body. A **reactant** is a substance that enters into a chemical reaction and is changed by it. For example, water is needed during digestion and energy production to break down starches into glucose. Remember that starch is a chain of glucose molecules bonded together. Water is needed to split the bonds in the starch chain. The elements of the water molecules are hydrogen and oxygen. These elements become part of the separate glucose molecules, **10-2**.

Transports Nutrients and Waste Products

Water is a solvent. **Solvents** are liquids in which substances can be dissolved. Water can dissolve most substances, including amino acids from proteins, glucose from carbohydrates, minerals, and water-soluble vitamins. These nutrients are dissolved in the water of digestive fluids. Then they are absorbed from the small intestine and transported through the blood to the cells. Blood is primarily made of water. Water-soluble proteins are attached to fatty acids and fat-soluble vitamins so the water-based blood can transport them, too.

The blood carries dissolved wastes away from the cells. Your kidneys filter wastes from your blood and form urine. Water also plays a role in removing wastes from the body through perspiration, exhaled water vapor, and feces.

Lubricates Surfaces

A **lubricant** is a substance that reduces friction between surfaces. Water is an excellent lubricant in your body. The water in saliva lubricates food as you swallow it. Throughout the digestive system, water acts like a lubricant to assist the easy passage

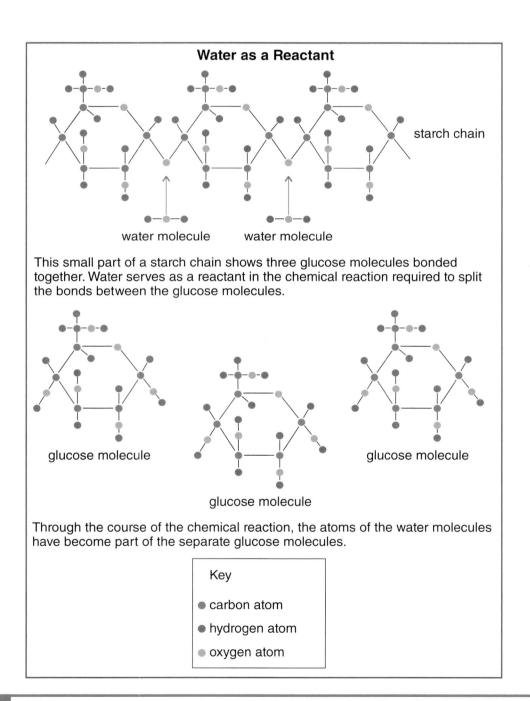

Water as a Reactant

starch chain

water molecule   water molecule

This small part of a starch chain shows three glucose molecules bonded together. Water serves as a reactant in the chemical reaction required to split the bonds between the glucose molecules.

glucose molecule

glucose molecule

glucose molecule

Through the course of the chemical reaction, the atoms of the water molecules have become part of the separate glucose molecules.

Key

● carbon atom

● hydrogen atom

● oxygen atom

10-2   Water serves as a reactant in many chemical reactions that take place in the body.

of nutrients. Tears lubricate your eyes. Fluids surround your joints to keep bones from rubbing against each other. Water also cushions vital tissues and organs to protect them from injury. For example, your spinal cord is protected by surrounding fluids.

Regulates Body Temperature

Another key function of water is to regulate your body temperature. Blood and perspiration are the body fluids responsible for this task.

Normal body temperature for most people is near 98.6°F (37°C). Temperatures that are above or below this by 5°F (2°C to 3°C) or more can cause serious health problems. For instance, the heat of high body temperatures can denature enzymes, which are proteins. This means when the body overheats, there is a slowdown in the chemical reactions promoted by enzymes in the body. Extremely high or low body temperatures can result in death.

Imagine you are riding a stationary bicycle. Although you are using only your leg muscles, your whole body becomes hot. This is because blood distributes body heat. Your body uses this distribution system to regulate body temperature.

Heat from your body is released into the air when blood flows near the surface of your skin. When you become warm, the blood vessels near your skin surface expand. This happens when you are exercising or have a fever. The expanded blood vessels allow more blood to flow near the skin surface, releasing heat into the air.

At the same time, your sweat glands begin producing perspiration. The perspiration transmits heat from your body through pores in your skin surface. The evaporation of water in perspiration helps cool your body, **10-3**. The slowed evaporation of perspiration is what causes you to feel uncomfortable when the humidity level is high.

When your body temperature drops, your body takes steps to conserve heat. It constricts the blood vessels near the surface of your skin. This restricts the amount of blood flowing near your skin surface, so less heat is lost.

Keeping Water in Balance

You can think of water balance at two levels. At the cellular level, there needs to be a balance between the water inside cells and the water outside cells. At another level, the body requires a balance between water intake and water loss.

Cellular Water Balance

Cells are like balloons that maintain their shapes. Like balloons, cells do not have an infinite ability to expand. If too much water flowed into a cell, it could burst. Conversely, if a

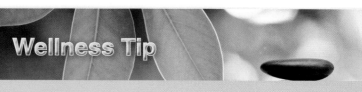

Wellness Tip

Bottled Water and Dental Health

For most people, fluoridated community water systems are the chief source of fluoride—an element that prevents tooth decay. Because most bottled waters have little or no fluoride, people who replace part or all of their drinking water with bottled water may be at greater risk for tooth decay. The next time you are thirsty, reach for the tap instead of a bottle.

cell did not contain enough water, it would collapse. However, the body has mechanisms that keep the balance of water inside and outside the cells fairly constant. These mechanisms keep cells from bursting and collapsing.

There are two categories of water in the body. **Intracellular water** is the water inside the cells. **Extracellular water** is the water outside the cells. Water can move freely across cell membranes. The concentration of sodium, potassium, and chloride particles inside and outside the cells determines the movement of water. Health experts call these minerals *electrolytes*.

Water Intake

Thirst is the body's first signal that it needs water. Therefore, if you feel thirsty you should drink liquids. Thirst goes away automatically when you consume liquids. Deciding how much to drink is a lifestyle choice you can make that affects your state of wellness.

How Much Water?

If you are like most people, you need to increase your fluid intake. The recommended adequate intake of water for females and males ages 14 to 18 is 2.3 liters and 3.3 liters. This represents about 2½ to 3½ quarts of liquids per day to replace lost body fluids. You meet your fluid needs through the liquids you drink and foods you eat. Liquids from milk, juice, soft drinks, coffee, and food supply the needed water. A small amount of water is produced in the body as a by-product of nutrient metabolism.

The color of your urine will help you determine if you are drinking enough water. Urine that is dark yellow indicates it is highly concentrated with wastes. This is stressful to your kidneys. When fluid intake is too low, the kidneys must work harder to

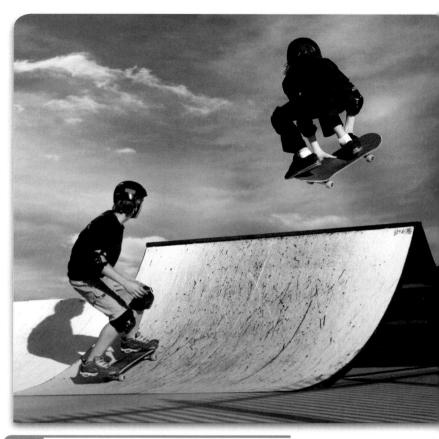

10-3 Perspiring during exercise helps reduce body temperature.

eliminate wastes. Light-colored urine shows you are drinking enough to keep wastes flushed out of your body. Drinking plenty of water while you are young may lessen your chances of kidney problems in later years.

Needs Across the Life Span

Some groups of people have above-average needs for water. An infant's immature kidneys are not as efficient as an adult's kidneys at filtering waste from the bloodstream. Therefore, infants excrete proportionately more water than adults to rid their bodies of waste. This increases their fluid needs, **10-4**.

Other groups who have above-average water needs include older adults, who lose some of their water-conserving abilities. Pregnant women need extra liquids because they have

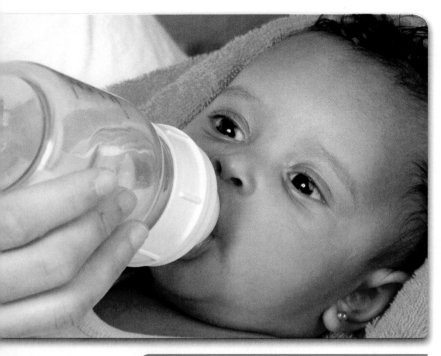

10-4   Infants need more water per unit of body weight than children and adults.

Math Link

Making Conversions

According to the Dietary Reference Intakes for water, the AI for 14- to 18-year-old males is 3.3 liters per day and 2.3 liters per day for females in this age range. Liters (L) and milliliters (mL) are metric system units used to measure volume. The following are common U.S. and metric system conversions:

1 L = 1000 mL
30 mL = 1 fl. oz.
8 fl. oz. = 1 cup
4 cups = 1 quart

1. Convert the AIs for 14- to 18-year-old males and females from liters to fluid ounces. (round up to one decimal)
2. Convert the fluid ounces to cups for both groups.

an increased volume of body fluids to support their developing babies. Lactating women need fluids to produce breast milk. People on high-protein diets require extra water to rid their bodies of the waste products of protein metabolism. A buildup of these waste products can cause kidney damage.

Older adults have the same need for fluids as young adults. The thirst mechanism of older adults can change and fluid intake can be affected. Some older adults choose to limit water intake if they have urinary inconti-nence problems. This requires medical treatment to avoid dehydration. Adequate fluid intake is necessary for continued good health through the aging years.

Supplying the Body's Water Needs

Drinking liquids generally supplies the greatest amount of fluids. Of course, plain water is a pure source of this vital nutrient. However, milk, soft drinks, juices, broth, tea, and other liquids also have high water content.

You may be surprised to learn foods supply almost as much of your daily water needs as liquids. Most foods contain some water. Some foods are higher in water content than beverages. As an example, summer squash is 96 percent water, whereas orange juice is only 87 percent water. Even foods that look solid are a source of water. For instance, bread is 36 percent water. Butter and margarine contain water, but cooking oils and meat fats do not, **10-5**.

Roughly 12 percent of your water needs are met through metabolism. When carbohydrates, fats, and proteins are broken down in the body, some water is released. Your body can then use this water in other chemical reactions.

Water Content of Common Foods	
Food	**Percent Water Content***
Lettuce	96
Salsa	92
Fat-free milk	91
Cola	89
Orange juice	87
Tomato soup	85
Apple	84
Potato	80
Egg	75
Milk shake	74
Tuna, water pack	74
Pasta, cooked	66
Chicken breast, roasted, skinless	65
Hot dog	54
Ground beef, lean	53
Pizza	48
Whole-wheat bread	38
Cheddar cheese	37
Butter	16
Chocolate chip cookie, homemade	6
Jellybeans	6
Corn flakes	3
Peanut butter	1
White sugar	<1
Corn oil	0
*percent of total weight	

10-5   Nearly every food contains some water.

Your sources of water replacement may vary greatly from day to day. When you eat many water-loaded fruits and vegetables, you may not drink as much liquid. When you eat dry foods, you are likely to consume more liquids.

Water Loss

Water losses, referred to as water output, occur naturally as you carry on regular activities throughout the day. On average, you lose about two to three quarts of fluid each day.

How does water leave the body? There are several paths. Most body fluids are lost through urine. Your kidneys regulate the amount of urine lost. Kidneys can retain some water, but they must also produce urine to rid the body of wastes.

The volume of your urine varies with the amount of water you drink. If you produce less than 2½ cups (625 mL) of urine per day, the urine will be concentrated with wastes. This increases the risk of kidney stones. *Kidney stones* are hard particles of mineral deposits that form in the kidneys. They can cause tremendous pain when they pass from the kidneys to the bladder and out of the body. A healthy urine output is one to two quarts per day or more.

You lose body water through three vehicles other than urine. Fluids are lost through your skin as you sweat. You lose moisture in your breath as you breathe. You have small losses through bowel wastes, too.

A number of factors can impact water losses. Environmental conditions, level of physical activity, medications, and health status can influence how much fluid is lost and needs to be replaced. Being aware of these factors can help you determine your fluid replacement needs.

Weather Conditions and Altitude

Hot and humid weather, as well as warm work or living environments can cause larger losses through sweating. Dry climates increase water losses through quick skin evaporation. Such climates include the atmosphere on airplanes and in buildings when heating systems are operating. The low oxygen pressure at high altitudes increases water losses for people not used to these altitudes. For example, people living in mile high areas breathe harder to draw more oxygen into their bodies. They have a greater output of water vapor and must focus careful attention on the need for fluid replacement. When the weather is hot, you should make an effort to increase your fluid intake.

Physical Exercise

Exercise causes increased water losses. The body's energy production takes place in the fluid environment of the blood and muscles. The release of chemical energy generates much heat. The heat must be removed by sweating to avoid dangerous increases in body temperature. Most fluid is lost through sweat. The more energy you expend, the more you sweat, and the more water you need, **10-6**. Vigorous exercise can cause the loss of a quart of water in an hour. Long distance runners, such as marathon runners, can lose up to 13 pounds of water weight during a 26-mile race. To help maintain the body's fluid balance, athletes should plan to consume adequate liquids before competition, during, and after competition.

Use of Diuretics

Using diuretics promotes water losses. **Diuretics** are substances that increase urine production. Doctors often prescribe diuretics for patients with high blood pressure or body fluid imbalances. Alcohol and energy drinks act as diuretics, too. For this reason, you need to use care when choosing liquids to replace body fluids. Coffee or soft drinks that contain caffeine may not be the best options for fluid replacement. Liquids, such as water, mineral water, or diluted fruit juices, may be better choices for restoring fluid losses. Distilled water has natural minerals removed and is not recommended to replace plain water.

Illness

Vomiting, diarrhea, bleeding, and high fever are all conditions that can cause fluid losses. Tissue damage caused by burns also affects the body's fluid balance. The more severe these conditions are, the greater the fluid losses will be. Medical supervision and treatment may be necessary to correct these fluid losses.

During illness, you may not always feel thirsty. However, drinking plenty of liquid is important to replace increased losses. Consuming fluids also helps flush the products of drug metabolism from your body.

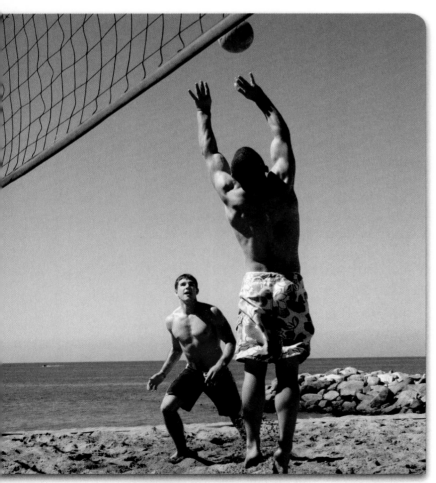

10-6   Exercise increases water losses as the body sweats to remove excess heat.

Fluid Imbalance

The thirst mechanism is not always a reliable indicator of fluid needs. During hot weather or heavy exercise, the body may lose a fair amount of fluid before signaling thirst. When the body either loses or takes in too much water, fluid imbalances result.

Effects of Water Loss

Because fluids make up a high percentage of your body weight, when you lose water, you also lose weight. Someone who wants to drop a few pounds may think this is good news. However, the weight you want to lose is fat, not water. Water weight is quickly regained when body fluids are replenished.

Even a small percentage weight drop due to water loss will make you feel uncomfortable. When you lose two percent of body weight in fluids, you will become aware of the sensation of thirst. Both the brain and the stomach play a role in making you aware there is a water imbalance. If you do not replace water losses, you may become dehydrated. **Dehydration** is a state in which the body contains a lower-than-normal amount of body fluids.

When dehydration occurs, the body takes steps to help conserve water. Hormones signal the kidneys to decrease urine output. Sweat production also declines. As the volume of fluid in the bloodstream drops, the concentration of sodium in the blood increases. The kidneys respond to the higher blood sodium level by retaining more water. These water-conserving efforts cannot prevent all fluid losses from the body. If fluids are not replaced, the damaging effects of dehydration will begin to take their toll.

Some older adults do not always recognize the thirst sensation. In cases such as these, it is important not to wait for the thirst signal to begin consuming liquids. Older adults may need to make a point of drinking even when they do not feel thirsty.

Replacing lost water is important for peak athletic performance. Athletic performance levels decline after a 3 percent loss in water weight. When water is lost from working muscles, blood volume decreases. The heart must pump harder to supply the same amount of energy. Mental concentration is affected as fluid losses increase. Some clear signs of dehydration are fatigue and lack of energy. Other symptoms may include dizziness, headache,

Case Study: Losing the Hydration Game

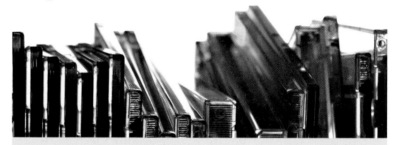

Taryn is a 15-year-old girl who lives in Denver, Colorado—also known as the "Mile High City." Taryn loves to spend many hours playing basketball outside in the summer months. It is hot, sunny, and dry in the summer. There is a water fountain in a building near the basketball court, but she does not bother to take the time to drink. Her friends tell her to bring a water bottle with her. She usually forgets the water and thinks it is not that important anyway. Sometimes she remembers on her way to the game and buys a can of soda from a vending machine.

Taryn is often disappointed with her game. She finds that she runs out of energy by mid-game and often gets a headache. She wants to improve so that she can make the high school team next year.

Case Review

1. What do you think is contributing to Taryn's disappointing performance on the basketball court?

2. Why do you think Taryn believes that water is not important?

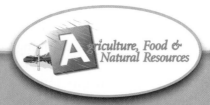

Hydrologist

Hydrologists often specialize in either underground water or surface water. They examine the form and intensity of precipitation, its rate of infiltration into the soil, its movement through the earth, and its return to the ocean and atmosphere. Hydrologists use sophisticated techniques and instruments to monitor the change in regional and global water cycles. Some surface-water hydrologists use sensitive stream-measuring devices to assess flow rates and water quality.

Education: A bachelor's degree is adequate for a few entry-level positions. However, most hydrologists need a master's degree for most research positions in private industry and government agencies.

Job Outlook: Employment growth for hydrologists is expected to be faster than the average for all occupations. Spurring this demand is the need for environmental protection and responsible water management.

muscle cramping, and reduced muscle endurance. A 10- to 11-percent drop in body weight due to water losses can result in serious organ malfunctions.

Can You Drink Too Much Water?

You may wonder if it is possible to drink too much water. The answer is yes. The result is a rare condition called **water intoxication**. Water intoxication is caused by drinking too much water and consuming too few electrolytes.

Athletes who sweat heavily can experience water intoxication. These athletes experience dehydration problems from the excessive sweating. As a result, an imbalance of blood-sodium concentration occurs. Sodium losses must be replaced to maintain an electrolyte balance. If the athlete drinks only plain water, the electrolytes are not replaced. If electrolyte levels stay low, early symptoms of water intoxication may appear such as headache and muscle weakness. Severe cases of water intoxication can cause death.

In some cases, there can be a psychological disorder of drinking excessive amounts of water on a daily basis. This can also cause a type of water intoxication by diluting the electrolyte imbalance.

The greatest danger of water intoxication is when infants with diarrhea and/or vomiting are given plain water. Diarrhea and vomiting pull electrolytes as well as water from the body. When fluid losses are excessive, electrolytes and fluids must be replaced. Electrolyte imbalance can happen to people of all ages. However, infants are at greater risk. They can lose body fluids more easily than people in other age groups.

Better Water?

In recent decades, sales of bottled and enhanced waters have increased dramatically. The cost of these waters can be several hundred times higher than the cost of tap water.

Bottled Water Versus Tap Water

Why do people buy bottled water? The reasons vary. Some think bottled water contains miracle minerals that promote health. Research does not confirm this. Others want the convenience of carrying bottled water when they are traveling or at work. For added convenience, they choose to buy the water rather than fill a safe, reusable bottle.

Many people claim bottled water tastes better than local water supplies. Dissolved minerals give water its taste.

Depending on where you live, the water from the tap may taste of iron deposits, sulfur, or other minerals. People who object to such mineral tastes may buy bottled water even though tap water is safe and clean.

Some bottled-water drinkers are concerned tap water contains contaminants. Purity of tap water depends on the area in which you live. Public drinking water is treated to meet federal health standards. Water from private wells is more likely to contain microorganisms. People who are concerned about the safety of their water can have it tested for the presence of contaminants.

Water sold in bottles is not always safer, cleaner, or purer than tap water. In fact, bottled water comes from the same sources as water from the faucet. Bottled water sold across state lines must meet the FDA federal standards for purity. Check the label for "IBWA" trademark. This organization supports the FDA regulations for purity and sanitation. Not all states enforce bottled water sanitation rules.

Some people choose to use filtration systems to treat their tap water at home, **10-7**. These systems vary in cost and require upkeep or filter replacement from time to time. They also vary in terms of what they filter from the water. Some systems remove certain harmful contaminants. Others may do little more than make water taste better.

Use of Fortified Water

Bottled sports, health, and energy drinks are a fast growing industry. **Fortified water** is plain water enhanced with specific nutrients or supplements intended to aid or improve health or energy outcomes. Examples of fortified waters include sports drinks and energy drinks.

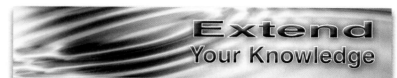

The Cost of Hydration

Make a list of drinks commonly enjoyed by teens such as bottled water, carbonated drinks, sports drinks, powdered drink mixed with water, fruit juices, and energy drinks. Gather information on the cost per gallon of the listed drinks. Use your family water bill to calculate the cost per gallon your family pays for tap water. Organize your findings in a table. Rank order the drinks by cost per gallon from most costly to least costly. Which drinks are most economical for hydration purposes?

Sports drinks are a beverage with added electrolytes and sweeteners intended to improve and sustain energy. There are many types of sports drinks available on the market shelf. Sports drinks may be high in added sugar and calories. The costs of these drinks vary and contents can be confusing. Sports drinks, used for fluid replacement, are recommended to be used sparingly. In cases where

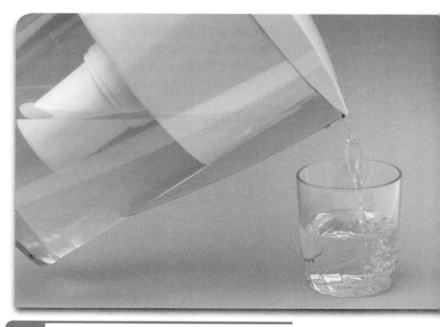

10-7 A water filtration system can help improve the taste and quality of tap water.

athletes sweat heavily such as long sports events or hot days, sports drinks may be helpful. However, simply eating foods that contain salt, such as pretzels, salty energy bars, or tomato juice may be sufficient, **10-8**.

Energy drinks contain added caffeine, vitamins, or herbal supplements intended to have a stimulant effect. Consumers need to know that commercially bottled fluids, called energy drinks, are classified as a food supplement. This means there is no Food and Drug Administration regulation for these drinks. There is no assurance of quality or purity of the drink. Long lists of ingredients on the label can mean there is greater chance for negative effects on the body. Energy drinks are not recommended for children, teens, or pregnant women.

The effect of fortified fluid use continues to be researched. What is beneficial and what is harmful to health is not clear. Moderation in use is one known key to good health. Reading the label to determine if the ingredients can be harmful or helpful is difficult but necessary.

Considering a Performance Enhancing Drink?
Check It Out...

✓ **Type of sugar**

Added sugars may slow absorption of the water. Look for a combination of sucrose and glucose, which are easily digested and absorbed quickly.

✓ **Amount of sugar**

Lower sugar concentration is easier to digest. Look for 6% or less (14 g or less sugar/8 oz. of water).

✓ **Amount of added salt**

Higher sodium content (100–200 mg sodium/8 oz. of water) for endurance athletes.

✓ **Added vitamins and minerals**

No research finds that energy levels or physical performance are improved by sports drinks with added vitamins and minerals. A daily vitamin may be more economical than vitamins supplied in bottled water.

✓ **Added protein**

Drinks with added protein may cause an upset digestive system and have not been proven to add health or performance benefits.

✓ **Added caffeine energy drinks**

Caffeine can elevate heart rate and blood pressure. Added caffeine may contribute to feelings of anxiety and edginess.

10-8   Make sure you know how the contents of an enhanced drink may impact your body before you consume it.

Reading Summary

Water is a vital nutrient you must replace daily. It is in every cell in your body and is the main component in all body fluids. Water makes up over half of your body weight.

Water performs a number of functions in the body. It plays a role in chemical reactions. It transports nutrients to cells and carries wastes away from cells. Water acts as a lubricant and helps regulate your body temperature, too.

The fluids in your body need to remain in balance. There needs to be a balance between intracellular and extracellular water. There also needs to be a balance between your total water input and output. You receive water through the liquids you drink and the foods you eat. You also get water as a by-product of metabolism. You lose body fluids through urine, sweat, vapor in your breath, and bowel wastes. Hot weather, warm environments, dry climates, high altitudes, and use of diuretics can all increase water losses. Illnesses and exercise increase water losses, too.

When you do not replace water losses, you can become dehydrated. Greater levels of fluid loss can cause a decrease in physical performance and a lack of mental concentration. An excessive drop in body fluids can result in serious organ malfunctions.

Bottled and enhanced waters are more expensive options for hydration than tap water. People buy bottled water for a variety of reasons including convenience, taste, and purity. However, bottled waters are not always safer or more pure than tap water. Enhanced waters have specific nutrients or supplements added that are intended to improve health or performance. Research is not yet clear on the benefit or harm from these fortified fluids.

Review Learning

1. Name five body fluids composed mainly of water.
2. How does water's function as a solvent play a role in human nutrition?
3. How does water help the body release excess heat?
4. What three minerals control cellular fluid balance?
5. Name three groups of people who have increased fluid needs.
6. Name three foods that are more than 50 percent water.
7. List four factors that impact water loss.
8. How does physical exercise increase water losses?
9. Describe the steps the body takes when it needs to conserve water.
10. True or false. Sports drinks are recommended to be used sparingly.

Critical Thinking

11. **Identify evidence.** Suppose you have a friend who decides to go on a weight-loss diet and is delighted to have lost two pounds in a day. You know this weight loss is likely due to water loss. What evidence can you give your friend to show that restricting food and fluids can negatively influence health?

12. **Compare and contrast.** With advertisers' push for bottled and fortified waters, people may be confused about what choices to make for good health. Compare and contrast the benefits of tap water to bottled and fortified waters.

Applying Your Knowledge

13. **Evaluate water consumption.** For one day, avoid all beverages except water. Evaluate your satisfaction with water as your primary source of fluids. Include your personal evaluation in a written report on the advantages and disadvantages of choosing only water as a beverage.
14. **Interview.** To find out what advice coaches give athletes regarding fluid intake before, during, and after a game or competition, interview a sports coach. Share your findings with the class.
15. **Research.** Learn how bottled water is regulated in your state. Prepare a fact sheet stating what to look for to be assured you are buying safe bottled water.
16. **Create a PSA.** Working in small groups, evaluate how the media influences people's choice of beverage for hydration. Prepare a public service announcement (PSA) promoting the merits of drinking tap water.

Technology Connections

17. **Internet search.** Using reliable Internet sources, learn how to make water safe to drink if you are camping and run out of drinking water. Prepare a flyer to share with others what you learn using desktop publishing software.
18. **Electronic presentation.** Use presentation software to prepare a report explaining how the body regulates the need for water. Use diagrams to show which body systems are involved in the thirst response.
19. **Research.** Find out what your state is doing about source water protection. Use the Internet to find your state's source water protection Web site. How does your state maintain the purity of tap water? Then check out the EPA Web site to learn more about what individuals can do to protect quality of their drinking water. Share your findings with the class members.
20. **Create a graph.** Use Internet resources to learn the percent body weight that water comprises for a baby, a teen male or female, an obese male or female, a person over age 80, and a competitive athlete. Prepare a bar graph using spreadsheet software to display the results. Summarize the differences for the class.

Academic Connections

21. **Social studies.** Locate the areas of the world where safe drinking water is scarce. What resources are needed to improve the situation? What agencies are helping to solve water shortage problems? Prepare a poster describing water needs around the world.

22. **Math.** Design a blind taste test comparing a variety of waters such as tap, bottled, and mineral water. Create a rating system and have class members rate each water type. Calculate and report the results of your taste test.

23. **Science.** Learn about the field of hydrology. Write a paper describing hydrology. What are the current issues in the field? What do hydrologists do?

24. **Speech.** The Great Lakes represent 18 percent of the surface fresh water on the planet. Research the Great Lakes Basin Compact to learn the purpose of the compact. Prepare a speech to share your findings with the class.

Workplace Applications

Using Computer Technology

As a teacher and wrestling coach, you are keenly aware about the importance of water to health and wellness. It has come to your attention that a number of athletes are limiting their water intake as they prepare for competition. Several wrestlers on the team became extremely dehydrated and sick during the last meet. You decide to e-mail a reminder to the athletes and their parents about the need for proper hydration. Draft a message about the importance of proper hydration before, during, and after a meet.

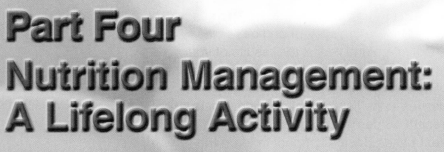

Part Four
Nutrition Management: A Lifelong Activity

Reduction

Reduction is accomplished by heating a flavorful liquid in order to decrease its volume through evaporation. This process intensifies the flavor of the liquid and results in a thicker product than the original liquid. The thicker, more flavorful liquid is used as a sauce to complement or improve dishes. Fats and starches are used to thicken most sauces. Reduction sauces are a healthier option since neither fat nor starch must be used.

Nearly any flavorful liquid can be used to create a reduction sauce. However, salty liquids become too salty after reduction and should not be used. For instance, use chicken stock that has no added salt for a reduction. Salt can be added to the finished sauce if needed. Another consideration when choosing a liquid for reduction is cost. A significant amount of liquid must be used to produce a small amount of reduction sauce. During the reduction process, a liquid may lose as much as 75 percent of its original volume. If the liquid you are reducing is expensive—for example, balsamic vinegar—the amount needed to produce a sauce for a typical meal could be quite costly.

Arrabbiata Sauce (6 servings)

Ingredients

- 3½ pounds ripe tomatoes, peeled and seeded
- 2 tablespoons olive oil
- 1 small onion, chopped
- 4 cloves garlic, minced
- ¼ teaspoon crushed red pepper flakes
- ¼ teaspoon dried basil
- salt and pepper to taste

Directions

1. Bring pot of water to boil. Prepare large bowl of ice water. Cut a small "X" on the bottom of each tomato. Place tomatoes in boiling water for about 1 minute. Remove tomatoes with slotted spoon and place in ice water. When tomatoes are cool enough to handle, core, peel, and squeeze out seeds. Chop tomatoes.
2. In a large pot over medium heat, cook onion and garlic in oil until soft. Stir in tomatoes, crushed red pepper, and basil. Bring to a boil, and then reduce to a simmer over low heat. Cook for 2 hours or until sauce reduces to desired consistency.
3. Add salt and pepper to taste. Serve over favorite pasta.

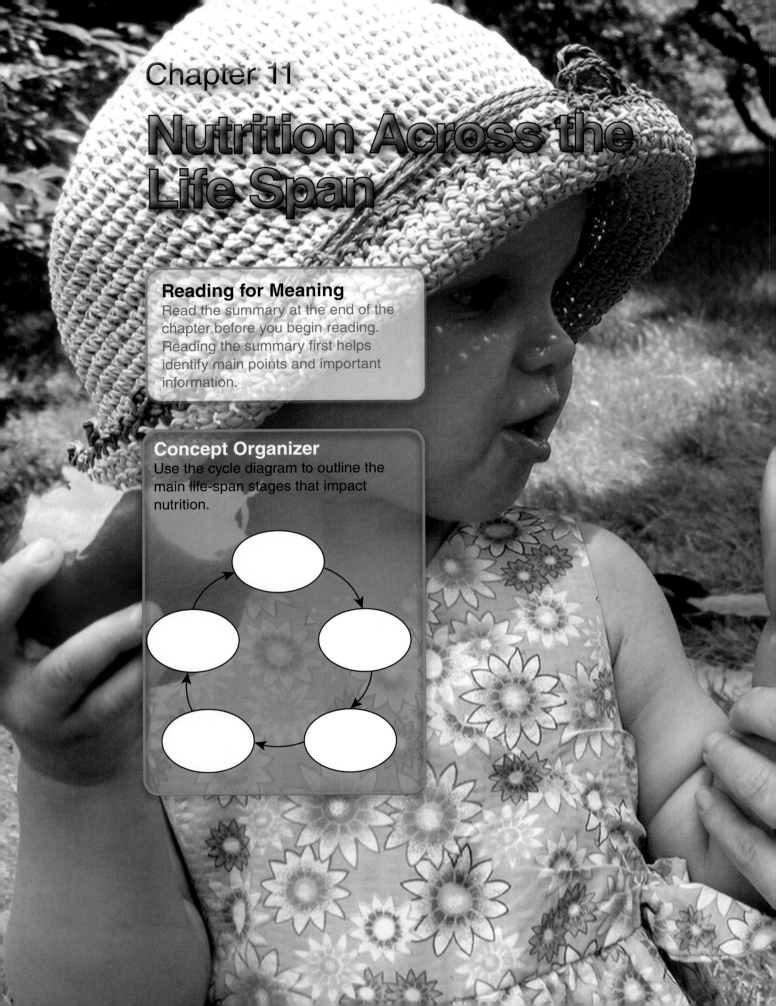

Chapter 11
Nutrition Across the Life Span

Reading for Meaning
Read the summary at the end of the chapter before you begin reading. Reading the summary first helps identify main points and important information.

Concept Organizer
Use the cycle diagram to outline the main life-span stages that impact nutrition.

Terms to Know

life cycle
fetus
lactation
low-birthweight baby
premature baby
trimester
pica
placenta
congenital disability
fetal alcohol syndrome (FAS)
infant
toddler
adolescence
puberty
growth spurt

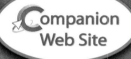

Companion Web Site

- **Print out the concept organizer at g-wlearning.com.**
- **Practice key terms with crossword puzzles, matching activities, and e-flash cards at g-wlearning.com.**

Objectives

After studying this chapter, you will be able to
- **explain** the relationship between the life cycle and nutrition.
- **conclude** health and nutritional needs specific to each stage of the life cycle.
- **evaluate** food choices to best meet nutritional needs at each stage of the life cycle.
- **recognize** the role of activity in nutrition and fitness through the life cycle.

Central Ideas
- Nutritional needs vary depending on a person's stage in the life cycle.
- Eating a variety of foods that supply essential nutrients and participating in age-appropriate fitness activities helps promote lifelong good health.

At the beginning of your life, you were smaller than the period at the end of this sentence. Then you grew. As an adult, you will be several million times bigger than you were at the start of your life.

The projected life span for an infant born today is between 75 and 80 years. During his or her life span, an individual's nutrition and fitness needs change. Although all humans need the same basic nutrients, certain stages of life may bring special nutritional concerns. This chapter will help you look more closely at nutritional needs as your body changes and you move through life.

Life-Span Nutrition

During an individual's life span, he or she progresses through a predictable pattern of changes called the *life cycle*. The **life cycle** is the series of growth and development stages through which people pass from before birth and until death. The life-cycle stages include pregnancy and lactation, infancy, toddlerhood, childhood, adolescence, and adulthood. These stages are often further subdivided to reflect significant developmental changes. Each person's development is unique and the stages may vary from person to person, **11-1**.

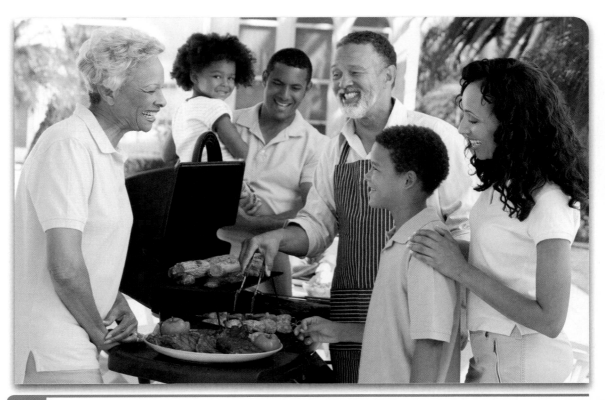

11-1   People need different amounts of nutrients in each stage of the life cycle.

Throughout their life span, people need adequate amounts of nutritious foods to build, repair, and maintain body tissues. The need for nutrients begins before birth. An unborn child's development depends on nutrients from the mother's bloodstream.

Each child's development is unique. Different parts of the body grow at different times and at different rates. However, there are predictable growth patterns. For instance, bone and muscle growth are most rapid in infancy and adolescence. Nutritional requirements are especially high during these periods. Rapid bone growth increases the need for calcium. Rapid muscle growth increases the need for protein.

Nutrient needs for adults decrease to a maintenance level. During the later years of life, the aging process affects nutritional status.

Some lifestyle choices such as participating in a sport or following a vegetarian diet can impact nutritional needs during the life cycle. These decisions contribute an additional level of nutritional need. However, these factors are choices that are not common to all individuals.

In addition to the life-cycle stages, a number of other factors influence the amounts of nutrients needed. These factors include body size and composition, age, gender, activity level, and state of health. These factors in combination with the demands of the life-cycle stage create a set of nutritional needs that are unique to each individual.

A relationship exists between an individual's nutrition and his or her life span. The quality of nutrition during each life-cycle stage can influence an individual's health during future stages and across the life span. When good nutrition practices begin early in life, chances for optimal health in the future are improved.

The following sections focus on the nutrients the body needs during the various stages of life, beginning with pregnancy and ending with older adulthood.

Pregnancy and Lactation

The life cycle begins in a woman's body. During pregnancy, a woman's normal body functions change to take care of the developing baby. After conception, nourishment from the mother's body is necessary to support growth. Two weeks after conception, the developing human is called an *embryo*. From nine weeks after conception until birth, a developing human is called a **fetus**. Following the birth of the baby, the mother's body begins producing breast milk. This is called **lactation**. The demands of pregnancy and lactation placed on a woman's body affect her nutritional needs.

Health Needs Before Pregnancy

Women should be in good health before becoming pregnant. When planning a pregnancy, a woman should see a medical professional who can evaluate the woman's health. The woman should visit a doctor again as soon as she thinks she is pregnant. The doctor needs to monitor the woman's health throughout the pregnancy. This type of *prenatal* (before birth) care helps reduce the risk of health problems for the mother and fetus. Prenatal care also increases a woman's chances of delivering a healthy baby.

A woman's weight before pregnancy should be appropriate for her height. Obstetricians advise underweight and

Wellness Tip

Preventing Infant Botulism

Infant botulism is caused by a spore called *Clostridium botulinum*. These spores are all around you—in the dirt, in dust, and in the air. Honey—pasteurized or unpasteurized—can be a source of these spores. To reduce the risk of infant botulism, do not feed honey or foods processed with honey (such as honey-coated cereals and honey graham crackers) to infants before one year of age.

overweight women to attain a healthy weight before becoming pregnant. This helps ensure good health for the women and their babies.

Women who enter pregnancy 10 percent or more below healthy weight face a greater risk of having a **low-birthweight baby**. This is a baby that weighs less than 5½ pounds (2,500 g) at birth. Low-birthweight babies have an increased risk of illness and death in early life. They are also more likely to have health problems that could affect them throughout life, **11-2**.

Women who are 20 percent or more above healthy weight are also more likely to experience problems during pregnancy. However, pregnancy is not an appropriate time for a woman to try to lose or maintain weight. A woman needs to gain a certain amount of weight for a healthy pregnancy and a healthy baby. A special diet plan can help an overweight woman achieve a healthful weight gain during pregnancy.

Both underweight and overweight women are at greater risk of giving birth to a premature infant. A **premature baby** is a baby born before the 37th week of pregnancy. Premature birth is the leading cause of death

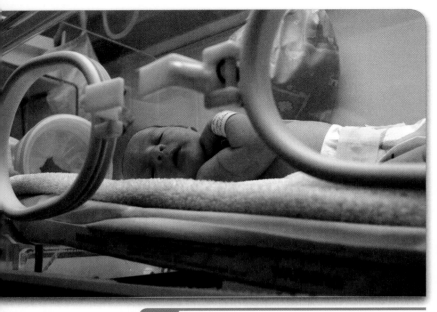

11-2   Low-birthweight babies have a higher risk for health problems at birth and throughout their lives.

among babies. Most premature babies have a low birthweight and are at risk for related health problems. Premature babies also have underdeveloped lungs. This increases their risk of respiratory problems throughout life.

Nutrient Needs During Pregnancy

You may know a normal pregnancy lasts about nine months. When describing prenatal development, doctors refer to trimesters. A **trimester** is one-third of the pregnancy period and lasts about 13 to 14 weeks. A pregnant woman's nutritional needs vary a bit from one trimester to the next. This is because nutrients are critical in varying proportions for different aspects of a baby's development.

A woman needs extra amounts of many nutrients during pregnancy. One of the best ways to prepare for these increased needs is to form healthful eating habits before pregnancy. This

approach benefits a woman in two key ways. First, a well-nourished female builds reserves of some nutrients. These reserves help her meet the increased nutrient demands of pregnancy and avoid deficiencies. Second, a woman who chooses a nutrient-dense diet knows which foods will increase her nutrient intake during pregnancy.

Pregnant women need extra protein to help build fetal tissue. They also need extra protein to support changes in their bodies, such as increasing their blood supply and uterine tissue. Many women already consume more than enough protein. Therefore, most women do not need to adjust their diets to meet the protein needs of pregnancy.

A pregnant woman needs increased amounts of most vitamins. Folate is especially important at the beginning of the first trimester. This vitamin aids the normal development of the baby's brain and spinal cord during the first few weeks of pregnancy. This is before most women know they are pregnant. Therefore, health experts recommend all women of childbearing age consume 400 micrograms of folic acid from fortified foods and supplements daily. During pregnancy, the recommendation is to consume 600 micrograms of synthetic folic acid from fortified foods or supplements in addition to sources obtained from eating a varied diet, **11-3**. Meeting this recommendation will reduce the number of babies born with damage to the brain and spinal cord.

Pregnant women have an increased need for vitamin B_{12}. This vitamin works with folate to make red blood cells. It occurs naturally only in animal foods. Therefore, women following strict vegetarian diets need to eat fortified foods or take supplements containing vitamin B_{12}.

Women have some increased mineral needs during pregnancy. They need extra zinc to support the growth and development of the fetus. They need more magnesium to promote healthy fetal bones and tissues. Pregnant women require increased amounts of iron to provide reserves the infant will need after birth. They also need iron because their growing bodies are making more red blood cells. Pregnant women need extra iodine, too. This mineral supports thyroid activity as basal metabolic rate increases in the second trimester.

The recommended daily intake for calcium does not increase during pregnancy. However, the calcium needed to form the baby's bones is pulled from the mother's bones. Therefore, it is critical that pregnant women consume the recommended 1,000 milligrams of calcium per day. This will help reduce the loss of minerals from their bones. Pregnant teens need 1,300 milligrams of calcium daily.

Hormonal changes affect the way a pregnant woman's body uses certain nutrients. For instance, when a woman is pregnant, her body absorbs and stores more calcium and iron. These changes help provide for some of an expectant woman's additional nutrient needs. However, many pregnant women have trouble meeting all their needs through diet alone. This is especially true for iron. Therefore, health professionals often prescribe vitamin and mineral supplements to help pregnant women meet their increased needs. Pregnant women should take supplements only with their doctor's recommendation.

A woman who fails to meet added nutrient needs during pregnancy can affect her health. She can affect the health of her baby, too. The woman may experience iron deficiency anemia. She is more

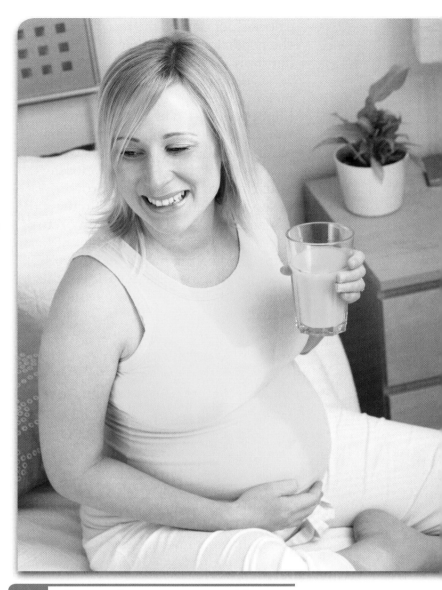

11-3 Pregnant women may want to make fresh orange juice part of their daily diets. It is a good source of folate.

susceptible to disease. She is even at an increased risk of death. Her baby is more likely to be born early or have a low birthweight. The newborn may not have the necessary nutrient reserves to draw on for growth. The baby may also be more susceptible to illnesses.

Along with extra nutrients, a pregnant woman needs extra calories to support fetal development. In the second trimester, an expectant woman needs to begin eating an extra 340 calories per day. In the third trimester, she needs to add another 110 calories to her daily diet.

Gaining enough but not too much weight during pregnancy is very important, **11-4**. The recommended weight gains result in the best chances of having a healthy baby. This weight reflects the weight of the developing fetus. It also allows for the growth of tissue and increase of body fluids in the mother, **11-5**. Most weight gain occurs during the second and third trimesters. With good eating habits and exercise, most women lose the majority of this weight within a few months after delivery.

Weight Gain During Pregnancy	
Prepregnancy Weight	**Total Weight Gain**
Underweight	28–40 lb. (12.5–18 kg)
Normal weight	25–35 lb. (11.5–16 kg)
Overweight	15–25 lb. (7–11.5 kg)
Obese	11–20 lb. (5–9 kg)

11-4 Guidelines for weight gain during pregnancy for both teens and adults are based on prepregnancy weight.

Accounting for Pregnancy Weight Gain	
Component	**Weight Gain**
Baby	7–8 pounds (3.2–3.7 kg)
Amniotic fluid	2 pounds (0.9 kg)
Placenta	1–2 pounds (0.5–0.9 kg)
Growth of uterus	2 pounds (0.9 kg)
Extra blood volume	3–5 pounds (1.4–2.3 kg)
Growth of breast tissue	1–2 pounds (0.5–0.9 kg)
Other body fluids	3–5 pounds (1.4–2.3 kg)
Fat stores and other body tissues	6–9 pounds (2.7–4.1 kg)
Total	**25–35 pounds (11.5–16.1 kg)**

11-5 Most weight gain occurs in the second and third trimesters.

Pregnancy and Physical Activity

A woman should follow a plan of regular exercise before, during, and after pregnancy. Physically fit women should stay physically active throughout their pregnancy. Staying active helps reduce stress, facilitates the process of labor, reduces the chances of gestational diabetes, and reduces the discomfort of pregnancy. Practicing fitness activities helps the mother lose excess weight after pregnancy and she begins to feel fit sooner after birth. Following a daily exercise program will also smooth the transition to active parenthood. A woman should speak with her doctor about what types of exercise to do during pregnancy.

Caution is advised regarding the kind of physical activity chosen by pregnant women. Avoid sports activity where there is a chance of falling or being hit. Sports with low impact activity are safest. This includes swimming, walking, stair climbing, rowing and light strength training. If there is a medical condition, professional advice should be followed. Drink plenty of fluid before, during, and after exercise.

Nutrient Needs During Lactation

After giving birth, a mother must feed her baby frequently to help it grow and develop. Nearly all health and nutrition experts strongly urge most mothers to choose breast-feeding over formula-feeding. Breast-feeding benefits the health of the baby and the mother, **11-6**.

In some situations, breast-feeding may not be recommended. For example, certain maternal diseases and medications can be passed through the breast milk and harm the baby. Some babies

Benefits of Breast-Feeding	
For Mothers	**For Infants**
• Promotes bonding • Faster return to prepregnancy weight • Saves money and time spent buying and preparing formula • Reduces environmental waste from formula bottles and cans • May reduce mother's risk for osteoporosis, and breast and ovarian cancers	• Promotes bonding • Best meets baby's nutritional needs • Enhances immune system • Easier to digest than formula • Reduces frequency of allergies and infections • May reduce future risk for chronic diseases such as obesity and diabetes

11-6   Breast-feeding benefits both the mother and baby.

are born with a disorder that prevents them from converting the monosaccharide (galactose) found in milk. The galactose builds up and causes serious damage to the baby.

Mothers who choose to breast-feed need even greater amounts of some nutrients than during their pregnancy. Their doctors may prescribe vitamin and mineral supplements to boost nutrients found in a nutritious meal plan. Besides vitamins and minerals, lactating women need increased amounts of protein. They also need generous amounts of fluids and extra calories to produce the milk that nourishes their babies. Lactating women should drink at least two quarts of liquids per day and consume additional nutrient-dense calories as recommended by their doctor. The Dietary Reference Intakes (DRI) provide nutrient recommendations for women who are pregnant or lactating. For women who are obese or sedentary, the recommendations for added nutrient-dense calories may be too high. For underweight adolescent mothers who are still growing, more nutrient-dense calories may be needed.

Case Study: A Healthy Pregnancy

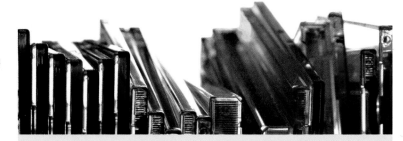

Hannah was excited to learn that her older sister, Jill, is pregnant. Hannah had health class last semester and learned a great deal about healthy pregnancies.

Jill and her husband do not like to cook. The couple usually eats at fast-food restaurants or microwaves frozen pizzas. Jill likes to read and play video games, but is not very active. Needless to say, Jill has gained weight since she got married and is now about 35 pounds overweight. Jill has decided she does not want to gain even more weight during this pregnancy and is putting herself on a weight-loss diet. She told Hannah that the vitamin supplement the doctor prescribed for her makes her sick to her stomach, so she is not going to take them.

This baby will be Hannah's first niece or nephew and she plans to be a good aunt. However, Hannah is already worried for the health of her sister and the baby.

Case Review

1. Why do you think Hannah is worried about Jill and the baby?
2. What would you do if you were Hannah?

Meals to Meet Nutritional Needs

Pregnant and lactating women are advised not to skip meals, especially breakfast. Eating regular meals and snacks provides them and their infants with a steady supply of needed nutrients.

Meals should offer a variety of nutritious foods. Whole-grain and enriched breads and cereals supply B vitamins and iron. Whole-grain products may also provide dietary fiber. Fruits and vegetables are good sources of vitamins, including the folate needed before and during early pregnancy. Fat-free and low-fat milk, soy milk, yogurt, and cheese provide protein and calcium. Limiting fat intake helps to reduce intake of problem amounts of cholesterol and too many calories. Lean meats, poultry, fish, and meat alternates furnish protein, iron, B vitamins, and zinc, **11-7**.

When planning meals, lactating women can include soups and fruit juices to help meet their fluid needs.

Both during and after pregnancy, women can select fruits, vegetables, peanut butter, and low-fat yogurt and cheese as nutritious snacks. However, foods that provide little more than fats and sugars should be limited.

Pregnant or lactating women who follow vegetarian diets have an extra challenge when meeting nutrient needs. They should discuss their food patterns with a doctor or registered dietitian. Including good food sources of protein, such as nuts, seeds, whole grains, legumes, and tofu is very important. Vegetarians must plan carefully to get enough iron, vitamin B_{12}, and folate for their important role in cell reproduction. Calcium, magnesium, iron, and zinc needs are high. Vegetarians may require supplements to meet their needs for iron. Vitamin B_{12} needs can be met by consuming supplements or fortified foods. Women who do not use dairy products may need calcium and vitamin D supplements as well. Protein supplements are not recommended and may be harmful.

11-7   Eating a variety of nutritious foods will help a woman meet the extra nutrient needs of pregnancy.

Special Dietary Concerns

Certain conditions and foods can create special dietary concerns during pregnancy. Women should discuss these concerns with their physician or a registered dietitian.

Women sometimes experience strange cravings during pregnancy that are not based on physiological needs. Most cravings are simply due to changed sense of taste and smell. They may also occur when women are low in some nutrients. Women who practice pica during pregnancy may have specific dietary concerns. **Pica** is the craving for and ingestion of nonfood materials such as clay, soil, or chalk. These substances do not deliver the nutrients she needs. They may interfere with the absorption of other nutrients the body needs or simply replace nutritious foods in the mother's diet. Eating these substances can have an adverse effect on the pregnancy.

Nausea, often called *morning sickness*, may be a problem during the first months of pregnancy. Some women have morning sickness throughout their pregnancies. Many women feel nauseated at times other than morning. To relieve nausea, pregnant women are advised to eat whatever they believe will make them feel better. For some women, this may mean salty foods; for others it may mean bland foods. Eating frequent small meals may also help ease this condition.

Sometimes nausea and vomiting are extreme. Persistent vomiting can result in dehydration and poor weight gain. This condition is a health risk for both the mother and unborn baby. A woman experiencing this problem should inform her doctor.

Another common condition during pregnancy is heartburn. Heartburn is a burning feeling in the chest and throat that results when substances in the stomach move the wrong way and up into the esophagus. To decrease symptoms of heartburn do not eat foods that make it worse, avoid lying down for one hour after meals, and eat small, frequent meals.

Constipation becomes a problem for many pregnant women, especially later in pregnancy. Hormones cause the intestinal muscles to relax, and the expanding uterus crowds the intestines. These factors decrease the rate at which the intestines are able to move waste through the body. The longer feces remain in the large intestine, the more water is absorbed from them. As feces lose water, they become hard, making bowel movements painful. Straining

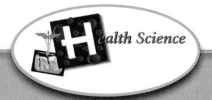

Lactation Consultant

A lactation consultant is a health-care professional with special training and experience in helping breast-feeding mothers and babies. These consultants may be on staff at a hospital or in a pediatrician's office, home health agency, or they may work in private practice.

Education: A Board Certified Lactation Consultant is required to take certain college-level classes plus a minimum number of hours working with breast-feeding mothers in a clinical setting. Many are registered or licensed in other health professions, such as nursing.

Job Outlook: There are far more mothers and babies that need help with breast-feeding than there are lactation consultants to work with them.

during bowel movements can increase the likelihood of developing hemorrhoids during pregnancy.

To avoid problems with constipation and hemorrhoids, pregnant women should be sure to drink plenty of fluids. Consuming an ample amount of fiber by choosing foods such as whole grains, fruits, and vegetables will help. Getting moderate daily exercise will also promote regular elimination.

Some women develop a form of diabetes or high blood pressure during pregnancy. These conditions can be serious and require careful monitoring by a doctor. They may also call for some dietary changes. Fortunately, these conditions often go away after delivery.

Certain foods are a cause for concern for pregnant women. Certain types of fish contain high levels of a heavy metal called *mercury*. Mercury can damage the fetal brain and nervous system. To limit exposure to mercury, the FDA cautions women who are pregnant or may become pregnant, and women who are breast-feeding to

- avoid eating shark, swordfish, king mackerel, or tilefish
- consume no more than six ounces per week of albacore (white) tuna
- check with local authorities about the safety of fish caught in local waters

Most artificial sweeteners have been found to be safe during pregnancy. However, there is still some concern about the safety of saccharin. Most health professionals believe artificial sweeteners are safe when used in moderation. One exception is individuals who have a hereditary disease that prevents their body from breaking down the compound found in aspartame. They should not use aspartame. The best advice is to check with your doctor and use artificial sweeteners in moderation or not at all. Instead, choose foods that are naturally sweet.

Pesticides may cause harm to unborn babies and children. Pregnant women should avoid contact with pesticides as much as possible. Wash and peel fruits and vegetables to remove pesticide residues. If pesticides must be applied in your home, remove all food and dishes from the area. Afterward, have someone else wash any food-contact surfaces.

Concerns Related to Teen Pregnancy

Pregnancy places extra stress on the body of a teenager. The adolescent body is still growing and, therefore, has large nutrient requirements. The nutrient needs of the fetus are then added to the teen's needs. Meeting these combined nutrient needs is very difficult for most teens, **11-8**.

Many adolescent women have poor diets. They fail to get enough calories, iron, folic acid, zinc, calcium, and vitamins A and D to help them grow to their optimum height and muscle development. Teens with poor nutritional status do not have the nutrient reserves needed to meet the demands of a developing fetus. If these teens lead an inactive lifestyle, they are not at an ideal level of physical fitness, either.

These factors place teens at a much higher risk of complications during pregnancy than adult women. Teens are more likely to have miscarriages and stillbirths. They are also more likely to have premature and low-birthweight babies. Their babies are at higher risk for health problems and death.

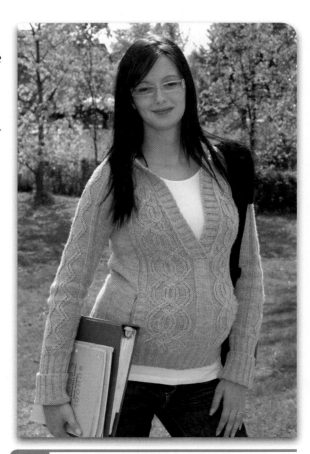

11-8　Pregnancy creates especially great nutrient needs for teenage women.

To help reduce risks, a teen needs to visit her doctor as soon as she thinks she is pregnant. Being aware of the first signs of pregnancy can help teens determine when to seek prenatal care. These signs include a missed menstrual period, fatigue, nausea, swelling and soreness in the breasts, and frequent urination.

A pregnant teen must carefully follow the advice of her doctor. She needs to select an adequate number of servings of nutrient-dense foods each day. She must also take any nutrient supplements her doctor prescribes. This type of diet provides the nutrients needed by the teen and her developing baby. It helps her achieve recommended weight gain during her pregnancy. Taking these steps improves a teen's chances of avoiding complications and delivering a healthy baby.

Drug Use During Pregnancy and Lactation

During pregnancy, an organ called the **placenta** forms inside the uterus. In the placenta, blood vessels from the mother and the fetus are entwined. Materials carried in the blood can be transferred between the mother and the fetus through the placenta. Oxygen and nutrients from the mother's blood-stream are delivered to the fetus. Waste products and carbon dioxide from the fetus are transported to the mother for elimination. Harmful substances such as alcohol and drugs from the mother's bloodstream can also be passed to the fetus through the placenta.

The term "drug" describes a broad range of substances. These include caffeine and nicotine. They also include alcohol, over-the-counter and prescription medications, and illegal drugs. It

is worthwhile to note here how these substances can affect pregnancy and lactation.

When a woman uses a drug, it enters her bloodstream. If she is pregnant, it can pass through the placenta to her unborn child. If she is lactating, the drug may be secreted in her breast milk. Therefore, any drug a woman uses affects not only her but also her baby.

Fetuses and infants have such little bodies that even a small amount of a drug can be harmful. They also have immature organs that cannot break down drugs efficiently. Therefore, the effects of drugs last longer in fetuses and infants.

Drugs present dangers to a fetus throughout pregnancy. However, they are of special concern during the first trimester of the pregnancy. This is the period when the vital organs and systems of the fetus are developing. Some drugs can also cause excessive bleeding during the last trimester of pregnancy. Some over-the-counter and prescription drugs are known to cause congenital disabilities. **Congenital disabilities** are conditions existing from birth that limit a person's ability to use his or her body or mind.

Doctors discourage pregnant women from using any types of drugs, even common nonprescription drugs, such as aspirin. Over-the-counter drug labels warn pregnant women to seek the advice of a health professional before using the product. A physician can recommend which over-the-counter drugs might be safe during pregnancy.

Caffeine is a stimulant found in colas and many other soft drinks, coffee, tea, and chocolate, **11-9**. Caffeine is in many over-the-counter and prescription drugs, too. Studies about the effects of caffeine on fetuses have led researchers to various conclusions.

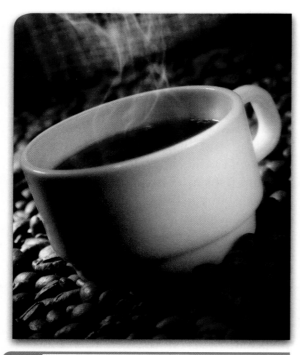

11-9   Many health professionals advise pregnant women to limit their use of coffee, tea, chocolate, soft drinks, and other products containing caffeine.

Further study is needed to settle the debate. However, many health professionals recommend that women limit foods and beverages containing caffeine during pregnancy. Health professionals also recommend limiting caffeine during lactation. This is because caffeine passes into breast milk and has been shown to cause irritability and restlessness in nursing babies.

Smoking is not healthy for anyone. However, health care providers especially caution pregnant women against smoking. A pregnant woman who smokes is more likely to have a low-birthweight baby. Cigarette smoking decreases the oxygen delivered to the fetus and can endanger its health. Also, smoking causes nicotine to circulate in the mother's bloodstream. The fetus can absorb this nicotine, which increases the risk of the fetus developing certain types of cancer in childhood.

Pregnant women should not drink alcohol, including beer and wine. Drinking even a small amount of alcohol during pregnancy can cause permanent damage to the fetus. A miscarriage or stillbirth may occur. Alcohol may damage the baby's developing organs such as the brain and heart. The head may not grow properly. The baby may die in early infancy or have intellectual disabilities. The baby may have sight and hearing problems, slow growth, and poor coordination. **Fetal alcohol syndrome (FAS)** is a set of symptoms that can occur in newborns whose mothers drink alcohol while pregnant. Babies born with FAS suffer its effects throughout their lives. A baby born with FAS could have some or all the following symptoms:

- brain damage and below-average intelligence
- slowed physical growth
- facial disfigurement, including a flattened nose bridge, small eyes with drooping eyelids, and receding forehead
- short attention span
- irritability
- heart problems

Mothers should continue to refrain from drinking alcohol during lactation. If a lactating mother drinks alcohol, the alcohol can reach the baby through the breast milk. This may cause the baby to have developmental problems.

Infancy and Toddlerhood

Infants and toddlers have special nutritional needs and problems. An **infant** is a child in the first year of life. Children who are one to three years old are often called **toddlers**. Nutritional care is very important during these periods.

Many parents receive nutritional advice from their children's doctors. Some doctors suggest parents consult a registered dietitian to better understand their children's unique nutritional needs.

Growth Patterns of Infants and Toddlers

Growth is more rapid during infancy than at any other time in the life cycle. The muscles, bones, and other tissues grow and develop at dramatic rates. A healthy baby's weight triples during the first year, **11-10**. The baby's length increases by one-half. That means a 7-pound, 20-inch newborn will be at least a 21-pound, 30-inch 12-month-old.

The pattern of growth changes during the toddler years. The muscles of the legs and arms begin to develop more fully. Bone growth slows, but minerals are deposited in the bones at a rapid rate. This helps make the bones stronger to support the increasing weight of the toddler.

Nutrient Needs of Infants and Toddlers

Infants and toddlers need the same variety of nutrients as adults. However, growing, active children have *proportionately* greater nutritional needs than adults. This means children require more of each nutrient per pound of body weight. For example, the Adequate Intake (AI) for calcium for a four-month-old infant is 200 milligrams per day. A 35-year-old adult needs 1,000 milligrams of calcium daily. Suppose the infant weighs 15 pounds and the adult weighs 150 pounds. This means the infant needs approximately 13 milligrams of calcium per pound of body weight. However, the adult requires only about 6.7 milligrams per pound of body weight. Proportionately, the infant needs more than twice as much calcium as the adult.

Infants born to healthy women who consumed adequate amounts of iron during pregnancy should have iron stored in their bodies. This stored iron should be enough to last until the

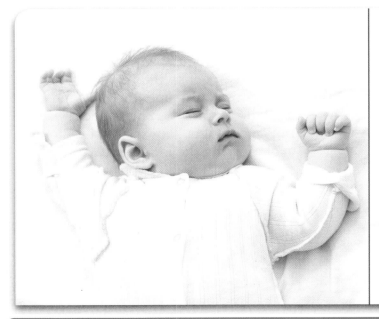
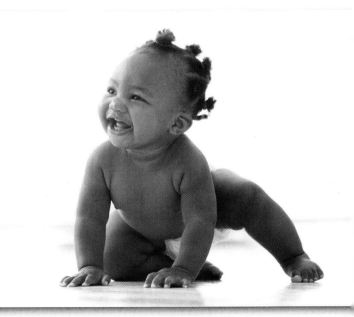

11-10   Babies grow and change rapidly during the first year of life.

infants are able to begin eating iron-fortified cereals. Infants also need high-quality protein to support the growth of muscles and other body tissues. An ample supply of calcium and phosphorous is essential for the development of teeth and bones. Breast milk or infant formula is designed to meet infants' needs for these and other nutrients. Breast milk or infant formula normally supplies enough water to replace fluid losses. If rapid fluid losses occur as a result of diarrhea or vomiting, then extra electrolyte fluid for infants may be necessary. Consult with the baby's doctor for special care.

Infants grow fastest in the first six months or so of life. Growth slows during the second six months, and it continues to slow through the toddler years. Toddlers still need proportionately more nutrients than adults, **11-11**.

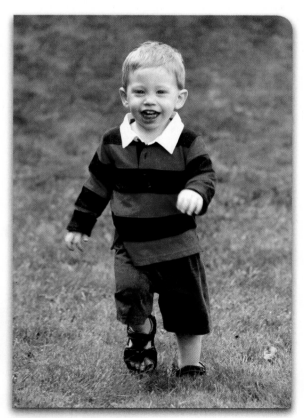

11-11   A toddler's diet must supply enough calories to support the toddler's high level of activity.

However, their proportional needs are smaller than those of an infant.

Feeding Schedule for Infants

Proper feeding of an infant is critical to ensure normal growth. During the first few weeks, babies need to be fed every two to three hours. They are just learning how to eat, and their digestive tracts are immature. Therefore, newborns can handle only small amounts of breast milk or infant formula at each feeding.

After the first few weeks, babies usually want to be fed at fairly regular times. Most babies require six feedings a day. Caregivers can plan a schedule to space feedings at four-hour intervals. Caregivers usually can reduce the number of daily feedings to five when the infant is around two months old. At around seven or eight months, four daily feedings usually are sufficient. By a child's first birthday, he or she can join family members for three daily meals with nutritious snacks in between meals.

Caregivers need to be flexible in following a feeding schedule. They need to remember a baby may be hungry at irregular times. Caregivers need to respect an infant's signs of hunger or lack of appetite. They need to feed the infant when he or she cries to indicate hunger. However, they should avoid forcing the infant to eat when signs of satisfaction appear. These signs include spitting out food or turning the head away from food.

Foods for Infants

Many nutrition experts view breast milk as the ideal food for infants, **11-12**. Human breast milk has a nutrient

Stages of Breast Milk

Stage	Time Frame	Characteristics
1st—Colostrum	First 3–5 days following birth	• creamy, yellow, thick milk • high in protein, vitamins, minerals, and antibodies
2nd—Transitional milk	Lasts about 2 weeks	• thinner, whiter milk • high in fat, lactose, and vitamins
3rd—Mature milk	Until baby is weaned	• 90% water for hydration • carbohydrate, protein, and fat needed for growth and energy

11-12   The stages that breast milk composition progresses through may vary slightly in length and timing for each mother.

composition that is specifically designed to nourish humans. During the first few months following birth, breast milk changes to meet the changing needs of the infant. Composition of breast milk is quite different from cow's milk and infant formulas. Formulas include more of some nutrients than breast milk. However, more is not necessarily better. The smaller amount of protein in breast milk is easier for babies' immature systems to digest. Babies absorb the smaller amount of iron in breast milk more fully than they absorb the iron in formula. Breast milk also contains antibodies not found in formula. These antibodies help protect babies against diseases.

The only alternative to breast milk recommended by the American Academy of Pediatrics (AAP) is iron-fortified infant formula. There are different types of these formulas including milk-based, soy-based, and some specialized formulas for specific health conditions. Most infants do well on milk-based formula, but some vegetarian parents may prefer to feed their baby a soy-based formula. The specialized formulas should only be used with a doctor's supervision. The nutrient composition of infant formulas must meet AAP standards. Iron fortification is important because an infant's iron stores at birth are enough to last only four to six months. A doctor can help parents find a suitable formula.

Vitamin D is another nutrient concern for infants. Doctors recommend that all infants get 600 IU of vitamin D every day. This includes infants who are breast-fed as well as those on formula. The need for vitamin D supplement should be discussed with a doctor.

Formulas are usually sold in ready-to-feed, powdered, or liquid concentrate forms. Formulas must be prepared according to the directions. Food safety must be practiced when preparing or storing infant formulas, **11-13**. Practicing food safety is also essential when breast milk is being pumped and stored for later use. Formula or pumped breast milk that is improperly handled can result in a foodborne illness for the infant. This can be especially harmful because a baby's immune system is not fully developed.

Babies should receive breast milk or iron-fortified formula for at least one year. Caregivers should not give babies cow's milk until they are one year old. It does not have enough iron and it has too much calcium.

Preparing Infant Formula
• Wash hands before preparing formula and feeding
• Clean bottles in the dishwasher or follow manufacturer's instructions
• Check that nipples are not clogged or torn. Discard any torn nipples.
• Mix formula according to directions on package and refrigerate until needed
• Use refrigerated formula within 48 hours
• Warm formula slowly in hot water. DO NOT boil or microwave formula. Test the temperature of the formula on your arm before feeding.
• Throw away any formula left in the bottle after feeding

11-13 Care must be taken during preparation and storage to ensure infant formula is safe and wholesome.

Caregivers should not add solid foods to infants' diets until they are four to six months of age. Before four months, infants have trouble swallowing such foods. In addition, their immature GI tracts can absorb whole proteins instead of just amino acids. This can greatly increase infants' risks of developing allergies. Also, infants' kidneys are immature and cannot handle the increased load of excreting wastes generated by solid foods. These wastes include sodium and certain other minerals. To rid their bodies of these extra wastes, infants must excrete more urine. Thus, eating solid foods before four to six months can cause dehydration.

Caregivers can watch for several signs to tell if infants are ready for solid foods. Infants should be able to sit with support. This provides a straight passage for solids to travel from the mouth to the stomach. Infants should no longer drool. This indicates they can control their mouths and tongues in a way that will permit swallowing of solids. Infants should double their birth weight. They should also show interest in eating solids by practicing chewing when they see others eating.

Infant cereals are usually the first solid foods added to a baby's diet.

These cereals provide iron in a form babies can easily absorb. After cereals, infants are usually given strained vegetables, then fruits. Many parents introduce fortified apple juice at this time as a source of vitamin C. Meats are generally introduced last. By the end of the first year, a baby's diet should include a variety of foods.

Caregivers should introduce only one food at a time. They should wait four to five days before introducing another food. This will help them identify food allergies and intolerances. Pediatricians usually recommend introducing infants to rice cereal first. It is the least allergenic. Wheat cereal is more likely to cause an allergic reaction. Therefore, it is usually introduced later. Egg white and orange juice can also cause allergic reactions if they are introduced too early. Pediatricians advise waiting until after a baby's first birthday to introduce these foods.

Caregivers should repeatedly serve new foods. This allows the baby to learn to accept the foods by growing used to their new flavors and textures.

Baby foods can be purchased from the supermarket or made at home. Commercially-prepared baby food is convenient and has a long shelf life. However, homemade baby food can be as nutritious as and less expensive than commercially-prepared baby food, **11-14**. When preparing baby food at home, steps must be taken to ensure that the food is

- prepared and stored using safe food practices
- an appropriate texture for the child
- nutritious
- prepared without added sugar, salt, or spices

Caregivers should avoid overfeeding infants to prevent the development of excess fat tissue. The amount of food infants willingly accept varies. The quantity consumed depends on age, sex, size, state of health, and characteristics of the food.

As infants develop teeth and the muscle coordination to chew, they can begin to eat mashed and chopped foods. They enjoy chewing crusts of hard bread, especially if they are teething. By the age of six or seven months, infants can pick up foods with their fingers. Holding foods with their hands helps prepare infants to hold spoons.

Feeding Problems During Infancy

Though their nutrient needs are high, infants have small stomachs. This is why they need frequent feedings.

Preparing and Storing Homemade Baby Food

Preparation

1. Select good quality, fresh food. Avoid using leftover foods.
2. Wash, peel, seed, or trim foods as needed. Remove fat from meat.
3. Cook food until tender. Cook protein foods until well done.
4. Use a food mill or blender to process foods to appropriate texture. Foods can also be pushed through a fine-mesh strainer with a spoon.
5. Add cooking liquid, water, or fruit juice to thin puréed food if needed.

Storage

Foods that are not eaten immediately after cooking should be stored in refrigerator or freezer. Do not let the food sit at room temperature.

To Refrigerate

1. Place food in clean container with lid.
2. Label and date food.
3. Refrigerate immediately.
4. Discard food after 24 hours.

To Freeze

1. Place baby food into clean container. (Clean ice cube trays can be used to freeze food into baby-size portions.) Cover tightly with lid, plastic wrap, or foil.
2. Label and date food.
3. Place in freezer immediately.
4. Discard food after one month.

11-14   Always wash hands, equipment, and work area before you begin to prepare food.

Premature infants need special attention. They have greater needs for calories and all the nutrients. Premature infants do not have the iron reserves full-term babies have. They may also have trouble sucking and swallowing.

Problems can arise when caregivers have inappropriate expectations about when and how babies should eat. For instance, it is unrealistic to expect an infant to consume every last drop of milk or spoonful of cereal. Infants will start eating less as their growth slows and their weight gain begins to taper off. Caregivers must be patient and understanding about such normal infant behaviors, **11-15**.

Caregivers should not be upset when a child rejects a food. Rejecting a food is one of the few ways a baby has of showing independence. The child may accept the food if caregivers offer it again a few days later.

Pediatricians do not recommend forcing children to eat. Pleasant, happy eating conditions help children form positive feelings toward food and eating.

Babies are not born with food dislikes—they learn them. Caregivers must be aware of how they communicate their likes and dislikes to an infant. When a caregiver acts negatively toward a food, a child will notice this response. As a result, the child may learn to reject that particular food.

Foods for Toddlers

Foods for toddlers should be cut into bite-sized pieces. Toddlers like foods they can pick up with their fingers. They also like colorful foods and soft textures that are easy to chew. Servings should be about one tablespoon of food for every year of age. The toddler's appetite should guide how much food he or she eats. Wait until the child asks for more food. The MyPlate food guidance system can be used to determine recommended amounts from each food group for older toddlers, **11-16**.

Foods from the dairy group continue to be an important part of the toddler's diet. Some of this milk may be served as cream soups, pudding, yogurt, and cheese. Milk provides calcium as well as needed protein and phosphorus. It also supplies vitamins A and D, riboflavin, and some of the other B vitamins. Whole milk and milk products are recommended during the first two years of life. Fat is needed for calories and the normal development of organs such as the brain.

The protein foods group contributes protein to a child's diet. Eggs, meats, peanut butter, beans, and peas are included in this group. Meat can be

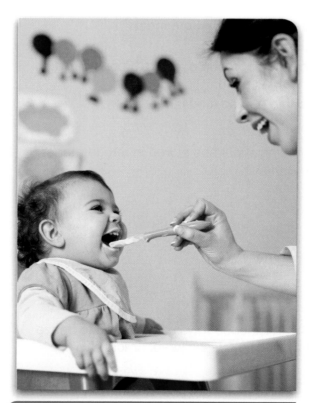

11-15   A caregiver's attitude when feeding a baby can affect the baby's response to the food.

My Daily Food Plan

Based on the information you provided, this is your daily recommended amount from each food group.

GRAINS 3 ounces	**Make half your grains whole** Aim for at least **1½ ounces** of whole grains a day
VEGETABLES 1 cup	**Vary your veggies** Aim for these amounts **each week**: **Dark green veggies** = ½ cup **Red & orange veggies** = 2½ cup **Beans & peas** = ½ cup **Starchy veggies** = 2 cups **Other veggies** = 1½ cups
FRUITS 1 cup	**Focus on fruits** Eat a variety of fruit Choose whole or cut-up fruits more often than fruit juice
DAIRY 2 cups	**Get your calcium-rich foods** Drink fat-free or low-fat (1%) milk, for the same amount of calcium and other nutrients as whole milk, but less fat and calories Select fat-free or low-fat yogurt and cheese, or try calcium-fortified soy products
PROTEIN FOODS 2 ounces	**Go lean with protein** Twice a week, make seafood the protein on your plate Vary your protein routine—choose more fish, beans, peas, nuts, and seeds Keep meat and poultry portions small and lean

Find your balance between food and physical activity Children 2 to 5 years old should play actively every day.	**Know your limits on fats, sugars, and sodium** Your allowance for oils is **3 teaspoons a day**. Limit extras–solid fats and sugars–to **140 Calories** a day. Reduce sodium intake to less than **2300 mg** a day.

Your results are based on a 1000 calorie pattern.   Name: _____

This calorie level is only an estimate of your needs. Monitor your body weight to see if you need to adjust your calorie intake.

11-16   This food plan is suitable for a two-year-old. *Credit: USDA*

ground or cut into small pieces depending on the number of teeth the toddler has for chewing. Nuts are a choking hazard at this age and should be avoided.

The fruit and vegetable groups provide toddlers with vitamins, minerals, and fiber. At least one fruit serving per day should be a good source of vitamin C. Foods rich in vitamin C include orange juice, strawberries, cantaloupe, and tomatoes. Dark green and deep yellow fruits and vegetables are important for vitamin A. Potatoes and other starchy vegetables provide carbohydrates.

Breads, cereals, rice, and pasta are included in the grain group. At least half of the grains in a toddler's diet should be whole grains. These foods supply carbohydrates, iron, and B vitamins to a toddler's diet.

Toddlers can be served three meals a day with some between-meal snacks. Snacks are very important for toddlers. They have small stomachs and cannot eat enough at mealtime to carry them through to the next meal. Caregivers may choose the kind and amount of snack food to complement the foods a toddler eats at mealtime. Snack foods should contribute nutrients, not just calories from sugar and fat. Caregivers should avoid giving toddlers cookies, candy, and soft drinks as regular snacks. Instead caregivers can offer fresh fruits, juices, milk, toast, and graham crackers. If snacks are eaten about two hours before a meal, they will not interfere with a child's appetite at mealtime.

Eating Problems of Toddlers

Several factors can lead to eating problems during the toddler stage. However, being aware of normal patterns of growth and development can help caregivers avoid many of these problems. Caregivers can help toddlers form food habits that promote good health and nutritional status.

Lack of teeth can be a source of eating problems for young toddlers. A one-year-old child may have only six to eight teeth. This can make chewing difficult and may lead to problems with choking. To make chewing easier, foods such as ripe fruit may be mashed into pulp or chopped into bite-sized pieces. To prevent choking, caregivers

should avoid feeding toddlers foods that contain seeds. Toddlers can also choke on nuts, corn, raisins, gristle in meat, marshmallows, pretzels, grapes, raisins, hard candy, and round slices of hot dogs and carrots.

Some caregivers view toddlers' messy eating habits as a problem. Toddlers learn by using their senses to explore their environment, and food is part of that environment. Toddlers may involve their whole bodies in the eating process. They mash food with their hands to see how it feels. They place food in their mouths to taste it and feel the texture. They drop food on the floor to see what happens when they let go of it. By the end of a meal, toddlers may have applesauce in their hair and peanut butter on their elbows. Understanding how toddlers learn will help caregivers develop patience during this stage.

A toddler's developing sense of independence can sometimes lead to eating problems. When toddlers become physically able to use a spoon, they usually want to feed themselves. This can be time-consuming and messy. When toddlers learn to talk, they begin to ask for the foods they want. They may not always ask for the most healthful foods. Caregivers should encourage these steps toward independence. Allowing toddlers to feed themselves helps them develop hand-eye coordination, **11-17**. Offer finger foods, or foods not used with an eating utensil, to encourage eating independence. Allowing toddlers to choose between two nutritious foods helps them learn decision-making skills.

A toddler's short attention span can be another eating problem. Toddlers are often easily distracted from eating. They may find it difficult to sit through a meal with their families. They may want to get down on the floor to play. Children need to have regular

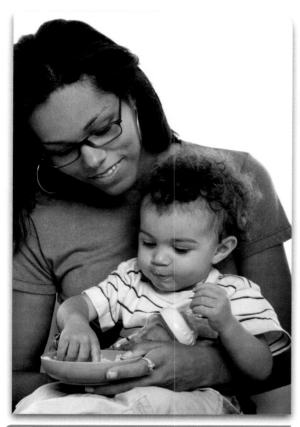

11-17 Young toddlers may make a mess when they feed themselves, but they are learning important skills.

mealtimes with few distractions. Turning off the television and keeping toys out of the eating area will help children focus on enjoying their food.

Picky eating is a common problem among toddlers. A child may not want to eat a certain food for many reasons. The food might be too hot, cold, spicy, or bland. The toddler may want a special plate or cup and will not eat without it. The child may be tired or excited about something. He or she may not be hungry because of eating a snack too close to mealtime. The toddler may be coming down with an illness. Sometimes a toddler simply rejects food because of the attention he or she can gain from the rejection.

At times, a toddler may eat all the food on his or her plate and want more. At other times, the toddler may eat only part of the food. Children's appetites vary. Appetite tends to increase during a growth spurt and slow when growth slows.

Parents often worry their toddler is not eating enough. Two indicators can assure parents a child is getting adequate calories and nutrients. These are normal growth and infrequent infections.

Caregivers need to make mealtimes pleasant experiences for toddlers. Caregivers should offer familiar foods children like in small, attractive servings. They can help children develop interest in new foods by expressing positive attitudes toward new tastes. Caregivers should not force children to eat or fuss over whether they are eating. After a reasonable amount of time, caregivers can simply remove any uneaten food.

Childhood

Nutritional needs change for children ages four to eight. Preschool and school-age children continue to eat the same basic foods they ate as toddlers. However, they need larger quantities to meet increasing energy needs.

Growth Patterns During Childhood

Growth rates vary among children. Every year brings unique changes. Illness, emotional stress, poor eating habits, and genetics can all affect growth patterns.

Growth is generally slower during childhood than it was in the first years of life. The chubby toddler becomes a taller, thinner preschool child. The child continues to grow and develop muscle control throughout the early school years.

Children are active during these years. Parents should encourage children to exercise through play activities. Exercise promotes wellness and helps children develop strong muscles and bones.

Nutrient Needs During Childhood

Preschool and school-age children need more total calories than infants and toddlers due to their larger body size. You can use the tools on the MyPlate Web site to create nutritious food plans, meals, and snacks for children.

The daily requirements for high-quality protein and many vitamins and minerals increase for children ages four and over. An adequate supply of nutrients allows for growth and maintenance of new body tissue. Children should eat a variety of nutritious foods to meet their nutrient needs. Children's diets should contain enough calories from carbohydrates such as whole-grain cereals, breads, and pasta to spare protein for tissue building.

Most health professionals believe the best source of vitamins and minerals for healthy children is from foods in their diet. A doctor may recommend vitamin supplements for children who are at nutritional risk. For example, a doctor may determine that a child who is underweight, on a restricted diet, has a chronic illness, or has multiple food allergies may benefit from vitamin supplements.

Meals for Children

Good meal plans for children include eating meals throughout the day. One important meal is breakfast, **11-18**. It should contain carbohydrates and a small amount of fat. It should

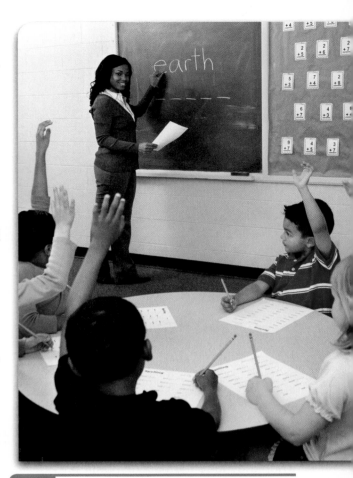

11-18   Eating a nutritious breakfast and lunch helps children stay alert and perform well in school.

provide at least one-fourth of the daily requirements for calories and protein. Children who skip breakfast may have trouble concentrating and performing well in school. They may also have trouble meeting their daily nutrient needs. A nutrient-dense lunch improves performance in school and provides energy for after-school activities.

Children can supplement meals with snacks to help meet nutrient needs. Healthful snacking is easier if the kitchen is stocked with nutritious foods. Parents should keep such items as fruits, yogurt, raisins, carrot sticks, and fat-free milk on hand. They should limit snack foods that have a high salt, sugar, or fat content, **11-19**.

Meal and Snack Pattern B

These patterns show one way a **1600 calorie MyPlate plan** can be divided into meals and snacks for a preschooler. Sample food choices are shown for each meal or snack.

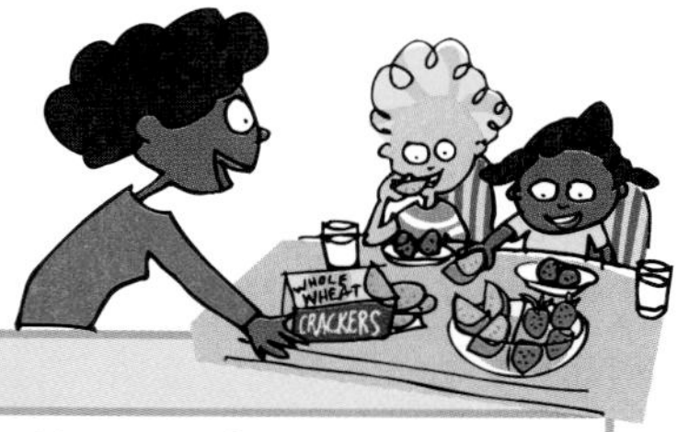

Notes for using the Meal and Snack Ideas.

Breakfast	Breakfast Ideas		
1 ounce Grains ½ cup Dairy* 1 ounce Protein foods	**Peanut-ty Toast** *1 slice whole wheat toast* *1 Tbsp peanut butter* *½ cup milk**	**Oatmeal made with Milk** *½ cup cooked oatmeal (¼ cup dry)* *made with ½ cup milk** *1 scrambled egg*	**Yogurt Parfait** *½ cup low-fat granola* *½ cup yogurt** *½ ounce finely chopped nuts*

Morning Snack	Morning Snack Ideas		
½ cup Fruit ½ cup Dairy*	½ small apple 1 string cheese*	**Fruit Smoothie** *½ cup frozen berries* *¼ cup milk** *¼ cup yogurt**	**Pear n' Puddin'** *1 medium pear* *½ cup pudding (made with* *½ cup milk*)*

Lunch	Lunch Ideas		
2 ounces Grains ½ cup Vegetables ½ cup Fruit ½ cup Dairy*	**Veggie Pita Pocket** *1 medium whole wheat pita* *½ cup romaine lettuce* *¼ cup mashed avocado* *2 Tbsp mashed kidney beans* *½ cup diced cantaloupe* *½ cup milk**	**English Muffin Pizza** *1 whole wheat English muffin* *¼ cup tomato sauce* *¼ cup mixed veggies* *3 Tbsp shredded cheese** *½ cup 100% fruit juice*	**Grilled Cheese Sandwich and Salad** *1 slice whole wheat bread* *3 Tbsp shredded cheese** *½ cup salad greens or lettuce* *¼ cup chopped tomato* *½ cup Mandarin oranges*

Afternoon Snack	Afternoon Snack Ideas		
½ cup Vegetables ½ cup Fruit 1 ounce Protein foods	**Veggie sticks with hummus** *½ cup zucchini or* *carrot "matchsticks"* *¼ cup hummus* *½ cup applesauce*	**½ cup oven-baked sweet potato "fries"** *¼ cup edamame (green soybeans)* *½ cup 100% fruit juice*	**Ants on a Log** *½ cup celery sticks spread with* *1 Tbsp peanut butter* *¼ cup raisins or mixed dried fruit*

Dinner	Dinner Ideas		
2 ounces Grains 1 cup Vegetables ½ cup Dairy* 3 ounces Protein foods	**Go Fish!** *3 ounces salmon filet* *½ cup onion* *½ cup cooked spinach* *1 cup egg noodles* *½ cup milk**	**Asian Stir-Fry on Rice** *1 cup vegetables (broccoli, mushrooms, bell pepper)* *3 ounces chicken breast* *1 cup cooked brown rice* *½ cup milk**	**Roast Beef with Baked Potato** *3 ounces roast beef* *½ cup baked potato* *½ cup green beans* *2 small slices French bread* *½ cup milk**

*Offer your child fat-free or low-fat milk, yogurt, and cheese.

11-19   This sample meal and snack pattern is appropriate for a 6-year-old boy who is active 30 to 60 minutes per day.

Too much snacking at the wrong times can spoil a child's appetite for regular meals. Caregivers can help children learn good snacking habits by offering appropriate amounts of snack foods. For example, caregivers can serve two graham crackers instead of offering children the whole box of crackers. They can give children a cup of plain popcorn rather than the bag.

Nutrition and Fitness Problems of Childhood

On the average, children today grow taller than children years ago. One reason for this is the availability of a healthful diet. However, children today are also more likely to be overweight or obese than their ancestors. Poor eating habits and lack of exercise are the main causes of childhood weight problems.

Caregivers play an important role in preventing weight problems among children. By providing healthful foods, caregivers can help children learn healthy eating habits. Children should be encouraged to drink water rather than sugar-sweetened drinks. Meals and snacks should be nutrient-rich foods. Caregivers can also limit the amount of time children spend in sedentary activities such as watching television or playing video games. Children should spend 60 minutes or more per day being physically active—riding bikes, playing ball, or doing chores. Caregivers must promote healthy choices by explaining to children why it is important to eat right, be active, and get enough sleep each night.

Dental caries is another problem related to nutrition that is common in childhood. The type of food and when it is eaten greatly affect the risk of dental caries. Sticky, carbohydrate-rich foods eaten between meals are the chief promoters of this problem, **11-20**. However, sound nutrition and dental health practices help develop and maintain healthy teeth and oral tissues. Caregivers can help children prevent tooth decay by teaching them about good eating and dental care habits.

Math Link

Calculating Equivalents

One study estimates that children between the ages of 8 and 18 spend an average of 6 hours per day in sedentary behavior such as watching TV, playing video games, or on the computer.
1. Calculate the equivalent of how many days per year these children participate in sedentary activity.
2. If one hour is spent participating in physical activity 5 days per week, how many days per year would that be? (Round to the nearest decimal place.)

Adolescence

Adolescence is the period of life between childhood and adulthood. You and others who are in this part of the life cycle are called *adolescents*. Adolescence is an important transition period. The body undergoes many changes during this time. Good food habits started in childhood need continued emphasis as your body continues to develop.

Growth Patterns During Adolescence

Puberty marks the beginning of adolescence. **Puberty** is the time

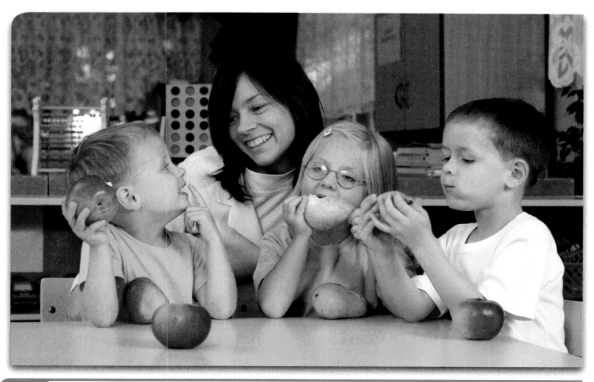

11-20 Caregivers can help children prevent dental caries by limiting sweet, sticky snack foods and encouraging children to brush after eating.

during which a person develops sexual maturity. This is the time when females begin menstruating. Hormonal changes cause secondary sexual characteristics to appear. For males, these characteristics include a deeper voice, broader shoulders, and the appearance of facial and body hair. Breast development and the growth of body hair are among the changes that occur in females. The onset of puberty occurs between the ages of 10 and 12 years for most girls. It occurs between the ages of 12 and 14 years for most boys.

Growth rates vary from person to person during adolescence. However, most adolescents experience a **growth spurt**. This is a period of rapid physical growth. Adolescents become taller as their bones grow. This increase in height is accompanied by muscle development and an increase in weight.

Body composition changes during adolescence. Well-nourished females develop a layer of fatty tissue that remains throughout life. Well-nourished males have an increase in lean body mass, which gives them a muscular appearance. When fully grown, males will have two times the muscle tissue and two-thirds as much fat tissue as females.

Nutrient Needs During Adolescence

Daily calorie needs in adolescence are higher than they are in late childhood. Specific needs vary with an adolescent's growth rate, gender, and activity level. The average caloric requirement for active 14- to 18-year-old females is roughly 2,300 calories a day. Males need more calories than females. This is partly because males have a higher percentage of lean body mass. The average daily requirement for active males 14 to 18 years old is about 3,100 calories. Teens of both sexes who are involved in intense physical activity have greater calorie needs. Likewise, teens who are less active have lower calorie needs, **11-21**.

Nutrient needs increase significantly for young people in the 9- to 13-year-old age group. Nutrient needs increase again for teens who are 14 to 18 years old. Teens in this group have needs equal to or greater than the needs of adults for most nutrients. Females need slightly smaller amounts of some nutrients than males.

Teens must consume adequate calories and nutrients to fulfill their growth potential.

Meals for Adolescents

The body functions better when it receives supplies of energy and nutrients at regular intervals throughout the day. A busy school, work, and social schedule may make you feel you do not always have time for regular meals. Some days you may skip breakfast. When you are in a hurry, you may be tempted to grab a candy bar instead of stopping for lunch.

You need to be aware of how irregular eating patterns can affect your overall wellness. Young people who skip meals tend to have more difficulty concentrating in school. They also become tired and irritable more easily and report suffering from more headaches and infections.

Eating a good breakfast replenishes your energy supplies after a night of sleep. Breakfast should provide about one-fourth of your daily nutrient and calorie needs. Any nutritious food helps get your body off to a good start in the morning. If you do not like cereal or eggs, try eating a peanut butter sandwich, yogurt, fresh fruit, or even pizza.

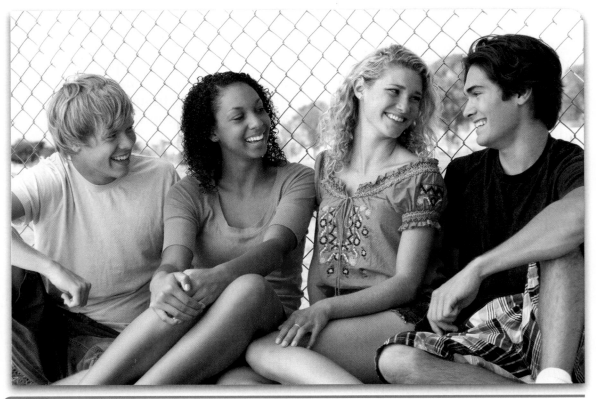

11-21   Growth is more rapid during adolescence than at any other life stage except infancy.

Eating at least two other meals throughout the day should allow you to meet your remaining calorie needs. Carefully choosing the recommended daily amounts from MyPlate should supply you with your nutrient requirements. Between-meal snacks can help provide some of these nutrients.

If you are like most teens, you probably eat some of your meals at fast-food restaurants. Foods such as pizza, hamburgers, and milk shakes provide nutrients, **11-22**. However, they also tend to be high in calories, sugar, fat, and sodium. Therefore, choose these foods in moderation. Balance them with other nutritious food choices throughout the day. Also consider ordering the salads, whole-grain pastas, fruits, and juices many fast-food restaurants now offer.

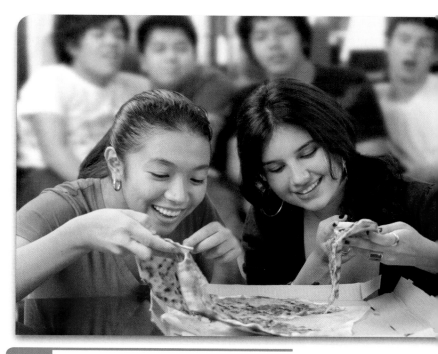

11-22 With careful selection and planning, fast foods can be part of a nutritious diet.

Nutritional and Fitness Problems of Adolescence

Teens often have a reputation for having poor eating habits. Many young people do not deserve this reputation. Surveys suggest many adolescents get enough of most nutrients. However, some adolescent nutritional problems exist.

Anemia is an iron-deficiency disease that often occurs during the teen years. Adolescents need increased amounts of iron to support growth of body tissues. After age 14, females require more iron than males due to losses through menstruation. Some doctors prescribe iron supplements to help adolescent females make up for a lack of dietary iron. Red meat, legumes, dark green leafy vegetables, and whole-grain and enriched breads and cereals are good iron sources.

Weight problems are common among adolescents. Teens who are overweight need to adjust their food intake and increase their activity level. Teens who are underweight are at the other end of the weight management spectrum. These teens need to consume excess calories and exercise to build muscle. Eating disorders are also a common weight problem among adolescents.

Smoking, consuming alcohol, and abusing drugs are habits that sometimes begin in adolescence. These lifestyle behaviors can affect nutritional status.

You need to be aware of the relationship between your diet during adolescence and your health as an adult. If your diet does not include enough calcium and vitamin D, your bones will not achieve maximum density. This lack of bone density will increase your risk of osteoporosis later in life. If you eat a diet high in sugar without proper dental hygiene, you are more likely to have dental caries. This increases your risk of gum disease and tooth loss in your later years. Eating a high-fat diet raises your chances of developing heart disease and some forms of cancer as an adult. Eating a healthful diet now can help prevent future health problems, 11-23.

My Daily Food Plan

Based on the information you provided, this is your daily recommended amount from each food group.

| GRAINS
10 ounces	**Make half your grains whole**
	Aim for at least **5 ounces** of whole grains a day
VEGETABLES
4 cups	**Vary your veggies**
	Aim for these amounts **each week**:
	Dark green veggies = 2½ cups **Red & orange veggies** = 7 cups
	Beans & peas = 3 cups **Starchy veggies** = 8 cups
	Other veggies = 7 cups
FRUITS
2½ cups	**Focus on fruits**
	Eat a variety of fruit
	Choose whole or cut-up fruits more often than fruit juice
DAIRY
3 cups	**Get your calcium-rich foods**
	Drink fat-free or low-fat (1%) milk, for the same amount of calcium and other nutrients as whole milk, but less fat and calories
	Select fat-free or low-fat yogurt and cheese, or try calcium-fortified soy products
PROTEIN FOODS
7 ounces	**Go lean with protein**
	Twice a week, make seafood the protein on your plate
	Vary your protein routine—choose more fish, beans, peas, nuts, and seeds
	Keep meat and poultry portions small and lean

Find your balance between food and physical activity	**Know your limits on fats, sugars, and sodium**
Be physically active for at least **150 minutes** each week.	Your allowance for oils is **11 teaspoons a day**.
	Limit extras—solid fats and sugars—to **650 calories a day**.
	Reduce sodium intake to less than **2300 mg** a day.

Your results are based on a 3200 calorie pattern.   **Name:** _____

This calorie level is only an estimate of your needs. Monitor your body weight to see if you need to adjust your calorie intake.

11-23   This is a nutritious meal plan for an 18-year-old male. How does your daily diet compare with this meal plan? *Credit: USDA*

Adulthood

Young men and women move from adolescence into adulthood. This phase of the life cycle lasts until death. It covers the largest number of years.

Nutritionists often divide adulthood into four stages. Early adulthood is the time from 19 through 30 years. By this stage, the rapid growth of adolescence has ceased and people's bodies have reached mature size. However, the bones are still storing calcium and increasing their density. Middle adulthood describes the years from ages 31 through 50. Some visible signs of aging begin to appear during this stage of life. Later adulthood includes people who are ages 51 through 70. Signs of aging become more apparent during these years. Older adulthood is over 70 years of age. People in this age group are more likely to develop special health and nutrition needs.

Signs of aging include graying hair, wrinkling skin, deteriorating vision, and slowing reflexes. These are natural changes that occur as the body gets older. However, many health problems that are more common among older people are not a natural result of aging. Research shows following a nutritious diet and exercising can help prevent such problems as heart disease and high blood pressure. This information has spurred many middle-aged adults to adopt good health habits. The earlier people make these habits part of their lifestyles, the more benefits they gain.

Nutrient Needs During Adulthood

Good nutrition is as important as ever during adulthood. The nutritional needs of adults are similar to those of adolescents. Adults need nutrients mainly to support vital body functions.

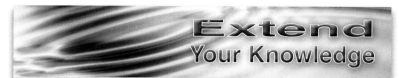

Fast Foods and Teens

It is estimated that one-fourth of teen calorie intake is from snacks. Frequently teens choose snacks high in saturated fat, sugar, and salt. Many teens do not get enough calcium, dietary fiber, iron, or vitamin A. What factors do you see that cause teens to choose snack foods high in calories and low in nutrients? Collect fast-food data sheets describing nutrient content of their menu items. Make a list of snack food choices that are higher in nutrients and lower in calories. Combine all the lists to create a master list for use by your peers.

Adult males need a bit more protein than adolescents. Because bones are no longer growing, adults need less calcium and phosphorus than adolescents. However, the Recommended Dietary Allowance (RDA) for calcium increases for women over age 50 and men over 70 years old. The RDA for vitamin D increases for adults over age 70. In addition, doctors often recommend calcium supplements for older women to help maintain strong bones. The RDA for vitamin B_6 increases for older adults as well. Iron requirements drop for women following menopause.

Calorie needs gradually decrease in adulthood. For many adults, this is due to a decrease in the amount of energy their bodies need to operate. However, energy needs can remain at the levels seen in early adulthood if a person exercises and maintains lean body mass. Older adults require fewer calories to maintain their body weight. Some older people become less active, which causes physical abilities to change. This lowers the need for calories even more. Many adults gain weight as they age because they fail to stay active and match their calorie intake to their calorie output.

Adult Food Choices

Some adults find it hard to change eating habits they established during childhood and continued in adolescence. In earlier life stages, people have high energy needs for growth. Some less nutritious food choices can fit more easily into diets at these stages. In adulthood, however, food choices need to be more nutrient-dense to meet nutrient requirements without exceeding calorie needs.

Many adults claim busy schedules and time pressures keep them from eating a nutritious diet. When they eat in a hurry, adults often choose foods that are high in fat, sugar, and sodium.

The sample menu in **11-24** would provide a nutritious diet for a healthy adult female. This menu includes foods that are nutrient dense. Adults who require more calories to maintain a healthy weight can increase the number and size of portions. Adults who need fewer calories to maintain a healthy weight are encouraged to increase their activity levels.

Nutritional and Fitness Problems During Adulthood

Maintaining a healthy body weight may be the biggest diet-related problem affecting adults today. Overweight has been linked with type 2 diabetes, heart disease, and gall bladder disease. Avoiding overweight is wise because losing weight is hard for most adults. Adopting a healthy lifestyle including a nutritious diet and regular, moderate physical activity can help older people avoid becoming overweight.

Sample Menu for an Adult Female

Breakfast
1 whole-wheat English muffin
    2 tsp. soft margarine
    1 Tbsp. jam or preserves
1 medium grapefruit
1 hard-cooked egg
1 unsweetened beverage

Lunch
White bean-vegetable soup:
    1 ¼ cup chunky vegetable soup
    ½ cup white beans
2-ounce breadstick
8 baby carrots
1 cup fat-free milk

Dinner
Rigatoni with meat sauce:
    1 cup rigatoni pasta (2 ounces dry)
    ½ cup tomato sauce
    2 ounces extra lean cooked ground beef (sautéed in 2 tsp. vegetable oil)
    3 Tbsp. grated Parmesan cheese
Spinach salad:
    1 cup baby spinach leaves
    ½ cup tangerine slices
    ½ ounce chopped walnuts
    3 tsp. sunflower oil and vinegar dressing
1 cup fat-free milk

Snacks
1 cup low-fat fruited yogurt

11-24 Adults need to choose foods that are rich in nutrients without being too high in calories.

Constipation is a problem for some adults. Getting regular exercise and choosing fiber-rich foods can help prevent this problem, **11-25**. Fruits, vegetables, legumes, and whole grains supply dietary fiber. Drinking at least six glasses of water a day can help prevent constipation, too.

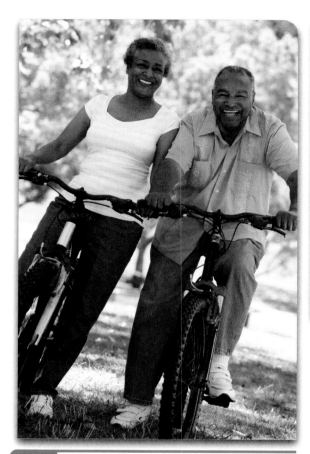

11-25 Remaining active can help adults over age 50 avoid problems associated with inactivity.

Many adult women fail to get enough calcium and vitamin D in their diets. This, along with hormonal changes of menopause and lack of weight-bearing exercise, increases their risk of developing osteoporosis. Eating the recommended number of daily servings of milk, yogurt, and cheese can help women meet their calcium needs. Some women may also need calcium supplements.

As people age, their ability to absorb several important nutrients decreases. In addition, they may fail to get enough nutrients in their daily meals. Vitamin D, folate, and vitamin B_{12} are of special concern in the later years. Some physicians recommend supplements for people in this age group.

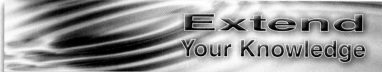

Aging and Life Expectancy in the United States

The percent of the U.S. population comprised of individuals age 65 or older is expected to be 19.6% by the year 2030. This represents over twice as many people in this age range as in the year 2000. This aging trend in the population is due to an increase in average life span and an increase in fertility in the two decades following World War II, known as the "Baby Boom." Find the report *65+ in the United States: 2005* on the U.S. Census Bureau Web site to learn more about this trend in aging.

Special Problems of Older Adults

You may have friends or relatives who are in their later years. Some of these older people may be healthy and active. Others may have serious health problems and be confined to their homes. Health status is just one of several factors that affect nutritional needs in older adulthood.

Doctors recommend modified diets to help treat many diseases, including heart disease and diabetes. However, many other health problems can affect nutrient needs. For instance, recovering from surgery and some illnesses increases the need for protein. Recovery also increases the need for some vitamins and minerals, especially vitamin C and zinc. Medications can affect a person's nutritional status, too. As an example, taking large daily doses of aspirin increases the rate of blood loss from the stomach. This can increase the need for iron. Older adults may want to consult a registered dietitian about how health problems and medications affect their nutrient requirements.

A number of factors can affect an older adult's desire and ability to eat. This, in turn, has an impact on the adult's nutritional status. A diminished sense of taste causes foods to seem bland to some older adults. Tooth loss may make chewing difficult. Digestive problems may result in stomach upset after eating.

Limited income and lack of mobility can have an impact on food intake for some older people. Older adults with low incomes may choose to limit their food expenditures. Others may have trouble getting to a food market and carrying home bags of groceries. Buying, preparing, and serving a pleasing variety of foods for one or two persons may be a difficult task, **11-26**.

Isolation is another factor that affects the appetites of some older adults. A number of older adults live alone. They may be separated from family members and friends. Living alone may decrease their motivation to prepare and eat nutritious meals.

Some senior citizens' centers offer meals to help older people who are troubled by loneliness. Home meal delivery services assist those who have difficulty getting out to shop for food. To stay healthy, older people should include physical activity in their everyday life. Even taking short walks throughout the day keeps muscles toned and improves blood circulation. A formal physical activity program may not be necessary, but joining a seniors' fitness program can be a motivator for staying healthy and active. Nutrition and fitness programs such as these help older adults maintain health through the years.

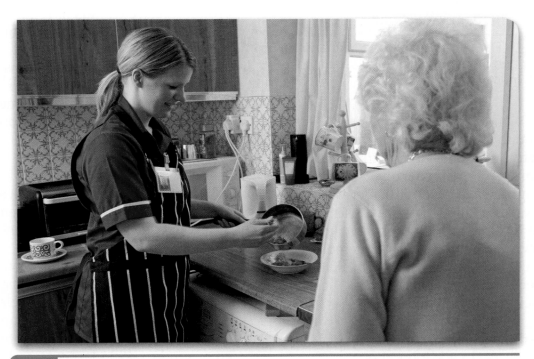

11-26 Older adults may benefit from help with meal preparation.

Reading Summary

The life cycle is divided into stages. People in each of these stages require the same basic nutrients. However, the amounts needed vary due to special nutritional needs associated with each stage.

Good health and nutritional status before pregnancy helps ensure the health of mothers and their babies. Women require extra calories and nutrients during pregnancy to meet the needs of the developing fetus. Pregnant teens have especially high nutrient needs to support their development as well as their babies' development. Women who choose to breast-feed their babies have increased nutrient needs, too. Eating a variety of nutritious foods is the best way to meet these needs. Smoking and using alcohol and other drugs during pregnancy may harm a developing fetus. These habits may also harm infants during breast-feeding.

Healthy babies grow rapidly during the first year of life. Toddlers, who are one to three years of age, grow more slowly. Infants and toddlers both need nutritious foods to support rapid growth. Breast milk or formula is the only food infants need for the first few months. Then a variety of strained foods are gradually added to the diet. Toddlers can eat small portions of most table foods. Being aware of normal infant and toddler development helps caregivers know what to expect when feeding young children.

Preschool and school-age children need more calories and nutrients each day than infants and toddlers. Healthful snacks can be an important source of nutrients for children at this age.

Bone and muscle growth are rapid during the adolescent growth spurt. Nutritional requirements are especially high during this period. Teens need to avoid poor eating habits, such as skipping meals or eating too many high-fat foods from fast-food restaurants. Such habits can cause nutritional deficiencies that may lead to health problems later in life.

By adulthood, the body has reached its mature size. Nutrient and energy recommendations for this age group are set at a maintenance level. However, many adults exceed these recommendations. This makes overweight the biggest diet-related problem affecting adults. A number of physical, emotional, and social factors can place an older adult's nutritional status at risk. Consuming a good diet throughout the life cycle contributes to a state of wellness.

Review Learning

1. What are the six major stages of the human life cycle?
2. What factors other than life-cycle stage influence the amounts of nutrients needed by an individual?
3. In what two ways will forming healthful eating habits before pregnancy help a woman during pregnancy?
4. True or false. Mothers who choose to breast-feed need even greater amounts of some nutrients than they needed when they were pregnant.
5. What are two factors that place teens at a higher risk of complications during pregnancy than mature women?
6. What are three symptoms that might occur in a baby born with fetal alcohol syndrome?
7. Explain the statement "Children have proportionately greater nutritional needs than adults."

8. Why should caregivers introduce only one food at a time to an infant's meal plans?
9. Describe two factors that can lead to eating problems during the toddler years. Give a suggestion for dealing with each factor.
10. What are four examples of healthful snacks for school-age children?
11. What are two problems related to nutrition that are common in childhood?
12. Why do adolescent males need more calories than adolescent females?
13. Give two examples of how nutritional patterns during adolescence can affect health in adulthood.
14. Why do calorie needs decrease in older adulthood?
15. List four factors that can affect an older adult's desire and ability to eat.

Critical Thinking

16. **Compare and contrast.** How are the nutrient needs of adolescents and adults similar and different?
17. **Predict consequences.** What health consequences might teens face later in life due to poor nutritional and fitness choices throughout the life span?

Applying Your Knowledge

18. **Interview.** Interview a pregnant woman to find out what nutritional advice she has received from health-care professionals. Report your findings in class.
19. **Evaluate menus.** Obtain school lunch menus from grammar, middle, and high schools. Evaluate whether each menu substantially meets the needs of the age group it serves. List any changes you would recommend.
20. **Snack lab.** Prepare two healthful snacks that would appeal to young children. Serve the snacks to a group of preschoolers and evaluate their reactions.
21. **Brochure design.** Investigate meal service and delivery programs that are available for older adults in your community. Design a brochure describing these programs.
22. **Oral history.** Conduct an oral history interview a healthy older adult you know about his or her diet and lifestyle. Ask what eating and activity patterns he or she believes have contributed to his or her well-being.

Technology Connections

23. **Game summary.** Play the Blast Off Game found on ChooseMyPlate.gov with a school-age child. In a brief report describe how effective the game was for teaching the importance of choosing a healthy food plan and getting exercise. Describe if the child enjoyed playing the game. What was fun about the learning experience?
24. **Compare food amounts.** Using ChooseMyPlate.gov, compare the daily amounts from each food group recommended for a young child to that for an adult. Include the recommended amounts for fats and oils.
25. **Web page design.** Design a page for your school's Web site on the importance of physical activity in the life of teens and their parents or care providers. List example types of physical activities that are appropriate for each of the age groups.

26. **Online survey.** Use an online survey tool to survey students about the number of soft drinks they consume daily. Compute a class average for the number of soft drinks consumed per day. Post your results so students can see how they compare to their peers.

27. **MyPlate plan.** Go to "Daily Food Plan" at ChooseMyPlate.gov. Enter the age of a child between the ages 6–11, the sex, and the activity level of your selected child. Enter the information on the activity part of the Web page. Develop food plan recommendations (amounts from specific food groups per daily) for the specific age of the child, sex, and activity level you have chosen.

Academic Connections

28. **Science.** With the help of a biology teacher, examine how bones physically change and develop. Prepare a poster showing what happens as a bone grows larger and denser. Explain how nutrition and physical activity affect the development of bones.

29. **Math.** Research and prepare cost estimates for breast-feeding versus bottle feeding for the first year of life.

30. **Social studies.** Take a field trip to an early childhood center that works with preschool children. Observe the children during snack time. Note the kinds of snacks served to the children. Record serving portions and food groups represented for each of the snacks. Summarize your findings and how they compare to recommendations.

31. **Science.** Use a reliable biology resource to outline the stages of human gestation. Investigate to learn the impact of nutrition at each stage.

32. **Speech.** Debate the following topic: Can nutrition help people live longer?

Workplace Applications

Solving a Problem

As a nutrition educator at a family fitness center, you work with multigenerational families who find it difficult to meet nutrition needs economically and efficiently.

One of your clients is a family with three children (ages 3, 7, and 12) whose parents hold full-time jobs. Living with them is a 75-year-old grandmother who has osteoporosis. Several nights per week involve a trip to the local fast-food drive through for the family meal. This is taking its toll on the family's budget and health. Write your responses to the following as you prepare to help this family:

- What appears to be the core problem for this family and what alternatives might solve it?
- How would you help the family develop an appropriate plan and take action on it?
- How would you help the family evaluate results?

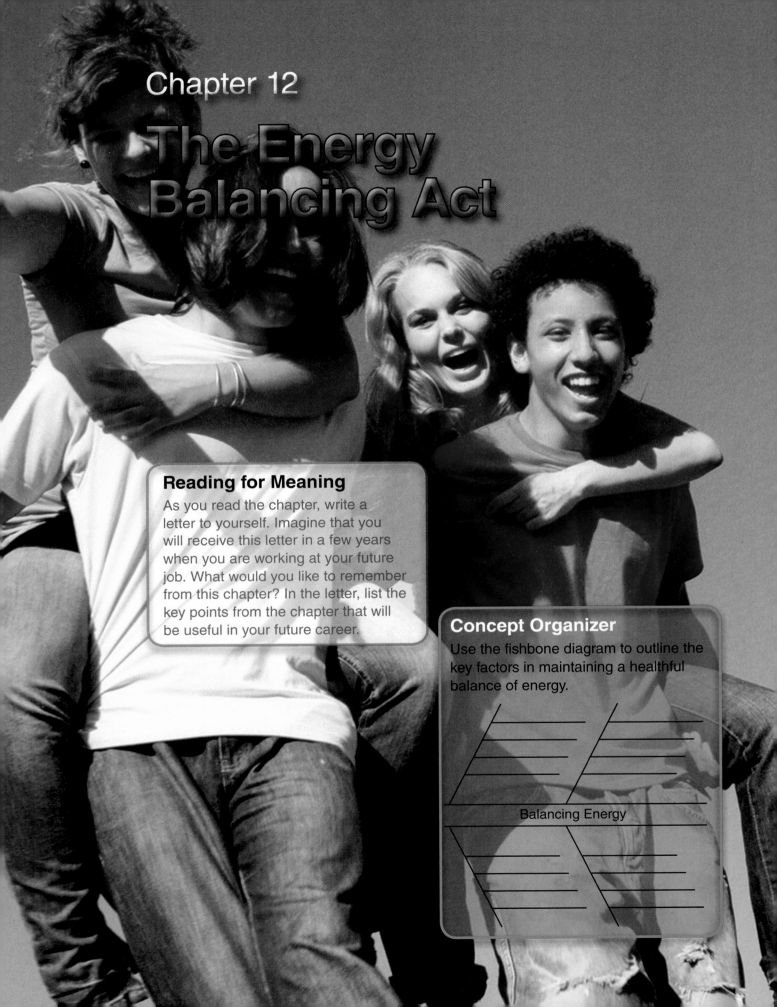

Chapter 12
The Energy Balancing Act

Reading for Meaning
As you read the chapter, write a letter to yourself. Imagine that you will receive this letter in a few years when you are working at your future job. What would you like to remember from this chapter? In the letter, list the key points from the chapter that will be useful in your future career.

Concept Organizer
Use the fishbone diagram to outline the key factors in maintaining a healthful balance of energy.

Balancing Energy

Terms to Know

energy
calorie density
Estimated Energy Requirement (EER)
basal metabolism
basal metabolic rate (BMR)
resting metabolic rate (RMR)
sedentary activity
thermic effect of food (TEF)
ketone bodies
ketosis
healthy body weight
body mass index (BMI)
overweight
obese
underweight
body composition
skinfold test
subcutaneous fat
bioelectrical impedance

Companion Web Site

- **Print out the concept organizer at g-wlearning.com.**
- **Practice key terms with crossword puzzles, matching activities, and e-flash cards at g-wlearning.com.**

Objectives

After studying this chapter, you will be able to

- **explain** how the amount of energy in food is measured.
- **calculate** the three components of your energy expenditure.
- **identify** the outcomes of energy deficiency and excess.
- **differentiate** between body weight and composition.
- **use** various tools to determine your healthy weight.

Central Ideas

- Balancing energy is important to maintaining a healthy weight throughout the life span.
- Maintaining a healthy weight occurs by making wise food choices and getting regular exercise to balance energy.

Your body is using energy as you sit and read this page. **Energy** is the ability to do work. There are many different forms of energy. You cannot create or destroy energy. However, you can change energy from one form to another. When you eat, you take in chemical energy stored in food. Your body changes this energy into mechanical energy when you move. Through various activities, your body also generates heat, which is another form of energy, **12-1**.

Understanding energy balance is the key to weight management. Balancing energy involves equating the amount of energy you take in (food) with the amount of energy you use (physical activities). The energy in foods is measured in calories. Therefore, the energy balance equation could be expressed as "calories in equal calories out," or calorie balance. When

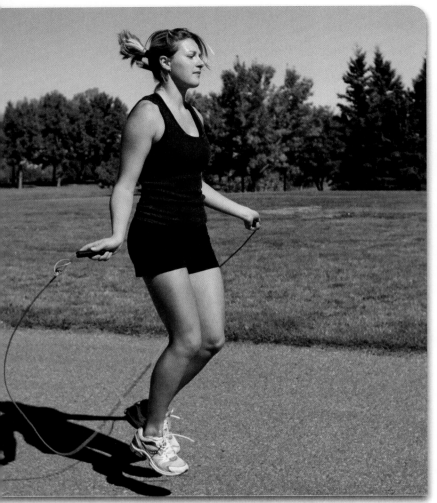

12-1   The body converts chemical energy from food into the heat and mechanical energy of physical activity.

energy in and energy out are in balance most every day, body weight does not change.

Balancing energy does not need to be complicated. This chapter will help you understand the relationships between calorie intake, use of energy, and weight gains or losses.

Energy Input

One side of the energy balance equation looks at the foods you consume. Three nutrient groups provide food energy—carbohydrates, fats, and proteins. (Although alcohol provides calories, it is not considered a nutrient. Alcohol is a drug.) For most people in the United States, approximately 43 to 58 percent of daily calories comes from carbohydrates. About 30 to 45 percent comes from fats, and about 12 percent comes from proteins. The metabolism of these nutrients is the source of chemical energy in your body.

Measuring the Amount of Energy in Food

Did you ever wonder how people know how many calories are in a spoonful of sugar? Researchers have determined the energy value of foods by burning them and measuring the amount of heat they produce. This technique for measuring energy is called *direct calorimetry* because it measures the heat produced directly by the food. To take this measurement, a piece of food is first precisely weighed. Then it is placed in a closed, insulated device called a *bomb calorimeter*. The chamber holding the food is surrounded by a container holding a kilogram of water. After the food is burned completely, the change in water temperature is accurately measured. Each degree of increase on a Celsius thermometer equals one calorie of energy given off by the food, **12-2**.

Through direct calorimetry, researchers have measured the calories in the wide range of foods listed in food composition tables. They have also determined the energy yield of one gram of a pure nutrient. As you have already learned, one gram of pure carbohydrate or protein yields 4 calories. One gram of pure fat yields 9 calories. This means fats produce more than twice the energy of the other two nutrients.

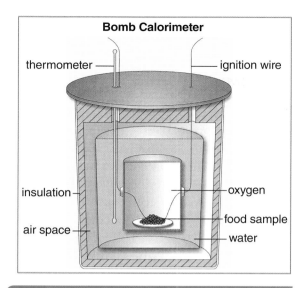

Bomb Calorimeter

thermometer — ignition wire

insulation — oxygen

air space — food sample

— water

12-2 A food's calorie value is a measure of the heat it gives off when it is burned in a bomb calorimeter.

Being aware of the calorie density of foods can help you balance energy. **Calorie density** refers to the concentration of energy in a food. Fats are a concentrated source of energy. Therefore, foods that are high in fat are calorie dense. On the other hand, foods that are high in water lack calorie density because water yields no energy. Comparing 100 grams of two foods will help you see the relationship between fat content and calorie density. Lettuce, which is high in water and contains no fat, provides 13 calories per 100 grams. Mayonnaise, which is low in water and high in fat, provides 714 calories per 100 grams. Mayonnaise is clearly the more calorie dense food.

The Dietary Reference Intake (DRI) for energy is called the **Estimated Energy Requirement (EER)**. The EER is the average calories needed to maintain energy balance in a healthy person of a certain age, gender, weight, height, and level of physical activity. Visit ChooseMyPlate.gov and use the Daily Food Plan interactive tool to learn your EER.

Energy Output

The other side of the energy balance equation looks at the calories you burn throughout the day. Researchers have determined you need energy for basal metabolism, physical activity, and the thermic effect of food. Together, these three factors account for the calories you expend each day.

Basal Metabolism

No matter how still your body is, even during sleep, internal activity continues, **12-3**. Your brain and liver use about 40 percent of your body energy when you are resting. **Basal metabolism** is the amount of energy required to support the operation of all internal body systems except digestion. Basal metabolism keeps your body alive when it is at rest. It includes the energy your body uses every day to breathe, circulate blood, and maintain nerve activity. Secreting

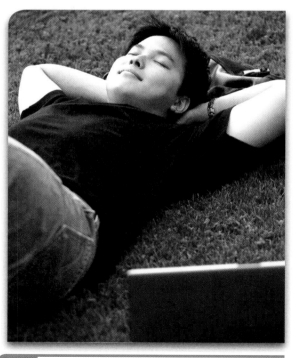

12-3 Even during sleep, the body needs energy to maintain the functions of its various systems.

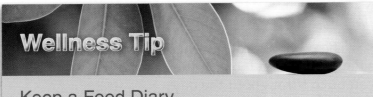

Wellness Tip

Keep a Food Diary

Keeping a food diary can help you evaluate your daily energy intake as well as your nutrient intake. Examine the number of calories per serving of foods listed in your diary. Those high in calories are energy dense.

hormones, maintaining body temperature, and making new cells are also part of basal metabolism.

The **basal metabolic rate (BMR)** is the rate at which the body uses energy for basal metabolism. In general, women require 0.4 calorie per pound (0.9 calorie per kilogram) of body weight per hour to support basal metabolism. Men require 0.5 calorie per pound (1.0 calorie per kilogram) of body weight per hour. An adult's daily basal energy needs can be estimated by substituting the appropriate factor into the same formula, **12-4**. You may be surprised at the amount of calories necessary to support basal needs. Basal metabolism is the largest part of energy output for most people.

Basal Metabolic Energy Needs

For Adult Women
weight in lb. x 0.4 calories/lb. = basal energy needs/hour
(weight in kg x 0.9 calories/kg = basal energy needs/hour)

basal energy needs/hour x 24 hours/day = basal energy needs/day

For Adult Men
weight in lb. x 0.5 calories/lb. = basal energy needs/hour
(weight in kg x 1.0 calories/kg = basal energy needs/hour)

basal energy needs/hour x 24 hours/day = basal energy needs/day

12-4   Basal metabolic energy needs are different for men and women.

Resting metabolic rate (RMR) is another method used to measure the body's resting energy expenditure. It can be used nearly interchangeably with BMR. The RMR measures are slightly higher. The difference stems from the method used to collect the data. RMR data is collected four hours after food has been eaten or significant physical activity. This is different from the BMR data collection method. The BMR data collection occurs after a 12-hour fast in a controlled environment for a specific time while the individual is resting. Since the RMR data is easier to collect, it is more frequently used as a research tool and in sports nutrition or health clubs to help determine caloric needs.

What Affects Your BMR?

A person's BMR is affected by many factors. Body structure, body composition, and gender affect BMR. A tall person will have a higher BMR than a shorter person. This is because the taller person has more body surface area through which heat is lost. *Body composition* refers to the percentage of different tissues in the body, such as fat, muscle, and bone. A person with a larger proportion of muscle tissue will have a higher BMR than someone with more fat tissue. This is because it takes more calories to maintain muscle tissue than fat. Males generally have a slightly higher BMR than females because males have more lean body mass and greater oxygen consumption for their body mass.

Temperature, both inside and outside the body, can affect BMR. Fever increases the BMR. Adjusting to cold or hot temperatures in the environment increases BMR, too.

The thyroid gland secretes the hormone *thyroxine*, which regulates basal metabolism. An overactive thyroid produces too much thyroxine and increases the BMR. Conversely, an underactive thyroid secretes less thyroxine and decreases the BMR. This is why a thyroid disease can affect a person's body weight.

The BMR tends to decline with age. There is an approximate five percent decrease in BMR every 10 years past age 30. People over age 50 must reduce their energy intake up to 200 calories per day to avoid weight gain. Older people who remain active and maintain lean body mass do not experience as much of a decline in BMR, **12-5**.

A very low calorie diet decreases the BMR about 10 to 20 percent. The body responds as it would during a famine. It makes adjustments to preserve life as long as possible. By lowering the BMR, vital functions can be maintained even when fewer calories are available. Someone restricting calories to lose weight will have a harder time reaching his or her goal due to this factor. Stress in people's lives raises BMR. Stress releases hormones that affect BMR.

The BMR is higher during periods of growth. Therefore, infants, children, and teens have a higher BMR than adults. Women have a higher BMR during pregnancy. Meeting the basal energy needs for growth and maintenance of cells is critical for body development. This is why infants, children, teens, and pregnant women should not reduce their calorie intake unless advised by a doctor. These groups of people need the nutrients provided by a variety of foods. If children and teens are having trouble balancing energy, increasing physical activity is a more healthful choice than reducing calories.

Some of the factors described are temporary. Fever and pregnancy temporarily increase BMR. When these conditions end, BMR drops back to its normal level.

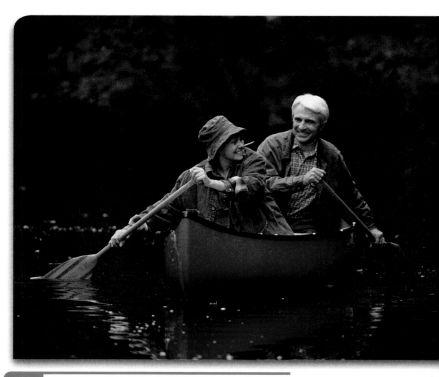

12-5   Staying physically active helps older people maintain a higher BMR.

Many of the factors that affect BMR cannot be changed. Therefore, the impact of these factors on the BMR cannot be changed either. However, basal metabolic rate can be changed by increasing muscle tissue. A regular exercise program helps develop muscle tissue and increase BMR. Generally, the

Math Link

Calculating Percent Basal Energy

Morgan is 26 years old and weighs 120 pounds. After keeping a food diary for several days, she learns she normally consumes about 2,000 calories per day.

1.   Calculate Morgan's basal energy needs.
2.   What percent of her calorie intake is used for basal energy?

greater the proportion of lean muscle tissue in your body, the higher your BMR will be.

Physical Activity

The second category of energy needs is the energy used for physical activity. Energy is needed to move muscles. Energy is also needed for the extra work of breathing harder and pumping more blood.

Energy output varies depending on body size. The larger the body size, the greater the amount of energy needed to make the muscles work. In other words, a 180-pound (82-kilogram) person burns more calories while walking than a 120-pound (55-kilogram) person walking at the same pace.

The actual amount of muscle movement also affects energy output. Therefore, more calories are burned if you swing your arms while walking than if you keep your arms still.

Sedentary activities are activities that require much sitting or little movement. Watching television, studying, working in an office, driving, and using a computer are all sedentary activities. People who do many sedentary activities need to make a point of including physical motion in their daily lives.

To burn more calories, look for more energy-intensive ways to complete daily tasks. For instance, take the stairs instead of an elevator. Swing your arms when walking. Stand rather than sit while waiting for someone. Walk or ride a bicycle instead of riding in a car. When you do drive, park the car away from your destination and walk the last block or two, **12-6**.

Determining Your Calorie Needs for Physical Activity

Researchers commonly measure the number of calories burned as a result of physical activity through *indirect calorimetry*. This measurement

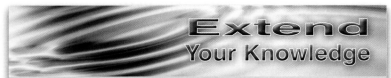

Extend Your Knowledge

"NEAT" Information

In addition to intentional physical activity, you expend calories through all the activities of daily living called NEAT (nonexercise activity thermogenesis). NEAT refers to the energy expended during those times when you are not sleeping, eating, or participating in planned exercise. For example, NEAT activities might include walking to school, using the keyboard, sitting in a chair, blow-drying your hair, or fidgeting while taking a test. The cumulative impact of energy expenditure due to nonexercise activities is believed to be a significant factor in a person's ability to maintain a healthy weight. Research to learn factors that might impact NEAT. What percent of an individual's energy expenditure might be from NEAT? What is the significance of NEAT on public health?

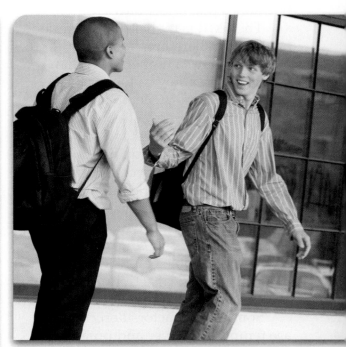

12-6   Walking instead of riding in a car can add more physical activity to your daily routine.

technique requires a person to wear an apparatus while performing a specific activity. The apparatus measures the person's oxygen intake and carbon dioxide output. (Oxygen consumption is required to burn calories. That is why you breathe harder when running or working hard.) The researchers then use mathematical formulas to convert the gas exchange into calories used.

Figure **12-7** lists ranges of calories used per hour for various common activities. These ranges include energy expended for basal metabolism as well as energy used for the activities. By comparing activities, you will soon know which ones are high energy users and which ones demand little energy. For instance, studying may seem like hard work. Unfortunately, studying burns no more calories per hour than watching television.

You can use Figure 12-7 to estimate how many calories you burn as a result of physical activity. Begin by keeping an accurate record of all your activities for one typical 24-hour period. Note the amount of time spent on each activity. Use the following formula to compute your approximate energy use for each activity:

calories used per hour × hours of activity = energy expended

Using this equation, you can calculate that you burn about 480 calories during 8 hours of sleep. You can also estimate that you use about 150 calories when you ride your bicycle for 30 minutes. Add the figures for all your activities in a 24-hour period to determine the total energy expended for the day.

Thermic Effect of Food

Your third need for energy is due to the **thermic effect of food (TEF)**. The thermic effect of food is the energy required to complete the processes of digestion, absorption, and metabolism. Think of it as the energy required to extract the energy from food.

Energy Cost for Various Physical Activities	
Activity	**Calories Used per Hour**
Sleep	60
Sedentary activities—reading, eating, watching television, sewing, playing cards, using a computer, studying, other sitting activities	80 to 100 (average 90)
Light activities—cooking, doing dishes, ironing, grooming, walking slowly, more strenuous sitting activities	110 to 160 (average 135)
Moderate activities—walking moderately fast, making beds, bowling, light gardening, standing activities requiring arm movement	170 to 240 (average 205)
Vigorous activities—walking fast, dancing, golfing (carrying clubs), yard work	250 to 350 (average 300)
Strenuous activities—running, bicycling, playing football, playing tennis, cheerleading, swimming, skiing, playing active games	350 or more

12-7   Body size and degree of muscle movement affect the specific number of calories a person burns through physical activity.

The thermic effect of food may depend slightly on the types and amounts of foods eaten. However, it generally equals 5 to 10 percent of your combined basal metabolism and physical activity energy needs. Remember the calorie ranges you used to calculate your energy needs for physical activity included basal metabolism. Therefore, simply multiply your calculated total energy expenditure for the day by 0.1 (10 percent). This will give you a reasonable estimate of energy used for the thermic effect of food. Someone burning 2,200 calories for physical activity and basal metabolism would spend about 220 calories for the thermic effect of food.

For most people, approximately 60 to 65 percent of energy output is for basal metabolism. About 25 to 35 percent is for physical activity. For athletes, a lower percentage of energy output is for basal metabolism and a higher percentage is for physical activity. Five to 10 percent of energy output is for the thermic effect of food, **12-8**.

Calculating exact total energy needs is difficult for a layperson. However, your estimates can help you determine whether you are balancing your energy input and output. If you are neither gaining nor losing weight, you are in energy balance. Maintaining weight means the calories you eat are balancing the calories you need for energy.

Energy Imbalance

Many factors can cause the energy equation to be out of balance. *Energy imbalance* occurs when a person consumes too few or too many calories for his or her energy needs. Over time, either of these conditions can lead to negative health consequences. In the short run, weight fluctuations are

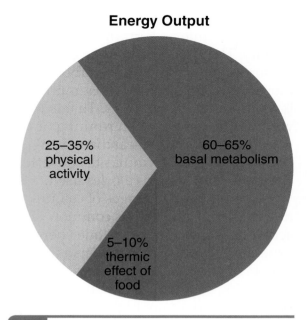

Energy Output

25–35% physical activity

60–65% basal metabolism

5–10% thermic effect of food

12-8   The majority of energy needs support basal metabolism, with a significant amount of energy also needed for physical activity.

normal. Small weight changes that can occur from one day to the next are mostly the result of water changes in the body.

A regularly occurring energy imbalance will cause a change in body weight. People who are trying to lose or gain weight intentionally create an energy imbalance in their bodies. People who pay little attention to their eating and activity habits may unintentionally create an energy imbalance.

Energy Deficiency

Energy deficiency occurs when energy intake is less than energy output. Several factors can result in an energy deficiency. In cases of poverty and famine, food sources may be too scarce to meet energy needs. Illness may depress appetite or hinder energy metabolism. Someone who eats a low-calorie diet purposely creates an energy deficiency.

The body responds to an energy deficiency in a number of ways. The body first uses energy from carbohydrates, fats, and proteins in food to meet its energy needs. If there is not enough food energy available, the body draws on stores of energy. The first store the body turns to is liver glycogen. This is the stored form of glucose from carbohydrates for use by nonmuscle tissue.

After about four to six hours, when glycogen stores are depleted, the body will draw on fatty tissue for energy. Weight loss will occur as fat is used. Unfortunately, the nervous system cannot use fat as a fuel source. It requires glucose, which cannot be obtained from fat.

The body can use amino acids from proteins in lean body tissues to make glucose to feed the nervous system. In order for the body to use this protein, however, it has to break down muscle and organ tissues. Muscle tissue is 75 percent water. Therefore, breaking down muscle proteins causes a rapid weight loss due to loss of body fluids. It also causes muscle weakness and can eventually lead to a number of dangerous health consequences.

When carbohydrates are not available, the body will take steps to limit muscle deterioration. It will slowly begin to use another method to feed the nervous system. The body will change fatty acids into compounds called **ketone bodies**. The nervous system can use ketone bodies to meet some of its energy needs. Ketone bodies reach the nervous system through the bloodstream. An abnormal buildup of ketone bodies in the bloodstream is a condition known as **ketosis**. This condition can be harmful because it changes the acid-base balance of the blood.

Carbohydrates are always important in the diet because they are the preferred fuel for nerve and brain cells

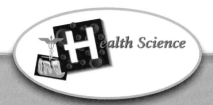

Health Science

Fitness Trainer

Fitness trainers lead, instruct, and motivate individuals or groups in exercise activities, including cardiovascular exercise, strength training, and stretching. They work in health clubs, rehabilitation centers, country clubs, hospitals, universities, resorts, and clients' homes. Fitness workers also are found in workplaces, where they organize and direct health and fitness programs for employees.

Education: Increasingly, most employers require fitness workers to have a bachelor's degree in a field related to health or fitness, such as exercise science or physical education. Some employers allow workers to substitute a college degree for certification, but most employers who require a bachelor's degree also require certification. Some workers receive specialized training if they teach or lead a specific method of exercise or focus on a particular age or ability group.

Job Outlook: Jobs for fitness trainers are expected to increase much faster than the average for all occupations. This is because more people are spending time and money on fitness. Likewise, businesses are also recognizing the benefits of health and fitness programs for their employees.

to function. Nutritionists do not recommend following very high-protein or very low-carbohydrate diets for extended periods of time. These diets cause muscle tissue to be broken down and large amounts of ketones to form. Instead, nutritionists suggest including enough carbohydrates in the diet to fuel the brain and central nervous system. Carbohydrate intake should also be sufficient to preserve muscle tissue. This will cause the body to use fat stores, not muscle, for energy. Weight loss will result from the loss of fat, not protein, **12-9**.

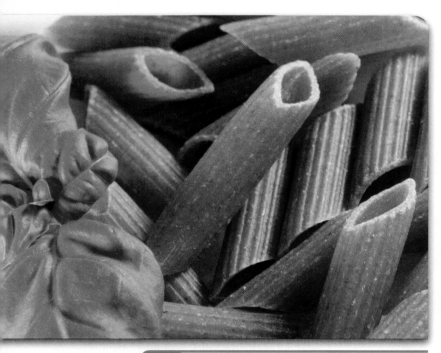

12-9 Including low-fat sources of carbohydrates in an energy deficient diet will result in weight loss without damage to body protein tissues.

Energy Excess

Energy excess occurs when energy intake is greater than energy output. Excess calories from carbohydrates, fats, proteins, and alcohol can all be stored in adipose tissue. The body can use this stored energy when there is not enough food intake to meet immediate energy needs.

If energy excess occurs on a regular basis, weight gain will result. An excess of 3,500 calories in the diet leads to 1 pound (0.45 kg) of stored body fat. The amount of weight and the speed with which it is gained depend on the degree of energy excess.

Most overweight people have gained weight slowly over a period of years. Consuming an extra 25 calories each day adds approximately 2½ pounds (1.2 kg) each year. Just this small energy excess could cause a healthy-weight 20-year-old to be 25 pounds overweight by age 30.

Excess adipose tissue, or where fat is stored, is a health concern. The greater the amount of fat carried on the body, the greater the risks for related health problems.

Determining Healthy Weight

There are health risks associated with too little and too much body fat. To avoid both sets of risks, you need to maintain a healthy weight. Body weight refers to the total mass of an individual measured in pounds or kilograms. **Healthy body weight** is body weight specific to gender, height, and body frame size and is associated with health and longevity. This may not be the weight at which you match the media image of a "perfect body." Instead, it is a weight at which your body fat is in an appropriate proportion to your lean tissue. Having a healthy weight reduces your risk of a number of serious medical problems.

There are several ways to determine whether your weight is healthy. You can use a mathematical calculation based on your weight and height. You can take measurements of your body fat, measure body composition, and assess body fat distribution patterns. Each of these methods has advantages and disadvantages. However, they can all be useful tools in helping you evaluate your weight status.

Using Body Mass Index

Federal guidelines define weight groups by **body mass index (BMI)**. This is a calculation of body weight and height. BMI relates to average relative body weight for height. BMI is most usable for people 20 years and older. BMI helps identify amounts of body fat and is associated with risk for disease. You can figure your BMI by dividing your weight in pounds by the square of your height in inches. Then multiply this figure by the constant 703. (When working in metric units, divide weight in kilograms by the square of height in meters. The result is the BMI. It does not need be multiplied by a constant.) Someone who is 5 feet 9 inches (1.75 meters) tall and weighs 145 pounds (65.25 kilograms) would calculate BMI as follows:

$$(145 \text{ pounds} \div 692 \text{ inches}) \times 703$$
$$(145 \div 4{,}761) \times 703$$
$$0.0305 \times 703 = 21.4 \text{ (rounded) BMI}$$

A chart that can help you easily find your BMI is shown in **12-10**. For adults, healthy weight is defined as a BMI of 18.5 to 24.9. An adult who has a BMI of 25 to 29.9 is said to be **overweight**. If an adult's BMI is 30 or more, he or she is identified as **obese**. With a BMI over 40, the person is extremely obese and at serious risk for other health problems. Medical attention is recommended. Any adult with a BMI below 18.5 is considered **underweight**.

BMI is not an appropriate weight evaluation tool for everyone. For example, body builders have excess muscle weight. For them, BMI is not an accurate gauge of overweight and obesity. Pregnant and lactating mothers, children, and frail elderly have unique BMIs because the amount of body fat normally changes with age and physical condition.

Definitions of weight categories based on BMI are less clear-cut for children and adolescents, whose bodies are still growing. They develop at different rates. Recommended BMI cutoffs to identify children and

Body Mass Index

Weight in Pounds

Height	90	95	100	105	110	115	120	125	130	135	140	145	150	155	160	165	170	175	180	185	190	195	200	205
4' 11"	18	19	20	21	22	23	24	25	26	27	28	29	30	31	32	33	34	35	36	37	38	39	41	42
5' 0"	18	19	20	21	22	23	23	24	25	26	27	28	29	30	31	32	33	34	35	36	37	38	39	40
5' 1"	17	18	19	20	21	22	23	24	25	26	26	27	28	29	30	31	32	33	34	35	36	37	38	39
5' 2"	17	17	18	19	20	21	22	23	24	25	26	27	28	28	29	30	31	32	33	34	35	36	37	37
5' 3"	16	17	18	19	20	20	21	22	23	24	25	26	27	28	28	29	30	31	32	33	34	35	36	36
5' 4"	15	16	17	18	19	20	21	22	22	23	24	25	26	27	28	28	29	30	31	32	33	34	34	35
5' 5"	15	16	17	18	18	19	20	21	22	22	23	24	25	26	27	28	28	29	30	31	32	33	33	34
5' 6"	15	15	16	17	18	19	19	20	21	22	23	24	24	25	26	27	28	28	29	30	31	32	32	33
5' 7"	14	15	16	17	17	18	19	20	20	21	22	23	24	24	25	26	27	28	28	29	30	31	31	32
5' 8"	14	14	15	16	17	18	18	19	20	21	21	22	23	24	24	25	26	27	27	28	29	30	31	31
5' 9"	13	14	15	16	16	17	18	19	19	20	21	22	22	23	24	24	25	26	27	27	28	29	30	30
5' 10"	13	14	14	15	16	17	17	18	19	19	20	21	22	22	23	24	24	25	26	27	27	28	29	30
5' 11"	13	13	14	15	15	16	17	18	18	19	20	20	21	22	22	23	24	25	25	26	26	27	28	29
6' 0"	12	13	14	14	15	16	16	17	18	18	19	20	20	21	22	22	23	24	25	25	26	26	27	28
6' 1"	12	13	13	14	15	15	16	17	17	18	19	19	20	21	21	22	23	23	24	25	25	26	26	27
6' 2"	12	12	13	14	14	15	15	16	17	17	18	19	19	20	21	21	22	23	23	24	24	25	26	26

12-10 This chart can help you determine your BMI.

adolescents who are overweight vary according to age and sex.

Measuring Body Composition

Analyzing your body composition is another way to judge your weight or, more importantly, health status. **Body composition** is a term used to identify the proportion of lean body tissue to fat tissue in the body. The *fat-free mass (FFM)* found in the body includes the water, protein, and minerals found in organs, muscle, and bone. A higher percent of FFM indicates stronger bones and a larger proportion of skeletal muscle tissue. As the percent FFM increases, the percent body fat decreases. According to the American Council on Exercise (ACE), body fat greater than 25 percent is considered excessive for young adult males. A more desirable fitness range is 14 to 19 percent. For women, over 32 percent body fat is excessive. A range of 21 to 24 represents fitness. Acceptable ranges for good health are 18 to 24 percent for males and 25 to 31 percent for females.

How is percentage of body fat determined? One of the most accurate ways for measuring body fat is underwater weighing. Breath is exhaled and the person is submerged under water.

The process is based on the principle that lean tissue is denser than fat tissue. A person with more lean tissue has a dense body. Water volume is measured to determine amount of body fat mass. A person with more body fat weighs less under water and is more buoyant. However, few people have access to an exercise physiology lab to have this test performed. Other acceptable, less expensive methods are available to provide data on body lean and fat mass composition.

A more common way to assess body composition is to do a **skinfold test**. This test uses a special tool called a *caliper* to measure the thickness of a fold of skin, **12-11**. An estimate is made about how much of the thickness is due to **subcutaneous fat**. This is the fat that lies underneath the skin, and it accounts for about half the fat in the body. Skinfold measurements are often taken on the thigh, upper arm, abdomen, and/or back. The amount of subcutaneous fat in these areas reflects the total amount of fat throughout the body. As people become more physically fit, body fat measurements will reflect more lean body tissue and less fat tissue.

A simple version of a skinfold test you can do at home is called the "pinch test." Grasp the skin on the back of your upper arm halfway between your shoulder and elbow. Pinch this fold of skin between your thumb and forefinger. Be sure to grasp only the fat, not the muscle. A distance between your thumb and forefinger of more than one inch (2.5 centimeters) may indicate a high percentage of body fat.

Another method for measuring body fat is **bioelectrical impedance**. This process measures the body's resistance to a low-energy electrical current. Lean tissue conducts electrical energy, whereas fat does not. The more fat a person has, the more resistance there is

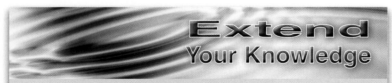

Learn Your Body Mass Index

Teens develop at different rates. Use the BMI Percentile Calculator for Child and Teen (age 2–20) located at the Centers for Disease Control and Prevention (CDC) Web site to learn your BMI and BMI-for-age percentile. Why is it important to know your percentile?

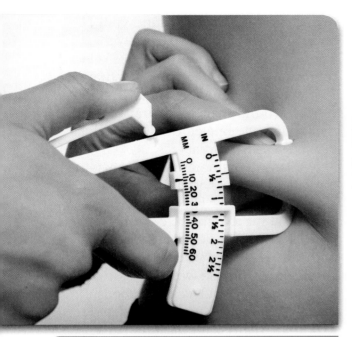

12-11 Skinfold measurement is an easy, inexpensive method for measuring body composition.

to the flow of the electrical current. The measure of resistance is then converted to a percentage of body fat.

Newer methods continue to be developed to give fitness trainers an indication of percent fat mass and fat-free tissue mass. For example, *infrared light beams* are being used to measure percent body fat. A fiber-optic probe is positioned at the mid-biceps (upper arm) and an electromagnetic radiation wave is sent out. This light beam is monitored as it enters subcutaneous fat and muscle. The reflection off the bone is read by the monitor. The amount reflected estimates body composition.

Measurements of body fat mass are estimates. The accuracy of the various methods used to measure percent body fat can differ significantly.

Location of Body Fat

Recent evidence suggests the location as well as the amount of body fat affects health. Fat stored in

Case Study: Healthy Weight— A Simple Matter?

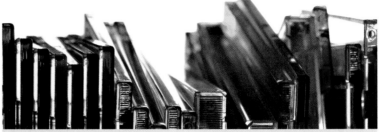

Jackie is 16 years old and barely 5 feet tall. After learning about the importance of maintaining healthy weight in her health class, she decided to learn more about her weight status. She used a BMI chart and discovered she is considered overweight for her age. Jackie knows being overweight increases her health risks. However, she is not experiencing any health problems now and feels alert and strong. She enjoys being active and is on her school's soccer team. She often lifts weights with her brother in the basement of their home.

Malia is Jackie's best friend. Malia hates to exercise, eats junk food all day, and is tall and thin. Malia told Jackie that her BMI is in the middle of the healthy weight range. Jackie doesn't understand how Malia could be healthier considering her lifestyle.

Jackie's family likes being outdoors, but they also enjoy celebrating good meals together. Cooking is a hobby that gives Jackie great satisfaction. Now, Jackie is convinced she must change her lifestyle to improve her health. She is afraid she will have to give up everything she enjoys.

Case Review

1. Is Jackie's assessment of her health and weight status complete and accurate?
2. Do you agree that Malia is healthier than Jackie?
3. What advice would you give to Jackie to help her stay fit and healthy?

the abdomen seems to pose a greater risk than fat stored in the buttocks, hips, and thighs. Fat around the waist increases the liver's production of low-density lipoproteins, which is a risk factor for heart disease.

Men and older women are more likely to accumulate fat in the abdominal area. They have what is sometimes referred

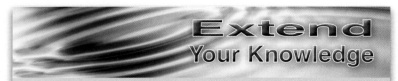

Normal-Weight Obesity

Researchers have found that more than half of American adults with normal-weight BMIs (18.5–24.9) have high body fat percents. Thus, the need for applying other assessment tools, in addition to just weight and BMI, can help determine an individual's health status. Adding other measurements of percent body fat and body fat patterns can be beneficial. Percent of body fat mass, not weight, is often considered a better measure of your health and fitness.

to as "apple-shaped" bodies. Younger women more often store excess fat in the hips and thighs. They have what may be called "pear-shaped" bodies. You may have limited control over where your body stores excess fat. However, if you maintain a healthy weight, your fat stores should not pose a health problem.

There are two methods used to help determine your fat patterning. These methods are applicable for fully grown adults. One method requires measuring the waist circumference. Waist circum-

ference is the distance around your natural waist (just above the navel). The goal for waist circumference is less than 40 inches for men, and less than 35 inches for women. People with more weight around their waist are at greater risk of lifestyle-related diseases such as heart disease and diabetes.

A second method uses the waist-to-hip ratio. This uses both the waist and hip measurements. Hip measurement is taken at the maximum circumference and includes distance around the buttocks. The waist value is then divided by the hip value. If a women's ratio is higher than 0.85 and a man's ratio is greater than 0.90, they are considered to be at higher risk for disease. These methods are not completely accurate, and recommended numbers can vary slightly from culture to culture. Consider these tools as another means to evaluate a person's healthy weight.

When you evaluate your weight, avoid media-promoted stereotypes of how you should look. Try not to be concerned about every pound on your body. Eat a nutritious diet and follow a program of regular exercise. These lifestyle choices will help you maintain your energy balance and support wellness, **12-12**.

Balancing Energy

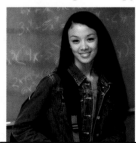

Energy In
(Calories eaten)
• what you eat
• how much you eat

Energy Out
(Calories used)
• basal metabolism
• physical activity
• thermic effect of food

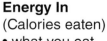 To balance the energy equation, the calories in the foods you eat must equal the calories you use each day.

Reading Summary

Balancing energy means matching the calories you take in from food with the calories you expend each day. You get food energy from carbohydrates, fats, and proteins. Knowing the calorie density of foods can help you balance energy.

You use energy for basal metabolism, physical activity, and the thermic effect of food. Basal metabolism is the energy needed to support basic body functions, such as breathing, blood circulation, and nerve activity. The rate at which the body uses energy for basal metabolism (BMR) is affected by many factors. Of the three basic energy need areas, you have the most control over physical activity. The longer and harder you exercise, the more calories you burn. The thermic effect of food is the energy needed for digestion, absorption, and metabolism.

If you consume too few or too many calories for your energy needs, you will be in energy imbalance. Energy deficiency occurs when there is not enough food energy available to meet the body's needs. Energy excess occurs when there is more food energy available than the body needs. Both energy deficiency and energy excess can lead to negative health consequences.

To avoid risks from too little or too much body fat, you need to maintain a healthy weight. You can estimate healthy weight using body mass index (BMI), fat measuring techniques, and assessing body fat distribution. Excess fat in the abdomen seems to pose a greater health risk than fat in the buttocks, hips, and thighs. You can maintain a healthy weight by balancing energy through wise food choices and regular exercise.

Review Learning

1. True or false. When a person eats food, his or her body uses it to create energy.
2. How much energy does a pure gram of each of the energy nutrients yield?
3. What are three internal body functions, other than breathing, blood circulation, and nerve activity, supported by the energy of basal metabolism?
4. What are known factors that affect a person's BMR? Name six.
5. Give three examples of ways to increase energy expenditure while completing daily tasks.
6. Explain how to estimate how many calories a person burns as a result of physical activity.
7. Which of the three areas of energy expenditure accounts for the smallest percentage of calories burned?
8. Why do nutritionists avoid recommending very low-carbohydrate diets?
9. How many excess calories are stored in 1 pound (0.45 kilogram) of body fat?
10. What resources are available to help you determine your healthy weight?
11. What is the relationship of BMI to body fat and health risks?
12. Why does fat stored in the abdomen pose a greater health risk than fat stored in the buttocks, hips, and thighs?

Critical Thinking

13. **Recognize points of view.** Some experts believe the thermic effect of food plays an insignificant role in total energy expenditure. Others believe the calories used for thermic effect can add up and contribute to leanness over a lifetime. Use Internet or print resources to research these views. What information appears to be relevant to energy use and healthful body weight? Why?

14. **Compare and contrast.** Compare and contrast the various methods for determining healthy body weight. Why is it beneficial to use more than one method in determining healthy weight?

Applying Your Knowledge

15. **Compare calories.** Collect Nutrition Facts panels from five food product labels. Calculate the percentage of calories from carbohydrates, fats, and proteins for each product. Determine which nutrient is providing the greatest source of energy. Share your findings with the class.

16. **Calculate basal energy.** Use the formula given in the chapter to compute your basal energy needs for one 24-hour period. Keep an accurate record of your activities for 24 hours. Note the amount of time spent on each activity. Use the formula given in this chapter and Figure 12-7 to compute your approximate energy use for each activity. (Remember the ranges in the chart include energy expended for basal metabolism as well as for the activities.) Calculate your total energy expenditure for the day. Then calculate your energy needs for the thermic effect of food. Finally, compute the percentages of your total energy expenditure used for basal metabolism, physical activity, and thermic effect of food.

17. **Bulletin board.** Make a bulletin board display illustrating how the body responds to an energy deficiency.

18. **Fitness calculations.** Calculate your body mass index. Find your waist and hip measurements and calculate your waist-to-hip ratio. Do a pinch test to evaluate your percentage of body fat. Assess whether your weight is healthy. Develop a plan to improve or maintain you weight status.

Technology Connections

19. **Food/activity diary.** Use the ChooseMyPlate.gov Web site and locate the "Daily Food Planner." Enter your age, sex, weight, height, and physical activity level to obtain your "Daily Food Plan" and recommended calorie level. Then click on the link to the "Meal Tracking Worksheet" and complete the worksheet for one day. Compare your worksheet to your Daily Food Plan. Are you in energy balance?

20. **Fitness e-pal.** Use a school-approved, global, social networking Web site to become an e-pal with someone from another country. Ask your e-pal what his or her country does to support good health of its citizens. Learn about the opportunities to participate in sports and other types of physical activities in his or her community.

21. **Technology research.** Use Internet resources to research ways technology is being used to measure body composition for professional athletes. Prepare a report using presentation software to share your findings with the class.

22. **BMR database.** Prepare a data base of information that may help a person (over the life span) improve their basal metabolic rate.

Academic Connections

23. **Math.** Use the formula from the chapter to calculate the BMI for a twenty-year-old woman who is 5′5″ and weighs 132 pounds. Check your answer with a BMI chart. Which category does she fall into?

24. **Speech.** Debate whether television viewing has a negative or positive influence on the health of teens.

25. **History.** Select a group of people to study who lived in the 19th century or earlier, such as medieval peasants, Victorian-era middle-class women, or child laborers during the Industrial Revolution. Compare the intensity of their daily work and life with that of an American high school student today. Prepare to discuss the detailed comparisons in small group discussions.

Workplace Applications

Using Leadership Skills

Imagine you are a fitness trainer at a rehabilitation facility that specializes in rehab for workplace injuries. You work closely with several physical therapists at the facility. A number of clients have expressed interest in a class you lead on learning how to balance their energy requirements for a healthy lifestyle. What topics would you use in the class? How would you help people develop a fitness routine for balancing energy? How would you use your leadership skills to motivate, inspire, and persuade your clients to make fitness and energy management a goal for life?

Chapter 13

Healthy Weight Management

Reading for Meaning

Find a magazine article from a reliable source on the Web that relates to this chapter. Read the article and write four questions that you have about the article. Next, read the textbook chapter. Based on what you read in the chapter, see if you can answer any of the questions you had about the magazine article.

Concept Organizer

Use the T-chart diagram to outline the main ideas of the chapter and one or more details supporting each idea.

Main Ideas	Notable Details

Terms to Know

weight management
habit
environmental cue
fad diet
crash diet
fasting
weight cycling

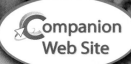

Companion Web Site

- **Print out the concept organizer at g-wlearning.com.**
- **Practice key terms with crossword puzzles, matching activities, and e-flash cards at g-wlearning.com.**

Objectives

After studying this chapter, you will be able to

- **summarize** health risks of obesity and underweight.
- **recognize** factors that influence a person's weight status.
- **estimate** your daily calorie needs and your daily calorie intake.
- **state** why some rapid weight-loss plans are dangerous and ineffective.
- **explain** guidelines for safe ways to reduce body fat.
- **list** tips for safe weight gain.

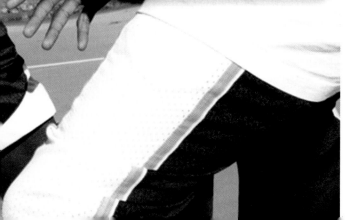

Central Ideas

- Healthy body weight and composition are important to health throughout the life span.
- Maintaining a healthy body weight involves eating a variety of healthful foods and having a moderate activity level.

Have you ever tried to lose or gain weight? If you have, you have much company. Millions of people every year take steps to try to adjust their weight. **Weight management** means attaining healthy weight and keeping it throughout life.

In this chapter you will be examining health risks associated with too much and too little body fat. You will identify factors that affect your weight status. You will also learn to follow the guidelines of good nutrition and exercise as you learn to manage your weight.

Healthy People Need a Healthy Weight

Reaching a healthy body weight and composition, and maintaining it throughout life are important wellness goals. Having a healthy weight can improve your total sense of well-being and reduce your risk of many diseases.

Instead of discussing *weight* management, it may make more sense to discuss *body fat* management. Not everyone who is overweight has excess body fat. Overweight can also be due to muscle development. Athletes, for example, often have high weights for their heights. However, the weight is due to muscle, not fat. This type of excess weight is not a health problem. Problems associated with overweight and obesity arise when the weight is due to excess fat rather than excess muscle, **13-1**.

With so much attention focused on overweight, problems associated with underweight are often overlooked. In the United States, the number of people who are underweight is much smaller than the numbers who are overweight. However, both groups are at increased risk of health problems.

Health Risks of Obesity

In the United States, overweight and obesity have become more common in recent years. Most alarming is the increase in overweight and obesity in children. Childhood obesity

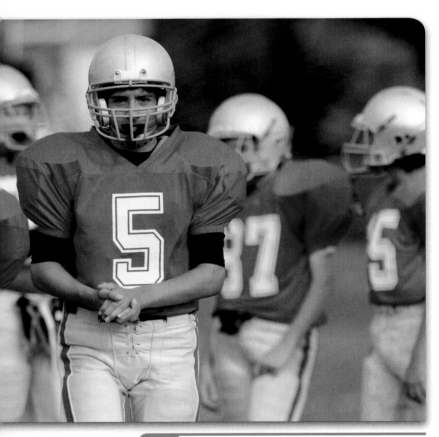

13-1   Athletes who are overweight due to a high proportion of lean muscle tissue may be considered healthy weight.

in the 1960s was about 4.5 percent. In most recent years, the rate of obesity in children is near 17 percent. Many more are overweight.

An adult with a body mass index (BMI) of 25 to 29.9 is considered *overweight*. A BMI score of 30 or more is considered *obese*. Currently, over 60 percent of the people in the United States have BMIs greater than 25. Obesity is linked to many health risks, **13-2**. For this reason, reducing the occurrence of obesity in the United States is a national health goal. The more excess fat a person carries, the greater the risks. When excess pounds are lost, positive health gains result.

Social and Emotional Health Risks

Obesity can be a source of social and emotional problems as well as physical ones—especially for children and teens. For years, mass media have overvalued a thin body as a standard of beauty. People are sometimes portrayed negatively simply because they are obese.

Some people can be very cruel to those who are overweight or obese. Childhood obesity can be particularly cruel as it relates to the development of their self-image. People who are obese may face isolation and discrimination in school. Adults may face difficulties at work and in other social settings. To add to the problem, excessive body fat may cause people to shy away from fitness activities.

Faulty media images and ill treatment from others add to stress among people who are obese. These factors can also cause people who are obese to form low opinions of themselves. People who are overweight often have the mistaken belief they are less worthy than people who have healthy body weights. Some weight-management

Health Risks of Obesity
• Heart disease
• Type 2 diabetes
• Cancers (endometrial, breast, and colon)
• Hypertension (high blood pressure)
• High total cholesterol or high levels of triglycerides)
• Stroke
• Liver and gallbladder disease
• Respiratory problems
• Osteoarthritis (a degeneration of cartilage and its underlying bone within a joint)
• Gynecological problems (abnormal menses, infertility)
• Complications during surgery and pregnancy

13-2 The Centers for Disease Control and Prevention (CDC) reports research findings relating overweight and obesity to increased risks for certain health conditions.

programs work to dispute this misconception. They use counselors to help clients realize that personal value is not based on body weight.

Health Risks of Underweight

Having too little body fat can have serious effects on health. Underweight people may lack nutrient stores. When fat stores are needed, such as during pregnancy or after surgery, underweight people may have problems. Underweight people may also feel fatigued and have trouble staying warm.

Severely underweight people are urged to gain body fat as an energy reserve. Females with low body fat may stop menstruating. A number of other health risks result from underweight due to eating disorders.

Factors Affecting Your Weight Status

Weight status refers not only to how much you weigh, but also to your ability to gain and lose weight. Your weight status is the product of many factors. A combination of these factors is responsible for the increase in overweight and obesity in this country.

Heredity is one factor known to influence how much and where you store body fat. What causes people to gain excess weight or maintain a healthy weight is very complex. There are factors inside your body (metabolic and hormonal) and factors outside your body (environmental and psychological) that influence your weight status. Your physical activity level also has a major impact on your weight.

Heredity

Genes set the stage for body shape. The size of bones and the location of fat stores in the body are inherited traits. Fortunately, healthy body weight can be found in a variety of body shapes. Heredity also affects basal metabolic rate, **13-3**.

The human body has a complex system of hormones that interact in many different ways. Some research indicates certain genes may be linked to obesity. These genes are believed to be connected to hormones that influence appetite and energy expenditure.

Two hormones involved in appetite regulation and energy expenditure are *leptin* and *ghrelin*. Leptin is produced in the body fat cells. As the number of fat cells in the body increase, more leptin can be produced. The circulating leptin enters the brain and triggers a

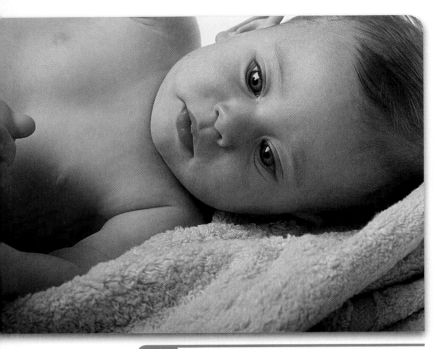

13-3 People are born with a genetic code that affects how their bodies will store fat throughout their lives.

reduction in appetite. However, people who are obese can become resistant to the hormone leptin. Appetite becomes hard to manage. More food is eaten than needed when leptin functions at a reduced level.

Ghrelin is a hormone produced in the stomach. People who are overweight produce higher levels of ghrelin. This hormone stimulates the appetite. Ghrelin also encourages fat

production and body growth. During periods of fasting, ghrelin is produced and hunger occurs. For people of healthy weight, ghrelin helps to stabilize body weight. People who are obese may develop a different sensitivity to ghrelin that promotes overeating.

These hormones may begin to explain why people differ in their tendency to gain weight. However, the genes linked to these hormones are not a recent development in humans and cannot be solely responsible for the rise in obesity. Other factors, such as calorie-dense foods and decreased activity, are likely contributing to the problem as well. Further research in the genetics and possible causes of obesity is still needed.

A family history of obesity does not necessarily destine a person to be obese. However, weight management may be more complex for people who inherit genes that promote obesity. Following a healthy lifestyle, increasing physical activity, and choosing nutritious foods will help overweight people work toward a healthy weight. Similarly, someone who has numerous thin relatives has no guarantee of a thin body. However, some people are genetically prone toward thinness. Their bodies store fat less readily than others. People who inherit this trait may find it hard to gain weight.

Heredity and genes play a role in making you special. They also help define what your health needs might be. Inherited traits can minimally impact your quality of life, and others may require a lifetime of medical attention.

Eating Habits

Weight trends within families are the result of more than just genetics. Eating habits affect weight status by influencing the "calories in" side of the

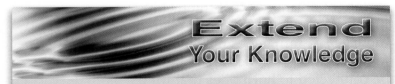

Diet or Lifestyle—Which Is It?

Find the feature "Healthy Weight—It's Not a Diet, It's a Lifestyle" on the Centers for Disease Control and Prevention (CDC) Web site. In a one page report explain why weight management is considered a lifestyle. Include a summary of what the CDC sees as a vision of the future for lifestyle changes.

energy balance equation. A **habit** is a routine behavior that is often difficult to break. For example, eating buttered popcorn at the movies can become a habit.

People begin to form eating habits early in life. Eating behaviors of children are based largely on the foods parents or caregivers offer them. They develop patterns in the kinds and amounts of foods they choose. They form habits related to when and why they eat, too.

Parents need to be aware that children and teens who are obese have an increased risk of becoming obese adults. Parents can plan meals and snacks around appropriate portions of nutritious foods. This will help children establish healthful eating habits that promote weight management. Children who develop eating behaviors based on good nutrition are more likely to practice healthful eating habits throughout life.

The common pattern of eating meals away from home contributes to weight problems. "Eating out" usually means choosing from a menu of foods that are high in fat, sugar, and calories. Portions are often "supersized" to appeal to consumers. Fast-food restaurants promote big portions which have little relationship to recommended amounts for healthy eating. In addition, the electronic age of television and computers often involves snacking on foods throughout the day in a mindless manner.

As children grow up, some of their eating habits are likely to change. During the teen years, people begin to have more control over what foods they eat. Busy schedules, peers, and weight concerns often influence food choices. Many teens form the habit of frequently eating fast foods that are high in fat and calories. Others adopt patterns of skipping meals.

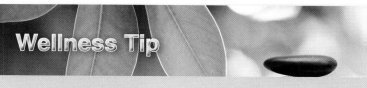

Wellness Tip

Eat to Maintain

Most health professionals would agree maintaining a healthy weight is much easier than reducing weight. This is important information to know as you establish healthful eating habits. Learning to maintain a healthy weight now will help you avoid the difficult task of taking off excess pounds at midlife.

Eating habits continue to change through adulthood. Work and family obligations often impact food choices and eating behaviors. Adults who commute to work may eat on-the-go. Adults with children sometimes develop the habit of finishing leftovers from their children's plates. These habits may lead to excess calories.

Environmental Cues

Some eating habits are responses to environmental cues. An **environmental cue** is an event or situation around you that triggers you to eat. The sight, taste, and smells of foods are common cues that stimulate eating. The time of day, such as lunchtime, is an environmental cue for many people. Social settings, such as parties, can be environmental cues, **13-4**.

Appetite and hunger usually work to make sure people eat enough to supply the fuel their bodies need. However, sometimes cues in the environment cause people to eat even when they are not hungry. For example, a vendor calling "Hot dogs!" may prompt you to eat at a ball game. This type of eating behavior often causes people to consume more calories than they need.

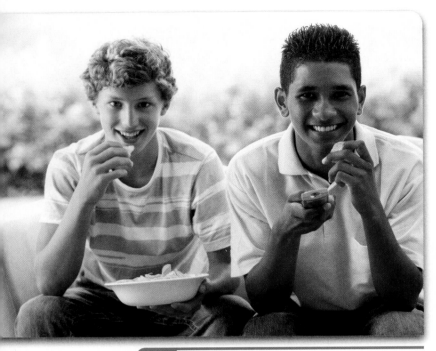

13-4 For many people, watching television is an environmental cue to eat.

Being aware of when and why you eat is important. This will help you realize when you are responding to environmental cues rather than hunger. Developing this awareness of your eating habits can help you avoid overeating. When a cue triggers eating, replace your eating response with a response that makes you feel good about yourself. For example, coming home from school may be an environmental cue to have a snack. Families can help provide healthy cues for you. Seeing fruit on the table, rather than cookies or chips, may be just the cue you need to make a healthier food choice. To avoid the sedentary habit of playing video games, you could change your response to this cue and go outdoors for a social game of basketball.

Psychological Factors

Have you ever noticed your emotions influencing when and how much you eat? Eating habits are sometimes responses to psychological factors. Boredom, depression, tension, fear, and loneliness may all lead to erratic eating patterns. Some people respond to such feelings by overeating—others respond by failing to eat.

Good nutrition can help you maintain good health, which is an important tool in handling emotional challenges. Try to notice which emotions affect your eating behaviors. Look for appropriate ways to deal with these emotions while following a nutritious diet. For instance, if you find yourself reaching for food when you are bored, consider going for a walk instead. This will promote your total state of wellness.

Activity Level

Physical activity levels affect weight status by influencing the "calories out" side of the energy balance equation. If you burn the same number of calories you consume, you will maintain your present weight. If you burn fewer calories than you consume, you will gain weight. If you burn more calories than you consume, you will lose weight.

One of the ways your body burns calories is through physical activity. As you become more active, you need more calories for energy.

For some people, an energy excess is the result of overeating. For many people, however, an energy excess is due to physical inactivity. Many people in today's society spend much time doing sedentary activities. They ride in a car instead of walking. They watch television, play video games, or use the Internet to connect with friends instead of taking part in physical activities, **13-5**.

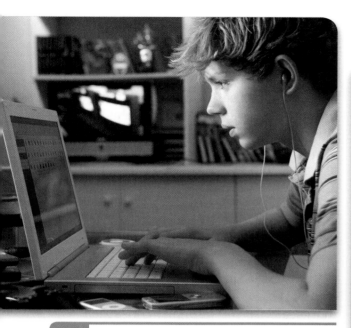

13-5 Students need to balance time spent in sedentary study with time spent in physical activity.

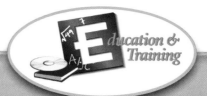

Sports Nutrition Consultant

Sports nutrition consultants work under contract with healthcare facilities or in their own private practice. They perform nutrition screenings for their clients and offer advice on diet-related concerns related to sports nutrition. Some work for wellness programs, sports teams, and coaches.

Education: Sports nutrition consultants need at least a bachelor's degree. Licensure, certification, or registration requirements vary by state.

Job Outlook: Applicants with specialized training, an advanced degree, or certifications beyond the particular state's minimum requirement should enjoy the best job opportunities. Employment is expected to increase.

Losing Excess Body Fat

People who are overweight due to excess body fat would improve their health by reducing their fat stores. Creating an energy imbalance is required for weight loss. Numerous strategies for accomplishing this goal are promoted in books and magazines. Some of these strategies are safe and effective, others are dangerous. Knowing some basic information can help overweight people make sound weight-management decisions.

People should consider several factors when thinking about beginning a weight-loss program. One factor is health status. Women should not try to lose weight during pregnancy. Nutritious foods and a minimum weight gain are required to ensure the health of a developing fetus. People who are ill should avoid restricting calories to lose weight. The body needs an adequate supply of nutrients to restore health.

Meeting these nutrient needs is difficult when calories are severely restricted.

Age is another issue to keep in mind when considering a plan to reduce body fat. Weight loss is not recommended for children and teens who are still growing. Losing weight could permanently stunt their growth. The recommendation for children and teens is to hold weight steady and grow into it. If a child is extremely obese, then health care supervision is needed.

People need to evaluate their motivation and body structure when considering weight loss. The main goal of weight management is good health. People who try extreme weight-loss methods to achieve an unrealistically slim appearance may put their health at risk. Remember, weight above a standard range is a health risk only if it is due to excess body fat. Weight due to muscle mass is not a cause for concern and does not indicate a need for weight loss.

People planning a weight-loss program should also consider how much emotional support they will have. Adopting new eating patterns is difficult. People who are most likely to succeed in a weight-management plan are those who receive encouragement. You may want to join a class or program to help with weight-management efforts. Your doctor or a registered dietitian can help you select a program that is right for you. Some people choose a partner to help support and encourage them. Talking to family members and friends before beginning a weight-loss program can help gain their support.

The Math of Losing a Pound of Fat

One pound (0.45 kg) of body fat stores roughly 3,500 calories of energy. To lose one pound (0.45 kg) of body fat, therefore, a person must create an energy deficit of 3,500 calories. Studies show maintaining weight loss is easier for people who spread this calorie deficit over one to two weeks. This means creating a calorie deficit of 500 to 250 calories per day.

You can create a calorie deficit by reducing calorie intake or increasing calorie needs. Fat loss occurs from the body as a whole. Fat loss cannot be targeted to a specific part of the body. However, muscle tone improves with exercise, which results in a "slimmer" appearance.

Before you can determine how to adjust your food patterns and exercise plan, you need to know your current energy needs. You also need to know how many calories you regularly consume.

Estimating Calorie Needs

Daily energy needs can be estimated based on BMR, physical activity, and the thermic effect of food. Another way to estimate your body's calorie needs is to visit ChooseMyPlate.gov and use the "Daily Food Plan" interactive tool.

Estimating Calorie Intake

A food diary is a record of the kinds and amounts of foods and beverages you consume over a period of time. Accuracy in recording is important. Record the information soon after eating. Your food diary can help you figure the number of calories you consume during an average day.

Counting calories is especially important during the early stages of trying to reduce calorie intake. Use food composition tables or diet analysis software to find the calorie values of each food you consume. Add your totals for each day. Then add your daily totals and divide by the number of days to find the average.

Math Link

Calculate Calories

Jill weighs 130 pounds. She swims after school three days a week for one hour each of the three days. She learned that swimming at a speed of 20 yards per minute uses 0.058 calories per pound of body weight per minute.
- How many calories per week does she use swimming?

Comparing Calorie Needs with Calorie Intake

You can figure what your daily calorie limit must be to achieve your weight-management goals. Compare your estimated energy needs to your average daily intake. If your intake is greater than your estimated needs, you probably have been gaining weight. Reducing daily calorie intake to make the numbers match will allow you to maintain your present weight. Reducing intake even further will result in weight loss.

Some people should avoid diets that restrict calories below the number needed to maintain a healthy weight. A lactating woman's body requires a high level of energy to produce milk. Children and teenagers need energy to support growth. Older adults will have trouble meeting their nutrient needs if calories are restricted, **13-6**.

Unsafe Weight-Loss Practices

People who do not like what the scale reads become prime targets for "quick and easy" weight-loss schemes. It seems to be human nature to want to tackle weight problems with fast solutions that require minimal effort. Unfortunately, no magic tricks exist for healthful weight loss. To avoid weight-loss schemes, you need to become aware of the gimmicks and tricks designed to encourage you to buy products.

Fad Diets and Other Weight-Loss Gimmicks

New weight-loss schemes turn up every day. Just turn the pages of any teen or sports magazine. You will likely find descriptions of eating plans promising rapid weight loss. Such plans

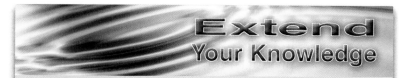

Extend Your Knowledge

What Are Your Cues for Eating and Exercising?

Keep a food and exercise diary for three days. Analyze your diary to learn the environmental cues and psychological factors that influence your eating habits and activity behaviors. What works to keep you eating and exercising in a healthy manner? What are problem areas? Write a behavior-change contract to help you move toward a healthier lifestyle.

that are popular for a short time are often referred to as **fad diets**.

Pills, body wraps, gels, and other weight-loss gimmicks are also widely available. These products are often advertised with words like *fast-working,*

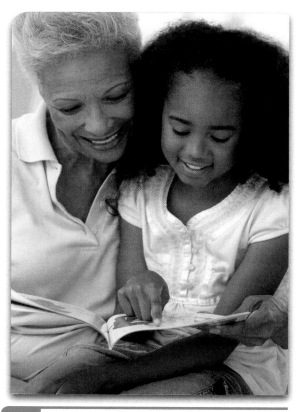

13-6 Older adults and children should not restrict calorie intake below the amount needed to maintain a healthy weight.

incredible energy, inexpensive, painless, and *guaranteed.* However, the advertising is often more effective than the products. Consumers spend millions of dollars on dubious weight-loss products every year.

You may read advice such as, "Eat all the protein you want, but avoid fattening carbohydrates." You might hear a plan like, "Eat only rice for 10 days, and you will lose a pound a day." With all the slick advertising, separating dieting truths from fallacies can be difficult.

Research on several kinds of anti-obesity pills reported that people still remained obese with the use of the drugs. The truth is anyone can make a claim about how to lose or gain weight. Many people who promote dieting schemes lack medical or nutrition training. These people may be more interested in your money than your health.

You may assume federal agencies will protect you from weight-loss frauds and the hucksters who promote them. However, the FDA and FTC take action only when false claims are made about particular products or foods.

The best way to deal with diet fads is to arm yourself with nutrition knowledge. Consult a registered dietitian or qualified nutrition educator if you have questions about the claims of a particular dieting scheme.

Dangers of Rapid Weight-Loss Plans

Weight-loss diets that provide fewer than 1,200 calories per day are sometimes referred to as **crash diets**. Such diets lack essential nutrients. MyPlate should be used to guide weight loss to ensure that recommended amounts from each food group are eaten, **13-7**.

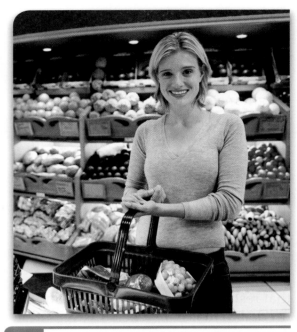

13-7   When on a weight-loss plan, it is important to include the recommended amounts from each of the food groups.

Fasting is a form of crash dieting. **Fasting** means to refrain from consuming most or all sources of calories. Fasting over an extended period can create health problems. Within 24 hours of beginning a fast, the body's carbohydrate stores will be depleted. After this, the body will slowly begin breaking down lean tissues, including muscles and organs, to produce energy. The body will also convert fatty acids from body fat into ketone bodies that can fuel the nervous system. An abnormal buildup of ketone bodies in the bloodstream, which is known as *ketosis*, can be dangerous. Ketosis affects the acid-base balance of the blood.

Ineffectiveness of Rapid Weight-Loss Plans

Crash diets seldom have long-lasting positive weight-loss results. Crash dieting may produce some dramatic initial weight loss. Most of this weight loss is due to fluid loss.

When the diet ends, fluid levels in the body readjust and water weight is quickly regained. Losing weight too fast will reduce glycogen stores used for energy and protein stores found in muscle mass tissue.

Fad diets often have several key drawbacks that keep them from being effective for weight loss. Very low-calorie diets trigger the body to lower BMR, which makes it harder to lose weight. Fad diet plans usually tell people exactly how much and what they can eat. This gives people no control over their food choices. Fad diets require eating patterns that are radically different from most people's normal eating habits. This causes many people to give up on the diet because they miss the foods they are used to eating. Fad diets teach people nothing about better eating behaviors. These diets are not designed to help people maintain their new weights. After completing the diet, most people return to their old eating habits and the lost weight quickly returns.

For some people, crash dieting leads to weight cycling. **Weight cycling** is a pattern of repeatedly losing and gaining weight over time. Weight cycling is sometimes referred to as the *yo-yo diet syndrome*. Following the diet, people begin to eat more than ever simply because they feel starved and deprived of food. Some people gain more weight than they lost by dieting. Discouragement over the lack of success in maintaining weight loss causes them to try another crash diet. This dieting cycle may be repeated many times throughout life, **13-8**.

Research indicates weight swings from year to year may be harmful to health. Emotional stress, physical fatigue, and food deprivation may create a greater chance of developing some diseases. Quality of life may be threatened.

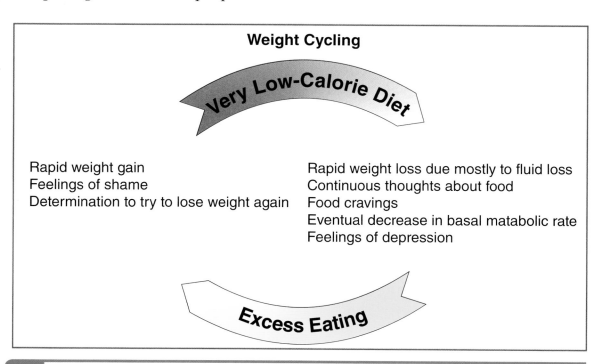

Weight Cycling

Very Low-Calorie Diet

Rapid weight gain
Feelings of shame
Determination to try to lose weight again

Rapid weight loss due mostly to fluid loss
Continuous thoughts about food
Food cravings
Eventual decrease in basal matabolic rate
Feelings of depression

Excess Eating

13-8   Failing to make permanent changes in eating and exercise habits causes some people to repeatedly lose and regain weight.

Safe Fat-Loss Guidelines

Weight-management experts often advise people not to think of losing weight as "dieting." Likewise, they suggest not viewing food as an enemy to fight. Instead, they recommend thinking of losing weight as managing calorie and fat intake. Foods do not need to be eliminated, but rather chosen with fitness and health in mind. Experts also remind people that food is meant to be enjoyed. It just needs to be enjoyed in moderation.

People with health problems should talk to a doctor before beginning a weight-loss program. A medical checkup is always recommended before children and teens go on a weight-management program. A checkup is also advised for people in other age groups who are trying to lose excess pounds.

Having correct information can help people be sure their weight-loss efforts are safe and effective. The following guidelines for reducing calories and changing eating habits promote wellness through the loss of excess body fat.

Evaluate Weight-Loss Plans Carefully

Evaluating a diet plan's effectiveness and related risks can be rather confusing. If a weight-loss plan sounds too good to you, be sure to read the information carefully. Always be wary of diet schemes that encourage unsound eating patterns. Registered dietitians can counsel people about sensible weight loss.

Choose a weight-management plan that is nutritionally sound. For greatest success, it should allow you to take off pounds slowly. It should also include a component of moderate exercise. A healthy weight-loss plan should
- provide all the nutrients your body needs
- be as close to your tastes and habits as possible
- keep you from being hungry or unusually tired
- allow you to eat away from home without feeling like a social outcast, **13-9**
- offer you a change in eating habits you can follow for the rest of your life

Avoid weight-loss plans that stress the eating of single food items. For instance, a diet that suggests eating only bananas does not reflect normal eating behaviors. Such a diet may be dangerous because it is not nutritionally balanced. Remember, a nutritious diet includes foods from all the major food groups in the MyPlate system.

Beware of plans that restrict which foods you can eat. This includes diet plans that stress eating mostly one macronutrient, usually protein. These

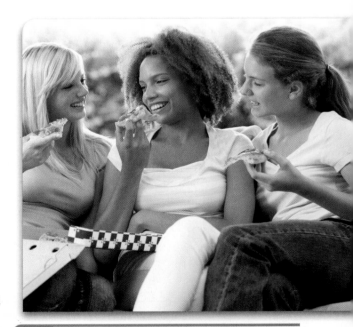

13-9   An effective weight-loss plan will allow people to feel comfortable in social settings while following it.

eating plans may lack important vitamins, minerals, and phytochemicals abundantly found in fruits and vegetables. In addition, high-protein diets may cause weakness, dizziness, and digestive disturbances. High-fat diets increase blood cholesterol levels and add to the risks of heart disease.

Avoid diet plans that require the use of pills. Many diet pills are ineffective and the long-term effects are unknown. No known pill can burn off body fat. Some pills can help suppress appetite or prevent fat absorption, but they cannot correct poor eating habits. Some diet pills may be addictive, others produce a variety of side effects.

Avoid weight-loss plans that suggest fasting or modified fasting. Liquid diets and other programs that are very low in calories may cause fatigue, irritability, nausea, and digestive upsets. They can also affect heartbeat rhythm and the acid level of the blood.

Be wary of weight-loss plans that promise large weight losses in a short time. Dieters who constantly follow the latest and greatest diet scheme often find only short-term successes. People who lose weight slowly are more likely to maintain a healthy weight once they reach it. Losing weight slowly also reduces health risks.

Through a combined eating and exercise plan, a person should attempt to lose no more than one to two pounds a week. Teens who are growing taller can modify this advice by maintaining weight throughout their growth. Gradual weight loss gives the body time to adjust. Remember, it takes time to gain excess weight. It will also take time to lose it without jeopardizing health.

Control Calorie Intake Through Planned Food Choices

Your food choices determine the number of calories you consume. The following suggestions for selecting foods may help you manage calories:

- Substitute low-fat or fat-free foods for foods higher in fat. Fat has the highest number of calories per gram. Therefore, cutting fat is a key way to reduce excess calories. For example, low-fat dairy products are lower in calories than whole-fat dairy products, **13-10**.

Case Study: Kim's Weight-Loss Plan

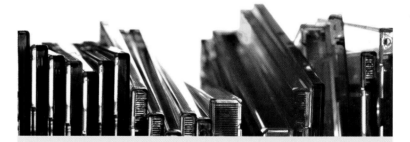

Kim is in a hurry to lose 24 pounds before the school dance. The dance is just three weeks away. She is determined to fit into her older sister's dress for the dance.

Kim found a diet plan on the Internet that she thinks is great. The diet is called the "M and M Diet" because all you can eat are marshmallows and meatballs. She tells her best friend, Keisha, that she has lost 10 pounds in only 10 days. Keisha and Kim have been friends since kindergarten and are on the same basketball team. Keisha has noticed that Kim has been crabby and has been tiring quickly during basketball practice. Keisha has seen Kim lose weight quickly like this many times before, but she always gains the weight back.

Case Review

1. Do you think this weight-loss plan will work for Kim long term?

2. If you were Keisha, what would you tell Kim?

Substitutions to Reduce Fat

Consider selecting:	Rather than:
Nonfat yogurt	Sour cream
Evaporated fat-free milk	Cream or nondairy creamers
Fat-free or 1% fat milk	Whole or 2% fat milk
Reduced-fat cheese	Regular cheese
Low-fat or nonfat dairy desserts	Ice cream
Two egg whites	One whole egg
Angel food cake, sponge cake, gelatin dessert, or fresh fruits	Butter cake, mousse, or fruit pie
Broth-based soups	Cream soups
Jams, jellies, or reduced-fat margarine in tubs	Butter, lard, or stick margarine
Bagels, English muffins, or toasted bread	Doughnuts, pastries
Pretzels, air-popped popcorn, or saltines	Chips or other fried snacks
Graham crackers, vanilla wafers, or gingersnaps	Buttery cookies

13-10 Substituting low-fat foods for high-fat foods is an easy way to cut excess calories from the diet.

- Eat more vegetables and whole-grain foods. Make them the main dishes instead of the side dishes in your menus.
- Choose fresh fruits as an alternative to high-fat snack foods and desserts.
- When eating out, choose steamed, baked, or broiled foods rather than fried items. Ask for sauces and salad dressings on the side. Consider splitting an entrée with a friend, or take part of your food home for a later meal.
- Select recipes that are low in fats most often. Substitute low-calorie ingredients when possible. For instance, you might sauté vegetables in broth instead of butter.
- Use healthy food preparation methods. For example, microwave or steam vegetables and season with lemon juice instead of butter and salt.

Following these basic guidelines will help you maintain good health and a healthy weight while enjoying a delicious diet.

Change Eating Habits

A food diary is a key self-monitoring weight-management tool. It can help you identify eating habits shaped by environmental cues and psychological factors. When completing your diary, list the time of day and where you eat. Also, note who you are with and what you are doing. Jot down how you are feeling at the time, too. This information can tell you as much as the list of what you consumed, **13-11**.

Analyze your completed food diary to see what you can learn about yourself. Do you snack while watching television? Do you eat after school? Do you skip any meals? Do you tend to eat more when you are alone or with friends? Answering questions like these may help you learn where and why you might be consuming excess calories.

Once you recognize problem eating behaviors, you can explore ways to change them. For example, you may realize the snack counter at the movies tempts you to eat. As a solution, you

					Food Diary			
Meal	*Amount*	*Food*	*Time*	*Location*	*People Present*	*Activity*	*Mood*
breakfast	1 medium	banana	7:00 a.m.	kitchen	Mom, T.J.	getting ready for school	grumpy
	2 slices	toast					
	2 tsp.	raspberry jam					
	1 cup	lowfat milk					
lunch	1 slice	cheese pizza	11:45 a.m.	cafeteria	Carla, Darnell	studying for test	nervous
	1 cup	tossed salad					
	2 tbsp.	French dressing					
	1 cup	lowfat milk					
	½ cup	chocolate pudding					
snack	8 oz.	apple juice	3:00 p.m.	locker room	Carla, Lilly, Cecilia	getting ready for basketball practice	excited
	1	granola bar					

13-11 Keeping track of the circumstances in which you consume food can help you identify problem eating habits.

may decide not to bring along extra money for snacks when you go to the movies. Your new habits should not be temporary adjustments until you lose a few pounds. View your eating and exercise habits as permanent changes that will help you maintain a healthy weight throughout your life.

Knowing how emotions affect your eating behaviors can help you manage these behaviors. You may find you eat when you feel lonely or bored. If so, prepare a list of activities you can do instead of eating when these feelings hit you. For instance, when you feel lonely, call a friend, **13-12**. If you are bored, try working on a hobby.

Modifying your behavior involves finding ways to change your response when overeating is a concern. For instance, suppose a friend invites you to an after-school study session at his home. The friend sets out a bowl of potato chips and dip. How can you change

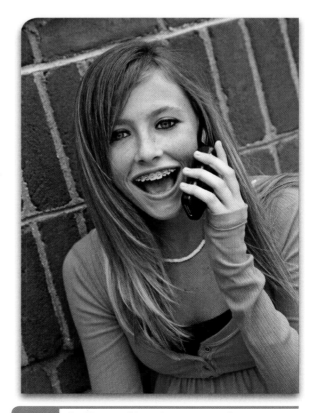

13-12 Calling a friend can be a fun way to take your mind off food when you are bored or lonely.

this environmental cue so you will not overeat? You could move away from the bowl of chips. This may prevent you from responding to their sight and smell. You might also bring some fruit or cut vegetables to share with your friend while you study. Eating a low-calorie snack can help satisfy your desire to nibble.

One way to change an eating habit is to write a behavior-change contract. This is an agreement with yourself about the methods you will use to reach a personal goal. Written contracts seem to work better than mental or verbal contracts. In the contract, write what you plan to do. You might write, "I will limit myself to no more than one soft drink each day." Your food diary can quickly show you if you are achieving your goal. After you reach one goal, you can celebrate success and move on to another goal.

Do not be discouraged if you fail to live up to your contract. You may have set a goal that was unrealistic. Evaluate the methods you are using and your ability to reach your goals. Rewrite your contract if necessary. With practice, you will be able to use behavior-change contracts to improve your eating habits.

Another technique some people find helpful for modifying eating habits is a point system. Give yourself a set number of points for healthful eating behaviors. For example, snacking on carrot sticks instead of corn chips might be worth a point. Skipping a rich dessert might be worth two points. After collecting a set number of points, treat yourself to a reward, like a movie or a new music download. Avoid giving yourself a reward that involves food.

Increase Levels of Daily Activity

Besides making careful food choices, you need to focus on your level of physical activity. Try to complete one hour a day of physical activity at a moderate and enjoyable pace. Many studies show people lose weight faster and maintain weight loss longer when they become more active. Exercise speeds the body's metabolism as body composition changes to a higher proportion of muscle. Exercise also curbs short-term hunger for some people.

Simply changing food habits is not enough for weight loss. Physical activity is an especially important weight-loss strategy for children and teens. Young people need energy from food to support their growth. With moderate daily activity, they can lose weight without reducing their intake of nutritious foods, **13-13**.

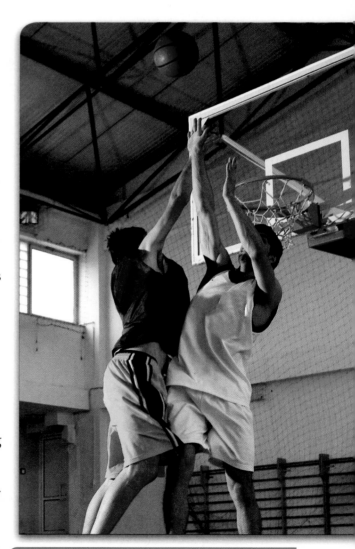

13-13 Physical activity plays a key role in reaching and maintaining a healthy weight.

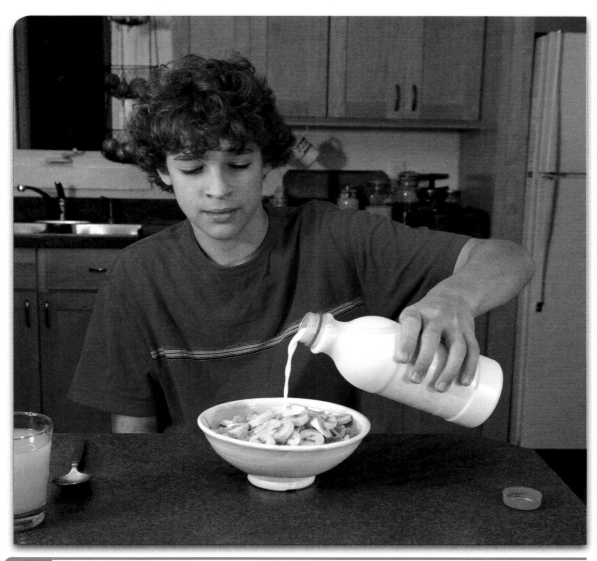

13-14   Teens who eat breakfast are more likely to be healthy weight.

Tips for Weight Loss

If you have trouble achieving or maintaining a healthy weight, try the following tips:

- Avoid eating a large amount of food at any one time of the day. Spread the day's calories over all your meals.
- Eat three to six planned meals throughout the day rather than eating haphazardly. Be sure to keep portion sizes at each meal moderate. This will help you avoid snacking binges.

- Make breakfast a habit. It gets you through the morning without experiencing extreme hunger. If you become exceedingly hungry, you are more likely to overeat, **13-14**.
- Keep a lean refrigerator and cupboard. Focus on stocking nutritious foods that are lower in calories. Select foods that make you feel full when you eat them. Carrots, apples, plums, whole-grain breads have food bulk to help you feel full. Keep foods that are high in calories and low in nutrients out of sight most of the time.
- Avoid eating after 7:00 p.m.

- Eat slowly. Lay your fork down between bites of food. You will feel full with less food.
- Avoid talking on the phone or watching TV while eating. This will keep you from associating these activities with wanting to eat.
- Before a meal begins, drink a glass of water. This may help you feel a little fuller, so you will eat less. Reduce amounts of soft drinks, sodas, or fruit punches that are calorie dense.
- Avoid feeling the need to finish leftover foods. Store leftovers promptly and eat them at another meal.
- Use a smaller plate to manage portion sizes. Moderate portions look larger on a small plate.
- Avoid taking second helpings of foods. Serve yourself one plate. Avoid having all the food placed in serving dishes on the table.
- When eating out, try to decide what you will have before other people order. Then stick with your decision. This will keep you from being swayed by the power of suggestion if other people order high-fat, high-calorie foods.
- Avoid weighing yourself more than once or twice a week. If you are following a healthful weight-loss plan, you will be losing no more than two pounds per week. Therefore, frequent weight checks are unlikely to show much progress and may result in discouragement.

Gaining Weight

For some people, managing weight means wanting to add pounds to body weight, 13-15. Health issues are not as severe for moderately thin people as for people with obesity. However, being underweight may hamper a person's ability to feel strong and healthy. Underweight may also increase a person's susceptibility to infectious diseases such as colds and flu. A BMI of 18.5 and under may indicate undernutrition or malnutrition. The causes of underweight should be medically determined. Anyone who has unexpected weight loss should have a physical exam. A doctor can make sure there are no health problems causing the weight loss.

Gaining weight is as hard for someone who is underweight as losing weight is for someone who is overweight. Healthy weight gain should be due to a combination of fat stores and muscle tissue. Some people seem to inherit a tendency to be thin. They have difficulty storing body fat. However, they can add muscle mass through strength training exercises, such as weight lifting.

As with weight loss, weight gain requires a plan. Gaining weight means consuming more calories than the body expends. The goal is to gain lean body mass, not simply fat tissue. To build lean body mass (muscle), exercise is necessary. Registered dietitians often recommend that people trying to gain weight consume 500 extra calories per day to gain an extra pound of body weight per week. Depending on your level of physical activity, 700 to 1000 calories extra may be appropriate. Of course, the source of these calories should be nutritious foods. Added calories will create an energy excess over what is needed for the increased level of activity.

A teen who has a distorted body image may be driven to build a very muscular body. When a teen perceives his or her body as too thin or lacking muscles, a harmful interest in shaping very large muscles may result.

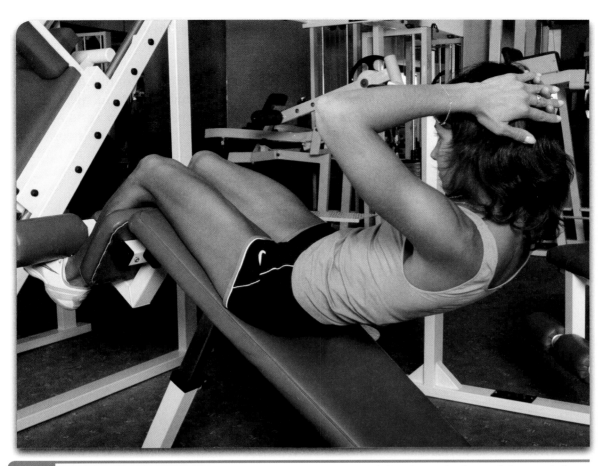

13-15 Exercises that build muscle are a required part of the formula for gaining weight.

Sometimes this leads to use of drugs and other harmful strategies for weight gain and muscle building.

People who are trying to gain weight need to avoid fads and gimmicks. Many body-building magazines and Web sites advertise products that promise to help people "bulk up" fast. These products may not provide a proper balance of nutrients. They will not help people establish long-term healthful eating habits. Some of these products may also have harmful side effects. Using a slow, steady approach to weight gain is the safest, most effective way to put on pounds. Gaining one-half to one pound per week is acceptable. A balanced diet with adequate protein will be necessary.

Tips for Weight Gain

People who are trying to gain weight can follow several suggestions for shifting their energy balance.

- Choose calorie-dense foods containing healthy fats such as the mono- and polyunsaturated fats found in peanut butter, olives, and nuts.
- Snack on dried fruits which are nutrient- and energy-dense choices.
- Add small amounts of calorie-dense toppings, such as salad dressings, croutons, and dessert sauces.
- Try eating bigger, more frequent meals. Protein supplements are not necessary. They can be expensive and sometimes harmful.

- Consume snacks between meals, such as sandwiches, puddings, and thick vegetable soups.
- Add juices, milk, and low-fat milk shakes as fluid sources that are higher in calories than water, **13-16**. Continue to drink plenty of water throughout the day.

- Limit bulky, low-calorie foods, such as leafy vegetable salads and clear soups.
- Avoid drinking extra fluids before eating or during your meal.
- Add a weight-lifting or resistance training program to help increase lean body mass and body weight.
- Get adequate amounts of rest.

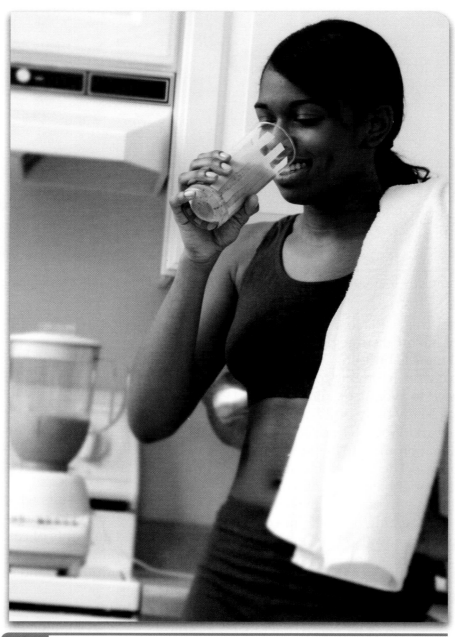

13-16 Shakes made with yogurt and frozen fruits are nutritious snack ideas.

Reading Summary

Weight management means reaching a healthy weight and maintaining it throughout life. People who are either under- or overweight are at increased risk of health problems.

Several factors affect your weight and your ability to put on and take off pounds. These factors include your heredity, eating habits, and level of physical activity. Environmental cues and psychological factors can influence your eating habits.

People who want to lose weight should first evaluate their health and consider their motivation. They need to estimate their current daily calorie needs. They also need to use a food diary to estimate their daily calorie intake. Comparing these two calorie figures can help them determine an appropriate daily calorie limit to maintain or lose weight.

To lose weight safely, people should avoid fad diets and other weight-loss gimmicks, which can be dangerous and ineffective. People trying to lose weight should carefully evaluate the nutritional quality of any weight-loss plan they are considering. Healthful weight loss involves controlling calorie intake through planned food choices. This may require modifying some eating habits. Effective weight loss also demands a plan of daily physical activity.

Weight gain can be just as difficult as weight loss. People who are trying to gain weight need to include more calorie-dense foods in their diets. They also need to follow a program of muscle-building exercise.

Review Learning

1. True or false. A person who is overweight may not have excess body fat.
2. What are five health risks for which people who are obese are at a greater risk?
3. What are two health problems associated with being underweight?
4. How does heredity affect a person's weight status?
5. Who has the greatest influence on eating habits formed early in life?
6. How can a person estimate his or her average daily calorie intake?
7. Why is a fasting diet plan dangerous?
8. What are two reasons fad diets may be ineffective?
9. What is a basic weight-management recommendation for a teenager who is overweight and still growing?
10. What information should be included in a food diary to help people identify factors that prompt them to eat?
11. What are general guidelines for losing body fat safely?
12. How many extra calories should a person who is trying to gain weight consume each day?
13. What are three tips for safe weight gain?

Critical Thinking

14. **Predict consequences.** What long-term consequences do you see as a result of rapid or ineffective weight-loss plans? Why do you think this is so?

15. **Analyze information.** Locate a description of a weight-loss plan in a magazine or online. Why does the plan sound appealing? How well does it follow the guidelines in this chapter for a healthy weight-loss plan? What characteristics might cause the plan to be dangerous or ineffective? How much potential do you think the plan has for long-term weight-loss success? Attach a copy of the weight-loss plan.

Applying Your Knowledge

16. **Weight survey.** Survey two adults who have tried to lose or gain weight at some time. Ask them to describe the diet plans they followed. How did they feel physically and emotionally while following the plans. Did they achieve their weight goals? If so, how long did they maintain their new weight? Compile your findings with those of your classmates. Write an article for the school newspaper about successful weight management.

17. **Food diary.** Find your daily calorie needs based on your activity level. Keep a food and activity diary for three days. Use food composition tables or diet analysis software to figure your average daily calorie intake. Compare your daily calorie needs with your average daily caloric intake. How do the actual and computed amounts compare? Consider healthy ways you can balance your energy equation.

18. **Weight-loss bulletin board.** Find advertisements for weight-loss products in magazines or online. Create a bulletin board display of the ads. Next to each ad, post your brief evaluation of the product's safety and effectiveness. Cite any research that is available to suggest the product sold is safe or effective.

Technology Connections

19. **Internet research.** Use print or Internet resources to research a specific health risk associated with obesity or underweight. In an oral report, explain how unhealthy body weight increases this particular health risk.

20. **Video clip.** Write a script for a video clip about safe weight loss geared to teens. Include tips for safe weight loss and gain. Include a list of lower-calorie food alternatives for high-calorie foods that are popular with teens. For instance, a broiled chicken sandwich would be a lower-calorie alternative for a double cheeseburger. Use a video camera (or digital camera with a video-clip option) to record active teens making healthy food choices. Share your video with the class.

21. **Compare Web sites.** Compare reliable Web sites for such organizations as Mayo Clinic, the CDC, and *WebMD* and compare information about how to safely gain weight and build muscle mass. How does the information from each site compare? Share your findings with the class.

Academic Connections

22. **Writing.** Perform research to learn what actions food manufacturers and restaurants are taking to improve the health of the foods they are selling. Discover the motivation for change. In your opinion, how do you think these changes will impact the companies? the health of consumers? Write a summary of your findings.

23. **Speech.** The incidences of obesity, heart disease, and diabetes are increasing among young adults. Debate the following topic: All high school students should be required to take an exercise and nutrition class as a requirement for graduation. Address how this might affect students, the school, and the community.

24. **Math.** Select two foods to compare such as raw baby whole carrots and potato chips. Using the serving size on each food's label, determine the weight of each food in grams using a food scale. Divide calories per serving (found on the label) by the weight in grams. Determine which food has the greater number of calories per gram. Identify other foods that have bulk (weight), but few calories per gram.

25. **Social studies.** Interview a psychologist to learn how behavior modification principles can be applied to weight-gain or -loss goals.

Workplace Applications

Setting Goals, Taking Action

Presume the supermarket you work for is participating in a community health fair that will take place in six months. You are on the planning committee for the exhibit. Your exhibit at the health fair will focus on providing information on healthful foods for weight management. Demonstrations for preparing healthful foods are also in-work. With your committee (several classmates), set the goals for your exhibit. How will you take action on these goals in your exhibit booth? Consider using the following links on the U.S. Department of Health and Human Services Web site: *Healthfinder* and the *WIN—Weight-Control Information Network*.

Chapter 14
Eating Disorders

Reading for Meaning

Arrange a study session to read this chapter with a classmate. After you read each section independently, stop and tell each other what you think the main points are of the section. Continue with each section until you finish the chapter.

Concept Organizer

Use the spider web diagram to identify types of eating disorders and details about the disorders.

Eating Disorders

Terms to Know

eating disorder
anorexia nervosa
bulimia nervosa
bingeing
purging
binge-eating disorder
female athlete triad
outpatient treatment
antidepressant

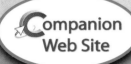

Companion Web Site

- **Print out the concept organizer at g-wlearning.com.**
- **Practice key terms with crossword puzzles, matching activities, and e-flash cards at g-wlearning.com.**

Objectives

After studying this chapter, you will be able to

- **identify** characteristics and health risks associated with three common eating disorders.
- **analyze** possible causes of eating disorders.
- **summarize** methods of treatment for people with eating disorders.

Central Ideas

- Eating disorders are a group of serious conditions characterized by dangerously abnormal eating patterns.
- A variety of factors cause the development of eating disorders.
- Treatments for eating disorders vary with the severity and characteristics of the disorder.

Have you ever overeaten at a buffet or skipped lunch to finish a school project? Neither of these behaviors may be the wisest choice from a nutritional standpoint. However, making an occasional unwise choice is not likely to risk your health. This is especially true if you balance such a choice with wiser choices throughout the day. By contrast, an individual who participates in abnormal eating patterns that focus on body weight and food issues may have an **eating disorder**. The emotional and physical problems associated with eating disorders can have life threatening consequences.

Characteristics of Eating Disorders

The three most common eating disorders are anorexia nervosa, bulimia nervosa, and binge eating disorder. Certain behaviors are typical of each disorder for males and females. Each can be harmful to health. As you study these disorders, you will note they are alike in a number of ways.

Eating disorders are most common among teenage and young adult women. However, people of both genders and other age groups can develop these disorders. Where thinness and body image is highly valued, disordered eating can emerge. Eating disorders commonly begin during the adolescent years. Many people who develop eating disorders share certain traits, **14-1**.

Common Characteristics of People with Eating Disorders

- Fear of becoming overweight
- Poor body image (see self as overweight)
- Low sense of self-worth
- Preoccupation with food
- Distorted feelings about hunger and satiety
- Feels guilty after eating
- Emotionally withdrawn from friends
- High achievement orientation
- High stress levels
- Secretive eating behaviors

14-1 Being familiar with these common characteristics may help you identify someone who is at risk of developing an eating disorder.

Anorexia Nervosa

Anorexia nervosa is an eating disorder characterized by the person refusing to maintain a minimal normal body weight. An individual with anorexia is likely to have a body weight 15 percent or more below recommended weight for age and height. Fear of weight gain is intense. Self starvation is extreme. Perceptions of body image and shape are distorted.

The severe food restrictions practiced by individuals with anorexia nervosa can lead to illness, and social and emotional problems. The focus becomes weight loss, how to avoid food, and feelings of dissatisfaction with body weight. Signs of these problems may include a tendency to withdraw from social events and a quiet, serious personality. Individuals with anorexia view losing weight as a way to solve their problems. The ability to control their weight gives them a sense of power they may lack in other areas of their lives. Anorexia is the third most common chronic illness among adolescents.

Today, the number of males with anorexia is growing. Ten percent of people diagnosed with anorexia nervosa are male. Males are more likely to concentrate on exercise as a way to lose body weight. Sometimes they choose to eat very low-calorie, low-fat diets that appear to be choices for good health, but actually are for weight loss. Many males avoid seeking treatment for eating disorders due to fear and shame. The belief that anorexia is a female problem may prevent males from seeking help. By the time an eating problem is identified and treatment is sought, the illness can progress to dangerous levels.

Most of the underlying psychological factors that lead to an eating disorder are the same for both men and women. Low self-esteem, a need to be accepted, depression, anxiety, an inability to cope with emotions, and personal problems are common. All the physical dangers and complications associated with eating disorders are the same regardless of gender.

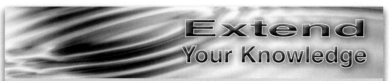

Extend Your Knowledge

When Is It No Longer Healthy Behavior?

Sometimes people are motivated by health, but the behaviors they adopt become unhealthy. *Orthorexia nervosa* is a term used to describe attempts to eat healthy that become so limiting that an individual's health is at risk. People who begin exercising to improve health or athletic performance may cross over into compulsive exercising. This disorder is known as *anorexia athletica*. Research online to find out more about these disorders. What are identifiable clues that behaviors cross the line and become potentially unhealthy?

People with anorexia place excessive emphasis on the shape and weight of their bodies. They may become consumed by unreasonable expectations about what they should look like and how much weight they should lose. They see themselves as fat even though they may be gravely underweight.

The onset of anorexia nervosa commonly begins in adolescence or during the early twenties, **14-2**. Less frequently, it may occur in the adult years. Anorexia may start as a diet plan to lose a few pounds. People with this disorder tend to be highly achievement oriented. They feel a sense of control and pride when they reach their weight goals. They enjoy compliments from others about how nice they look. This inspires them to diet further to reach new, lower weight goals. As this dieting pattern continues, people with anorexia become more intent on losing weight. Feelings of pride turn into strong self-criticism. "I feel good about reaching my weight goal" becomes "I'm too fat. I have to lose more weight." Dieting becomes a life-threatening obsession. However, these individuals are usually unaware they have an eating disorder. Thus, denial becomes a serious obstacle to treatment.

Specific behaviors may vary from person to person. Skipping meals is a common behavior with anorexia. When they do sit down for a meal, individuals with anorexia are likely to eat very little. Instead, they might simply move the food around on their plates. Others will eat only in private. Some people with anorexia choose to take laxatives or diet pills to lose weight. In addition to dieting, excessive exercise is used to control weight and body shape. They may jog, swim, or do aerobics for hours each day. However, the desire to be thin rather than the desire to maintain good

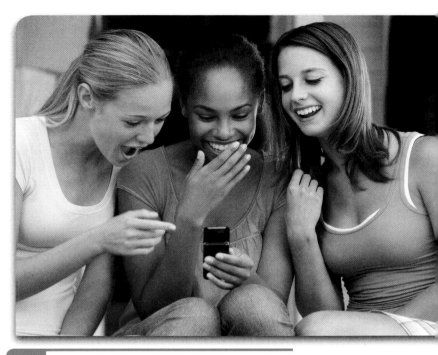

14-2 Young women are the population group most likely to develop anorexia nervosa.

health is what motivates their workouts. People with anorexia often wear baggy clothes to hide their overly thin bodies.

As anorexia nervosa develops, physical symptoms appear. A very low-caloric intake leads to a large drop in weight as a key symptom. Low body weight and body fat cause females to develop amenorrhea, or the cessation of menstrual periods. The disease causes stress, which may take the form of restlessness or irritability. Loss of insulation from the layer of body fat under the skin causes people with anorexia to feel cold. The body adapts to this loss of insulation by growing a covering of fine hair to trap heat. Rough, dry skin and hair loss are two other symptoms resulting from poor nutrient intake.

Anorexia nervosa takes a toll on health in many ways. Normal growth and development will slow down or halt. Muscle tissue wastes away along

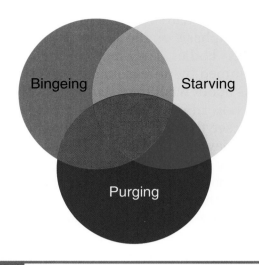

14-3 Patterns of behavior may overlap for people with eating disorders. A person may be involved in one, two, or all forms of disordered eating behavior.

with body fat. Blood pressure and pulse rate drop and the body organs begin to shrivel. Bone density decreases and symptoms of osteoporosis may occur. Some people with anorexia die from starvation. Others fall into a deep depression and the risk of suicide increases.

Bulimia Nervosa

Some people suffer from an eating disorder known as **bulimia nervosa**. This disorder involves two key behaviors. The first is **bingeing**, which is uncontrollable eating of huge amounts of food in a relatively short period of time. The second is an inappropriate behavior to prevent weight gain. For many people with this disorder, the second behavior is **purging**. This means clearing the food from the digestive system. People with bulimia may purge by forcing themselves to vomit. Some abuse laxatives, diuretics, or enemas to rid their bodies of the food.

Instead of purging, some individuals use excessive exercise or periods of fasting to prevent weight gain. Some people alternate between bulimic and anorexic behaviors, **14-3**.

People with this disorder repeat the cycle of bingeing and purging at least twice a week. Some repeat the cycle several times a day. Once the cycle begins, it is hard for many people to stop.

A person with bulimia often comes from a family and social group where weight and appearance are important. He or she usually possesses a low self-esteem.

As with anorexia, people with bulimia are always thinking about food. When bingeing, they consume thousands of calories in a few hours. Binge foods are often high in fats and carbohydrates. During a binge, someone might eat a whole cake, a dozen donuts, and an entire carton of ice cream. Choices about which foods and how much to eat are not related to hunger and satiety. Eating behaviors are out of control.

People with bulimia realize their eating patterns are not normal. They binge and purge in secret because they do not want others to be aware of their behavior. If a person with bulimia has a fairly average body size, others may not notice the problem for a long time.

Serious health problems are associated with bulimia nervosa. As the disorder becomes established, damage to the body becomes more severe and more difficult to reverse. Repeated vomiting can cause glands in the throat to swell. Acids from the stomach burn the esophagus. In addition, the acid can destroy tooth enamel. Vomiting can also cause a loss of water and minerals from the body. This can result in dangerous fluid and electrolyte imbalances. Problems with heart and liver damage can develop as a result of bulimia. The disorder can be fatal.

Binge-Eating Disorder

Binge-eating disorder is another eating disorder that involves repeatedly eating very large amounts of food. People with this disorder rapidly overeat until they are uncomfortably full. However, they do not engage in a follow-up behavior to prevent weight gain.

People who binge eat are likely to have problems with excess weight as their eating gets out of control. They tend to feel guilty about overeating. They may also have ongoing feelings of frustration and rejection.

People with this disorder are likely to drop out of weight-loss programs due to emotional stress. While in a program, they might lose weight. Without specific treatment for their disorder, however, they are apt to begin bingeing again after completing the program. As a result, lost weight is quickly regained.

Other Eating Disorders

Many forms of eating disorders exist. Not all fit the definition of anorexia nervosa, bulimia nervosa, or binge-eating disorder. Disordered-eating behaviors may show up in people who are too concerned about their body shapes. People with eating disorders may strictly limit their food choices to only a few foods. They may binge, purge, and/or fast from time to time. These behaviors can be harmful to health and may develop into specific eating disorders.

Probable Causes of Eating Disorders

The probable causes of eating disorders are complex and may be intertwined. A single factor may not lead to problem eating patterns. However, when several factors occur together, an eating disorder may be triggered, **14-4**. Exact reasons people develop eating disorders remain a puzzle.

Math Link

Calculating Percentages

It is estimated that 2.6% of the U.S. population has an eating disorder. Of those individuals with an eating disorder, 90% are women. If the population of the United States is 309,220,471 people, solve the following:

1. Calculate the estimated number of people with an eating disorder.
2. Calculate the estimated number of women with an eating disorder.

Probable Causes of Eating Disorders

Social Influences

- Media emphasis on thinness
- Unrealistic social perception that thinness is the source of success and happiness

Psychological Influences

- A need for control
- Poor self-esteem
- Need for acceptance and approval
- Unrealistic self-expectations
- Depression
- Inability to cope
- Family and social stresses

Genetic Influences

- Hormonal imbalance
- Other medical causes

14-4 The probable causes of eating disorders might be social, psychological, or genetic in nature.

Theories

One theory of eating disorders says social pressure to be thin prompts people to form unhealthful dieting patterns. Much of this pressure comes from the media. Most of the models and stars on television and in movies and magazines are thin. The few overweight people that appear in the media are often portrayed as dull and dowdy. Thin celebrities shape society's concept of beauty. Many people feel they must be thin to be attractive and successful. They measure their self-worth by their body weight. This compels them to diet. However, they do not grasp the reality that most body types can never fit the model image. They may not realize photos of models are often digitally altered to eliminate inches and imperfections. When one diet program fails to produce the unrealistic body size they desire, many people try other diets. This pattern eventually leads some people to develop eating disorders.

Another theory about what causes eating disorders suggests there may be a genetic link. Studies indicate certain chemicals produced in the brain may prompt people to overeat sweet, high-fat foods.

Evidence suggests typical family patterns may be involved in the development of eating disorders, too. Family members of patients with eating disorders often show overt concern with appearances and high achievement. They may lack communication skills. They may also show a tendency to avoid conflicts within the family.

Risk Among Teens

The theory about social pressure to be thin points to emotional factors that may trigger eating disorders. Teens are especially vulnerable to such feelings as rejection, worthlessness, and guilt. Their lives are in a state of physical, social, and emotional change as they approach adulthood, **14-5**. They seek reassurance from others. Some teens assume their appearance is the reason for any feelings of rejection they sense from others. They may feel worthless if they are overweight. They develop feelings of guilt because they cannot achieve society's standard of beauty.

Emotional change during the teen years may also create out-of-control eating patterns. Facing the challenges of physically growing up and separating from family and friends creates much stress for many teens. They may feel powerless over their lives. Such feelings lead some teens to become emotionally dependent on food. They use food as a source of comfort. They may also see food as one aspect of their lives

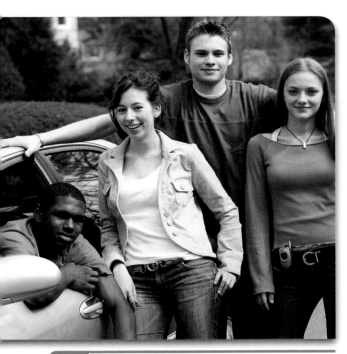

14-5 Teens feel social and emotional pressure to maintain a desired body shape and image.

over which they can have control. Such views of food can be harmful.

Not measuring up to society's body image makes some teens reluctant to eat in public. Simply enjoying a piece of pizza with a friend may result in feelings of low self-esteem. These teens may fear their friends will think they lack self-control for not turning down the pizza. Such fears may prompt these teens to eat alone. This can lead to a pattern of secretive eating, which is part of disordered-eating behavior.

Risk Among Athletes

Some groups of teens are more susceptible to eating disorders than others. Athletes are often at risk because many coaches focus on body weight during training. For instance, a wrestler knows he or she must compete within a weight class. A gymnast is told his or her body size will affect balance. Constantly trying to achieve

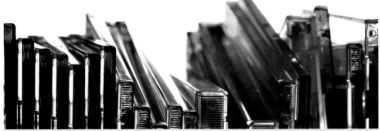

Case Study: The Model of Self-Esteem

Kathy is a 17-year-old high school senior and an excellent student. She wants to become an actress some day. Kathy takes great care in the way she presents herself. She spends much time on her clothes, hair, and makeup. Her body weight is healthy, but she sees herself as needing to look and be better. Kathy constantly thinks about food. Some days she doesn't eat at all in order to maintain her weight. Other days she cannot seem to stop eating. She eats when no one sees her. She quickly eats as much as she can. Sometimes she makes herself vomit. Kathy finds that she is unhappy with herself most days.

Kathy likes hanging out with her best friend, Abby. Kathy thinks Abby has it made. Abby doesn't obsess about her weight and figure like many girls their age. And Kathy has never heard Abby remark on someone else's appearance the way many girls do. Abby is easy to be around. Kathy has never heard Abby complain about her body—she seems very happy with the way she looks. Kathy feels better about herself when she is around Abby. Abby often admires Kathy's intelligence and her speaking ability. She assures Kathy that she will be great at whatever she decides to do.

Case Review

1. Why do you think Kathy feels better when she is with Abby?

2. Who do you think has healthier self-esteem? Why?

and maintain weight goals for their sports may lead athletes to develop eating disorders.

Males who compete in low-weight oriented sports such as jockeys, wrestlers, and runners are at an increased risk of developing an eating disorder. The pressure to succeed, to be

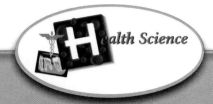

Clinical Psychologist

Clinical psychologists work with the assessment, diagnosis, treatment, and prevention of mental disorders. They are trained to use a variety of approaches aimed at helping individuals, and the strategies used are generally determined by their specialty. Clinical psychologists often interview patients and give diagnostic tests in their own private offices. They may design and implement behavior modification programs. Some clinical psychologists work in hospitals where they collaborate with physicians and other specialists to develop and implement treatment and intervention programs.

Education: A master's or doctoral degree and a license are required for most psychologists. Licensing and a doctoral degree usually are required for independent practice as a psychologist.

Job Outlook: Employment of psychologists is expected to grow as fast as average. Job prospects should be the best for people who have a doctoral degree from a leading university in an applied specialty, such as counseling or health. Master's degree holders will face keen competition.

the best, to be competitive and to win at all costs also places weight issues as a top concern. Combine these issues with any other pressures in their lives, such as family problems, friendship issues, or emotional or physical abuse, can help to contribute to the onset of disordered eating.

Athletes who train intensely may skip meals to train longer and harder. This can become the start of an eating disorder. Wrestlers in weight class events may choose to participate in a class below their normal weight. Disordered-eating patterns may be used to get to the desired weight class. During the off-season, athletes may gain back the weight. As the next season

approaches, they may choose harmful ways to lose the weight once again. This is a form of weight cycling that is dangerous for health and performance. The sports governing organizations do not approve of using harmful methods to "make weight."

Female athletes may be more prone to eating disorders than the general population. Performance stress and the desire to look perfect add to the desire to be slim. A girl may choose a particular sport to support or hide her eating disorder.

Coaches and trainers may advise an athlete to lose weight. Most students want to please their coaches. If you are given advice to lose or gain weight, ask for the necessary information on how to do so safely and effectively. The team may have access to a registered dietitian who knows your sport and can assist with helping you set realistic and attainable goals. Losing or gaining weight alone does not guarantee better performance. Realistic goals and body composition must be considered. Weight changes following good nutrition and use of appropriate training guidelines will offer long term performance success, **14-6**. Disordered eating among female athletes has become quite common. In fact, it is one of a trio of health problems many female athletes face. The second problem is amenorrhea. Amenorrhea has been linked with mineral losses from bone tissue. This leads to the development of the third health problem—osteoporosis. This set of medical problems has been given the name **female athlete triad**.

One part of female athlete triad leads to another. The combination of the three disorders poses a greater threat to health than each of the individual disorders. A female athlete trains hard and eats little to maintain a weight goal. This causes her to stop

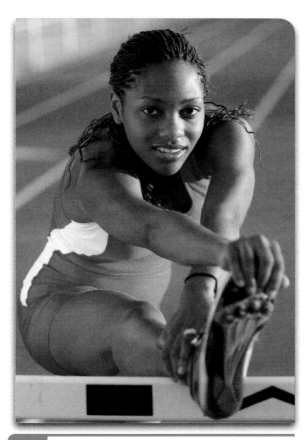

14-6 A female athlete must maintain a nutritious diet to avoid health problems associated with female athlete triad.

menstruating. The resulting hormonal imbalances cause her to lose bone mass. This puts her at greater risk of training and performance fractures. Lack of nutrients in the diet and minerals in the bones slows healing of fractures. This causes sports performance to deteriorate, which may foster feelings of low self-esteem and perpetuate the disordered-eating behaviors. If this cycle of problems continues, the young woman is at serious health risk.

What Help Is Available?

People need professional help to overcome eating disorders. Without medical care, people with eating disorders can suffer long-term health problems or even death. Treatment programs vary depending on the factors that led to the eating disorder. However, treatment must focus on the psychological roots of the disorder as well as its physical symptoms. The treatment is highly personalized and varies with each eating disorder.

The recovery rate for people with eating disorders is much higher if they get early treatment. Family and friends can help get someone with an eating disorder into a treatment program. However, they must recognize that an eating disorder is not just a passing phase.

Treatment for Anorexia Nervosa

Treatment for anorexia nervosa is neither quick nor simple. Therapy for this eating disorder can take many years.

Several approaches are used to treat anorexia. In some treatment programs, only the client is treated. In other programs, the family also becomes involved in the treatment. Sometimes programs require clients to stay in a hospital or treatment facility.

The first step in treatment is to attend to the physical health problems the disorder has caused. Care should be provided by a doctor trained in treating eating disorders. National help organizations can refer clients to treatment programs in their region, **14-7**.

Once a patient's physical condition has been stabilized, he or she can begin to accept psychological help. Clients explore attitudes about weight, food, and body image. They learn to think about and accept what a healthy body weight means. They receive nutrition counseling to help them gain weight and form healthful eating habits. They

Resources for People with Eating Disorders

- Eating Disorder Referral and Information Center
- National Association of Anorexia Nervosa and Associated Disorders (ANAD)
- National Eating Disorders Association (NEDA)
- Binge Eating Disorder Association (BEDA)

14-7 These organizations can provide information about eating disorders.

find out how to view their body shapes more realistically. They develop suitable exercise programs. As patients receive help to improve their self-images, their overall health also improves.

Clients are taught to build new controls into their lives. They practice verbal skills that help them relate better to their family members and friends. They learn stress-management techniques to use when responding to their emotions.

Family support helps ensure a patient will stick with a recovery program. Many professionals advise family therapy to improve relationships among all the family members.

Getting early treatment for anorexia improves the chances for healthy outcomes. Some people recover fully from anorexia nervosa. Most who recover do well in school and work. However, some with this disorder continue to have problems. Studies show about 20 percent of adults who have a history of anorexia nervosa remain underweight. They may still struggle with bouts of low self-esteem and weight-image distortion.

Treatment for Bulimia Nervosa

As with anorexia, people with bulimia should be treated by health care professionals with specialized training. These professionals know how to fit treatment programs to the needs of the individual. Treatment for young patients often includes family members. Therapy for older patients may involve only the individual. In both cases, support from family members and friends is vital to the success of the treatment.

Unless a case is severe, people with bulimia usually receive **outpatient treatment**. This is medical care that does not require a hospital stay. Sometimes physicians prescribe **antidepressants** as part of a treatment program. These are a group of drugs that alter the nervous system and relieve depression. They may be used to help the client control mood swings and avoid bingeing. Drugs can help control behavior. However, they cannot cure the mental problems at the root of an eating disorder. The use of antidepressants also involves risks and side effects. Doctors should discuss these issues openly with clients before prescribing medications, **14-8**.

Support groups can provide people recovering from bulimia with information and encouragement. However, these groups cannot replace therapy.

Some studies show treatment helps about 25 percent of people with bulimia stop bingeing and purging. With or without treatment, however, many people with this disorder have relapses. Relapses most frequently take place during periods of stress or change. Counseling can help individuals prepare for and manage stressful events and thus avoid a relapse.

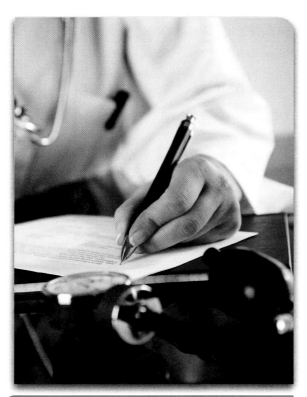

14-8 Prescription medication cannot cure bulimia nervosa, but it is sometimes helpful in the treatment of this eating disorder.

Treatment for Binge-Eating Disorder

Like other eating disorders, binge-eating disorder requires treatment that focuses on emotional issues as well as eating problems. Counseling usually involves helping people with this disorder learn how to like themselves. It helps the clients analyze how their personal beliefs affect their actions. It gives clients the emotional tools to take control of their eating behaviors.

Treatment programs teach weight-management facts. They encourage people who binge eat to seek a healthier weight and form better eating habits. Therapy and the support of friends can help people with this disorder make sound lifestyle choices in many areas.

Seeking Professional Services

Treatment for an eating disorder is likely to require the services of a team of health care professionals. If the disorder has affected physical health, a medical doctor will be part of this team. A psychologist can help a patient deal with the emotional issues at the root of the disorder. In most instances, a registered dietitian will become part of the team. He or she can help the patient form healthful eating habits. An exercise specialist may help the patient plan a moderate exercise program. A treatment center may be recommended where the client is admitted for a period of time.

All these professionals should have special training in handling eating disorders. Some regions may not have many qualified professionals. However, most health care providers can refer patients to specialists or clinics that are equipped to address eating disorders.

For treatment to be effective, a client needs to feel comfortable with the members of the health care team. A concerned friend or family member can help someone with an eating disorder find out about a treatment program. He or she can call to ask about treatment methods, fees, and insurance coverage. If everything sounds agreeable, the friend or family member can schedule an appointment. He or she can go with the client to a screening interview. This face-to-face meeting will help the client decide if he or she feels at ease with the health professionals. Having a positive feeling about the treatment program will help the client recover from his or her disorder, **14-9**.

Questions to Ask a Therapist Before Treatment Begins
• How long have you been working with clients who have eating disorders?
• What are your professional credentials for treating people with eating disorders?
• What is your treatment philosophy?
• What types of treatment have you found most effective in treating eating disorders?
• What is your success rate in treating people who have eating disorders?
• What type of affiliations do you have with other support services, such as registered dietitians, physicians, hospitals, clinics, educational programs, and community-based support groups?
• Do you provide family as well as individual counseling?
• How long does treatment generally last?
• Are you available for consultation if an emergency should occur?

14-9 Asking a professional counselor these questions can help someone with an eating disorder evaluate a treatment program before beginning therapy.

Helping a Friend with an Eating Disorder

What can you do if you suspect a friend has an eating disorder? The person may not admit he or she has a problem. Your friend may even get angry if you suggest he or she has a disorder.

Do not give up on your friend. Tell the person you are very concerned about him or her. If your friend is not receptive to your concern, you can seek help. Talk to a counselor or to your friend's parents. Tell them about the symptoms you have spotted that concern you.

You can also take steps to help prevent people from developing eating disorders. Be careful when encouraging someone to lose weight. Emphasize your acceptance of the person regardless of his or her weight. Show concern for the person's health and well-being. Encouragement, support, and acceptance may be just what your friend needs to help him or her reach healthy weight goals.

Reading Summary

A person with anorexia nervosa starves himself or herself. Someone with bulimia nervosa engages in out-of-control eating. He or she then takes drastic steps to avoid weight gain. People who binge-eat also go on uncontrollable eating sprees. These disorders all have psychological aspects. They can all lead to severe health consequences.

The causes of eating disorders are complex. Theories propose a range of explanations. Eating disorders are most common among teens and young adults. People who take part in sports or other activities where weight goals are rigid are most at risk.

Treatment for an eating disorder should be sought as soon as a problem is identified. Treatment must focus on the needs of the individual. It must address both psychological and physical characteristics of the disorder. This type of treatment generally requires the help of several professionals. Physicians, registered dietitians, and psychologists may all be part of the clinical team.

Review Learning

1. List five psychological factors that might lead to eating disorders in men and women.
2. How does anorexia nervosa affect a person's health?
3. Why are others often unaware when someone has bulimia disorder?
4. What is the main difference between bulimia nervosa and binge-eating disorder?
5. Explain the theory that social pressure leads to eating disorders.
6. Why are athletes at greater risk of developing eating disorders?
7. True or false. Treatment for eating disorders must focus on both psychological and physical aspects of the problem.
8. What factors contribute to successful recovery for people with eating disorders?
9. What factors are likely to trigger a bulimic relapse?
10. Name three health professionals who might be part of a treatment team for someone with an eating disorder. Explain the role each professional would play in the treatment.
11. How can a person help prevent others from developing eating disorders?

Critical Thinking

12. **Cause and effect.** What characteristics about eating disorders do you think might make people with diabetes prone to developing eating disorders? What effect might an eating disorder have on a person with diabetes?
13. **Analyze behavior.** Suppose you have a friend who has either gained or lost a significant amount of weight in the past several months. What actions would you take to help your friend?

Applying Your Knowledge

14. **Journal entry—food.** Write a journal entry answering the following questions about your feelings toward food:
    a. How do I use food to reward or punish myself?
    b. What strong emotions might cause me to eat when I am not hungry?
    c. How do I feel about being hungry?
    d. How do I feel about myself when I eat too much at a meal or exercise excessively?
    e. How do I feel about myself when I turn down a snack or dessert?
    f. How do I feel about eating in front of other people?
    g. How do I feel about other people who eat too much food?
15. **Journal entry—exercise.** Write a journal entry answering the following questions about your feelings toward exercise:
    a. How do I use exercise to reward or punish myself?
    b. What strong emotions might cause me to exercise for unusually long periods of time?
    c. How do I feel about myself when I exercise excessively to keep myself thin?
16. **Resource list.** Use the Internet to make a list of resources in your community for people with eating disorders. Then contact the resources and request information about eating disorders. Organize the materials you receive along with your list into a resource folder. Distribute resource folders to the nurse and counselors at your school.

Technology Connections

17. **E-mail question.** Formulate a question you or a friend has about eating disorders. Submit your question electronically to an eating-disorder expert such as found on the National Eating Disorders Web site.
18. **Electronic presentation.** Based on information learned on national-eating disorder Web sites, prepare an electronic presentation on common myths about eating disorders. Dispel the myths with accurate information about the illness. Share with the class.
19. **Digital storybook.** Use desktop-publishing software to write and illustrate a short story for children. Include age-appropriate font, graphics, and artwork. The theme of the short story is that beauty comes in different shapes, forms, and sizes. The book should emphasize how to appreciate your body. After your instructor's review, read your story to a group of young children. Reflect on any questions they have as a result of your story.

Academic Connections

20. **History.** Choose a year in history before 2000. Research how under- and overweight people were portrayed in the media that year. Find out what movie and television stars were popular. Investigate how models were used to advertise products in magazines and newspapers. Compile examples for presentation. Prepare an opinion paper about the media's role in shaping society's concept of beauty.

21. **Writing.** Interview a person who is recovering from an eating disorder. If you are unable to interview someone, read a case history of a person with an eating disorder from the Internet or a library resource. Write a summary of your interview or reading describing how the eating disorder affected the person's life.

22. **History.** Learn about the history of eating disorders. When were the first cases diagnosed? Why were the terms used for the disorders? Who coined the term? Prepare a one-page summary of your findings.

Workplace Applications

Practicing Integrity

As a person who navigates life by firmly adhering to a strong code of ethics, you find yourself facing an ethical dilemma. A friend from school and work confides in you about her struggle with an eating disorder and makes you promise not to tell anyone about it. You've noticed over a period of time that your friend's productivity at work is declining. You are concerned about her health and life. You are wondering if you should talk with your friend's parents or the school counselor about the symptoms of her condition. What should you do? What is the best way to practice integrity in this situation?

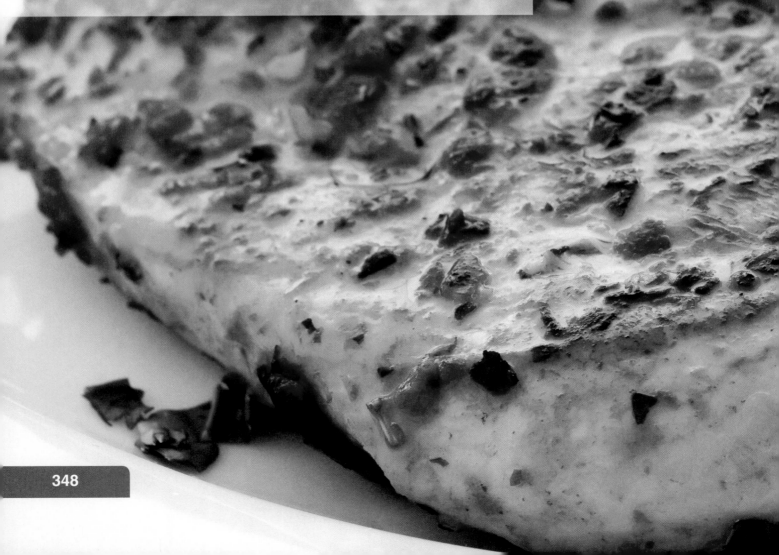

Part Five
Other Aspects of Wellness

Marinating

Marinating is a technique used to add flavor to meats and poultry before cooking. Food is soaked for a period of time in a liquid called a *marinade*. The marinade usually includes an acidic liquid such as a citrus juice or wine vinegar. Herbs and spices are added to the marinade for additional flavor. Marinades often include oil as well. The food can be marinated in the refrigerator for as little as 30 minutes or as long as 24 hours. Remove food from marinade before cooking. Marinade should be disposed of if it was used for raw meat, poultry, or fish. Shake off excess marinade before cooking. Marinated foods are often grilled or broiled.

Fruits and vegetables can also be marinated. Often these preparations are served cold as desserts or salads. Cooked pasta can be added to vegetables to create marinated salads.

Marinated Chicken Breasts (4 servings)

Ingredients

- ¼ cup cider vinegar
- ¾ teaspoon dried thyme
- ¾ teaspoon dried oregano
- ¾ teaspoon dried rosemary
- 3 tablespoons whole-grain mustard
- 2 cloves garlic, crushed
- ½ cup canola oil
- 4 chicken breasts, boned and skinned

Directions

1. Mix the vinegar, herbs, mustard, garlic, and oil in a resealable bag. Add chicken to bag, seal, and shake to coat with marinade. Refrigerate until ready to cook.
2. Preheat grill to medium-high. Remove chicken from marinade allowing excess marinade to drip off before placing on grill. Cook chicken until it reaches 165°F.

Chapter 15

Staying Physically Active: A Way of Life

Reading for Meaning
Describe how this chapter relates to information you've learned in another class. Make a list of the similarities and differences.

Concept Organizer
Use the KWHL chart to note details about staying physically active throughout the life span.

K What I Know	W What I Want to Learn	H How I Can Learn More	L What I Have Learned

Terms to Know

physical fitness
aerobic activity
*Physical Activity Guidelines for
  Americans*
posture
cardiorespiratory fitness
anaerobic activity
muscular endurance
strength
flexibility
power
agility
balance
coordination
speed
reaction time
heart rate
resting heart rate
maximum heart rate
target heart rate zone

Companion Web Site

- **Print out the concept organizer at g-wlearning.com.**
- **Practice key terms with crossword puzzles, matching activities, and e-flash cards at g-wlearning.com.**

Objectives

After studying this chapter, you will be able to

- **state** various examples of personal physical activity goals.
- **explain** the benefits of physical activity.
- **recall** the health and skill components of physical fitness.
- **measure** resting heart rate.
- **determine** your target heart rate zone.
- **identify** four keys to a successful exercise program.
- **plan** a personal exercise program.

Central Ideas

- Staying active for a lifetime involves setting goals for a fitness program and taking action on the plan.
- An active lifestyle promotes good health and wellness.

What is your daily routine like? Do you ride in a bus or car to get to and from school? After school, do you spend time studying and talking to friends on the phone? Do you watch television, play video games, text friends, or spend hours on your computer? Does relaxation for you mean reading a book? Many teens would answer "yes" to these questions, indicating they may have formed a pattern of inactivity. If this pattern describes your life, this chapter will help you learn why and how you can make some changes.

Physical inactivity, especially among teens and adults, is a national health concern in the United States. Many people lack physical fitness due to inactivity, **15-1**. **Physical fitness** is a level of physical condition in which all body systems function together efficiently. Physical activity is necessary for becoming physically fit.

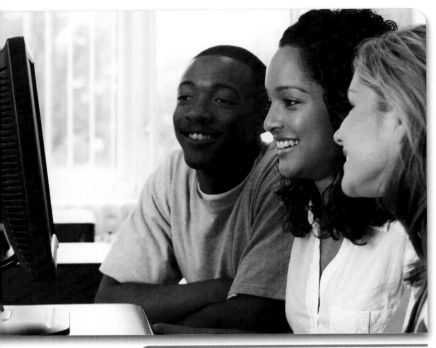

15-1 A physically inactive lifestyle causes many teens to lack physical fitness.

Goals for Physical Activity

Most people who are active or who want to become active have one of three main goals for physical activity. They want to achieve good health, total fitness, or peak athletic performance. The kinds of activities you do and the way you do them will be affected by which goal you choose.

Good Health

Most experts agree physical activity plays a key role in achieving and maintaining good health. Nearly everyone can be at least moderately active, regardless of age or physical limitations. The health benefits of physical activity outweigh the risks. Many activities that promote good health are free and require no special equipment.

To achieve the goal of good health, most of your daily activity should be aerobic. **Aerobic activities** use large muscles and are activities done at a moderate, steady pace for fairly long periods. *Aerobic* means with oxygen. Aerobic activities improve heart and lung health. Certain types of exercise improve bone health. Physical activities involving impact with a hard surface—such as running or jumping—stimulate bone growth and strength. Muscle strengthening exercises also increase bone strength. If you have been relatively inactive, a moderate level of activity would be a good place for you to start.

In 2008, the U.S. Department of Health and Human Services established the *Physical Activity Guidelines for Americans*. The ***Physical Activity Guidelines for Americans*** specify amounts and types of exercise that individuals at different stages of the life cycle should do to achieve health benefits, **15-2**. These guidelines can be followed to meet your goal for good health.

You may be surprised how easy it is to include more activity in your lifestyle. Physical activity does not need to occur all at once, but it does need to be in addition to the light-intensity activities of daily life. Light-intensity activities include standing, walking slowly, and lifting light objects. Your goal can be met with health-enhancing physical activities that fit into your daily routine. For instance, you could spend 15 minutes riding your bicycle to school and another 15 minutes riding home. Then take your dog for a brisk 15-minute walk and spend 15 minutes shooting baskets in the driveway with friends. By the end of the day, you have accumulated a total of 60 minutes of activity.

Physical Activity Guidelines for Americans

Children and Adolescents (6–17 years)

- Should do 1 hour or more of physical activity every day.
- Most of the 1 hour or more of physical activity should be either moderate- or vigorous-intensity aerobic activity, and should include vigorous-intensity physical activity at least 3 days per week.
- Part of the daily physical activity should include muscle-strengthening activity on at least 3 days per week.
- Part of the daily physical activity should include bone-strengthening activity on at least 3 days per week.

Adults (18–64 years)

- Should do 2 hours and 30 minutes a week of moderate-intensity, or 1 hour and 15 minutes a week of vigorous-intensity aerobic physical activity, or an equivalent combination of moderate- and vigorous-intensity aerobic physical activity. Aerobic activity should be performed in episodes of at least 10 minutes, preferably spread throughout the week.
- Additional health benefits are provided by increasing to 5 hours a week of moderate-intensity aerobic physical activity, or 2 hours and 30 minutes a week of vigorous-intensity physical activity, or an equivalent combination of both.
- Should also do muscle-strengthening activities that involve all major muscle groups performed on 2 or more days per week.

Older Adults (65+ years)

- Older adults should follow the adult guidelines. If this is not possible due to limiting chronic conditions, older adults should be as physically active as their abilities allow. They should avoid inactivity.
- Older adults should do exercises that maintain or improve balance if they are at risk of falling.

15-2   Physical activity is important to the health of Americans at all ages.

Many household tasks can count as part of your daily physical activity. Pushing the lawn mower, shoveling snow, and raking leaves all require a moderate amount of physical effort. You can judge the intensity of your physical activity by using a scale of 0 to 10 based on your personal capacity for activity, or fitness level. For instance, an activity you rate 5 or 6 on your scale is considered moderate intensity. An activity you rate at 7 or 8 is considered vigorous intensity, **15-3**. As your fitness level improves, your scale will change. For example, a level of activity you once considered vigorous intensity, you may now experience as moderate intensity.

Total Fitness

Once you start feeling the benefits of being more active, you may become like a rolling wheel picking up speed. The better you feel, the more active you will want to be. After a while, you may want to change your goal to try to achieve total fitness. You may also become more interested in other aspects of your health. Many people who start exercise programs develop an interest in nutritious eating and other healthful lifestyle behaviors.

Most of this chapter focuses on the goal of developing total fitness. You will learn what total fitness means.

Examples of Aerobic Activity Intensity Levels		
Type of Physical Activity	**Age Group**	
	Children/Teens	**Adults**
Moderate-intensity aerobic	• Hiking • Skateboarding • Bike riding (<10 mph) • Brisk walking • Pushing lawn mower • Raking leaves	• Brisk walking (>3 mph, but not racewalking) • Water aerobics • Doubles tennis • Bike riding (<10 mph) • Ballroom dancing • General gardening
Vigorous-intensity aerobic	• Bike riding (>10 mph) • Martial arts • Sports such as soccer, basketball, or swimming • Cross-country skiing	• Singles tennis • Racewalking, jogging, running • Aerobic dancing • Swimming laps • Heavy gardening

Source: 2008 Physical Activity Guidelines for Americans, U.S. Department of Health & Human Services

15-3   The intensity of an activity can vary depending on the amount of effort you put into it.

You will learn the benefits an exercise program can have for your body and your life. You will also study what makes a good exercise program. If you follow the ideas discussed here, you can look forward to enjoying an improved sense of well-being.

Peak Athletic Performance

A third goal for some physically active people is to reach their highest potential in sports performance. Achieving this goal requires a good level of overall fitness. It also requires intense training designed to develop specific sports skills. For instance, the football team does drills to build speed. A gymnast does exercises intended to develop balance. A tennis player's workouts are devised to strengthen coordination.

Athletes who truly want to be the best in their sport spend many hours each week in training. They know there is always room for improvement. They also know they will not continue to improve if they do not practice nearly every day.

The Benefits of Physical Activity

Becoming physically active at any level can positively affect your total health and performance. Not only will you feel physical benefits, but your mental health will improve, too. These benefits can have positive short-term and long-term effects.

Improved Appearance

One benefit of physical activity that inspires many people to exercise is improved appearance. Exercise can positively affect your appearance by altering your posture, movements, and weight.

Exercise can help you develop strong back and abdominal muscles, which are necessary for maintaining good posture. **Posture** is the position of your body when you are standing or sitting. Having erect posture when standing helps your clothes hang properly so you will look your best. Having erect posture when sitting helps you look and feel more alert. Having good posture also helps you avoid back problems.

Many teens go through a stage when they feel clumsy and awkward. You will find exercise can help you move more gracefully, 15-4. Agility, balance, and coordination developed through exercise will be reflected in all your movements.

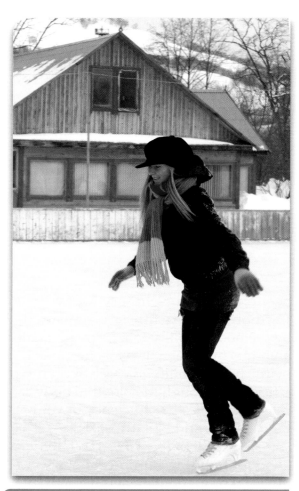

15-4 The balance and agility you develop through activities like ice skating will be reflected in all your movements.

Exercise burns calories. This is good news for people who are overweight. Thirty minutes of moderately intense activities will burn about 200 extra calories. This may not seem like much. When you multiply the calories burned over an extended period, however, the results are impressive. For instance, doing 30 minutes of moderate exercise five days a week will burn about 52,000 extra calories per year. That is nearly 15 pounds of body fat. Those who combine their exercise program with a low-fat diet that is moderate in calories can lose even more weight.

People who do not have weight problems should not overlook the benefits exercise can have for them. Over a lifetime, many people experience a slow weight gain by eating an extra 75 to 150 calories per day. An exercise program could easily burn up these excess calories and help keep weight at a healthy level throughout life.

Disease Prevention

Exercise can help reduce the risk of developing several diseases. These include osteoporosis, coronary heart disease (CHD), diabetes mellitus, and stroke. Physical activity and exercise boost your immune system. Exercising regularly helps your body balance hormones to protect cells from damage that may lead to some cancers. Exercise is not guaranteed to increase your life span, but it can improve your quality of life. It can help you have the energy you need for daily work and leisure activities.

Improved Mental Outlook

For many people, exercise creates a feeling of well-being. Adolescents who exercise regularly state they have improved self-control, self-esteem, and body image. They also report greater alertness and better school performance.

Although exercise does not solve problems, it helps relieve tension. When exercising, your thoughts focus on the physical activity rather than school or family pressures, **15-5**. Following a workout, you are likely to feel mentally refreshed. You will be more prepared to cope with day-to-day problems. For adults, exercise can help reduce feelings of depression. For older adults, the benefits of daily exercise include improved cognitive functioning. Regular physical activity can help to maintain or enhance various aspects of perception, thinking, and reasoning in older adults.

15-5   Exercise can relieve tension and improve mental outlook.

What Is Total Fitness?

Is a weight lifter who has difficulty running a mile physically fit? How would you rate the fitness of a distance runner who can only manage two push-ups? Total fitness involves more than being strong or fast. There are many aspects to physical fitness. Someone who has athletic skill will not necessarily be fit in all areas. However, striving for at least a moderate level of fitness in each area will promote good health and athletic performance.

Health Components of Physical Fitness

Five major components are used to measure the impact of physical fitness on your health. They are cardiorespiratory fitness, muscular endurance, strength, flexibility, and body composition. Being fit in each of these areas reduces your risk for certain health problems, including heart disease and certain cancers. It also improves your body's ability to perform its various functions.

Cardiorespiratory Fitness

The greatest sign of good health is cardiorespiratory fitness. **Cardiorespiratory fitness** is measured by the body's ability to take in adequate amounts of oxygen. It is also evaluated by the body's ability to carry oxygen efficiently through the blood to body cells. It involves the efficiency of your lungs, heart, and blood vessels.

Aerobic activities are especially good for building cardiorespiratory fitness. Throughout an aerobic activity, your heart and lungs should be able to supply all the oxygen your muscles need. Health benefits increase as your intensity of exercising increases. The goal of aerobic exercise is to increase your heart and breathing rates to safe levels for an extended time. Most fitness experts recommend holding these raised levels for 20 to 60 minutes to get the most cardiorespiratory benefits. Walking, jogging, in-line skating, bicycling, and swimming laps are examples of aerobic activities, **15-6**.

Anaerobic activities are activities in which your muscles are using oxygen faster than your heart and lungs can deliver it. Anaerobic fitness means you are able to lift or move objects forcefully as required for use in every day activities. Anaerobic activities use short, intense bursts of energy that make you feel like you need to catch your breath. Muscles rely on a limited supply of glucose and energy is released quickly. For example, sprint events and sports such as football, baseball, tennis, or a 100-meter race are anaerobic activities. They cannot be sustained long enough to help you increase cardiorespiratory fitness. This is because you must stop often during anaerobic activities to catch your breath. Anaerobic activities can help you build strength, power, and speed.

Muscular Endurance

Muscular endurance refers to your ability to use a group of muscles over and over without becoming tired. For instance, muscular endurance allows you to use your leg muscles to continuously pedal a bicycle throughout an hour-long ride. Muscular endurance helps you perform physical activities comfortably. It also enables you to remain active for extended periods.

Some people have more endurance in one muscle group than in another. For instance, people trained as runners are bound to have developed endurance in their leg muscles. However,

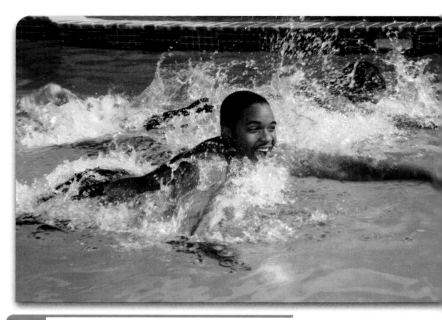

15-6   Using the muscles of the arms and legs while breathing rhythmically makes swimming an excellent aerobic activity.

they may find it hard to swim several laps without their arms tiring. This is why it is important to work on developing all your muscle groups. Hiking, rowing, skating, and gymnastics can help you develop muscular endurance.

Strength

Strength is the ability of the muscles to move objects. It is usually measured in terms of how much weight you can

Math Link

Calculating Resting Heart Rate

The resting heart rate averages between 60 and 80 beats per minute. Jack, a nonathlete, has a resting heart rate of 70 beats per minute. His friend, Joe, runs cross country and has a resting heart rate of 40 beats per minute. Joe's stronger heart pumps more blood with fewer beats.

- How much faster is Jack's resting heart rate than Joe's?

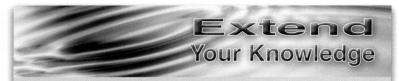

Extend Your Knowledge

Building a Better Body

Interview a number of body builders. Learn what motivates their interest in body building. Is their focus to increase muscle strength, endurance, or both? Compare their answers to recognized benefits for increasing muscle strength. Are the body builders' reasons different from benefits identified in this chapter?

lift. You move your body by contracting your muscles. Having strong muscles will allow you to move your body more efficiently. Developing strength can also help you avoid some sports injuries. Obviously, weight training is an excellent activity for developing strength and lean muscle mass, **15-7**.

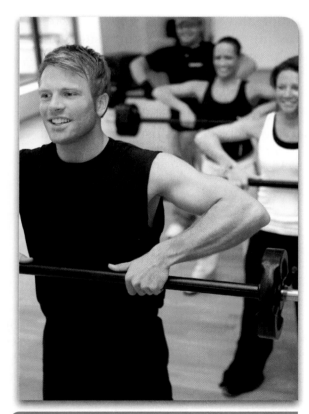

15-7 Using muscles to lift weights helps develop strength.

Flexibility

Flexibility is the ability to move your joints through a full range of motion. Joints are the places in your body where two bones meet. Elbows, knees, shoulders, hips, and ankles are all examples of joints. A high degree of flexibility helps prevent injury to muscles that control movement of the joints.

Females generally have the potential for greater flexibility than males. Stretching exercises can help increase flexibility.

Body Composition

Body composition is the percentage of different types of tissues in the body. High body fat percentage is a risk factor for a number of diseases. Therefore, body composition is a component of total physical fitness.

If you are at or below a healthy weight, you may ask, "Do I really need to exercise?" The answer is "yes." Everyone at all ages needs to be physically active. As described earlier, physical activity has many benefits besides helping people maintain a healthy weight. It is an essential component in maintaining overall good health and fitness.

Remember, weight is not a reliable indicator of body composition. Someone who has a large percentage of lean body tissue may be overweight according to his or her body mass index (BMI). However, he or she is not overfat.

Exercise helps the body burn fat and build muscle. Glucose is the body's chief source of energy. After about 20 minutes of aerobic activity, however, the body begins to use fat for energy. Doing activities that increase muscular endurance and strength helps build muscle tissue. Increasing the proportion of muscle mass in the body raises the basal metabolic rate (BMR), thus helping to burn even more calories. Along with a low-fat diet, exercise is a key factor in achieving and maintaining a healthy body composition.

You will not see changes in body composition after a single workout. Over time, however, you will notice an increase in lean body tissue and a decrease in body fat. Cross-country skiing, racquetball, soccer, and other aerobic exercises are among the sports that are especially good for controlling body fatness, **15-8**.

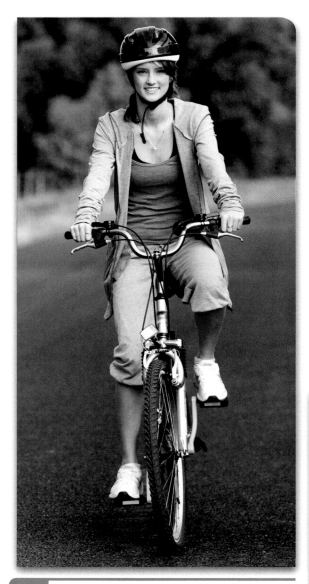

15-8   Biking helps maintain a healthy body composition because it builds muscle while burning fat.

Skill Components of Physical Fitness

There are six skill components of physical fitness. They are power, agility, balance, coordination, speed, and reaction time. For some people, strength in these components seems to come naturally. However, most people can work to improve their ability in these areas.

Having a high level of the various skill components can improve your performance in certain sports. You are more likely to take part in activities when you are confident in your performance. Therefore, developing your skill components can motivate you to be active. This, in turn, can bring you the benefits that come from an active lifestyle.

Skill-related fitness can benefit you in everyday activities as well as sports. For instance, having good balance, agility, and coordination can help you avoid accidents. Older people who have these skills are less likely to fall and experience the problems of injury.

If you lack some of the skill components, keep in mind many activities do not require all of them. Such activities include walking, bicycling, and swimming laps. Maintaining an active lifestyle, regardless of the type of activity, is the key to a positive health status.

Wellness Tip

Sanitizing Sports Equipment

If you work out at the school gym or a fitness center, be sure to sanitize your sports equipment before and after use. To prevent disease transmittal, use sanitizing wipes or solution and wipe down such surfaces as handles for treadmills, stationary bikes, stair climbers, and rowing machines; floor and wall exercise mats; free weights; weights and lifting bar; and lifting benches.

Power

Power is your ability to do maximum work in a short time. It requires a combination of strength and speed. People need power to excel in some sports activities, such as football and many track and field events. Lifting or stacking boxes and pushing a child on a swing are everyday activities that require power.

As muscles get stronger, they also become more powerful. Joining a softball league or shooting baskets in the gym can help you develop power.

Agility

Agility is your ability to change the position of your body with speed and control. Agility is an advantage in many sports. It is important to everyday living, too. An agile player can easily move down a sports field in and among other players. Agility can also help you weave through a crowded shopping mall. Downhill skiing, soccer, modern dance, and rope jumping can help develop agility, **15-9**.

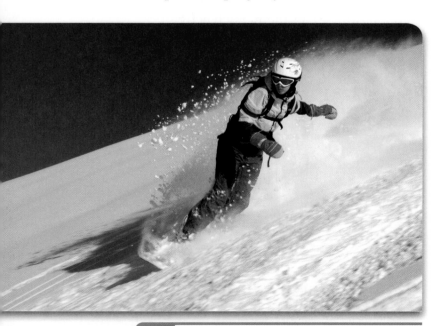

15-9   Controlling his body as he speeds down a slope helps this snowboarder develop agility.

Balance

Balance is your ability to keep your body in an upright position while standing still or moving. Balance requires concentration on the task, coordination, and muscle control. Practice is needed to improve balance skills. Some sports, such as gymnastics and dancing, require athletes to have sensitive balance to excel. A good sense of balance can also help anyone avoid falls and feel more graceful. Ice skating and bicycling can help you develop balance.

Coordination

Coordination is your ability to integrate the use of two or more parts of your body. Many sports require coordination of the eyes and hands or the eyes and feet. Many daily tasks require these types of coordination, too. A football player needs good coordination to catch a pass. You need coordination when chopping vegetables for a salad to avoid cutting off your fingers. A soccer player needs coordination to maintain possession of the ball when dribbling down the field. You need coordination to avoid tripping over objects and stepping in puddles. Bowling, golf, volleyball, and tennis are all activities that help develop coordination.

Speed

Speed is the quickness with which you are able to complete a motion. Obviously, athletes who compete in sprint events need speed. You use speed in daily tasks when you hurry through chores or run to catch a bus. You might consider a class in judo or karate to help you develop speed. Handball, table tennis, and roller skating are also activities that will help you build speed.

Reaction Time

Reaction time is the amount of time it takes you to respond to a signal once you receive the signal. In most physical activities, your response will be some type of movement. A soccer goalie needs good reaction time to block a ball headed for the net. A driver needs to be able to react to changes in traffic. Playing baseball, basketball, football, or softball can help you strengthen your reaction time, **15-10**.

How Fit Are You?

You can assess yourself in each health and skill component of physical fitness through a variety of simple tests. For example, the *President's Challenge on Physical Fitness* can be found on the Internet and offers instruction on how to test your ability in several areas of fitness. You are likely to find you are strong in some components but weak in others. To be totally fit, you should be moderately strong in all the health components. You can set goals to improve in your weaker areas. Building strength in each of the health areas will also help you develop more of the skill components.

Later in the chapter you will read about how to plan an exercise program and stay motivated to follow it. Following the guidelines outlined will help you plot a strategy for improving your total fitness.

Exercise and Heart Health

Physical inactivity is a risk factor for coronary heart disease (CHD). As higher levels of physical fitness are achieved, the risks of death from heart disease decline.

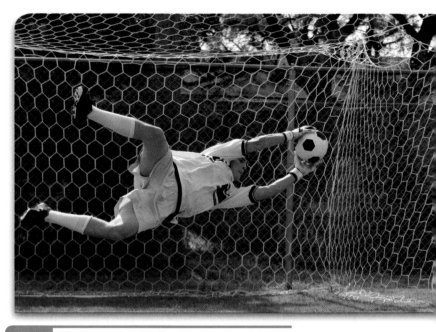

15-10 Responding to their opponents' movements requires goalies to have good reaction time.

Exercise affects the cardiovascular system (the heart and blood vessels) in several complex ways to improve overall heart health. Remember that exercise helps develop cardiorespiratory fitness. One indication of this type of fitness is a slower heartbeat. The heart beats slower because it is able to work more efficiently. It pumps more blood with each beat. This improved efficiency puts less strain on the heart muscle.

Another way exercise affects heart health is through its impact on blood lipids. A high level of low density lipoproteins (LDL) indicates a high risk of CHD. A high level of high density lipoproteins (HDL) indicates a low risk of CHD. Regular exercise—especially when combined with a diet low in saturated fat and cholesterol—reduces LDL and increases HDL. These changes in blood lipid levels lower the risks of coronary heart disease.

Exercise improves heart health by lowering blood pressure. Exercise also encourages the formation of extra branches in the arteries of the heart. This increases blood flow and allows the heart to work more efficiently.

Measuring Your Heart Rate

Your heart rate is an indication of the effect physical activity is having on your heart. Your **heart rate**, or pulse rate, is the number of times your heart beats per minute.

You can measure your heart rate by finding your pulse and counting the beats. When measuring your heart rate, always use your index and middle fingers, never your thumb. Heart rate is usually measured in one of two places: the wrist or the neck. At your wrist, slide the fingers of one hand along the thumb of your other hand to your wrist. You should feel your blood pulsating when you apply gentle pressure. You should be able to feel a similar pulsating in your neck. Put your two fingers just to the left or right of your Adam's apple. Using the second hand on a watch or clock, count the beats for 15 seconds. Then multiply the number of beats by four to find the number of beats per minute.

Another way to count your heart rate is to count the number of beats in six seconds. Then add a zero to the number to figure the number of beats per minute. In other words, 7 beats in six seconds equals a heart rate of 70 beats per minute.

Your heart rate will vary depending on your level of activity. The harder you work out, the faster your heart will beat.

A **resting heart rate** is the speed at which your heart muscle contracts when you are sitting quietly. An average resting heart rate for a moderately fit teen or adult is about 70 beats

per minute. As mentioned above, improved cardiorespiratory fitness results in a slower heartbeat. Someone who has been training for several months may have a resting heart rate of about 60 beats per minute, **15-11**.

Maximum heart rate is the highest speed at which your heart muscle is able to contract. Maximum heart rate is related to age. It is higher for a younger person than for an older person. You

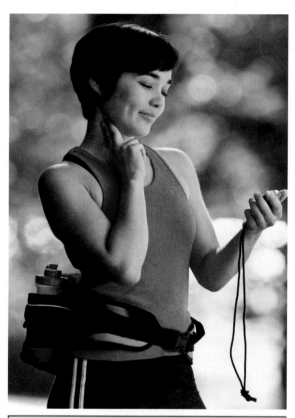

Measuring Resting Heart Rate	
Heart Rate (beats per minute)	**Fitness Rating**
<59	Excellent
60–69	Good
70–79	Average
80–89	Fair
>90	Poor

15-11   As cardiorespiratory fitness improves, resting heart rate will drop because the heart is working more efficiently.

can calculate your maximum heart rate using the following formula:

220 – your age = maximum heart rate

A 16-year-old using this formula would calculate his or her maximum heart rate to be 204 beats per minute (220 – 16 = 204). A 50-year-old would calculate his or her maximum heart rate to be just 170 beats per minute (220 – 50 = 170).

Exercising Your Heart

The heart is a strong muscle. Like your other muscles, your heart needs exercise. Measuring your heart rate can help you see if you are giving your heart enough exercise.

For good exercise, your heart needs to beat faster than its resting rate. However, it should not beat so fast that it is unsafe. You should never try to reach your maximum heart rate. Instead, you should try to exercise within a safe **target heart rate zone**. This is the range of heartbeats per minute at which the heart muscle receives the best workout. Your target heart rate zone is 60 to 90 percent of your maximum heart rate. A 16-year-old would calculate target heart rate zone as follows:

Maximum heart rate:
  220 – 16 = 204 beats per minute

  204 × 0.6 = 122 beats per minute
  204 × 0.9 = 184 beats per minute

Target heart rate zone:
  122 to 184 beats per minute

When you begin an exercise program, count your heart rate frequently during your workouts. This will help you decide whether you are pushing yourself too little or too much. Your initial goal should be to keep your heart rate at the low end of your target zone. As your fitness improves, you should be keeping your heart rate closer to the high end of your target zone, **15-12**.

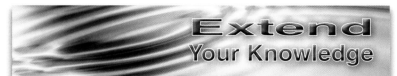

Facts About Resting Heart Rate

The American Heart Association reports that the best time to measure your resting heart rate is in the morning, after a good night's sleep, and before you get out of bed. The heart beats about 60 to 80 times a minute when at rest. Resting heart rate usually rises slightly with age. It is usually lower for physically fit people, often lower than 65 beats per minute. Resting heart rate is used to determine one's training target heart rate. The heart rate adapts to changes in the body's need for oxygen, such as during exercise or sleep.

Keys to a Successful Exercise Program

Beginning an exercise program can be hard for some people. You need to feel sure rewards will follow. Talk with people who exercise regularly. Ask them what benefits they have noticed as a result of being physically active. Their answers may inspire you to begin an exercise program that includes more than just daily lifestyle activities.

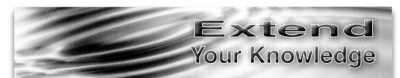

How Does Your Heart Rate?

Measure your resting heart rate after sitting for 30 minutes or more. Record your resting heart rate. After taking a leisurely walk for 10 minutes, measure and record your heart rate. Measure and record your heart rate after a brisk 10-minute-walk. Were the results what you expected? Determine your resting heart rate fitness rating using guidelines provided in this chapter. (If your results are consistently high, you should consult your health-care provider.)

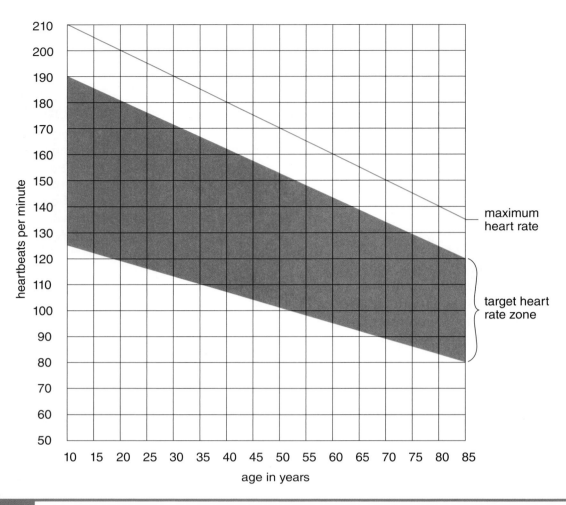

15-12 For a good cardiorespiratory workout, keep your heart rate in your target zone when exercising.

Researchers have identified some factors that help people stick with their exercise programs. These factors include written goals, enjoyable activities, a convenient exercise schedule, and knowledge of personal fitness level. Consider these factors as you plan a program for yourself.

Put Fitness Goals in Writing

Your physical fitness efforts are most likely to be effective if you set some specific goals for them. Your long-term goal may be to achieve and maintain total fitness. For most people, however, trying to fulfill such a big goal would be overwhelming. You need to break this goal down into smaller, more manageable goals.

Begin by identifying which component of fitness you want to improve first. Then think about activities that can help you improve in that area. Review the choices of activities presented in **15-13**. Select activities that are of interest to you. Make a specific plan to include those activities in your weekly routine.

One way to stay focused in your exercise program is to write down your fitness goals. Start with one specific and attainable goal. Your goal might read "I will improve my cardiovascular fitness until my pulse drops to 100 beats per minute following a three-minute

Building Health Components of Fitness

Health Component of Physical Fitness	Activities
Cardiorespiratory Fitness	Aerobic dancing, bicycling, cross-country skiing, hiking, in-line skating, rope jumping, rowing, racquetball, soccer, swimming
Muscular Endurance	Backpacking, calisthenics, cross-country skiing, football, gymnastics, ice skating, in-line skating, mountain climbing, rowing, swimming, weight training
Strength	Backpacking, ballet, football, gymnastics, walking, weight training
Flexibility	Aerobic dancing, ballet, calisthenics, gymnastics, modern dance
Body Composition	Aerobic dancing, bicycling, cross-country skiing, handball, hiking, in-line skating, mountain climbing, racquetball, rope jumping, rowing, soccer, swimming, walking

15-13 Choose activities you enjoy that will help you develop health components of fitness in which you are weak.

step test." Then list specific steps for achieving your goal. You might write "I will bicycle for 30 minutes after school on Monday and Thursday. I will skate for 30 minutes after school on Tuesday and Friday." You might want to write your goal and the steps for achieving it as a personal exercise contract. Post a copy of the contract in a spot where you will see it several times a day.

Your chances for success are much better if you write down what you accomplish. Keep a record of when you exercise and for how long. You will be less likely to skip an exercise session if you know it will show up on your record. You will feel good about yourself when you see how faithfully you are following your exercise contract. Be sure to praise yourself for your success.

Fitness goals take time to achieve. However, you should see some signs of improvement within a few weeks, **15-14**. If you have been following your contract and do not see improvement, evaluate your exercise plan carefully. You may

need to revise the steps you are using to reach your goal. You may also want to consider seeing a fitness counselor. When you achieve your goal, congratulate yourself for a job well done. Then set a new goal and begin working toward it.

Choose Activities You Enjoy

Physical activity should be fun, not a chore. If you choose activities you enjoy, you are more likely to stick with your exercise program. You may enjoy outdoor activities such as hiking and canoeing. Perhaps you like the competition of team sports. Maybe you prefer such partner sports as tennis or handball that you can play with a friend. No matter what activity you choose, the important point is to be active.

Variety can help keep an exercise program enjoyable. You may become bored following the same exercise routine day after day. Doing different types of activities can keep you from

Personal Exercise Contract

Goal

I will improve my cardiovascular fitness until my pulse drops to 100 beats per minute following a three-minute step test.

Action Plan

I will do one of the following activities at least five days a week.

Progress—Week 1

Activity	Sunday	Monday	Tuesday	Wednesday	Thursday	Friday	Saturday
Bicycle 30 minutes	✓						
Skate 30 minutes							✓
Swim 20 laps			✓		✓		
Walk 30 minutes				✓			

Progress—Week 2

Activity	Sunday	Monday	Tuesday	Wednesday	Thursday	Friday	Saturday
Bicycle 30 minutes							✓
Skate 30 minutes		✓				✓	
Swim 20 laps			✓		✓		
Walk 30 minutes	✓						

15-14 Using a personal exercise contract can motivate you to stick with an exercise program to meet your fitness goals.

getting into a rut. Different activities also help develop different components of fitness. This will help you reach your long-term goal of achieving a good level of total fitness. If you enjoy anaerobic activities, try to include some aerobic activities in your exercise program, too. Also remember to choose activities that focus on different large muscle groups. For instance, you might try rowing to develop upper body strength and jogging to build leg muscles.

Although your exercise program should meet your personal fitness needs, you do not need to exercise alone. Working out with friends or family members can make a fitness program more fun. Doing activities with other people can also help you stay motivated, **15-15**. On a day when you are tempted to cancel your workout, a friend can encourage you to get going.

Choose a Convenient Time

Scheduling physical activity at a convenient time will increase your likelihood of following through with your exercise program. You may want to work out first thing in the morning to get your day off to a good start. You might have some free time after school when you can enjoy activities with friends. Perhaps you would rather exercise at night before going to bed. It does not matter when you exercise as long as you do it.

Once you find an exercise time that is convenient for you, make it a set part of your daily schedule. This will help you form a habit that is easy to follow.

Know Your Fitness Level

For your exercise program to be successful, you need to know your fitness level. In striving to meet your goal for total fitness, resist the temptation to begin working out too hard too soon. This increases your risk of fatigue and injury and, thereby, increases your likelihood of discontinuing your fitness program.

Before you begin an exercise program, measure your level of fitness in each of the health components. Ask a

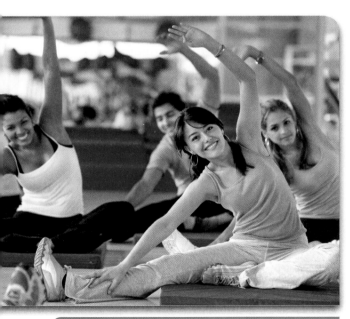

15-15 Exercising or playing sports with a friend can make physical activity more fun.

fitness counselor or health or physical education teacher for information about self-assessment exercises. Also review the checklist in **15-16** to see if you need to seek medical advice before you start exercising. If you are in good health, you can begin a sensible exercise plan.

Case Study: Jake's Fitness Goals

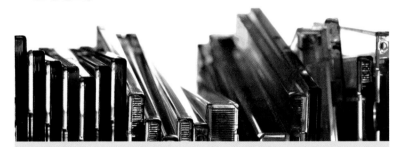

Jake stopped playing soccer two years ago. He hasn't been active in any sports since then. He spends much of his free time studying and playing video games. Lately, he has noticed that his muscle tone is gone and he can't run up the stairs as easily as he once could. Yesterday in gym class, he was winded just a few minutes into a game of basketball! Jake decides he needs to take action before his fitness level gets any worse.

That night, Jake sets the alarm on his clock for one hour earlier in the morning. Even though he hates exercising in the morning, he is determined to start his new fitness plan first thing the next day. His fitness plan is to run three miles and lift weights before school every morning.

When the alarm goes off the next morning, Jake hits the snooze button four times before he finally drags himself out of bed. He throws on some clothes and sets off for a run. Jake is out of breath and begins to walk after running just two blocks. He is so discouraged that he turns around and goes home. By the time Jake showers and has breakfast, he is running late and misses the bus for school. As his mom is driving him to school, Jake decides being fit just isn't worth the trouble.

Case Review

1. How do you think Jake felt after deciding to give up on his fitness plan?

2. Why do you think Jake's new fitness plan failed?

3. What suggestions would you give to Jake about improving his fitness plan?

Proceed with Caution If...

_____ your doctor said you have a heart condition, such as a heart murmur.

_____ your doctor said you have high blood pressure or cholesterol.

_____ you have a medical condition, such as type 1 diabetes, that might require special attention in an exercise program.

_____ you have pain in your joints, arms, or legs that could be made worse by physical exercise.

_____ you weigh 25 or more pounds above healthy weight.

_____ you often feel faint or have periods of dizziness.

_____ you experience pain or shortage of breath after moderate physical activity.

If you have any chronic conditions or symptoms, seek the advice of a health-care provider to determine the types and amounts of activity appropriate for you.

15-16 If any of these statements applies to you, see your doctor before starting an exercise program.

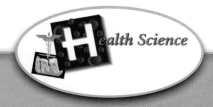

Health Science

Personal Trainer

Personal trainers work one-on-one or with two or three clients, either in a gym or in the clients' homes. They help clients assess their level of physical fitness. Personal trainers also help clients set and reach fitness goals. They demonstrate various exercises and help clients improve their exercise techniques. Trainers may also advise clients on lifestyle modifications outside of the gym to improve their fitness.

Education: Although the education and training required depends on the specific type of personal training, employers increasingly require fitness workers to have a bachelor's degree. This degree is generally in a field related to health and fitness, such as exercise science or physical education. Some personal trainers often start out by taking classes to become certified. Then they may begin by working alongside an experienced trainer before being allowed to train clients alone.

Job Outlook: Jobs for fitness workers are expected to increase much faster than average for all occupations. Aging baby boomers, one group that wants to stay healthy and fit, will be the main driver of employment growth for personal trainers. With fewer physical education programs in schools and parents' growing concern about childhood obesity, parents are often hiring personal trainers for their children.

Gaining physical fitness is a building process. It involves three key factors—frequency, intensity, and duration.

- *Frequency* is how often you exercise.
- *Intensity* is how hard you exercise.
- *Duration* refers to how long an exercise session lasts.

Begin your exercise program with moderate frequency, low intensity, and short duration. You might start by exercising three times a week. Keep your pulse at about 60 percent of your maximum heart rate for 20 minutes. As you notice improvements in your state of fitness, gradually increase the frequency, intensity, and duration of your exercise. Compete with yourself to achieve new, higher-level goals. Try increasing your frequency to five to seven days per week. Build your intensity up to 70 or 80 percent of your maximum heart rate. Extend the duration of your workouts up to 60 minutes.

Being aware of your fitness level can protect you from injuries caused by too much stress on your body. Exercise should not be painful. You need to learn to tune in to what your body tells you. Burning muscles and feeling as if you cannot catch your breath are signs you are working too hard. These symptoms may occur more rapidly as you increase your speed, exercise in heat or high humidity, or grow tired. If you experience these symptoms, you need to slow down your exercise pace.

Following basic safety precautions can help you avoid other types of injuries when exercising. Know how to use equipment and use it correctly. Wear protective gear, such as helmets and body pads, when appropriate. If you will be exercising outdoors, be prepared for the environmental conditions, **15-17**. If you are injured, follow first-aid practices and seek prompt medical attention if necessary.

Planning an Exercise Program

Your exercise program should include three phases for each workout session. You need a warm-up period, workout period, and cooldown period.

Warm-Up Period

On a cold morning, a car engine needs to warm up before you start driving. In a similar way, your muscles need to warm up before you start exercising. Warming up prepares your heart and other muscles for work. Many people ignore this important phase of an exercise program. If you do not warm up, you may be more likely to end up with sore muscles or an injury.

The warm-up period should last about 5 to 10 minutes. Begin by gradually increasing your heart rate. Some people choose a slow jog for this purpose. If you will be swimming or bicycling, you can simply start the activity at a slow pace. Gradually increase to a moderate pace to bring your heart rate near your target zone.

Following your heart warm-up, warm up the muscles you will be using in your workout. Do a series of gentle stretches, but avoid bouncing motions. Your movements should resemble those you will use in your exercise activity. If you will be playing tennis, slowly move

---

Preparing for Environmental Conditions

- Use caution when exercising in hot, humid weather. High temperatures combined with high humidity increase the risk of heat exhaustion and heatstroke. Wait until temperatures have cooled or choose to exercise in an air-conditioned facility. Be sure to drink plenty of water before, during, and after exercise.
- Use caution when exercising in extremely cold weather. Cold temperatures can cause frostbite and a drop in body temperature. If you feel cold, stop the activity and get to a warmer place.
- Use caution when exercising on wet, icy, and snow-covered surfaces.
- Move indoors at the first sight of lightning.
- Allow the body time to adjust to the lower air pressure before exercising vigorously in high altitudes (over 5,000 feet).
- Avoid exercising in areas that have high levels of fume exhaust from cars and industry. Polluted air can cause headaches, painful breathing, and watery eyes.

15-17 Following these recommendations can make your exercise activities safe and rewarding.

your arms as though you are making broad forehand and backhand strokes. Make these motions several times with empty hands. Then pick up a tennis racquet and repeat them several more times. After a brief warm-up session such as this, you will be ready for a more vigorous workout, **15-18**.

Workout Period

The workout period is the main part of your exercise program. It should last at least 20 minutes. During this time, do activities that will help you develop the health components of fitness. When choosing activities for your workout period, remember the keys for success you read about earlier in the chapter.

Cooldown Period

Never sit down or enter a hot shower immediately after exercise without a cooldown period. The body needs to slowly return to its pre-exercise state.

During exercise, your heart pumps extra blood to your muscles to meet their increased demand for oxygen and energy. The action of your muscles keeps blood circulating back to the heart. If you stop muscle action too quickly, the extra blood temporarily collects in your muscles. This reduces the amount of oxygen-rich blood available for the heart to pump to the brain and dizziness results.

The cooldown period should last about 10 minutes. You can use the same activities for your cooldown as you used for your warm-up. A slow jog will help reduce your heart rate and allow the muscles to push more blood toward the heart. Some stretching exercises will help prevent muscle cramps and soreness by loosening muscles that have become tight from exercise.

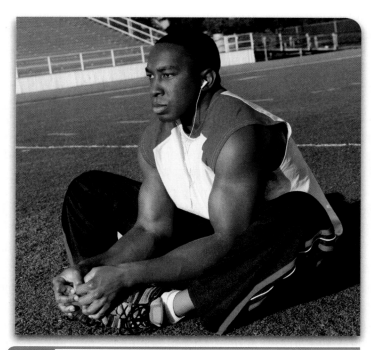

15-18 Stretching before a workout helps warm up muscles and prepare them for activity.

Reading Summary

Physical activity is needed for physical fitness. The kinds of activities you do and the way you do them will help you reach different fitness goals. To achieve good health, you can follow the *Physical Activity Guidelines for Americans*. Physical activity can also help you achieve the goals of total fitness or peak athletic performance.

Physical activity has several key benefits. It improves your appearance by helping you develop good posture, graceful movements, and healthy weight. It reduces the risk of several diseases, including coronary heart disease. Physical activity can also help improve your mental outlook.

Through physical activity, you develop the five health components of physical fitness. They are cardiorespiratory fitness, muscular endurance, strength, flexibility, and healthy body composition. Physical activity can also help you build six skill components that will improve your sports performance. The skill components of physical fitness are power, agility, balance, coordination, speed, and reaction time.

Exercise benefits heart health in several ways. It helps strengthen the heart muscle, improves blood lipid levels, and lowers blood pressure. Measuring your heart rate can help you see how exercise is affecting your heart. To give your heart the best workout, try to stay within your target heart rate zone when exercising.

There are several keys to a successful exercise program. Put your fitness goals in writing. Choose activities you enjoy and do them at a convenient time. Also, be sure to keep your workouts in line with your fitness level.

Each exercise session should have a warm-up, workout, and cooldown period. The workout period should last at least 20 minutes. You will find physical activity is a lifestyle choice with lifetime benefits.

Review Learning

1. What physical activity guidelines should teens follow for achieving good health?
2. What are three ways physical activity can improve appearance?
3. What types of activities are good for building cardiorespiratory fitness?
4. Which health component of physical fitness is demonstrated by an ability to repeatedly use muscles without tiring?
5. List four skill components of physical fitness and give an example of an activity that would help develop each component.
6. Why does someone with a high level of cardiorespiratory fitness have a slower heartbeat than someone who is less fit?
7. Where is heart rate usually measured?
8. What is the maximum heart rate for a 30-year-old man?
9. What percentage of the maximum heart rate is the target heart rate zone?
10. Why is an exercise program more likely to be successful if a written record of exercise sessions is kept?
11. What are two advantages of varying the activities in an exercise program?
12. What are the three key factors involved in gaining physical fitness?

13. True or false. Burning muscles are a sign of a good workout.
14. What is the purpose of the warm-up period of an exercise session?
15. Why might skipping the cooldown period at the end of an exercise session result in dizziness?

Critical Thinking

16. **Identify factors.** What factors impact your motivation to develop and maintain a personal exercise program? What can you do to overcome such obstacles?
17. **Assess outcomes.** Establish a personal exercise plan. Assess the outcomes of following through with your plan at two-week intervals throughout this course. What changes do you see in the health components of physical fitness? skill components?

Applying Your Knowledge

18. **Poster activity.** Create a poster illustrating activities that help develop the five health components of physical fitness.
19. **Rank fitness factors.** List 10 sports on a sheet of paper. Rank the importance of each skill component of physical fitness for each sport. Compare your list with the rest of the class.
20. **Calculate target heart rate.** Measure your resting heart rate. Compute your maximum heart rate and your target heart rate zone.
21. **Exercise contract.** Write a personal exercise contract. Identify a specific, attainable fitness goal and list the steps you intend to follow to achieve it. Follow the contract for three weeks. Then evaluate the strengths and weaknesses of your plan. Revise the plan to address weaknesses.

Technology Connections

22. **Exercise video.** Search the Centers for Disease Control (CDC) Web site for the *Physical Activity for Everyone* videos. Select one and watch one of the video exercise activities. With a partner, create your own video demonstrating this exercise for the class. Use a video camera or digital camera equipped with video capabilities.
23. **Electronic presentation.** Use at least three Internet resources to prepare an electronic presentation about physical activity targeted at a specific age group. Possible presentation ideas include parents building more exercise into the daily activities of their children, teens helping teens stay fit, or fitness activities for older adults.
24. **Activity graph.** Identify the calorie content for your favorite fast-food item. Then select five physical activities of varying intensity. Use Internet resources to learn how many calories per hour each activity burns. Use spreadsheet or graphing software to prepare a bar graph comparing the amounts of time each activity must be performed in order to expend the calories supplied by the fast-food item.

25. **Fitness test.** Identify an adult friend, parent, or grandparent who is interested in assessing his or her fitness level. Search the Internet for the *President's Challenge Adult Fitness Test*. Use the computer to help your adult volunteer determine their fitness score. Work with your volunteer to create a fitness plan to improve their fitness level.

26. **Electronic activity journal.** Create a list of tips for increasing physical activity in your life. Visit the physical activity section of ChooseMyPlate.gov for ideas. Keep an electronic physical activity journal to record your progress. After one week, evaluate how useful the tips were to you. Add, delete, or change your physical activity tips based on your evaluation.

Academic Connections

27. **Writing.** Prepare an appealing flyer on the importance of physical activity. Address your flyer to the needs for physical activity for a particular life-cycle stage. Share your flyer with a community group where people of that age group gather.

28. **Speech.** Prepare an oral report on the causes and treatment of common sports injuries. Discuss how warm-up and cooldown sessions may be related to the injury prevention.

29. **Science.** Select one muscle or group of muscles and research how it works and is used by physically fit people. Present your findings to the class. Use a diagram of the muscular system to show the location of the particular muscle(s) in the human body. As part of your presentation, demonstrate one stretch or physical activity that benefits this muscle.

30. **Reading.** Locate and read the CDC's position statement on youth's need for physical activity. Write a summary including five key points that you identify as important to future health of adolescents in the United States.

Workplace Applications

Using Organizational Skills

As part of an ongoing health and wellness program at your workplace, you have been put in charge of organizing a voluntary lunchtime exercise program for employees. With an hour for lunch, 30 minutes can be devoted to daily exercise. Using the information on the 2008 *Physical Activity Guidelines for Americans* Web site, organize exercise activities centered on cardiorespiratory, endurance, strength, and flexibility. Be sure to allow time for adequate warm-up, workout, and cooldown periods. Note that some of the activities on the plan can be done by employees on their own before or after work. Include ideas for keeping employees motivated to participate. Share your plan.

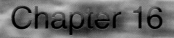

Chapter 16

Eating for Sports Performance

Reading for Meaning

After reading the chapter, outline the key points and compare your outline to the text. This will help you retain what you have read and identify what you need to read again.

Concept Organizer

Use the T-chart diagram to note the main ideas and supporting details for planning meals for athletes in training.

Meals for Athletes in Training	
Main Ideas	Supporting Details

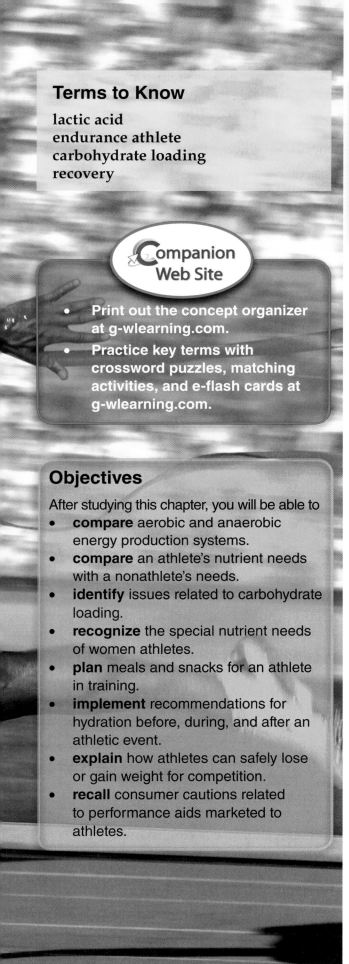

Terms to Know

lactic acid
endurance athlete
carbohydrate loading
recovery

Companion Web Site

- **Print out the concept organizer at g-wlearning.com.**
- **Practice key terms with crossword puzzles, matching activities, and e-flash cards at g-wlearning.com.**

Objectives

After studying this chapter, you will be able to

- **compare** aerobic and anaerobic energy production systems.
- **compare** an athlete's nutrient needs with a nonathlete's needs.
- **identify** issues related to carbohydrate loading.
- **recognize** the special nutrient needs of women athletes.
- **plan** meals and snacks for an athlete in training.
- **implement** recommendations for hydration before, during, and after an athletic event.
- **explain** how athletes can safely lose or gain weight for competition.
- **recall** consumer cautions related to performance aids marketed to athletes.

Central Ideas

- Athletes have a greater need for energy and some other nutrients than nonathletes.
- Athletes must consume adequate amounts of carbohydrates, vegetables, fruits, protein, fat, and water to meet their training and competition needs.

Sports activities are an important part of everyday life. Sports are relaxing, fun, and available for people of all ages and both sexes. These activities provide health and wellness benefits for all who take part. They promote self-esteem and build physical skills. Through teamwork, sports also help people grow socially and emotionally.

Athletes often have an intense desire to excel. Team and partner sports are competitive. The focus is on beating an opponent. Individual sports present athletes with a challenge to surpass their previous best performance.

The drive for peak performance has led some athletes to seek a winning edge through their diet. Their search has fostered the spread of nutrition myths and misinformation. This chapter will help you sort the facts from the fallacies. You will learn which diet choices can make a difference in how well you perform.

Fueling Muscle for Performance

Where do muscles get the energy needed to fuel activity? As you know, carbohydrates and fats are the main sources of energy for the body. These nutrients are found in the foods you eat and your body's stores of fat and glucose. However, the body must first convert these nutrients into an energy source that can be used by the muscle. This energy is produced either in the presence or absence of oxygen. An aerobic energy production system supplies energy in the presence of oxygen. Anaerobic energy production systems supply energy in the absence of oxygen. Each of these systems has benefits and drawbacks. The body uses them in combination to maximize the benefits.

The anaerobic energy production system is the first to supply energy when your body begins an activity. The first seconds of an activity are fueled by the very small but essential supply of energy that is stored in the muscle ready for immediate use. At the same time, the system begins converting the glycogen that is stored in the muscle to glucose. The glucose is then rapidly converted to an energy source the muscle can use, **16-1**.

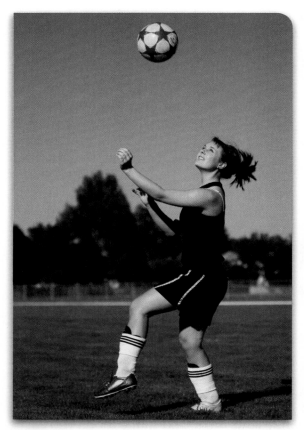

16-1 Soccer players' muscles are fueled by both aerobic and anaerobic energy production systems.

The anaerobic system supplies energy quickly, but cannot sustain this rate of energy production for long. Therefore, the body turns to the aerobic energy production system for fuel. The aerobic system is slower to respond to the body's need for energy because it requires the presence of oxygen. The oxygen must be inhaled and transported through the blood to the muscle, which takes time. However, this system can supply energy to the body for hours. Unlike the anaerobic system, the aerobic system can access and utilize the energy stored in fat as well as that found in glucose.

In the absence of oxygen, an incomplete breakdown of glucose results in a buildup of a product called **lactic acid** in the muscles. The lactic acid changes the body's acid-base balance. As a result, you experience a burning sensation and fatigue in the muscles. For example, a cross-country athlete running at a pace that is too fast becomes out of breath. When this occurs, the athlete may need to slow down to allow breathing to catch up with the need for oxygen. As breathing improves, the needed oxygen is delivered to the bloodstream and the acid-base balance is restored.

Both energy production systems can become more efficient with the use of appropriate training methods. For example, the anaerobic system can be improved with training that involves performing high-intensity exercises less than ten seconds in duration separated by brief rest intervals. When hockey players train with repeated sprints across the ice and rapid direction changes, they are trying to improve their anaerobic energy systems.

Some sports require athletes to use their muscles for long periods. These **endurance athletes** may be involved in sports such as marathon bicycle and foot races or distance swimming. Endurance athletes may require sustained muscle efforts for several hours at a time. You might wonder how they can extend their muscle performance to avoid exhausting their glycogen stores and "hitting the wall." Improving the efficiency of the aerobic energy system is a goal for these athletes. Endurance athletes train to improve the ability of their heart and lungs to deliver oxygen to their muscle. Increased oxygen in the muscle improves the muscle's ability to use glucose. This allows the body to use more fat for fuel and conserve glycogen. Trained muscles also become more tolerant of lactic acid. Thus, soreness and fatigue will not occur as quickly, **16-2**.

Both the aerobic and anaerobic energy systems are always in use by the body. However, the nature of the activity and the fitness of the athlete influence which system is supplying more energy.

The Nutrient Needs of an Athlete

What should an athlete eat to ensure that his or her muscles are supplied with the energy needed to perform? What foods will improve his or her performance? Should some foods be avoided before and during athletic participation?

The typical athlete burns many calories through exercise. The number of calories athletes use is determined by their body weight and the types of activities they are doing. The length of the exercise period also affects the number of calories used. People who weigh more, burn more calories during a given activity. More calories are burned because more energy is required to move a greater body mass. More vigorous activities require more energy than less active sports. For instance, running requires more energy than jogging, **16-3**. The longer the workout lasts, the more calories are burned.

Math Link

Calculating Calories Burned

Use the chart shown in Figure 16-3 to calculate the approximate number of calories burned if a 175-pound athlete played racquetball for 1½ hours.

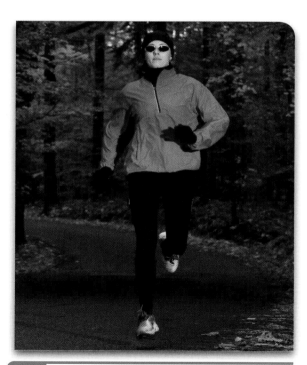

16-2 Marathon runners, who compete in 26-mile races, must train intensively. This improves their muscles' use of glucose and tolerance of lactic acid.

How Many Calories Do Athletes Burn?					
Activity	Calories Burned per Minute				
	100 lb. (45 kg)	125 lb. (57 kg)	150 lb. (68 kg)	175 lb. (80 kg)	200 lb. (91 kg)
Aerobic dance	6.0	7.6	9.1	10.6	12.1
Baseball	3.1	4.0	4.7	5.5	6.3
Basketball, recreational	4.9	6.2	7.5	8.7	10.0
Bicycling, 10 mph	4.2	5.3	6.4	7.4	8.5
Canoeing, 4 mph	4.4	5.5	6.7	7.8	8.9
Dancing, active	4.5	5.6	6.8	7.9	9.1
Football, vigorous touch	5.5	6.9	8.3	9.7	11.1
Golf, carrying clubs	3.6	4.6	5.4	6.4	7.3
Hockey	6.6	8.3	10.0	11.7	13.4
Horseback riding	2.7	3.4	4.1	4.8	5.4
Ice skating	4.2	5.2	6.4	7.4	8.5
Jogging, 5.5 mph	6.7	8.4	10.0	11.7	13.4
Racquetball	6.5	8.1	9.8	11.4	13.0
Roller skating	4.2	5.3	6.4	7.4	8.5
Running, 8 mph	9.7	12.1	14.6	17.1	19.5
Skiing, cross-country, 4 mph	6.5	8.2	9.9	11.5	13.2
Skiing, downhill	6.5	8.2	9.9	11.5	13.2
Soccer	5.9	7.5	9.0	10.5	12.0
Swimming, crawl, 35 yd./min.	4.8	6.1	7.3	8.5	9.7
Table tennis	3.4	4.3	5.2	6.1	7.0
Tennis, recreational singles	5.0	6.2	7.5	8.8	10.0
Volleyball, recreational	2.9	3.6	4.4	5.1	5.9
Walking, 4 mph	4.2	5.3	6.4	7.4	8.5
Wrestling	8.5	10.6	12.8	14.9	17.1

Note: The energy costs in calories will vary. Values are approximate. Factors that influence calorie needs include wind resistance, ground levels, weight of clothes, and other conditions.

16-3 Locate the column closest to your weight for an activity you enjoy. Multiply the calories burned per minute by the number of minutes spent in the activity to figure total energy expenditure.

An athlete who burns more calories through exercise than he or she takes in through food will lose weight. An athlete is more physically active than a nonathlete and, as a result, uses more daily calories. Therefore, the athlete needs to consume more calories to maintain a healthy body weight.

The *Dietary Guidelines* recommend 45 to 65 percent of calories should come from carbohydrates. Competitive athletes should aim for 60 to 65 percent because carbohydrates are the major fuel source for energy. Between 20 and 25 percent of calories from unsaturated fats is recommended. The remaining 10 to 15 percent of the calories athletes consume should come from protein. Athletes have a greater need for more calories when training is intense and long. Most athletes can meet their energy needs by eating extra calories from a wide selection of nutritious foods.

Athletes may need slightly more protein than nonathletes to build and maintain muscle tissue. Athletes also use some protein to meet energy needs. Protein-rich foods provide the amino acids you need to build and repair tissue. Most diets adequately meet the protein needs of athletes. Athletes can usually meet their protein needs without making major diet modifications.

Many foods provide protein. A slice of bread and ½ cup (125 mL) of cooked vegetables each provide about 2 grams of protein. A cup (250 mL) of milk provides 8 grams. A 3-ounce (84 g) cooked portion of meat or poultry provides about 26 grams of protein.

Teen females who follow the MyPlate system consume about 91 grams of protein per day. Teen males who follow MyPlate consume about 116 grams of protein daily. These amounts of protein are more than enough even for teen athletes.

Wellness Tip

Balance Your Protein

Because protein is important to building and repairing muscle, maintaining a good balance is important. Americans tend to eat enough protein; however, they often eat it only once or twice per day. For optimal performance, try balancing your protein throughout the day. Evenly divide your protein foods between breakfast, lunch, dinner, and snacks.

Protein supplements are not necessary. In fact, they may interfere with peak performance. If you fill your stomach on protein calories, you may not be getting enough carbohydrates to produce energy for your muscles. Also, excess protein causes a person to urinate more often, which could contribute to dehydration. The greatest amount of muscle growth occurs when protein intake is about 15 percent of daily food intake.

Carbohydrate loading is a technique used to trick the muscles into storing more glycogen for extra energy. Its use was intended to improve the performance only of endurance athletes. Carbohydrate loading involves eating a diet moderate in carbohydrates for a few days. Then during the three days before a sports event, an athlete consumes a high-carbohydrate diet. The increase in carbohydrates is coupled with a decrease in training intensity.

Some problems have occurred for athletes practicing carbohydrate loading. These problems have included water retention, digestion distress, muscle stiffness, and sluggishness. Athletes with chronic diseases such as diabetes are especially likely to have problems.

Case Study: Plan for Peak Performance

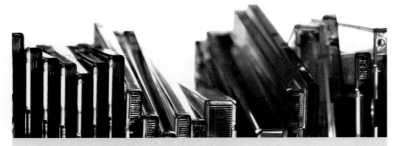

Nick is an aspiring athlete. He is 15 years old and wants to become a professional hockey player. He practices on the ice for hours several times a week. He was recently recruited by a league in his home town. After his first practice with the team, Nick decides he needs to make some changes. During practice, Nick found that he became winded much sooner than his teammates and was often lagging behind on sprint plays. He also felt that he was being outmuscled. Nick decides he needs a plan to improve his performance on the ice.

The first part of Nick's plan involves building strength. His goal is to increase the size of his muscles. Nick decides the best way to build muscle mass is to increase the amount of protein in his diet. He has heard guys talking about protein powder so he buys some. He begins drinking protein shakes and eating three eggs per day. He also increases the serving size of protein foods at his normal meals. Nick finds that he is often too full to eat the bread, potatoes, or rice from his meal.

The other part of Nick's plan is to begin running. He sets his alarm an hour earlier than usual and runs two miles before school most mornings.

After following his plan for four weeks, Nick is a little disappointed with the results. He has not noticed much change in his muscle size. Although he doesn't seem to get winded as quickly, he still seems to be lagging behind on the fast plays. In addition, Nick is disappointed because, despite his plans to improve his performance, he feels less energetic most of the time.

Case Review

1. Are you surprised by the outcomes Nick is experiencing with his plan? Why?

2. What would you do differently if you were Nick?

For most athletes, attempts to increase glycogen stores are not needed. If you are in a daily vigorous exercise program, eat a carbohydrate-rich diet. Include a rest day in your schedule now and then, too. Such rest days will help build up the glycogen stores you need.

Athletes need to plan their diets around a variety of foods rich in vitamins and minerals. These nutrients are important for the conversion of carbohydrates, fats, and protein to energy. They promote growth and aid in nerve and muscle function. Minerals such as calcium help maintain strong bones. Athletes can boost calcium intake by choosing dairy products such as low-fat milk, yogurt, and cheese. Protein, vitamins, and other minerals are also supplied by dairy products.

Vitamin and mineral supplements are an added expense and usually not necessary. However, some athletes may need a supplement. For example, a vegetarian athlete who avoids all dairy foods, fortified soy milk, and dark leafy vegetables would need a calcium supplement. When a supplement is advised, athletes do not benefit from those that provide more than 100 percent of the RDAs or AIs. A multiple vitamin and mineral formula will meet most athletes' needs.

Some athletes need more energy than they can comfortably consume through food. These athletes may find it helpful to consume energy in concentrated forms, such as dried fruits. Drinking high-energy liquids, such as yogurt shakes, may also be easier than eating solid foods, **16-4**. Supplements and special "power" foods are generally not needed and have not been shown to improve performance.

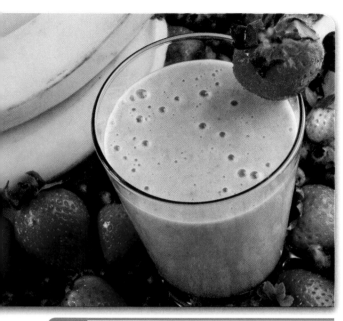

16-4 A high-energy fruit shake can provide an athlete with needed calories in a form that is easy to consume.

Nutrient Needs of Women Athletes

A healthy diet is important to all athletes. However, women athletes have nutritional needs that are uniquely affected by their gender. The most common nutritional issues for women athletes relate to bone health, iron deficiency, amenorrhea (absence of menstrual periods), and eating disorders.

Women's bone health deteriorates when too little calcium is in the diet. When girls and women restrict their calorie intake to maintain weight for athletics, a healthy diet is often not achieved. Eating too few foods high in calcium and foods fortified with calcium can result in deficiency. Teen girls need 1300 milligrams of calcium per day for calcium retention and bone mineral density. The health consequences of too little calcium can be poor formation of bone structure, athletic stress fractures during exercise, and osteoporosis in later life.

Many women do not get enough iron in their diet. Women with heavy menstrual cycles have increased loss of iron. When blood is lost, iron is lost and anemia can result. Symptoms of iron deficiency for athletes include fatigue and breathlessness. Anemia reduces athletic performance. If performance declines and cannot be explained in other ways, such as too much stress or lack of sleep, then iron-deficient anemia should be considered. Iron-rich foods, such as meat, fish, and poultry, help athletes meet their iron needs. Iron is also available in grains, peas, lentils, nuts, dark-green leafy vegetables, and nuts. A supplement may be recommended to improve blood levels and performance.

Women who practice intensive exercise for long periods of time may experience disorders with their menstrual cycles. Young athletes may experience delay in the onset of menstruation beyond the normal ages of 11 to 15 years. Low weight and body fat are related to the menstrual cycle abnormalities. Women gymnasts who have very low amounts of body fat and weight have delayed *menarche*, a term used to describe when menstrual cycles begin. *Amenorrhea*, or loss of a menstrual cycle, has negative consequences. Production of important hormones involved in the development of strong bones is reduced. With amenorrhea, bone density can become extremely low. Tendon injuries and stress fractures become an increased risk.

Female athletes may feel pressured to maintain a low weight for their height and age. With such emphasis on body weight, eating disorders can emerge. Maintaining low weight for particular sports, such as figure skating, long distance running, and cheerleading, creates health-related issues for females, **16-5**. Effective

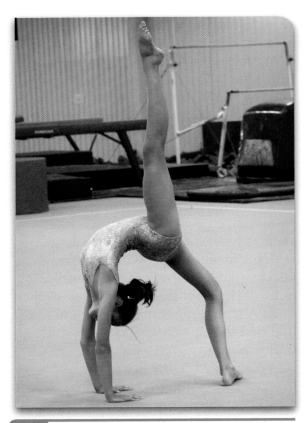

16-5 Although weight goals may be stressed in a sport such as gymnastics, female athletes should maintain 18 to 24 percent body fat.

coaches put less pressure on women to be thin. They give more encouragement for balanced eating. This helps avoid problems that interfere with a female's normal physical development.

Planning Meals for the Athlete in Training

Sports nutritionists will tell you that healthy eating provides athletes (and nonathletes) with the foundation for peak performance. Meeting the athlete's energy needs through caloric intake and getting the necessary fluid replacements is critical for athletes. Performance is at stake.

Maintenance Eating Patterns

Choosing to eat meals and snacks on a regular basis throughout the day keeps your body fueled for activity. Hydrating before, during, and after exercise is necessary to keep performance levels high. If you skip a meal and become too hungry, you may end up making poor food choices. Staying fueled throughout the day with nutritious foods and adequate fluids helps you follow an eating plan that supports your exercise activities. Keep in mind that healthy eating is essential for optimal performance.

Plan to eat breakfast to avoid an energy crash later in the morning. Skipping breakfast can reduce your energy levels for your workouts. Some people report feeling drained in energy for the rest of the day.

Practice selecting nutritious snacks between meals. Snacks can make up 20 to 50 percent of your day's calories. These additional small meals add nutritional benefits and boost your energy. Be sure to plan snacks that add valuable nutrients and needed energy rather than nutrient-poor calories. Choose foods such as fruits, whole-grain bagels, popcorn, low-fat cheese, nuts, or vegetables.

Good nutrition is critical to top level performance. Special sports nutrition products and supplements do not provide the same level of nutritional benefits that a healthy, well-planned meal pattern can supply.

Meal Management for Athletic Events

Meal and snack management for athletes is all about how food intake affects digestion and use of energy for top performance.

Pre-Athletic Activity Meals

The goals of the pregame meal should be to provide appropriate amounts of energy and fluid. The meal should also help the athlete avoid feelings of fullness and digestive disturbances.

Very large meals before competition should be avoided. They require too much energy to digest. This does not mean you should go hungry. Hunger makes you feel tired and sluggish. For most sports events, the best diet plan includes a high-carbohydrate meal within 3 to 4 hours before competition. Avoid the high-protein, high-fat steak dinners that were once training table standards.

Carbohydrates have been found to have positive effects on performance. However, very sweet carbohydrates such as syrups and candy bars can cause water to pool in the gastrointestinal tract. Discomfort and diarrhea may result.

Athletes should avoid bulky and fatty foods on the day of competition. High-fiber foods such as whole-grain breads and large portions of fresh fruits and vegetables should be limited. Also, avoid French fries, bacon, sausage, and other foods high in fat. Instead, choose foods such as bread, rice cakes, potatoes, juices, or other high-carbohydrate, low-fat foods, **16-6**.

Foods you have never eaten before are not recommended at pregame time. You cannot be sure how they will make you feel.

For some athletes, mental attitude can be just as important as the foods eaten. Suppose an athlete always eats

Pregame Meals		
Foods	**Calories**	**Carbohydrate (grams)**
Pregame Breakfast		
Orange juice	112	27
Cornflakes with milk	152	30
Banana	104	27
Toast with jelly	103	22
Hard-cooked egg	78	1
Total	549	107 (78% of calories)
Pregame Lunch		
Pasta with meatless sauce	404	73
Roll	85	14
Applesauce	52	14
Fat-free milk	86	12
Total	627	113 (72% of calories)
Pregame Snack Ideas		
Bagel or crackers	Yogurt	Pretzels
Apples or bananas	Dried fruit	Low-fat granola
Popcorn	Pudding	

16-6 A pregame meal, eaten 3 to 4 hours before a competition, should be rich in carbohydrates and moderate in calories.

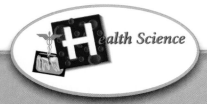

Athletic Trainer

Athletic trainers specialize in the prevention, diagnosis, assessment, treatment, and rehabilitation of muscle and bone injuries and illnesses. As one of the first health-care providers on the scene when injuries occur, they must be able to recognize, evaluate, and assess injuries and provide immediate care when needed.

Athletic trainers try to prevent injuries by teaching people how to reduce their risk for injuries. They also advise people on proper equipment use, exercises to improve balance and strength, and home exercises and therapy programs.

Applying protective or injury-preventive devices—such as tape, bandages, and braces—is another responsibility. Athletic trainers may work under the direction of a licensed physician or other health-care provider. They may discuss specific injuries and treatment options with a physician or perform evaluations and treatments as directed by a physician.

Education: A bachelor's degree is required for most jobs as an athletic trainer. Program education occurs both in the classroom and in clinical settings. Courses may include human anatomy, kinesiology, physiology, nutrition, and biomechanics. For college and university positions, athletic trainers may need a master's or higher degree to be eligible. Because some high school positions involve teaching along with athletic-trainer duties, a teaching certificate or license could be required.

Job Outlook: Employment is projected to grow much faster than average. Job prospects should be good in the health-care industry and in high schools, but expect competition for positions with professional and college sports teams. Employment is expected to grow for athletic trainers because of their role in preventing injuries and reducing health-care costs.

pizza before a competition. For this athlete, it may be psychologically important to eat pizza to be ready to win. Follow the pattern that works best for you.

Snacks Before an Athletic Event

Snacks before exercise and pregame meals are planned to provide appropriate amounts of energy and fluid. Snacks are necessary to maintain energy. If your exercise takes place after school or work, you may not have the time for a meal before you are scheduled to perform. If there is a pregame meal, avoid overeating to avoid feelings of fullness and digestive disturbances. Frequent smaller meals are better before performance events. Snacking on foods before you exercise can help to boost your energy levels.

Most athletes can tolerate a carbohydrate snack, such as a banana, an hour before physical exercise. The energy from the snack will be useful during the activity. However, if the activity is very intense, such as a time trial for a track event, you may be more comfortable competing with an empty stomach. Each athlete must learn what works best for his or her body in a given situation.

Eating During an Athletic Event

Eating small amounts of food during a long sports event can improve performance. A sports event that lasts two hours or more is considered long. For example, athletes like to eat small amounts of peanut butter crackers, fig bars, peanut butter and jelly sandwiches, or date snacks during triathlon events. Generally, the goal is to consume about 30 to 100 grams of carbohydrates per hour providing about 120 to 400 calories. Each athlete must learn what foods his or her body can tolerate without digestive disturbances. Any digestive discomfort will interfere with performance. Athletes can determine the energy source that works best for them by trying different foods during trial events. Foods in liquid form, such as food gels, high-nutrient shakes, and other energy drinks, may be easier to digest.

Fluid replacement is essential for avoiding dehydration and impaired performance, **16-7**. Some nutritionists recommend increasing salty foods in the diet for several days before an event. This depends on how much salt you tend to lose in sweat. Sports drinks are useful for long races such as marathons and triathlons. These drinks provide water, carbohydrates, and sodium.

Post-Athletic Event Nutrition

Recovery is the phase after exercise when glycogen stores are replenished

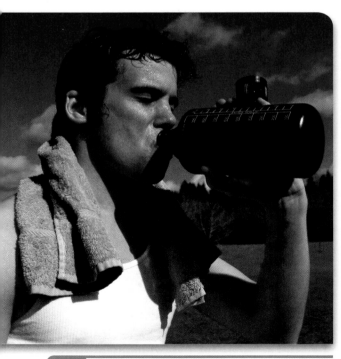

16-7 Athletes should maintain hydration for optimal performance.

to pre-exercise levels. Intense exercise takes a toll on your body. Training and competition cause physical and emotional stress to your body. Glycogen stores are depleted. Essential vitamins and minerals may be low or depleted. Recovery and relaxation are important goals. Following an event, you will recover faster if you consume both carbohydrates and protein. Eating within 30 minutes after an activity provides the best opportunity for replenishing muscle glycogen, body water, and electrolytes. Whole foods and water can supply essential nutrients. The most important nutrients to include in recovery nutrition are

- water
- a carbohydrate with a high glycemic index that enters the bloodstream quickly
- a source of high-quality protein
- sodium

Recovery drinks may be helpful if your body does not tolerate solid foods after an event. If you prefer recovery drinks, be sure to read the ingredients list. In some cases, nutrients are added that are not useful for recovery.

After two hours, have a meal of mixed carbohydrates, fats, and protein. Hydration continues to be important. Light, straw-colored urine is an indication that your fluid intake is adequate. Plan for adequate sleep to help your body fully recover.

Once the training season ends, you need to reduce calorie intake. If you continue with the snacks and extra foods you consumed to maintain weight during training, you will begin to gain weight. Balancing energy output with energy input may require adjusting your eating pattern.

Eating Away from Home

Athletes often travel to participate in sporting events. Sometimes the activity may require that you travel hours or even days at a time. Meal schedules may be irregular. Athletes may be tempted to skip meals. Drinking enough water may be difficult if water is not carried by the athlete. Good food sources of carbohydrate may be harder to find. Fast-food restaurant menus feature many high-fat, high-protein foods. These foods are often low in carbohydrates, calcium, and vitamins A and C. When carbohydrates are inadequate, glycogen stores become depleted. Without enough water, dehydration may occur before an event begins. The effect is reduced energy levels and performance.

The traveling athlete can improve performance by planning to include carbohydrates in the meals before an event. Choose restaurants that serve carbohydrate-rich foods such as pasta, burritos, baked potatoes, fruits, vegetables, and low-fat milk, **16-8**. These foods are common, inexpensive, and easily prepared by restaurants. The following tips will help you select nutrient-dense meals at restaurants:

- Choose grilled sandwiches, hamburger or cheeseburger, or turkey subs on a whole-wheat bun. Avoid high-fat condiments such as mayonnaise.
- Resist the temptation to order double burgers, large fries, and super-sized sodas.
- Limit high-fat salads and dressings, such as potato salad, marinated pasta, and vegetable salads when eating at salad bars. Go easy on high-fat toppings such as cheese and bacon.
- Request gravies, sauces, and salad dressings served on the side.
- Order pasta with tomato-based sauces and avoid cream or butter sauces.
- Choose salsa instead of sour cream or guacamole.
- Order stir-fried and steamed vegetables with rice or vegetarian pizzas with whole-wheat crusts.
- Avoid such deep-fried foods as fried fish, egg rolls, fried tortillas, and potato chips.
- Look for menu items that are steamed, boiled, broiled, roasted, or poached.

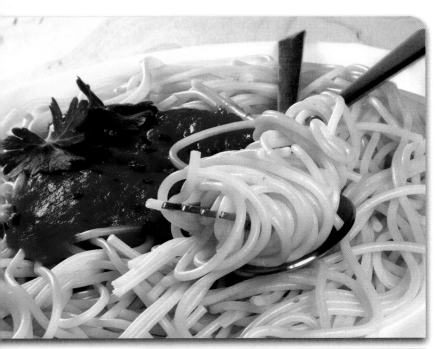

16-8 Many restaurants offer carbohydrate-rich spaghetti on the menu.

The Athlete's Need for Fluids

Drinking enough fluids may be the most critical aspect of sports nutrition. If fluid levels drop too low, dehydration results. Symptoms of dehydration include headache, dizziness, nausea, dry skin, shivering, and confusion. Dehydration also causes increases in body temperature and heart rate. Clearly, dehydration can impair performance.

Performing athletes may not feel thirsty because exercise masks the sense of thirst. Sweating during moderate exercise causes you to lose about 1 quart (1 L) of water per hour. If the workout is vigorous, a loss of 2 to 3 quarts (2 to 3 L) of water per hour may result. Therefore, athletes need to drink regardless of whether they feel thirsty.

Athletes can lose four to six pounds of water weight during a sports event. To determine how much water you lose, weigh yourself before and after an event, **16-9**. If you lose more than 3 percent of your body weight, your performance will deteriorate. For example, a 150-pound (67.5 kg) person should not lose more than 4½ pounds (2 kg) during an athletic activity.

To avoid dehydration, athletes should drink water before, during, and after an event. Specific fluid hydrations and replacement recommendations are dependent on an athlete's size, intensity of the physical activity, and temperature of the environment. All athletes need to be aware of fluid replacement guidelines. The National Athletic Trainers' Association (NATA) recommends the following guidelines for training and competition for athletes:

- 2–3 hours before event, consume 17–20 ounces (500–600 mL) fluid
- 10–20 minutes before event, consume 7–10 ounces (200–300 mL) fluid
- every 10–20 minutes during event, consume 7–10 ounces (200–300 mL) fluid
- within 2 hours following event, consume 20–24 ounces (600–700 mL) fluid for every one pound lost through sweat

Athletes lose water during exercise even when the air temperature is comfortable. Water losses are greater when exercising in hot, humid weather. This makes heat cramps and

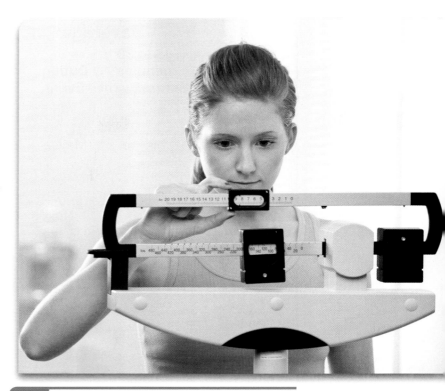

16-9 Weigh yourself before and after an activity to determine the amount of water loss.

heat exhaustion more likely. When exercising in these conditions, watching fluid replacement is even more critical.

Water is the preferred liquid for fluid replacement during a sporting event, **16-10**. Cool water (50°F–59°F) helps lower body temperature and water empties from the stomach more quickly than any other fluid. The carbohydrates in some sweetened drinks can pull water from the body into the digestive tract causing cramps. The carbohydrates in most sports drinks are designed to be easily absorbed to prevent such cramping. Even so, if you choose a sports drink, you may want to dilute it with water or ice. Caffeine may increase body water loss. Alcohol is a depressant, has a diuretic effect, and is unhealthy for recovery. They should be avoided during physical activity.

Athletes also lose sodium when they sweat. Most athletes get enough

Beverage Choices for Athletes				
Beverage	15 to 30 minutes Before Event	During Event	After Event	Reason
Water (cool)	Yes	Yes	Yes	Best fluid for your system; regulates body temperature
Special sports drinks	Maybe	Maybe	Yes	Depends on content; may be high in sugar, which slows fluids in emptying from the stomach; salt content may be too high
Carbonated soft drinks	No	No	No	Carbonation may cause problems during an event and sugar may prevent fluids from quickly emptying the stomach
Fruit juices	No	No	No	Sugar content is high; does not promote complete rehydration
Coffee/tea	No	No	No	Caffeine pulls water from the body through increased urination; makes the heart work harder
Fat-free milk	No	No	Yes	Too difficult to digest for fluid use
Alcohol	No	No	No	Undesirable, does not help performance, dehydrates cells and decreases muscle efficiency

16-10   What is the best drink before, during, and after an athletic event?

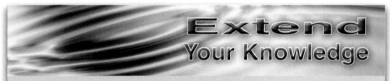

A Better Sports Drink?

Select two sports drinks and compare their ingredient lists and nutrition facts panels. Calculate the cost per 8-ounce serving of each product. Summarize the differences and special advertised benefits of the two different drinks. Visit the manufacturers' Web sites for each drink. What claims do they make about the effects of their products on athletic performance? Summarize your findings in a brief report comparing the ingredients and benefits of each of the two products.

sodium from the foods they eat. However, endurance athletes who compete in events lasting four or more hours may lose excessive amounts of water and sodium. These athletes may benefit from a sports drink that contains sodium, chloride, and potassium. Salting food a bit more liberally will also help them meet sodium needs.

Salt tablets are not recommended to replace sodium lost during physical activity. They worsen dehydration and impair performance. They can also irritate the stomach and may cause severe vomiting. This is especially true when fluid intake is not adequate.

Weight Concerns of Athletes

Achieving optimum weight can positively affect your athletic performance. What is optimum weight? The answer depends on your percentage of body fat, or your body composition.

Knowing your percentage of body fat suggests whether you need to lose extra fat and/or build more muscle mass. Too much body fat increases energy needs. Energy needed for performance ends up being used to move excess body weight. Too little body fat makes you lose body heat too fast. Energy needed for competition ends up being used to maintain body warmth.

Lean body mass is especially valued by some athletes, such as gymnasts, distance runners, and body builders. For other athletes, such as discus throwers and baseball players, body composition may not matter as much, **16-11**. Most male athletes do well with 10 to 15 percent body fat. An acceptable level for most female athletes is 18 to 24 percent body fat. Most females stop menstruating when body fat drops below 17 percent.

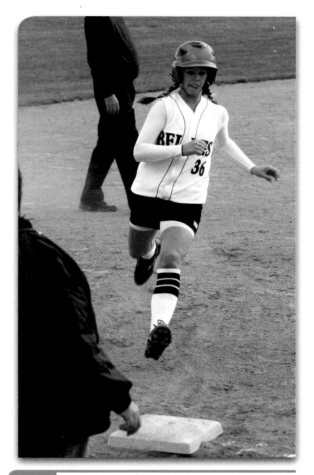

16-11 Body composition is not a critical factor for softball players.

Losing Weight for Competition

Athletes in some sports, such as wrestling, boxing, and weight lifting, compete in specific weight classes. Some of these athletes use harmful methods to try to reduce their body weight quickly to compete in lower weight classes. They may try to skip meals or refuse to drink fluids one or two days before competition. Some use laxatives, diuretics, and emetics (substances that induce vomiting) to rid their bodies of food and fluids.

Such practices can weaken an athlete's endurance.

Crash dieting can also harm an athlete's health. Severely restricting calorie intake while vigorously training can interfere with normal growth. The body will use energy to fuel activity rather than to support growth.

The best time to diet is before the official training season begins. Athletes need to weigh themselves well before the start of their sports season. Then they will have ample time to reduce body fat and reach weight goals in a healthy manner before they begin competing.

Gradual weight loss is the best way to reduce pounds. Athletes need to set realistic goals for weight loss at a maximum of two pounds per week. Athletes who lose weight faster than this are probably losing more than fat. They will be losing body fluids and muscle mass, too.

To lose one pound of body fat, an athlete needs to consume 3,500 fewer calories than he or she expends. However, the athlete needs an adequate supply of nutrients to maintain strength and stamina while trying to lose weight. Most teen male athletes need at least 3,000 calories per day. Teen female athletes need a minimum of 2,200 calories daily. These amounts need to come from nutritious foods that provide the full range of vitamins and minerals. Eating more complex carbohydrates while reducing fats in the diet can help athletes limit calorie intake. Increasing energy expenditure by moderately extending workouts will help athletes gradually reach their weight goals.

Athletes who are trying to lose weight should work with a registered dietitian. (Many coaches do not have adequate nutrition training to supervise an athlete's weight loss.) A dietitian can make sure athletes are meeting their daily calorie and nutrient needs for growth and training.

Gaining Weight for Competition

Some athletes, such as football and hockey players, want to gain weight or "bulk up." Their goal is to gain size as well as strength. A large body mass will make them seem more formidable to their opponents, **16-12**.

For many athletes, gaining weight is difficult because they burn so many calories through long, hard workout

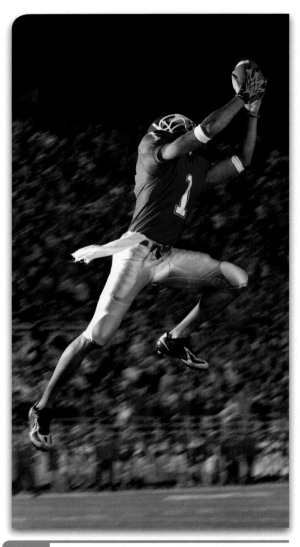

16-12 Football players require strength, power, and body mass to be effective in their sport.

sessions. Experts recommend athletes choose nutritious foods to add an extra 2,500 calories to their weekly intake. Some athletes may need to consume 5,000 or more calories per day to meet this recommendation.

High-fiber foods such as salads and whole-grain breads and cereals are not emphasized in a weight-gain plan. These foods will cause an athlete to feel full too quickly. Athletes should include moderate amounts of monounsaturated and polyunsaturated oils because they are calorie dense. However, they should avoid saturated fats because of their link to heart disease.

Athletes who are trying to gain weight may wish to reduce the length and intensity of their regular workout sessions. They may also want to increase their rest and sleep time. These efforts will decrease the number of calories athletes burn for energy. However, an athlete's weight-gain program must include exercise, particularly weight training. An athlete's weight-gain goal is to add muscle, not fat. Muscle size cannot be increased by consuming more calories. Weight gain without training will be fat gain, not muscle gain.

Athletes who consume coffee, tea, and colas should decrease their use of these products when trying to gain weight. The caffeine in these products tends to increase metabolic rates. Reducing caffeine consumption will help athletes burn fewer calories.

Modifying eating and exercise patterns will help athletes gain about 1 to 2 pounds (0.5 to 1 kg) per week. Athletes trying to gain weight should work with a registered dietitian.

Harmful Performance Aids

Perhaps you have wished there were a special drink or pill that would make you stronger or faster. If only you could find some magic key to success, you would be sure to win—right?

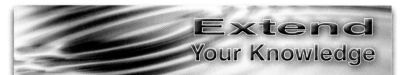

Extend Your Knowledge

Wrestling with Safety

Contact a national association for youth sports, such as the National Federation of State High School Associations (NFHS) or the National Alliance for Youth Sports (NAYS). List the rules and regulations for wrestler's hydration level requirements and body fat percentage. Find out the association's official position on weight requirements for competition among adolescent athletes.

Unfortunately, there is no special food, drink, or pill that will safely make an athlete stronger or faster. Likewise, no safe methods exist to add muscle weight quickly. Schemes promoted to build muscle mass fast are often frauds. Some can negatively affect performance and health. They can even interfere with normal growth and development. The health effects of drugs and other substances can produce a range of symptoms. Mild symptoms include headache and nausea. Severe symptoms include liver disease, stroke, and death, **16-13**.

New "performance enhancers" appear on the shelves of health food stores every day. The sales pitches are creative, and the claims often sound miraculous. However, as a careful consumer and serious competitor, you must evaluate claims carefully. Keep in mind that if a claim sounds too good to be true, it probably is. A planned program of supervised training and nutritious eating is the safest, most effective key to peak performance.

Harmful Effects of Performance Aids

Performance Aid	Reasons Used	Harmful Effects
Anabolic steroids	A male sex hormone used to build strength and add muscle mass	Liver disorders, kidney disease, growth disorders, decreased level of HDLs (good cholesterol) and increased level of LDLs (bad cholesterol), high blood pressure, sexual problems, reproductive disorders (men-affects the production and functions of testosterone; women-growth of facial hair, baldness, menstrual irregularities, aggressiveness), unusual weight gain or loss, rashes or hives
Bee pollen	Used to improve overall athletic performance	Has no proven beneficial effects on performance, serious harm to those with certain kinds of allergies
Caffeine	A stimulant to the central nervous system used to increase endurance during strenuous exercise	May increase fluid losses; increases heart rate; can cause headaches, insomnia, and nervous irritability
Carnitine	An amino acid supplement used to strengthen endurance	Can cause muscle cramps, muscle weakness, and loss of iron-containing muscle protein
Human growth hormones	Used to build muscle and shorten recovery time	Thickening of bones, overgrowth of soft body tissues, possibility of grotesque body features
Pangamic acid (sometimes called vitamin B_{15})	Used to improve efficient use of oxygen in aerobic exercises	Ruled illegal by the Food and Drug Administration, unsafe for humans
Bicarbonate of soda or soft drinks (soda loading)	Used to avoid muscle fatigue	A form of doping, no confirmed benefits for game performance
Vitamin supplements	Used to feel better and provide a competitive edge	False promises, promotes "pill popping," costs more than food sources, individual becomes less concerned about eating a nutritious diet

16-13 These performance aids may appear to be quick fixes, but they may actually be harmful to your health.

Reading Summary

Carbohydrates and fats are the main sources of energy for the body. The body uses both anaerobic and aerobic production systems to convert the nutrients into energy the muscles can use. In the absence of sufficient oxygen, the body's acid-base balance is changed. As a result, you experience a burning sensation and fatigue in the muscles.

Athletes have greater needs for energy and some nutrients than nonathletes. However, they can usually meet their calorie and nutrient needs through diet.

Athletes have high-energy needs to fuel their activity in training and competition. Most of this energy should come from carbohydrates in the diet. The diet should also provide moderate amounts of protein and fat. Athletes need vitamins and minerals to help metabolize the energy nutrients. Athletes need plenty of fluids before, during, and after sports events to avoid dehydration. Water is the preferred body fluid during vigorous exercise. Eating a high-carbohydrate diet a few days before an endurance event increases glycogen stores in the muscles. Athletes should avoid foods high in fat and fiber at pregame meals.

Reducing excess body fat and increasing lean body mass improves performance in many sports. However, weight adjustments should be gradual. They should occur before the start of an athlete's training season. Body fat should stay within recommended limits.

Review Learning

1. Why does the body not use fat for energy during anaerobic activity?
2. True or false. Endurance athletes train to improve their anaerobic energy production systems.
3. What are three factors that affect the number of calories an athlete burns through activity?
4. Why are protein supplements not recommended for building muscle tissue and fueling activity?
5. Describe the type of athletic activity that is most likely to benefit from carbohydrate loading.
6. Explain two tips for planning a pregame meal for an athlete.
7. List nutrients that are important to recovery after an athletic event.
8. How much liquid should an athlete consume after an event to replace fluid losses from the body?
9. What percentage of an athlete's body should be fat?
10. Why is exercise an important part of a weight-gain program for an athlete?
11. Why should athletes who are trying to lose or gain weight for competition consult with a registered dietitian?

Critical Thinking

12. **Analyze decisions.** Presume you have decided to train for a triathlon that involves running, biking, and swimming. What decisions do you need to make regarding your meals for training and competition?

13. **Identify evidence.** After a week of practice with the new lacrosse team at your school, you have discovered this new sport takes a lot of endurance and upper-body strength. You want to build muscle strength quickly and a friend suggests a new "performance enhancing" supplement he found at the health food store. What evidence would you look for to determine whether this is a safe supplement? Why is healthful eating and an effective exercise plan the best way to get your desired results?

Applying Your Knowledge

14. **Athlete interview.** Interview an athlete in your school about what foods he or she eats before a sports event. Learn the reasons behind the food choices. Write a brief comparison of the athlete's practices with the recommendations for pregame meals made in this chapter.

15. **Menu evaluation.** Obtain menus from two restaurants you are likely to eat at when participating in an event away from home. Use the guidelines in this chapter to select foods that would benefit your athletic performance. Circle or highlight your menu choices.

16. **Create a sports drink.** Prepare your own sports drink using ingredients you have at home. Find a formula using a sports nutrition resource or on the Internet. List the function of each of the ingredients for athletic recovery.

17. **Runner interview.** Interview a distance runner living in your community. Learn the training methods and nutrition practices he or she uses to prepare for events. What are his or her trusted resources for training and nutrition information?

Technology Connections

18. **Electronic presentation.** Use presentation software to prepare a lesson discussing the relationship between a nutritious diet and athletic performance. Ask the coach of one of your school's athletic teams and a nutrition instructor or foodservice director to provide feedback. Then share the presentation with a group of younger athletes.

19. **Internet research.** Research and create a list of reliable, accurate Web sites for sports nutrition information. Provide the list to your school's athletic director for inclusion in information packets for athletes and their parents.

20. **Digital lesson.** Prepare a five-minute classroom lesson using a digital projector to explain a specific topic discussed in this chapter. Share your mini lesson with the class.

Academic Connections

21. **Social studies.** Research public health concerns regarding the need for further federal regulation of energy drinks. Prepare a summary of your findings.

22. **History.** Learn about the dietary practices of Olympic athletes from past to present. Write a paper sharing your findings.

23. **Math.** Select five of your favorite sports or physical activities. Use resources from this chapter or online to determine how many calories per minute are burned during that activity. Calculate the total calories burned during 45 minutes of each activity (use the same reference weight for each calculation). Display your results using a bar graph.

Workplace Applications

Using Writing Skills

As a health writer for your local newspaper, it has come to your attention that there is high use of some performance aids among high school athletes at area high schools. Your current assignment is to write a full-page public service announcement that captures student attention and warns athletes about the harmful effects of these performance aids. In your research, be sure to identify certain performance aids students are using and the harm these aids do to the human body.

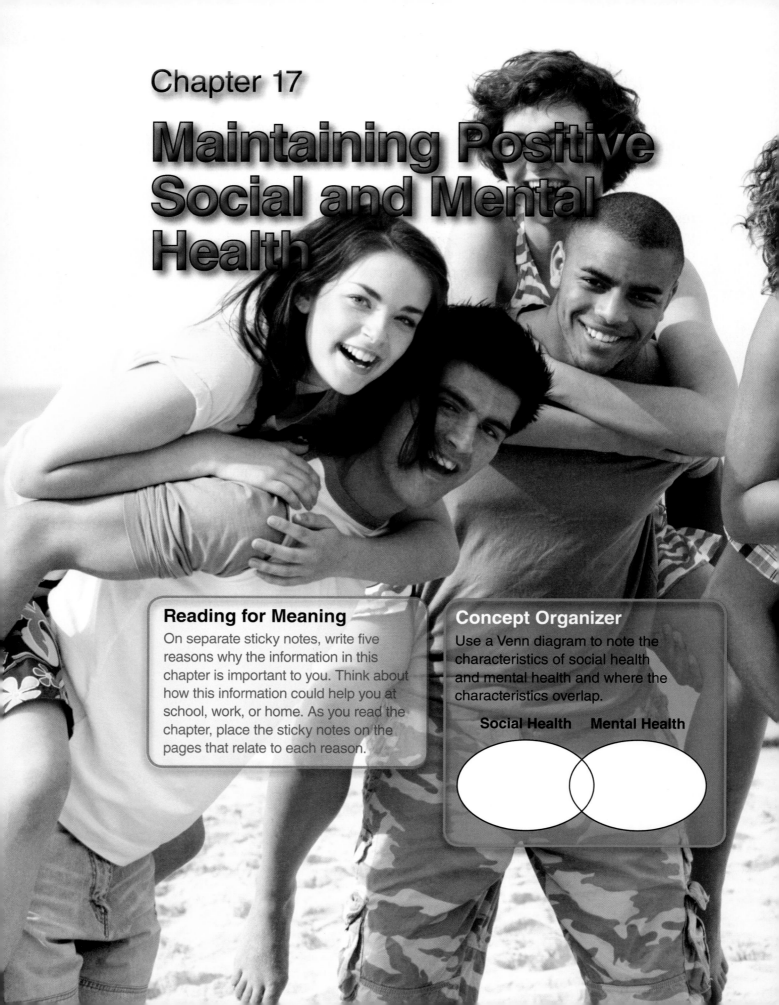

Chapter 17

Maintaining Positive Social and Mental Health

Reading for Meaning

On separate sticky notes, write five reasons why the information in this chapter is important to you. Think about how this information could help you at school, work, or home. As you read the chapter, place the sticky notes on the pages that relate to each reason.

Concept Organizer

Use a Venn diagram to note the characteristics of social health and mental health and where the characteristics overlap.

Social Health   **Mental Health**

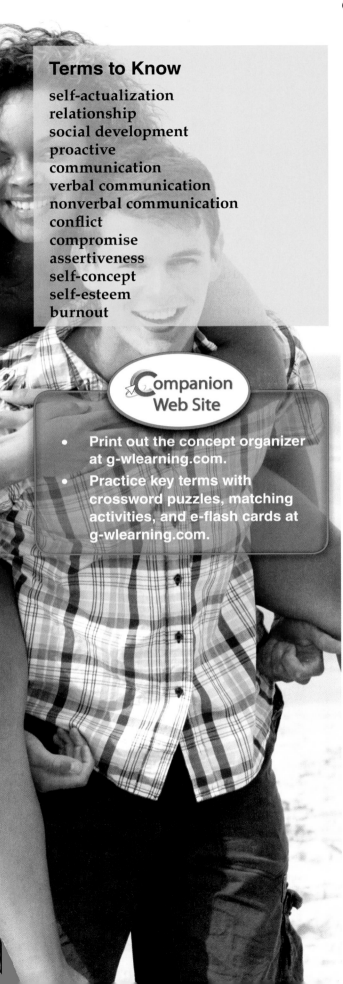

Terms to Know

self-actualization
relationship
social development
proactive
communication
verbal communication
nonverbal communication
conflict
compromise
assertiveness
self-concept
self-esteem
burnout

Companion Web Site

- **Print out the concept organizer at g-wlearning.com.**
- **Practice key terms with crossword puzzles, matching activities, and e-flash cards at g-wlearning.com.**

Objectives

After studying this chapter, you will be able to

- **determine** the order in which a person will typically strive to meet specific human needs.
- **recall** characteristics of a socially healthy person.
- **explain** techniques for promoting positive social health.
- **summarize** how self-concept is related to mental health.
- **identify** strategies for promoting positive mental health.
- **analyze** the relationships between nutrition, exercise, and physical and mental health.
- **create** a self-management plan to make a positive life change.
- **recognize** a situation that might require the help of a mental or social health care professional.

Central Ideas

- Positive social health and mental health is important to total wellness.
- Developing effective social skills and learning to maintain balance in life positively impact social and mental health.

Have you ever felt torn when you and your friends were on opposite sides of an issue? Has there been a time when you felt overwhelmed by more school assignments than you had time to complete? Have you skipped meals because your work and after-school practice schedule was too hectic for you to find time to eat? These situations often cause teens to lose sleep, and make poor food and exercise choices. They may even begin to feel physically ill. If this sounds familiar, you may not be surprised to learn your social and mental health can affect your physical health, **17-1**.

In this chapter, you will learn that your interactions with others and your mental state are important aspects of wellness. You will discover how communication skills can help you relate to others. You will also study strategies that will help you improve your social and mental health.

Basic Human Needs

As a human being, you have basic needs. The degree to which these needs are met affects your state of physical, social, and mental health. When your human needs are met, your potential for achieving a high level of wellness greatly improves.

Abraham Maslow, a psychologist, proposed a theory that human needs form a *hierarchy*, or a ranked series. He grouped needs into five basic levels. He believed people must meet their needs at the lowest level first, at least in part. Until they address these needs, people cannot focus on needs at the next level. Maslow's theory can be represented as a triangle, which has a base

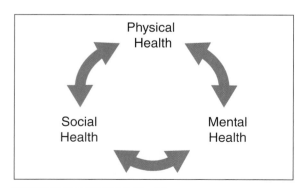

17-1 Physical, social, and mental health affect one another. When positive gains are made in one area, an individual often senses positive outcomes in the other two areas.

broader than the peak. This suggests needs shown at the base of the triangle provide a foundation for healthy growth and development, **17-2**.

Physical Needs

The first level of needs in Maslow's hierarchy is made up of physical needs that are basic to survival. These include needs for oxygen, water, food, shelter, clothing, and sleep. You are likely to have trouble thinking about much else until these needs are met to some degree. For instance, think about sitting in a football stadium when a terrible storm suddenly begins. Watching the game is likely to become less important than finding some way to meet your basic need for shelter.

Safety and security needs, which form the second level in the hierarchy, also affect physical health. You need to feel protected from physical harm. You also need to feel financially secure. When these needs are threatened or not met, your state of total health is jeopardized. For instance, safety needs are not being met if you are being driven by someone who has been drinking alcohol. Until you get out of this situation, your life is at risk.

Social Needs

If basic physical and security needs are adequately met, it will be possible to fulfill needs for love and acceptance. This third level of the hierarchy affects social health. These needs stem from a human desire to experience positive connections with people. All people need to know others care about them. Everyone needs to feel wanted as a member of a group. You may feel loved when a parent expresses concern about you. Perhaps you feel acceptance when a friend invites you to join in an activity.

Levels of Human Needs

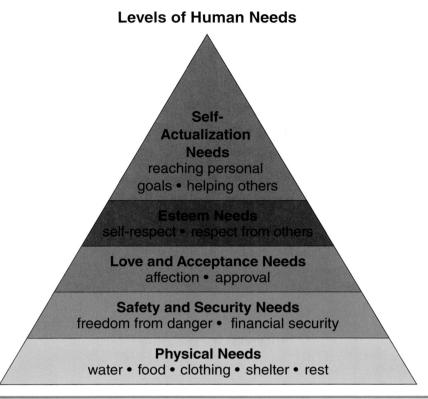

Self-Actualization Needs
reaching personal goals • helping others

Esteem Needs
self-respect • respect from others

Love and Acceptance Needs
affection • approval

Safety and Security Needs
freedom from danger • financial security

Physical Needs
water • food • clothing • shelter • rest

17-2 The needs at the base of Maslow's hierarchy must be at least partially met before addressing needs at the next level.

This group of needs also includes your need to be able to show love and acceptance for others. Loving others helps you feel good about yourself.

Another set of social needs falls at Maslow's fourth level in the hierarchy. This level includes needs for esteem. You need to feel others value you as a person. You must also value yourself. When others recognize your achievements or ask for your opinion, they are helping to address this need. When you congratulate yourself on a job well done, you are showing self-esteem.

Mental Needs

The peak of Maslow's hierarchy relates to mental needs. These are needs for people to believe they are doing their best to reach their full human potential.

Maslow referred to this as **self-actualization**. Meeting needs at this level involves more than facing and managing daily tasks. It requires you to work at the peak of your abilities. People who do volunteer work are often addressing their need for self-actualization. They find the experience rewarding and feel they are helping others.

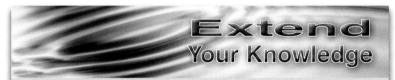

Extend Your Knowledge

Homelessness and Physical Needs

Visit a local homeless shelter or interview a shelter director. Learn how people respond to their life situation when their physical needs are not met. How are social and mental health impacted for individuals who are homeless? Prepare a concept map with "homelessness" in the center and diagram the connecting lines to other events that occur as a result of homelessness. Consider effects related to safe environments, access to healthy food, and other physical issues that result from becoming homeless.

The need for self-actualization expands as you pursue it. Meeting this need is a lifelong process. After achieving one goal toward self-actualization, you need to set new goals. Few people reach a point where they feel they have reached the highest level of achievement in every area.

What Is Social Health?

The degree to which your social needs for love, acceptance, and esteem are met affects your social health. Social health is reflected in your ability to get along with the people around you. It is measured by the quality of your relationships, **17-3**. **Relationships** are the connections you form with family members, friends, and other people.

People enrich their lives as they build relationships with others. They learn what types of interactions meet their social needs. They learn how to interact with people from other cultures who may have different values than their own. As you learn more about what is important to you, you are enabled to form stronger relationships.

Socially healthy people enjoy making new friends and keeping old ones. People who have good social health generally have certain traits that help them relate to others. Such traits include patience, empathy, courtesy, respect, and selflessness. Socially healthy people exhibit these traits through their daily words and actions when they are around others. They can share thoughts and ideas while showing respect for others' needs.

Social Development

One sign of social health is positive social development during childhood and adolescence. **Social development** is learning how to get along with others. It involves more than forming close personal relationships. It involves being able to act appropriately in all kinds of situations that involve people. Not talking in a movie theater, thanking a clerk for help, and raising your hand in class are social skills. As populations become more diverse, social skills are used to communicate effectively with people from different ethnic or economic backgrounds. Having such skills may not be enough to help you form close friendships. However, these skills should help you feel more at ease in social settings.

Food encounters are often used as a way to build social connections. Have you felt included when you are invited to a pizza party? At social gatherings food becomes a symbol of welcoming hospitality. Teen parties usually include favorite foods and beverages. The mere

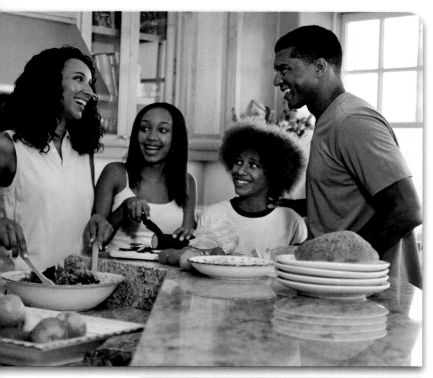

17-3 Sharing activities, such as meal preparation, is one way to build relationships.

presence of food often suggests fun, relaxation, and a time to get to know each other. You learn how to interact with friends informally.

Another example of how food can become a focus for social development is with school or community garden projects, **17-4**. Even young children can learn the importance of group cooperation and social responsibilities while planting and growing food in a common area. "Many hands make light work" is a quote that expresses the benefit of working together. Children learn from each other and from adults who model cooperative behaviors.

Like children, teens tend to model the conduct of their peers. Peers who model inappropriate social actions can have a negative effect on social development. Teens who learn to recognize and reject inappropriate behavior can protect their social health status.

Adult relationships involve getting along with coworkers as well as friends and family members. Job success depends on achieving social competence. Skills developed early in life can help people reach career advancement goals as adults.

People in Your Social Circle

For most people, the closest and most continuous relationships occur within families. These relationships begin at birth as family members respond to a baby's needs. A family that demonstrates care and respect for each of its members displays signs of positive social health, **17-5**.

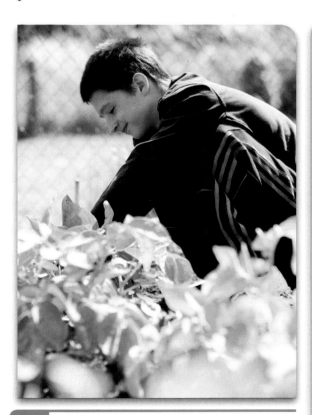

17-4 Community garden projects give teens the opportunity to demonstrate cooperation and responsibility.

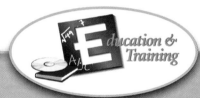

School Counselor

School counselors provide students with career, personal, social, and educational counseling. They help students evaluate their abilities, interests, talents, and personalities to develop realistic academic and career goals. Counselors often work with students who have academic and social development problems or other special needs.

Education: A master's degree usually is required to become a licensed or certified counselor, although requirements for counselors are often very detailed and vary by state.

Job Outlook: Employment for educational, vocational, and school counselors is expected to grow faster than the average for all occupations. Expansion of the responsibilities of school counselors also is likely to lead to increases in their employment. For example, counselors are becoming more involved in crisis and preventive counseling—helping students deal with issues ranging from drug and alcohol abuse to death and suicide.

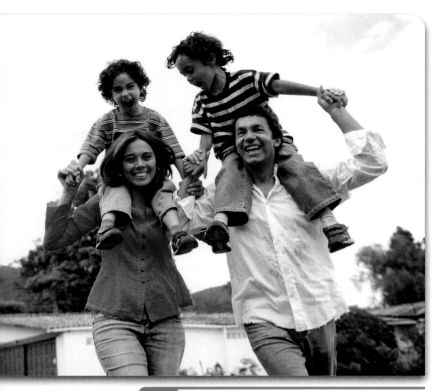

17-5 Much early social development occurs within the family unit.

Sharing friendships is an important way to achieve social health. Friends provide people with a source of shared fun and companionship. You feel free to exchange joys and sorrows with a friend. Most importantly, friends can help you work through problems and give you feedback on ideas. As your friends provide this type of support for you, you can provide it for them. This two-way interaction makes friends a valuable source of self-discovery. Beyond family members and friends, your social connections can expand through Internet communications, travel, media, and group activities. You face new social challenges as you include people from other cultures in your social network. As you interact with others, they influence your thoughts and feelings and you influence theirs. Sharing friendships is an important way to achieve social health.

Be proactive when choosing a circle of friends. Being **proactive** is taking steps in advance to deal with anticipated situations. Select friends who support your choice to live a healthy lifestyle. Avoid friends who encourage you to participate in destructive behaviors. If your friends support your interests in good health and fitness, you will find extra motivation to make health promoting choices.

Promoting Positive Social Health

You can take steps to build positive relationships that will meet your social needs. Many experts would agree that an ability to share ideas with others is the most important social skill. With this skill, you can solve problems with others and make your needs known to them. You can also express care for others and work with them to achieve goals.

Develop Communication Skills

Communication is the sending of a message from one source to another. Two basic types of communication are used to convey messages. **Verbal communication** uses words. It may be spoken or unspoken. Speaking to someone and writing a letter are both examples of verbal communication. **Nonverbal communication** transmits messages without the use of words. Posture, facial expressions, tone of voice, and symbols are nonverbal ways of communicating. When verbal and nonverbal communication both send the same message, communication is clear.

You need effective communication skills to be able to clearly exchange ideas with others. These skills can greatly affect your relationships and, thus, your social health. The following guidelines will help you plainly and openly communicate your ideas with others:

- Know what you want to say.
- Speak clearly and loudly enough to be understood.
- Avoid using slang terms that may not be familiar to your listener.
- Avoid sending nonverbal signals that contradict your spoken message, such as rolling your eyes when giving a compliment.
- Use specific words to convey your exact meaning.
- Maintain eye contact when you are communicating with someone in person.
- Be honest.

The increasing use of e-mail, text messaging, and other electronic communication makes clear communication skills more important than ever, **17-6**. A message containing errors or inaccurate information could end up making a bad impression on people all over the world in a matter of seconds.

You need to learn how to write effectively. Take time to select the right words and construct clear sentences. Use a writing style that conveys your intended tone. Be sure the message you send cannot be interpreted as offensive to another person or group of people. For informative writing, keep sentences short. Sentences that are long and use technical terms are harder for people to read and understand. Following these suggestions will help you represent yourself well as you use written communication to build personal relationships.

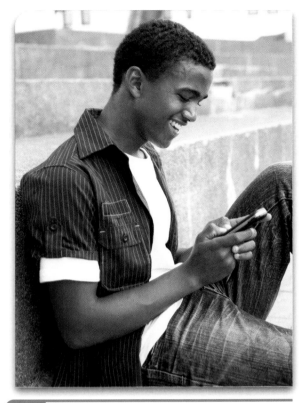

17-6 Electronic communication is more difficult because there are no nonverbal cues exchanged.

Resolve Conflicts

A **conflict** is a disagreement. Conflicts tend to arise between people in social situations. Perhaps someone has blamed you for something you did not do. You may have gotten into an argument with a good friend. You cannot eat normally because of the stress. These are examples of conflict.

If you do not handle conflicts carefully, they can grow. A conflict that gets out of hand can eventually destroy a relationship, **17-7**. This is why an ability to *resolve*, or settle, conflicts is important for maintaining good social health. You can use your communication skills to help you resolve conflicts.

Handling conflicts as soon as possible helps keep them under control. However, you should wait until you have a chance to talk about the problem

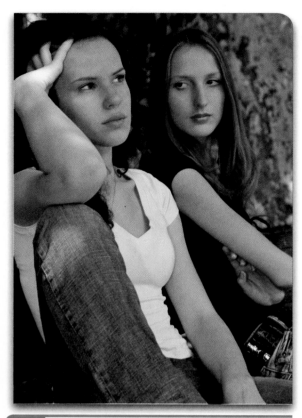

17-7 Ability to resolve conflicts is an indication of good social health.

privately. Airing your disagreement publicly is likely to make the other person uncomfortable and defensive.

Stay focused on the facts related to the problem. Try not to bring emotions into your discussion. Also avoid becoming sidetracked by other issues. Explain why you are unhappy with the person's actions, not why you are unhappy with the person.

Use "I" messages to state how you feel and why you feel that way. This allows you to take ownership of your feelings. In contrast, a "you" message blames your feelings on someone else. Compare the following examples:

- "I feel uncomfortable when we arrive late for our exercise class. I would appreciate your help in getting there on time."
- "You embarrass me by making us late for our exercise class. You better start getting us there on time."

The "I" statements in the first example are likely to evoke a more positive response from the other person.

Try to monitor your voice. Tone of voice greatly influences the quality of a conversation. A loud, angry voice will cause the other person to feel as though he or she is being attacked.

Do not simply criticize what is wrong with a situation. Explain what could be done differently. Suggest a plan that might work better. Describe why you think this solution would work. Stay flexible as you discuss various solutions to the problem. The other person may also have some good ideas. Together you may be able to reach a **compromise**. This is a solution that blends ideas from two differing parties.

Practice Assertiveness

Learning to be assertive will help you develop positive social health. **Assertiveness** is a personality trait. It is the boldness to express what you think and feel in a way that does not offend others. It is different from aggressiveness and goes beyond passiveness, **17-8**. To

Social Behavior Patterns		
Passive	Assertive	Aggressive

17-8 Assertiveness is the ability to express a personal point of view without offending others. You are neither passive nor aggressive in your words and actions.

be aggressive is to express your feelings in a way that is pushy and offensive. To be passive may mean failing to express your feelings at all.

Assertiveness allows you to take steps to reach desired outcomes. It allows you to feel actively involved in the decisions that must be made. It gives you the courage to ask important questions and locate necessary resources to achieve your needs and interests.

Assertiveness can help you feel more confident in socially challenging situations. You will be able to say no when an activity does not agree with your personal values and beliefs. You will be able to turn down offers to join in activities that do not fit into your schedule. You will be able to pursue opportunities that are important to you.

You can practice assertiveness if it does not come naturally to you. Make a point of expressing your opinions to others. Be firm when asking for what you want. However, if the answer is "no," let go of the issue. Avoid becoming angry, demanding, and argumentative. (This would be aggressive behavior.) Do not be afraid of your position or feel you must defend it. (This would be passive behavior.) Just state your feelings calmly and openly. In most cases, people will respect your honesty.

When you encounter someone who is aggressive, your most assertive response is to simply get away. You will not be able to reason with someone who is out of control. To protect yourself from potential violence, you need to remove yourself from the situation.

Be a Good Listener

Communication involves listening as well as speaking. You need to listen carefully to be sure you understand

Case Study: Social Health on the Menu

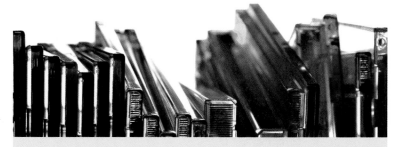

Mia and her friends decide to go out to eat after play practice. The group goes to a nearby fast-food restaurant. They each stand in line to place their orders. Mia is the last person to arrive at the table with her food. The rest of her group has ordered fries, sodas, milkshakes, and cheeseburgers. When they see Mia has a grilled chicken sandwich (no mayonnaise), nonfat milk, and a small salad on her tray, they begin teasing her. They tell her she eats like an old person and ask if her mom ordered her meal for her. They laugh and wonder if she is trying to get extra credit with the health teacher.

Case Review

1. Why do you think Mia's friends are reacting to her food choices in this manner?

2. How could Mia respond in an assertive manner without endangering the friendship of the group?

the message someone else is sending. Try restating information that has been shared. Ask questions about any points that are not clear. These steps allow you to confirm that you have correctly understood what the other person said.

Good friends are good listeners. You know you can rely on them and they can rely on you. Friends need to be understanding and sensitive about how you feel at any given time. Friends show signs of caring, too. They must show you they value your feelings and words as much as their own. At the same time, you need to offer others the same qualities you desire in a friend. Friends listen carefully to what each other is saying, **17-9**.

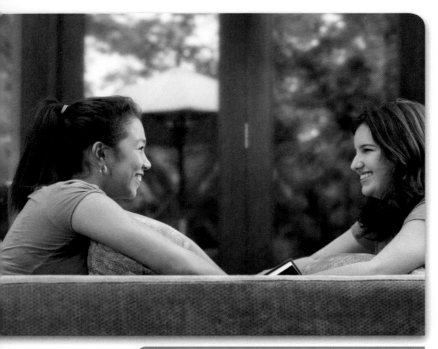

17-9 Friends will support your ideas and listen to your thoughts without criticism.

Be a Team Member

To be a socially healthy person, you must be able to be an effective member of a group. You must be willing to participate in teamwork. Teamwork is the effort of two or more people toward a common goal. Teamwork is often required to solve complex problems or complete involved tasks. For instance, making a parade float for a school club would require teamwork among club members.

Each person can contribute unique talents, giving the project balance and completeness. A club member with artistic skill could design the float. Someone with consumer skills could buy the supplies. A member who has construction skills could help build the float. Completing the project successfully would be much more difficult without the addition of each person's special abilities. By helping and encouraging one another, team members can accomplish more as a group than they can individually.

What are the characteristics of an effective team or group member? Groups who work together effectively have members who

- focus on the team goals
- show willingness to compromise
- value the importance of each person's job to the team's success
- cooperate and offer help when needed
- treat each person as a valued member by seeking his or her ideas and opinions

What Is Mental Health?

Most health care professionals agree that people's mental health reflects the ways they see themselves. People with positive mental health feel comfortable with their work and family lives. They can usually adapt to the demands and challenges they must face each day. Mentally healthy people also seek positive ways to meet their physical and social needs, **17-10**.

Mentally healthy people are not always smiling and happy. They sometimes have periods of fear, insecurity, and loss of control. These are normal emotional events. However, people with good mental health have learned to deal effectively with their emotional ups and downs.

Mentally healthy people have also learned how to react positively to major life events. They may become distressed after an emotional crisis, such as losing a job or ending a relationship. They may feel uneasy about a lifestyle change, such as a move to a new community. However, they find ways to control and reshape the effects of these emotional upheavals. They focus on improving the conditions they can change.

Characteristics of Positive Mental and Social Health

Positive mental and social health may be reflected in someone who

- maintains a positive self-image
- respects and takes good care of self
- finds pleasure in life; is happy and active most of the time
- shows awareness of personal thoughts and feelings and can express them in positive ways
- works to meet daily problems and challenges
- is not afraid to face problems and is willing to seek help when crises arise
- plans for achieving future goals
- enjoys humor and can laugh at self
- knows how to end personal relationships that are hurtful
- shows interest in learning and growing from mistakes and can accept criticism
- tolerates frustration without undue anger
- works well in group situations
- continues to work with an individual or group even when his or her ideas are rejected
- develops talents and abilities to their fullest
- enjoys positive interpersonal relations with people of both sexes
- genuinely likes people and shows interest in meeting new people
- considers the needs and rights of others when expressing personal needs and rights
- respects differences in appearances, race, religion, interests, and abilities

17-10 People who display many of these characteristics tend to have positive views of themselves and strong relationships with others.

Mentally healthy people are likely to view life's challenges as opportunities for growth. When an event occurs, they identify the issues involved. They think clearly about their goals. Then they search for solutions to resolve the problem. If a situation becomes too overwhelming, mentally healthy people are not afraid to ask others for help.

Self-Concept and Mental Health

Your **self-concept** is the idea you have about yourself. It is how you see your behavior in relation to other people and tasks. Part of having good mental health is having a positive self-concept. You have a realistic view of

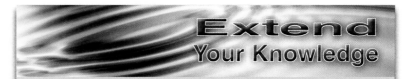

Extend Your Knowledge

Community Programs to Support Social and Mental Health

Develop a proposal for a community-based program to promote better social or mental health among the residents in the community. State the overall goal of the program. Give reasons why this program is needed and how it will achieve the goal. Provide a brief description of how the program would operate, who would oversee it, and the population served by it. Estimate the cost to start and maintain the program for one year. Find two references from literature or professionals in the field to support your program goals and cost estimates.

yourself and the events in your life. You realize most situations have pluses and minuses.

Through your early social interactions with family and friends, you begin to develop a concept of who you are. Your self-concept is often a reflection of the way you believe other people see you. If other people focus only on your strengths, you may form a *negative self-concept*. This means you have an inaccurate picture of yourself. You fail to realize you have faults as well as gifts. You are also likely to form a negative self-concept if other people dwell on your failures. You may not recognize you have both positive and negative qualities. If other people acknowledge both your strengths and weaknesses, you are likely to form a *positive self-concept*. This means you have an accurate picture of yourself. You understand you have abilities as well as shortcomings.

As you grow and change, your self-concept can change. Feedback from family members, friends, teachers, and community leaders may reinforce your self-concept, **17-11**. It may also cause you to reevaluate and redefine your self-concept. This is part of human growth over the life cycle.

Good mental health is also linked with having a high level of self-esteem. **Self-esteem** is the worth or value you assign yourself.

Like your self-concept, your self-esteem is affected by the people around you. When people give you the impression you do not matter, they can decrease your level of self-esteem. For instance, picture your teachers never calling on you when you raise your hand. Imagine your family members ignoring your opinions. Think about your friends always interrupting you. Over time, these actions may cause you to feel worthless.

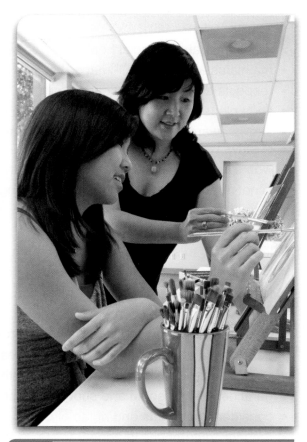

17-11 Feedback from people in your life helps you develop an accurate self-concept.

A person who has low self-esteem may feel helpless to make decisions. He or she may not feel deserving of good fortune. This person may be easily influenced by peer pressure.

When people express the opinion that you are worthwhile and important, they help build your self-esteem. For example, a teacher may say you did a good job on your science report. Your parents may show pride when you make a mature decision. Your friend may thank you for your loyalty. These types of positive feedback help you feel good about yourself.

With a high level of self-esteem, you will feel like a capable, secure, and creative person most of the time. You care about how situations will affect you. This helps you recognize negative peer pressure. It also empowers you to resist pressure urging you to take part in activities that could be harmful to you. A high level of self-esteem enables you to set goals and take actions to achieve them. Your self-esteem grows as you accomplish tasks that are important to you.

Promoting Positive Mental Health

You can take steps to promote good mental health. Having positive mental health can help you meet your mental needs. A realistic view of yourself can point you in the direction of activities that move you toward self-actualization.

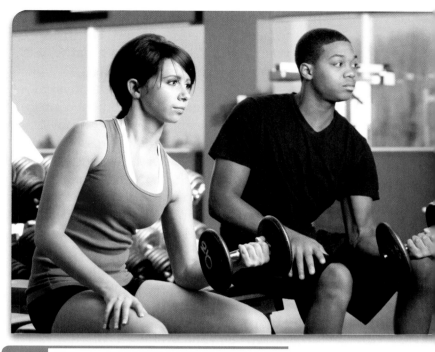

17-12 Surround yourself with people who support your nutrition and fitness goals.

Surround Yourself with Supportive People

Having good social health can boost your mental health. You need to surround yourself with people who will fulfill your needs to feel loved, accepted, and valued. Such people will help you build a positive self-concept and a high level of self-esteem. Their love and support will help you develop the confidence you need to succeed. They will show support for the nutrition and fitness goals you choose.

Try to connect with encouraging friends and adult role models, **17-12**. These supportive people can help you build on your strengths and learn from your mistakes. Avoid people who always send negative messages to you.

Keep in mind that healthy relationships involve giving as well as receiving. Just as you need support from others, others need support from you. When you encourage others, you are playing an important role in helping to fulfill their social and mental needs.

Remember that you need to be supportive of yourself. Encouragement from others will not go very far if you have a poor opinion of yourself. Try to avoid negative thoughts about yourself. Concentrate on using your strengths and improving your weaknesses.

The connection between social health and mental health goes both ways. When you have good mental health, you will find it easier to attract people who meet your social needs. Other people will be drawn to your positive outlook. They will appreciate your realistic view of yourself.

Protect Your Physical and Mental Health

Your physical health affects your mental health. When you feel physically well, you have the energy you need to face your problems. You have the strength to look for positive ways to help yourself feel good. For instance, you may find exercise is a great way to beat negative emotions.

Mental health also affects physical health. Feeling mentally content contributes in significant ways to good physical health. Feeling sad and depressed affects food choices and exercise activities. When someone feels down for a long period of time, he or she can lose interest in fitness. The immune system can become suppressed and physical health may deteriorate. When people are in a good state of mental and physical health, their bodies can fight disease more effectively.

The connection between nutrition and physical health is clear. Understanding of the link between diet and mental health is growing. The research that specifically looks at nutrition and mental health is still in its infancy. Consider the following ways to improve your physical and mental health with nutrition:

- *Eat breakfast to benefit mental health.* Performance and learning behaviors noticeably improve when individuals begin the day with breakfast.
- *Drink adequate fluids to protect against dehydration.* Dehydration affects your ability to think clearly and concentrate.
- *Eat meals on a regular basis to promote calmness and satisfaction.* A hungry person can feel irritable and restless.
- *Choose foods that are digested slowly and are a good source of fiber to moderate swings in blood sugar levels.* Mood and energy swings can be associated with big fluctuations in blood sugar levels that result from eating foods high in sugar and other simple carbohydrates. Include more fruits, vegetables, and whole grains in your diet, **17-13**.

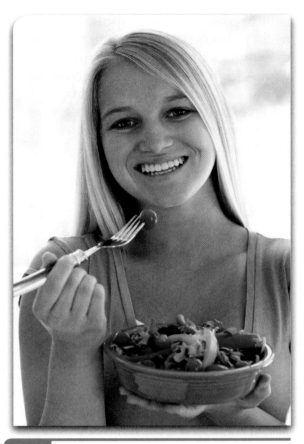

17-13 Salads can be a good source of fiber and nutrients.

- *Include high-quality proteins every day to supply all the amino acids needed for brain function.* Protein intake can affect brain function and mental health. Many of the neurotransmitters in the brain are made from amino acids. When these indispensable amino acids are missing from the diet, there is evidence of mood lowering effects, increased anxiety, loss of concentration, and fatigue.
- *Select foods and beverages rich in vitamins, minerals, and omega-3 fatty acids to support healthy brain function and a positive mental outlook.* Researchers have observed the prevalence of mental health disorders increases as the nutritious quality of food and beverage choices deteriorates. Deficiencies of

certain vitamins or minerals can result in damaged brain cells and reduced memory, problem-solving abilities, and brain function.

- *Consume sufficient calories to support the energy needs of a developing body and brain.* Developing fetuses and young children are susceptible to brain damage from malnutrition. Decrease in brain size, poor growth, and weak, brittle bones are some of the risks of eating disorders during a growth phase. Balanced nutrition is vital for reaching full brain development.

Knowing there is a relationship between body and mind highlights the importance of protecting your physical health. Make a point of eating healthful foods. Be sure to get enough rest and exercise. Avoid harmful substances, too. By following these guidelines, you will be caring for your mental health as well as your physical health.

Maintain Balance in Your Life

Have you ever been so busy going out with your friends that you barely have time to see your family? Have you ever been so involved with a school project that you forgot to eat a meal? From time to time, many people get excessively focused on one area of their lives. As a result, they lose touch with other areas. Their lives lack balance.

Balance refers to a sense of proportional distribution given to life's roles and responsibilities. A lack of balance can have a negative effect on mental health. People whose lives are out of balance may find themselves feeling emotionally exhausted. They are likely to experience **burnout**. This is a lack of

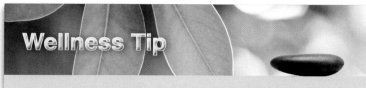

Wellness Tip

Teamwork—Benefits More Than Social Health

Effectively working as part of a team not only promotes positive social health, but has other benefits, too. Teamwork is considered an important job skill and can help you achieve career success. You can develop teamwork skills by taking an active role in school and community group projects.

energy and motivation to work toward goals. Burnout causes a reduced sense of personal accomplishment.

Maintaining balance requires you to step away from yourself. Look at your life from an outsider's point of view. This will help you see how your daily actions affect the quality of your whole life. It will help you get a better perspective of what really matters to you in the long run.

Balance comes from devoting an appropriate amount of time and energy to each of your roles. These roles may include family, school or job, and community roles. Each demands your personal attention, **17-14**.

While dividing your time among all your roles, do not forget to save some time for yourself. You need to take care of your physical, social, and mental needs. You need to allow yourself the time to select nutritious foods and get adequate amounts of rest and exercise. You need to take the time to relax and enjoy hobbies and friends, too. Taking this time for yourself makes you feel more prepared to face all your roles and responsibilities.

How Do You Divide Your Time?

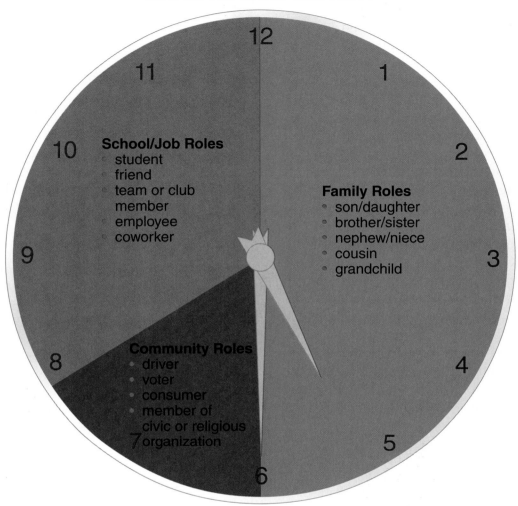

School/Job Roles
- student
- friend
- team or club member
- employee
- coworker

Family Roles
- son/daughter
- brother/sister
- nephew/niece
- cousin
- grandchild

Community Roles
- driver
- voter
- consumer
- member of civic or religious organization

17-14 Promoting positive mental health involves allotting an appropriate amount of time to each of your roles.

Math Link

Calculating Percentage

Keep an activity log for one day. Determine the number of hours spent in each of your various life roles. Roles may include family, school, job, community, personal, and other roles you may identify.

1. Calculate the percent of time you spent in each role.
2. Create a pie chart to display your results.

Making Positive Life Changes

Perhaps you have a desire to improve your social and/or mental health. You have read several suggestions for helping you reach this goal. However, following these suggestions may require you to adopt some new behaviors. Making such changes in your life can be difficult. It involves conscious and responsible efforts.

Using a self-management plan can make this change process easier. A *self-management plan* is an action-oriented tool for making a positive behavior change. It involves carefully analyzing goals, priorities, and choices. It requires you to identify options before making and acting on decisions. A self-management plan involves the following steps:

1. List your strengths.
2. List your "needs improvement" behaviors.
3. Prioritize your "needs improvement" behaviors.
4. Clarify your goal.
5. List your alternatives for achieving your goal.
6. Evaluate the pros and cons of each alternative.
7. Make a choice and act on it.
8. Evaluate the outcomes of your choice.

As you read about each step in the self-management plan, begin to prepare a plan of your own. This will allow you to clearly see the step-by-step actions you intend to take. It will help you monitor your progress. It will also enable you to reward yourself when you achieve successes.

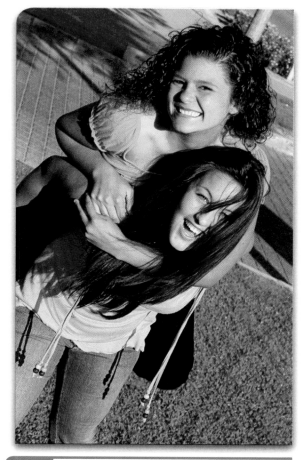

17-15 Relaxing with family and friends can help you feel refreshed and ready to face responsibilities.

List Your Strengths

Most people have experienced many successes in life. No one has a life full of failures. Begin your self-management plan by examining your strengths in the health area you want to improve. For example, suppose you want to improve your social health. Your current social strengths may include your honesty as a friend and your cooperative attitude when working on a team.

List Your "Needs Improvement" Behaviors

Identify health-related behaviors you feel you need to improve, **17-15**. You might believe being assertive is one of your weaker social skills. Maybe you feel you often hesitate to express your needs to others. As a result, your wishes go unnoticed. You might also feel you have trouble resolving conflicts. Perhaps you do not tell other people when you disagree with them. Instead, you allow negative feelings to build up until you have an outburst of temper.

Prioritize Your "Needs Improvement" Behaviors

After you have identified the "needs improvement" behaviors, you must narrow your focus. You are less likely to be successful if you scatter your attention in too many directions. Look at the list of behaviors you identified in the second step. Rank your list, placing the behavior that concerns you most at the top. You may believe assertiveness will help you resolve conflicts. Therefore, you decide to put "being more assertive" at the top of your "needs improvement" list.

Clarify Your Goal

Now that you have identified your main area for self-improvement, shape it into a specific goal. This will give you a sense of direction. State your goal in writing, using concrete, measurable terms. When possible, include a time frame for meeting your goal. Be realistic about what you can achieve.

Try to break your goal down into manageable subgoals. For example, your main goal is "I want to be more assertive." This is a broad goal. A measurable subgoal might be "I will ask one question or state one opinion every day." Another subgoal might be "I will not apologize when I have to say 'no' to an activity," **17-16**. You can easily see how well you are achieving these specific subgoals. This will give you motivation to continue working toward your main goal.

As you are clarifying your goal, decide how important it is to you. Ask yourself if you are willing to do what it will take to create a change. Also consider how the achievement of your goal will affect others. For example, how will your goal to be more assertive affect your family?

List Your Alternatives

For each subgoal you have identified, list all the ways you can think of to achieve it. Usually there will be more than one choice available. For example,

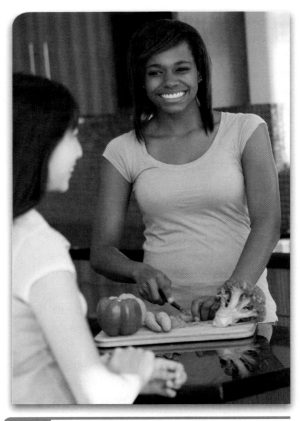

17-16 If your goal is to improve your overall health, a subgoal might be to increase vegetables in your diet.

to learn how to boldly ask questions and state opinions, you could attend an assertiveness workshop. You might read a book about expressing yourself with confidence. You could ask advice from someone who has an ability to speak out. You could also ask a trusted friend to help you practice asking questions and stating opinions. All these choices have the possibility of helping you develop assertiveness skills.

You may want to do some research to become aware of different alternatives for reaching your goal. The more options you know about, the more likely you will be to find one that will work for you. Use the Internet or your community library to gather information. Seek the advice of a school counselor or someone else who may be knowledgeable on the subject.

Evaluate the Pros and Cons

Identify as many advantages and disadvantages as you can for each alternative on your list. For example, an assertiveness workshop has the advantage of helping you gain new skills quickly. However, it may have the disadvantage of being costly. Weigh the pros against the cons for each alternative. Cross off any options on your list that have more drawbacks than benefits.

Think about how each alternative will affect your resources, including time, money, and physical energy, **17-17**. Also consider the results of choosing one alternative over another. Choosing one option can often remove other options. If you spend your money to attend a workshop, you can no longer use that money to buy a book.

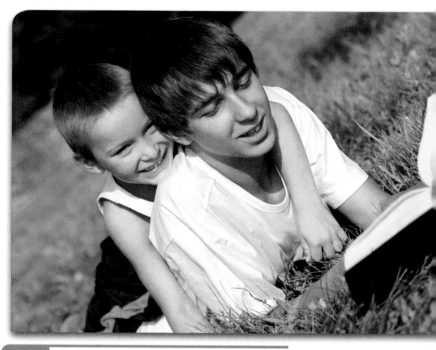

17-17 Choosing to spend time with a younger sibling will benefit his self-esteem and your own.

Make a Choice and Act on It

After comparing your various alternatives, choose the one that seems to suit you best. Then act on your choice. Suppose you decide to read a book on expressing yourself with confidence. Go to a bookstore or library. Find a book on this topic that seems engaging. Buy or check out the book and read it. Then start following the worthwhile advice from the book in your daily interactions with others.

Evaluate Outcomes

Evaluation is an ongoing process throughout a self-management plan. For example, in the first step, you evaluate your behaviors related to a particular type of health. This is an informal evaluation that occurs mainly in your head.

As a final step in a self-management plan, you need to do a more formal evaluation. Putting your evaluation in writing can help you think about how your chosen action helped you meet your main goal. You will be able to see whether following the advice from the book truly helped you become more assertive.

The following questions may help you evaluate the outcomes of your self-management plan:

- Am I satisfied with the results of my choices and actions?
- Do I feel better about myself than I did before?
- Is my health status better now than it was before?
- Do my friends and family show support of my newly developed behaviors and skills?
- Does my overall quality of life seem to be improved?

Answering no to any of these questions may indicate you did not choose the best way to improve your health. Try to view this situation as a chance to learn more about yourself. This will help you make better choices in the future.

If you can answer yes to each of these questions, your self-management plan worked for you. You took the necessary steps to make a change that helped you grow mentally and/or socially. Your physical health is also bound to improve as a result of your actions.

Seeking Help for Social and Mental Health Problems

Positive social and mental health are key parts of your total state of wellness. Many people find the methods described earlier helpful for improving these two health areas. However, some people have social and mental health problems that cannot be solved through self-help techniques. Such problems require the help of mental and social health care professionals, **17-18**. A nutrition counselor will help a person make and maintain dietary changes.

Mental and social health problems can occur for many reasons. Some are the result of specific crisis events, such as divorce, death of a person close to you, or school relocation. Other problems arise out of long-term situations, such as emotional neglect or substance abuse. No matter what is causing the problem, the important point is to find needed help.

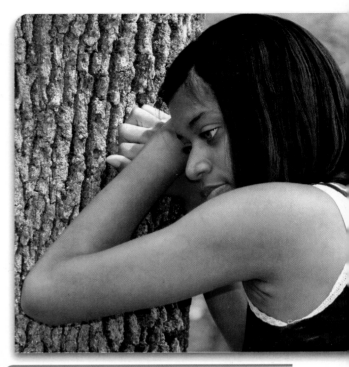

17-18 If mental or social conflicts are too stressful, you may feel unable to solve problems alone. Professional counselors are available to help teens in conflict.

A physician can recommend professionals who can help people with social or mental problems. A professional will begin by helping a client define the problem. Treatment may involve individual, family, or group therapy. Therapy often focuses on helping clients develop the social and mental tools they need to help themselves. Questions about a person's typical food intake may be asked. Treatment for some clients also involves medication.

Helpful therapists can convey interest, understanding, and respect to clients. They offer advice and support to help clients improve their mental and social health. However, the clients are responsible for making needed behavior changes.

Reading Summary

Your social and mental health play large roles in your wellness. These health areas are interrelated with your physical health.

All three health areas are affected by the degree to which your needs are met. You can group basic human needs into five levels. You have needs for physical survival, safety and security, love and acceptance, esteem, and self-actualization. Needs at each level must be at least partly met before you can focus on needs at the next level.

Your social health refers to your ability to form quality relationships with others. Your social health is influenced by your development of social skills as you grow up. It is also affected by the people in your social circle, especially family members and friends.

You can take steps to promote positive social health. One of the most important steps is to develop communication skills. Having these skills will help you resolve conflicts. You also need to practice assertiveness in social situations. Developing the qualities of a good friend and team member will help you build more positive relationships, too.

Your mental health is reflected in the way you see yourself and in the way you react to life events. Having good mental health involves having a positive self-concept and a high level of self-esteem.

As with social health, you can take steps to promote positive mental health. Surrounding yourself with supportive people can help you build a positive self-concept. Protecting your physical health will give you the strength to tackle problems that come your way. Maintaining balance among your various roles will help you avoid strain on your mental health.

A self-management plan can help you make positive life changes that will promote good social and mental health. However, some problems may seem too big for you to handle through self-management. In such cases, you may need to seek help from mental and social health care professionals.

Review Learning

1. Give examples of four physical needs that are basic to survival.
2. Explain why meeting the need for self-actualization is a lifelong process.
3. What are three traits that help people with good social health relate to others?
4. What are five guidelines for clear, open communication?
5. What are five tips for resolving conflict?
6. Which of the following would be an assertive way to express an opinion?
   A. Anyone who would buy that CD is an idiot. That music stinks.
   B. I would not buy that CD. I don't like that type of music.
   C. I'm not sure how I feel about that CD. What do you think?
   D. I would not buy that CD because I already have a lot of CDs. Besides, my mom says that music gives her a headache.
7. Describe how positive self-concept is formed.
8. Explain the two-way relationship between physical and mental health.

9. Give three examples of activities commonly associated with each of the following types of roles: family, school or job, and community.
10. Why should a person prioritize "needs improvement" behaviors when preparing a self-management plan?
11. What are three resources a person should consider when evaluating alternatives for reaching a life-change goal?
12. What is the final step in a self-management plan?
13. What is often the focus of professional therapy for social and mental health problems?

Critical Thinking

14. **Draw conclusions.** Your values and actions work together to balance life's roles and responsibilities. Draw conclusions about how your values impact life roles and responsibilities and your ability to maintain balance.
15. **Make inferences.** Why do you think some people avoid seeking professional help for social and mental health problems that are greater than those resolved through self-help techniques?

Applying Your Knowledge

16. **E-mail sharing.** To practice your written and electronic communication skills, connect with an e-mail partner in a family and consumer sciences class from another school. Ask what projects your partner is engaged in for his or her classes. Share information about the projects you are doing for your classes.
17. **Role-play assertiveness.** Write a brief description of a situation that would require assertiveness skills. In a small group, role-play the situation to practice using assertiveness skills. Video-record your role-play and invite your classmates to evaluate your use of the skills.
18. **Bulletin board.** Make a self-esteem bulletin board. Cover the board with plain paper and invite classmates to write esteem-building phrases on it. Discuss how these phrases relate to human needs in Maslow's hierarchy.

Technology Connections

19. **PSA video.** Using video-editing software to produce a public service announcement for a topic related to social and mental health.
20. **Web-page flyer.** Research the Internet for self-esteem building activities. Create a flyer using a desktop publishing program. Post the flyer on your class's Web page.
21. **Internet research.** Perform an Internet search for mental and social health services available in your community. List the locations, contact information, and costs for the various types of available services.

Academic Connections

22. **History.** Research and write a paper about Abraham Maslow. Discuss what led him to the development of his hierarchy of human needs theory.

23. **Social studies.** Develop a questionnaire to measure how working families balance their daily lives. Learn how much time is allotted to family, work, community, and other roles by each member of the family. Ask respondents to rate their satisfaction with the balance in their lives. Ask them to provide helpful tips they use to maintain balance in their lives. Survey at least two working parents of young children. Compile the class findings into an article for the school or local newspaper.

24. **Speech.** Prepare a five-minute speech on the effects of good nutrition on brain development and function.

Workplace Applications

Using Management Skills

Presume you have just started a new job. In your previous job, you were overworked and life was out of balance—and you developed many habits that were not good for your physical, social, and mental health. You know you need to make some changes. Use the steps in the self-management plan to create a step-by-step plan for making positive behavior changes to improve your social and mental health.

Chapter 18
Stress and Wellness

Reading for Meaning

Imagine you are a business owner and have several employees working for you. As you read the chapter, think about what you would like your employees to know. When you finish reading, write a memo to your employees and include key information from the chapter.

Concept Organizer

Use the graphic to identify factors that relate to the effects of stress on health, managing stress, and preventing stress.

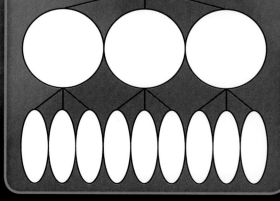

Stress

Terms to Know

negative stress
distress
positive stress
stressor
life-change events
daily hassles
fight or flight response
biofeedback
support system
progressive muscle relaxation
self-talk

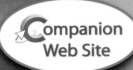

Companion Web Site

- **Print out the concept organizer at g-wlearning.com.**
- **Practice key terms with crossword puzzles, matching activities, and e-flash cards at g-wlearning.com.**

Objectives

After studying this chapter, you will be able to

- **recognize** potential sources of stress in your life.
- **summarize** the effects of stress on physical and mental health.
- **explain** how recognizing signs of stress, using support systems, relaxing, and using positive self-talk can help you manage stress.
- **use** strategies to prevent stress.

Central Ideas

- Stress is a part of life and can be both positive and negative.
- Stress can impact your physical, mental, and social health.
- Learning to prevent and manage stress can help reduce the impact of stress on total wellness.

How would the following events affect you physically and emotionally?

- Your teacher announces there will be a unit test in two days, and you have not yet read the chapters.
- You and your dating partner had a major disagreement last night and now you have no date for the prom.
- Varsity basketball tryouts are tomorrow afternoon, and making the team has been your goal for years.
- You were invited to be a bridesmaid in a cousin's wedding. She has not offered to pay for the dress, and you cannot afford it.
- High school graduation is in four months. You are excited, but undecided about your plans for the fall.

Each situation described above can produce stress. Stress is the inner agitation you feel when you are exposed to change. Many people associate stress with the feeling of being tense.

All people experience daily stress throughout their lives. Some stress is good for you and some is bad. In this chapter you will learn to recognize when stress can be positive. You will also read about how to manage the stress that can harm your state of wellness.

Stress Is Part of Life

To understand how stress can affect your life, you will need to examine the kinds of stress. You will also need to be aware of what causes stress and how your body reacts to it, **18-1**.

Types of Stress

Most people are aware that some stress in their lives tends to motivate them to achieve and perform well. They also know stress can be negative. Both types of stress impact social, emotional, and physical performance.

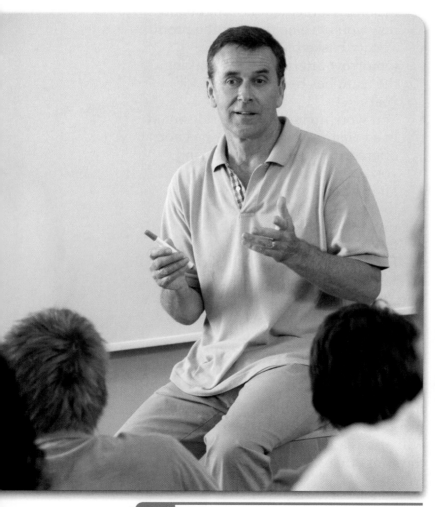

18-1 The announcement of an upcoming test may cause students to experience stress.

Negative Stress or Distress

When you see an event or situation as a threat to your well-being, you are likely to feel negative stress. **Negative stress**, or **distress**, is harmful stress. Negative stress can reduce your effectiveness by causing you to be fearful and perform poorly. If a classmate threatens to tell a teacher you cheated on a test, you will probably feel negative stress. Fear over whether the teacher will confront you about cheating may keep you from focusing on class material. This, in turn, may keep you from doing well in the class.

Another time distress can occur is when you experience a number of minor changes within a short period. For instance, suppose you have a job and are regularly scheduled to work from six to nine on Thursday evenings. On Wednesday, your manager calls and asks you to work on Friday evening instead of Thursday. This change in your schedule might not seem like a problem. However, imagine it occurred on the same weekend your best friend from out of town was planning to visit you. Suppose you have no car available to get to work. Now, your work schedule, your visiting plans, and your travel arrangements are all being changed at the same time. This many changes can cause distress.

Distress can result when one change continues to affect you for a long time, too. In the previous work example, suppose your manager asked you to make Friday your regular night to work. The first week, the Friday schedule might not bother you. However, imagine you missed seeing a movie with your friends on the second Friday. On the third week, you had to turn down a party invitation because of your job. On the fourth week, you had to skip going to a basketball game. By this time, the negative stress caused by the change in your work schedule is probably starting to build.

Positive Stress

Stress is not always bad. **Positive stress** motivates you to accomplish challenging goals. For example, athletes often feel positive stress when they are competing, **18-2**. The atmosphere during practice may not always prompt athletes to excel. At times, practice can feel like drudgery, and some athletes must push themselves to keep working. However, the atmosphere changes when opponents, fans, and officials are present. Athletes' response to this change in atmosphere is a form of positive stress. This stress of competition is the force that spurs athletes to give their best performance. They are inspired to achieve the goal of winning. The ability to turn a negative stress situation into positive stress is a wellness behavior that can be learned and practiced.

Causes of Stress

A source of stress is called a **stressor**. It is a change in circumstances that produces feelings of agitation and discomfort. Stressors can be physical, such as a change in your daily routine. Stressors can also be emotional, such as an increase in the amount of pressure you feel at school. A stressor is what begins the stress response.

Some researchers refer to major stressors that occur to people as **life-change events**. These are situations that can greatly alter a person's lifestyle. Death, divorce, remarriage, legal problems, and sudden unemployment are examples of life-change events. The kind and number of life-change events a person experiences directly affect his or her stress level.

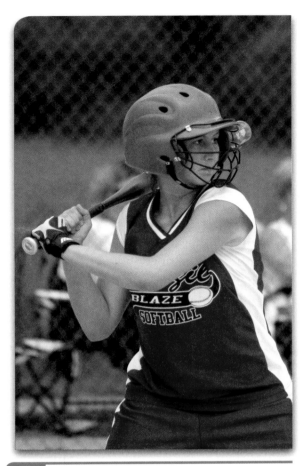

18-2 The positive stress of competition helps athletes work toward the reward of winning.

Not all the stress people experience comes from life-change events. Minor stressors that produce tension are often known as **daily hassles**. Long lines, heavy traffic, and misplaced belongings are common daily hassles. These types of persistent annoyances can strain a person's body, mind, and relationships. The result is negative stress, **18-3**.

Teens have many stressors in their lives. They face the physical changes associated with body growth and hormonal influences. Teens may also encounter emotional and social changes in relationships with family members and friends. Taking more challenging classes and making decisions that affect the future can create mental changes for teens, too.

Common Stressors	
Life-Change Events	
Death of a family member	New baby in the household
Parents' divorce or separation	Pregnancy
Personal injury	Moving
Change in health of family member	Outstanding personal achievement
Loss of a job and financial resources	Parent loses or changes job
Death of a close friend	Change in schools, church, clubs, sports activities
Daily Hassles	
Misplacing or losing items	School/job responsibilities
Concern about physical appearance	Change in sleeping habits
Arguments in the household	Loneliness
Difficulties with friends	Peer pressure
Trouble with boyfriend/girlfriend	Uncertainty of the future
Decision making	Money concerns

18-3 What other stressors could you add to these lists?

Most people can manage one or two stressors at a time. However, life seems to present an overload of stressors to some people. For example, when a divorce occurs, family financial resources may become stretched to the limits. To help, a teen may get an after-school job. The job involves pressure to perform well. It also takes time away from schoolwork, which leads to stress over grades. Over time, the snowball effect of one stressor adding to another can damage a person's physical, social, and emotional well-being.

The Body's Response to Stress

Your body goes through three stages when responding to a stressful event. These stages are alarm, resistance, and exhaustion.

To understand these three stages, imagine you just started a job in a fast-food restaurant. It is dinnertime and a long line of people is forming at your counter. Customers are reeling off orders, coworkers are bustling around, and children are crying in the background. You are trying to listen to orders, make change, package food, and keep the line moving. Suddenly one of your coworkers bumps into you. Your initial *alarm* response may include fear of spilling the food you are carrying. You may also feel mad at the coworker and discouraged about the delay in filling the customer's order.

These emotional responses during the alarm stage are coupled with physical responses. Inside your body, hormones are being released into your bloodstream. These hormones will cause your heart rate and blood pressure to increase. You will start breathing faster. Your face may flush, and you are likely to perspire. You may feel the muscles in your arms, legs, and stomach becoming tense. Your hearing will sharpen and your eyes will widen. All these reactions indicate your body is gathering its resources to conquer danger or escape to safety. This reaction to stress is often called the **fight or flight response**. You can choose to strike out (*fight*) or flee the situation (*flight*). This response is automatic and fast and more common when physical threat is perceived, **18-4**.

The next stage of the body's response to stress is *resistance*. During resistance, your body will give full effort to cope with the situation. Your whole body is engaged in fighting against the condition. In the resistance stage, continuous effort is made to cope with the stress. Then, as the line of customers at your counter becomes shorter, your stress level will subside. Your body systems begin to return to their prestress state. You may stop perspiring and your arms, legs, and stomach may begin to relax.

However, if the rush of customers continues for several hours, your body may never have a chance to recover. In this case, you will progress to the third response stage of *exhaustion*. Physical and mental fatigue are a part of this stage. You may feel tired and have a hard time thinking clearly. Your inner resources to resist and adapt to stress are gone.

Suppose you experience this kind of stress every evening at work. Soon your body will automatically become tense each day as you begin your shift. After months of working under these stressful conditions, tensions may begin to spill over into other areas of your life. You may find you are becoming less and less able to handle minor daily stressors. Over time, your body will begin to show signs of weakness. If lifestyle changes and stress reduction methods do not occur, physical illness may follow.

Case Study: Daily Hassles or Major Stressors?

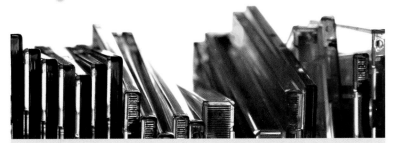

Kayla was enjoying high school. She got along well with her classmates and was getting good grades. Kayla's life was going well until a boy in the grade ahead of her began to make life difficult. Several times he bumped into her, causing her to drop her books in the hallway. He tried to get her attention and sometimes made her late for classes. He even text-messaged her asking when they could meet. People began to tease her about her new "boyfriend." Kayla did not want the boy's attention, much less to be his girlfriend! He constantly behaved rudely around her friends. One day, the boy wrote a nasty message about her in the boy's restroom. When Kayla learned about it, she didn't know what to do. Now Kayla was so worried that she felt sick. She was stressed out!

Case Review

1. Do you believe Kayla is experiencing a major stressor?

2. How do you think Kayla should handle this situation?

Physical Responses to Stress

- Pituitary releases hormones
- Eyes widen and pupils dilate
- Hearing sharpens
- Muscles tense
- Breathing speeds up
- Digestion slows down
- Blood pressure increases
- Heart races
- Sweat gland activity increases
- Blood contents change
- Adrenaline secreted
- Immune system suppressed

18-4 The fight or flight response will trigger certain physical reactions.

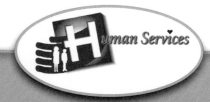

Group Exercise Instructors

Group exercise instructors conduct group exercise sessions. They lead, instruct, and motivate people in a variety of aerobic, stretching, and muscle conditioning exercises. Many instructors choose music and choreograph a sequence of exercise routines to the music which many participants find fun and relaxing. This conditioning of the body helps reduce the effects caused by stress and other health conditions. They demonstrate different positions and moves and carefully observe students to make sure they are doing the exercises correctly to avoid injury. Group exercise instructors are responsible for making classes motivating and safe while ensuring the exercises are not too hard for participants.

Education: Entry-level group fitness instructors may not be required to have certification; however, most organizations generally require group instructors to become certified. Achieving certification from a top organization is important. The National Commission for Certifying Agencies accredits reputable certification organizations (see their Web site). Once certified, continuing education is a requirement to keep certification. Some certifying organizations require an associate's or bachelor's degree in an exercise-related field.

Job Outlook: Demand for group exercise instructors is expected to remain strong at health clubs and fitness centers. Instructors with a degree in a fitness-related subject will likely have better opportunities because people will view them as having higher qualifications.

Effects of Stress on Health

Stress can affect your health. A continuous high level of negative stress can weaken body systems and increase your risks for certain diseases. Stress can also tax your emotional well-being. The type of personality you have can affect the degree to which stress impacts your health.

Effects on Physical Health

Over time and without your awareness, too much stress can damage your physical health. Some researchers believe stress may be the greatest contributor to illness in the modern, industrialized world.

You read earlier about physical reactions triggered by the release of stress hormones into your bloodstream. You breathe harder and faster to bring more oxygen into your body. Your heart beats more rapidly to quickly pump that oxygen out to the muscles. Your liver releases glucose and fat cells release fat into the bloodstream. Your blood pressure increases to speed the glucose and fat to the muscles for use as energy. All these reactions are intended to prepare your body to take action. Your muscles are getting ready to either defend you against the source of stress or run from it.

Many sources of stress in today's society do not require a physical battle or escape to safety. For instance, you may feel stress about auditioning for a part in the school play. However, dealing with this stress will not involve fighting or running from the director of the play. Therefore, the increase in your heart rate and blood pressure serve only to strain your heart and blood vessels. The extra fat released into your bloodstream may accumulate in your arteries. You can see how these results of stress can increase your risk for coronary heart disease, hypertension, and stroke.

Effects on the Immune System

Your body's immune system helps protect you from getting diseases. During periods of stress, your immune system defenses can become lowered. This may explain why you feel run-down after a long siege of stress.

During these times, you may find you have decreased resistance to infections, such as colds and flu. For example, during midterms or finals, you may be very worried about passing the tests. When the tests are over, your immune system may be so depressed you develop a cold.

Effects on Sleep Patterns

When stress hormones are released into your bloodstream, you are likely to experience heightened awareness. Your sense of sight and hearing becomes keener. Your mind may be racing with thoughts of the stressor and how to address it. You may have reached the exhaustion stage of the stress response. However, your increased level of mental activity can keep you from falling asleep quickly. It can also prevent you from enjoying a sound, peaceful sleep that will refresh you, **18-5**. This lack of rest can add to your stress and further depress your immune system.

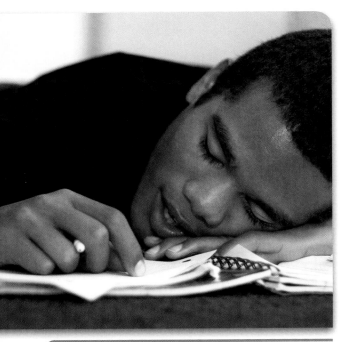

18-5 If stress causes you to lose sleep, you may be too tired during the day to fulfill school responsibilities. This, in turn, may cause you to feel more stressed.

Effects on Eating Habits

When stress hormones are circulating in the bloodstream, the body treats digesting food as a low priority. The body focuses its resources on the needs of the muscles and nerves rather than the digestive system.

Stress often affects people's eating habits and emotional responses to food. This is why stress is sometimes a factor in body weight problems. During emotional stress, some people nibble foods nervously. Others binge, which involves eating excessive amounts of food in a short time. Eating may seem to relieve their feelings of frustration. Some people cannot eat when under stress. They do not feel hungry because they are so focused on the source of stress. Others may experience upset stomach. Stress can also contribute to the development of anorexia nervosa and bulimia nervosa.

Eating habits affected by stress may change your nutritional status. Eating out of boredom or tension may cause you to eat excess calories. Weight gains can lead to overweight. Not eating because you are too excited, nervous, or worried, may cause you to lose weight and feel tired and cranky. Eating disorders can compound the effects of stress.

Math Link

Computing Average Heart Rate

Measure and record your heart rate every hour for eight hours. Compute your average heart rate for the eight hours.

Effects on Emotional Health

Too much stress can make you irritable, tense, and anxious. You may reach a point where you lack the strength to keep preventable sources of stress out of your life. When this happens, worry can overtake productive thinking, **18-6**.

Many social and emotional problems for teens can be related to undue amounts of stress in the family. Reports of substance abuse and suicide are often tied to an inability to cope with high stress levels. For adults, stress at work as well as in the family can take a toll on emotional health. Many cases of adults who abuse or abandon family members are linked to stress.

Personality Factors and Stress

Research has found health outcomes may be more related to your reaction to stress than to its cause. Many factors determine how you respond to the stressors in your life. These include heredity, experiences, and outlook, **18-7**.

Each person has different attitudes toward a given stressor. What may be stressful to one person may not be stressful to another. For instance, one student may agonize over getting a C on a test. Another student might be pleased to do that well. A third student may see it as an opportunity to do better next time. Also, events that

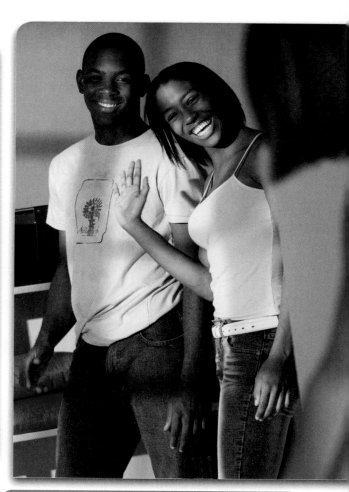

18-6 Stress at school may make you feel isolated and overwhelmed.

18-7 Positive attitudes can help people prevent stress from affecting their health.

cause stress may vary from one time in your life to another. Getting bitten by a mosquito can seem fairly stressful to some children. However, many adults would scarcely notice a mosquito bite.

Your reactions to stress depend partly on your personality type. Personality type refers to your general way of looking at life. You may have heard people refer to type A and type B personalities. People with type A personalities can be divided into two groups—hostile and nonhostile. People in both groups tend to be driven to achieve goals. However, people in the hostile group tend to be impatient, angry, and pushy. They easily become irritated over stressful events. People in this group are at greatest risk for stress-related health problems. People in the nonhostile type A group are less aggressive than hostile type A people. They are also less likely to become upset over stressful events. People with type B personalities are fairly relaxed and easygoing. Like nonhostile type A personalities, type B personalities are able to adapt to stress fairly well, **18-8**.

More important than your personality type is your attitude. If you approach problems as opportunities rather than threats, you are more likely to feel positive stress. Taking the following positive approaches toward life may help you have an easier time dealing with stressors:

- Look at new ideas and problems as exciting and challenging. Try not to feel threatened.
- Show a commitment to your work while showing a willingness to help others along the way.
- Take charge of your life, making decisions that will get you closer to your goals.
- Accept life's change with optimism rather than seeing it as a source of stress.

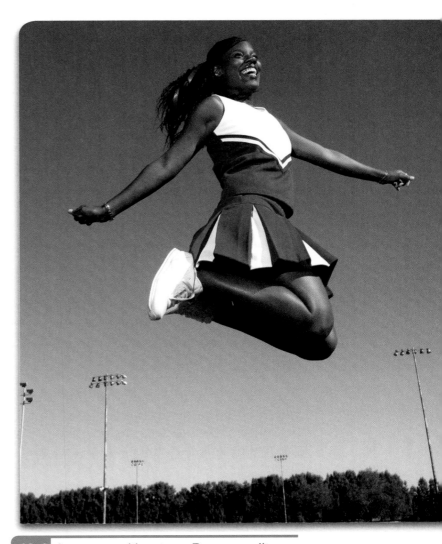

18-8 A person with a type B personality might find performing in front of others easier than a person with a type A personality would.

- Maintain positive health practices, taking good care of yourself.
- During times of personal crisis, talk openly with family members and friends.
- Be willing to seek the support of others. Do not wait for others to ask what is wrong.

Failing to react to life's events with these attitudes can create and promote excess personal stress. Excess stress can damage your mental and physical health. Stress can also hurt your relationships with family members and friends.

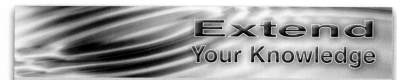

Personality, Stress, and Health

Research the relationship between personality types and stress responses. Ask the school counselor for references identifying literature on personality types. How does personality type affect the risk of health problems? Summarize your findings with a poster presentation.

Managing Stress

You cannot avoid all stress. However, you can learn to manage it. Most healthy, productive people search for ways to manage the stress in their lives. Stress management provides them with opportunities for personal growth. Viewing stress as positive allows people the chance to be creative. Learning how to adapt to negative stress helps people rationally deal with the changes that occur throughout life.

You can use a number of techniques to help you manage stress. Begin by learning to recognize the signs of stress. Rely on available support systems. Learn how to relax and use positive self-talk.

The key is to choose the methods that most easily fit into your lifestyle. Combine a variety of methods for greatest effects on total health. Be sensitive to other techniques that seem to help you relax.

At the very least, learning how to lessen the negative effects of stress can help you enjoy life more. At best, you can reduce your risks of disease and improve your state of wellness.

Wellness Tip

Laughter—Medicine for Stress

Have you ever noticed how good you feel after a good, hearty laugh? Research shows that laughter is an excellent source of stress relief. Not only does a hearty laugh reduce levels of stress hormones like *adrenaline*, it also increases beneficial hormones like *endorphins*. The next time you feel stressed or frustrated, laugh about the situation instead of worrying over it, watch a funny movie or your favorite cartoon, read a joke book, or join some friends for an evening of fun and laughter.

Recognize Signs of Stress

Identifying the warning signs of stress in your life is an important first step in stress management. Your emotions, behaviors, and physical health may all give you clues that negative stress is starting to take a toll. Frustration, irritability, and depression are common emotional signs of distress. Withdrawing from friends, grinding your teeth, and forgetting details are behaviors that may warn you of negative stress. Headaches, upset stomach, and fatigue are health indicators that you may have too much stress in your life.

You can learn to read your body's stress signals through biofeedback. **Biofeedback** is a technique of focusing on involuntary bodily processes in order to control them. Using biofeedback involves being aware of such conditions as your breath and pulse rates. Hard breathing or a rapid pulse rate may be a sign of distress. When you realize you are breathing hard or your pulse is racing, you will know you may be under stress. Then you can make a conscious effort to relax and bring your breathing and pulse back to normal levels. Through biofeedback, you may be able to avoid a headache or calm a nervous stomach caused by stress.

When you become aware that you are experiencing stress symptoms, try to determine what is causing them. Then you can take steps to either deal with or eliminate the source of the stressors.

If signs of stress occur on a regular basis, you may need to increase your stress management efforts. This will help you avoid the harmful effects of stress.

Use Support Systems

You need to identify people who can be part of your support system in times of stress or crisis. A **support system** is a person or group of people who can provide you with help and emotional comfort. Family members and friends can listen and offer insights to problems. School counselors, social workers, and psychologists can give their professional opinions about how to deal with stressful situations.

You must be willing to turn to these people when you are feeling overwhelmed. Your support system cannot help you if you do not access it, **18-9**.

Remember that you are part of other people's support systems. In this role, you can support people who are under stress by being a good listener. You may need to encourage others to talk about situations that are bothering them. If they are not ready to talk, do not pressure them. If they want to talk, however, be ready to listen attentively. Maintain eye contact and do not inter-rupt. Avoid offering advice unless someone asks you for it. Many times, people are not looking for advice. They simply want someone to listen to and understand their problems.

You may sometimes need to seek the help of an adult on your friend's behalf. Someone who mentions suicide is at great risk. Someone who talks about drinking or getting high to handle stress may also need professional help.

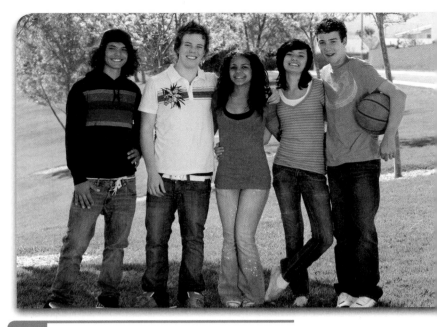

18-9 Friends can give support and comfort during times of stress.

Parents, teachers, guidance counselors, and members of the clergy can provide assistance when a friend is in potential danger.

Learn How to Relax

Learning how to play and see the joys of living will help relieve stress. Set aside time to enjoy leisure activities with your friends and family. Different people find different activities relaxing. For you, leisure may be listening to music, reading a book, or enjoying your favorite hobby. For someone else, playing sports or working out may be more relaxing. Learn to know when you need to take a break from work and other demands.

Relaxation Techniques

Besides enjoyable activities, you can use some techniques to help you relax when you begin to feel excess stress, **18-10**. One of these techniques is deep breathing. This involves pulling slow, regular breaths deep into the lungs.

Stress and Tension-Fighting Exercises

- Close your eyes and concentrate on breathing slowly. Imagine you are going down stairs in a 15-story building. Each time you exhale, you have reached a lower floor. When you reach ground level, resume normal activities by inhaling and counting to three.

- Close your eyes. Think of a beautiful scene and imagine you are there. Is it your last vacation spot or a favorite spot in your home? Spend a moment looking and enjoying every detail. Listen to the sounds. Can you smell the good smells?

- Sit up straight. Let your chin fall to your neck as you exhale. Inhale and move your head back slowly. Pretend you are trying to touch the back of your neck with your head. Then pull your shoulders up and try to touch them with your ears. Release your muscles and relax. Do your neck and back muscles feel relaxed?

- Take a deep breath. As you do, scan your body for tense muscles. Check out each group: face, neck, shoulders, arms, abdomen, legs, and feet. Seek out the tense ones. As you exhale, relax all that are tense.

18-10   These relaxation exercises are easy to do, even in public places such as a classroom.

Then you release each breath in a long, controlled exhale. Deep breathing calms the whole body. It forces you to slow down and focus on something other than stressors. You can use this breathing technique almost anywhere. You might be driving in heavy traffic, standing in a long line, or sitting in class before a test. A few minutes of deep breathing in any of these situations can help you feel more relaxed.

Another technique sometimes used to reduce stress is **progressive muscle relaxation**. This method involves slowly tensing and then relaxing different groups of muscles. Begin with your feet. Then gradually work your way up the body to your legs, midsection, hands, arms, shoulders, neck, and face. Tense each muscle group, hold for five seconds, then release. Try to clear your mind of all thoughts, focusing only on your muscle groups. As you release the tension in your muscles, you will also be releasing stress. This technique will probably work best in a setting where you can be alone for a few minutes. You may find listening to quiet music while you perform this technique helps you relax further.

Use Positive Self-Talk

Self-talk refers to your internal conversations about yourself and the situations you face. Unfortunately, self-talk for many people is filled with negative statements, such as "I'm stupid. I'll never be able to figure out how to solve this problem." This type of self-talk is harmful. It drains your emotional energy and produces stress. You begin to feel awful because you tell yourself how incompetent you are.

Positive self-talk, on the other hand, is beneficial and helps reduce stress, **18-11**.

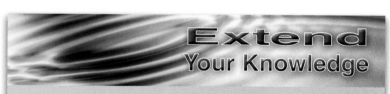

Extend Your Knowledge

Stress Reduction

Talk to a counseling psychologist or therapist to learn what stress reduction techniques they recommend for their clients. Teach your classmates two ways to reduce stress while taking an hour-long exam. What techniques can be used to feel more relaxed when giving a speech to a group?

Positive Self-Talk	
Instead of saying...	**Try saying...**
• Everything I do must be perfect.	• I will do the best I can.
• If I want it done right, I must do it myself.	• I can delegate tasks to others.
• My life is running me.	• I can take control of my life.
• I must not fail.	• I will try my best.
• I feel life is treating me unfairly.	• I will get through hard times—better days are ahead.

18-11 Try using positive self-talk to relieve stress.

This type of self-talk is filled with statements such as "I'm as smart as the next person. If I take my time, I'm sure I'll be able to figure out how to solve this problem." As you substitute positive statements for negative ones in your self-talk, you will build your confidence. When you feel positive about your abilities, you can more effectively deal with life's stressors.

a paper to write, and an after-school job. Having too little time to handle all the tasks you need to do can produce stress.

The overwhelming feeling of facing a number of tasks can be paralyzing. You may not know where to begin. You might feel there is no point in starting work because you will never be able to

Preventing Stress

Perhaps the best stress management technique is to prevent stress from occurring in the first place. You cannot stop all sources of stress. However, addressing the root causes of stress can go a long way toward improving your overall well-being. Root causes include lack of time, physical illness, fatigue, and substance abuse. Using time wisely and staying physically fit can help you keep many situations from turning into stressors. Eating nutritiously and getting enough sleep will help you prevent stress, too.

Learn to Manage Your Time

One key cause of stress for many people is poor time management, **18-12**. Imagine you have three tests tomorrow,

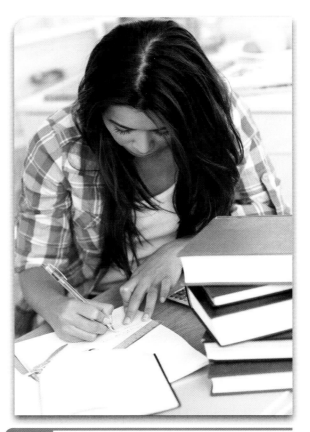

18-12 Failing to manage time effectively can be a source of stress for students.

complete everything. Overcoming your fear and taking action is the only way to eliminate this source of stress.

Using some time management strategies can help you avoid the stress of having too little time. You may want to study how you currently use your time by keeping a time-activity diary. Record how you spend the minutes of your day. Study your results.

As you review your time-activity diary, do you see periods when you could be using time more efficiently? Perhaps you could double up on some tasks, such as making a phone call while washing dishes. Maybe you could spend less time watching television or looking for misplaced items.

Use what you learn from your time-activity diary to plan a time schedule. The best way to handle important tasks is to place them on a numbered list. Keep the list in sight. Assign a priority to each one. Decide how many minutes and hours you will need to complete it. Write a schedule showing when you plan to do each task. Schedule the tasks with the highest priority first. This will give you some idea of what you can accomplish in one day. You may not have time to do everything, but using a schedule should help you do the most important tasks.

Do not forget to schedule time for leisure as well as work. Without taking time to relax, your efforts to complete tasks may become less efficient. For example, you may have trouble focusing on your studies if you become tense and tired from studying too long. Taking a short break can refresh you and help you work more effectively, **18-13**.

Realize you do not need to do everything perfectly. Also keep in mind you do not need to do every task yourself. When possible, delegate responsibilities to other people.

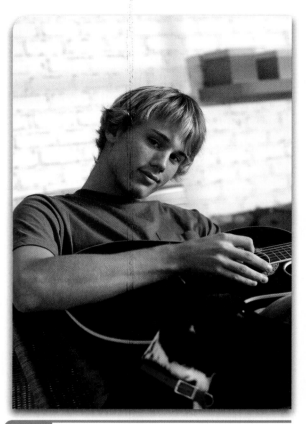

18-13 Taking short breaks during study time will help you feel more energized when you are working.

When other people request your time, examine their requests. If you have a chance to learn or do something new, you may want to accept the opportunity. This may mean giving up an existing event in your schedule. For instance, going to a book signing of your favorite author may mean skipping a movie with your friends. You may need to turn down requests that interfere with achieving higher priority goals. Avoid adding to your level of stress by overloading your schedule.

Cross items off your schedule as you accomplish them. This will give you a feeling of success. The stress of your schedule should lessen with each task you complete.

Eat a Nutritious Diet

Health problems can be a major source of stress. Therefore, steps you take to maintain good health are also steps for preventing stress. Eating a nutritious diet is one such step.

Eating right means following the recommendations of the MyPlate system on a day-to-day basis. Regularly choose the appropriate amounts of healthful, nutrient-dense foods. Limit snacks that are high in fat, sugar, and sodium. Also drink plenty of liquids to replenish body fluids and keep kidneys functioning properly.

You may have seen stress formula nutrient supplements on store shelves. Stress causes the release of hormones that trigger nerve reactions. However, a high stress level does not increase your need for nutrients involved in hormone synthesis and nerve functioning. On the other hand, if stress is prolonged, it can negatively affect your diet, exercise, and sleep. In this case, it can deplete your nutrient stores and increase your risk of disease. Unfortunately, taking vitamin and mineral supplements will not reduce your stress level. If you eat a healthful diet, you will be getting the nutrients your body needs to respond to stressful situations.

Stay Physically Fit

Staying physically fit can help you prevent stress. Your body and mind must work together to solve problems. Regular physical activity helps you stay healthy. It gives your body the strength to respond more efficiently to stressful situations. Physical activity refreshes your mind, too. It gives you the renewed energy to think more clearly about solutions to problems.

Physical activity also helps relieve stress when it occurs. You can work out frustrations and release tensions through movement. When your body is giving you signs of stress, plan an activity break. Participate in a favorite sport. Walk, swim, jog, skate, bicycle, or do some other activity. While your body is moving, your mind is less likely to be focused on your problems, **18-14**. After your activity, you may find you are able to face troubles with a clear mind and new insights.

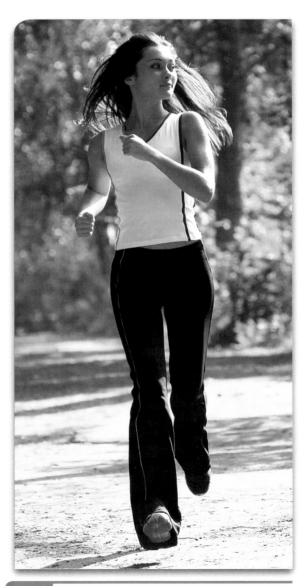

18-14 Physical activity is a positive alternative for managing stress.

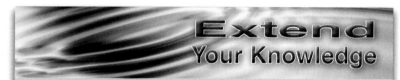

Can Medication Reduce Stress?

Ask a pharmacist or a medical professional about the name of a drug commonly prescribed to treat stress disorders. Research the literature on the drug. Is it effective? How does the drug work? Does it have side effects? Do nondrug treatments work just as well? Write a report on your findings.

Get Adequate Rest

Like staying fit and eating well, getting enough rest will help you prevent stress by guarding your health. Most people need at least seven to eight hours of sleep each night. Getting enough sleep can make you more alert, less irritable, and better able to manage stressful situations. When you have adequate sleep, you awaken feeling refreshed and ready to start your daily tasks.

Avoid Substance Abuse

Avoiding substance abuse is a key way to prevent stress. People who think alcohol and other drugs relieve stress are mistaken. These substances only temporarily mask the symptoms of stress. At the same time, they create a huge new source of stress for people who abuse them.

The use of alcohol and other drugs can cause stress by creating physical and mental health problems. Substance abuse can be a tremendous source of tension in relationships with others. It can also add to stress by increasing the possibilities of fights, accidents, and arrests.

No technique exists for preventing all sources of stress. Likewise, no strategy will instantly eliminate any stressors that creep into your life. However, being aware of stressful situations will help you take action to manage stress before it gets out of hand. Being aware of how stress can affect your health will prompt you to try to manage stress before it builds.

Reading Summary

Everyone experiences stress in their lives. Some forms of stress are negative and can harm your physical and emotional health. Other forms of stress are positive. They can motivate you and make your life exciting. The causes of stress vary from person to person. They can range from daily hassles to life-change events. The body responds to stress in three stages that each involves a number of specific reactions.

Stress can affect health in a variety of ways. Physical health outcomes include effects on the immune system as well as effects on sleep patterns and eating habits.

Effects of stress on emotional health are often exhibited as irritability and anxiety. Your reactions to stress, which are partly a factor of your personality, determine how stress will affect you.

You can take steps to manage stress. Learning to recognize your body's initial signs of stress can help you deal with stressors quickly. Using support systems, relaxation techniques, and positive self-talk can help you reduce the impact of stress.

You can prevent some sources of stress from creeping into your life. Learning to manage your time can help you avoid much stress. Staying physically fit, eating a nutritious diet, and getting adequate rest are also keys to keeping stress at bay. Avoiding substance abuse is an important stress prevention step, too.

Review Learning

1. Describe two types of situations that can cause negative stress.
2. List three life-change events and three daily hassles that are common sources of stress.
3. What are the three stages of the body's response to stress?
4. What are three internal physical reactions that occur when the body releases stress hormones?
5. How can stress affect the body's immune system?
6. How can the effects of stress on sleep patterns further add to stress?
7. What are three eating habits or emotional responses to food that can be triggered by stress?
8. What are four positive approaches toward life that may help people deal with stressors?
9. Give one example each of an emotional, behavioral, and physical sign of stress.
10. List three people who may be part of a person's support system.
11. Describe two relaxation techniques people can use when they begin to feel excess stress.
12. Which of the following is *not* a time management strategy that would help avoid stress?
    A. Delegate responsibilities.
    B. Use a time-activity diary.
    C. Prioritize tasks.
    D. Remove leisure activities from the schedule.

13. True or false. Physical activity can help a person both prevent and manage stress.
14. True or false. Taking stress formula nutrient supplements has been proven to help reduce a person's stress level.
15. Why are alcohol and drug use a poor choice for stress management?

Critical Thinking

16. **Identify cause and effect.** With a partner, create a list of positive and negative stresses that many teens face today. What are the causes of each stressful situation? What effects impact the individual as the result of each stressful event? Share your answers with the class.
17. **Assess outcomes.** Perform two of the relaxation techniques described in the chapter. Write a brief assessment stating which technique you found more effective. What were the beneficial outcomes of using this technique? Explain.

Applying Your Knowledge

18. **Stress diary.** Keep a stress diary for one day. Every time you feel stress, write down the source of the stress. At the end of the day, organize your list into two groups—stressors you can and cannot change. For each stressor you can change, jot down steps you can take to reduce the source of stress.
19. **Pair exchange.** Practice changing negative self-talk into positive self-talk. Working in pairs, list 10 common negative self-talk statements. Take turns suggesting how to turn each statement into positive self-talk.
20. **Bulletin board.** Prepare a bulletin board showing ways to manage and prevent stress. Use the Internet for more information. Use pictures to convey such concepts as relaxation, nutritious food, physical activity, hobbies, and time management.

Technology Connections

21. **Electronic presentation.** In teams, create an electronic presentation on stress-reduction strategies for freshmen to use to cope with the stressors of entering high school.
22. **Daily activity log.** Use a spreadsheet software program to create a daily activity log. Headers should include time of day, activity, and emotional state (for example, alert, flat, tired, energetic, etc.) Use your log to reflect on how you spend your time and what you value as important. Place a star in front of time-waster activities. Use this information to assess your time management.
23. **Photo essay.** Use a digital camera and desktop publishing software to create a photo essay of stress busters for use by students at your school. Identify resources for students who experience difficulty dealing with stress.

24. **Music playlist.** Create a relaxing playlist using music downloads or create and record your own restful music using open source software for recording and editing sounds. Be sure to use reliable music download sources to avoid copyright violations.

Academic Connections

25. **Math.** Prepare a pie chart showing how you spend the hours of a typical school day. The chart should illustrate the portions of the day dedicated to sleep, study, class time, exercise/sports, meals, personal needs, and recreation/leisure. Shade the areas in your chart that you would like to change by either adding more hours to that activity or subtracting hours.

26. **History.** Write a paper on the history of the identification of personality types. Find out how personality types were named. One theory, as developed by Carl Jung, states that each person is wired with different behavioral tendencies. Describe the origins of this theory. How useful is the theory today? Is it supported by current research?

27. **Writing.** Keep a personal journal of your worries and concerns. Be sure to journal at least three days a week. Include the source and reasons for the worry. After you make an entry, reflect on your level of stress. Do you find that writing down your concerns is helpful for reducing your stress and anxiety? After a few weeks of journaling, review your entries. Can you detect any patterns or gain insights about your sources of stress?

28. **Language arts.** Interview your parents, guardians, or grandparents to learn more about their stressors in life. Find out what techniques they use to manage stress. List commonly mentioned adult stressors. As a class, generate a list of stress-management strategies adults and older adults use. Evaluate each strategy to determine if it is healthy.

Workplace Applications

Taking Initiative

Imagine it's five years in the future and you are starting your first full-time job. Your new employer is a digital media developer, and you know the work is fast-paced and demanding. You've watched some family members and friends suffer the effects of workplace stress on their health and wellness over the years. Your goal is to maintain health and wellness by developing a plan for handling workplace stress. Investigate and evaluate the resources on the National Institute for Occupational Safety and Health link on the Centers for Disease Control Web site. Then write your plan for preventing job stress.

Chapter 19

Drug and Supplement Use and Your Health

Reading for Meaning

Read the list of terms at the beginning of the chapter. On a separate sheet of paper, write what you think each term means. Then look up the term in the glossary and write the textbook definition.

Concept Organizer

Use the fishbone diagram to outline types of misused and abused drugs. Add details as needed.

Drug Misuse and Abuse

Terms to Know

drug
medicine
ergogenic aids
prescription drug
side effect
over-the-counter (OTC) drug
generic drug
food-drug interaction
drug misuse
drug abuse
illegal drug
addiction
withdrawal
psychoactive drug
stimulant
amphetamine
tolerance
overdose
secondhand smoke
smokeless tobacco
depressant
cirrhosis
alcoholism
inhalant
narcotic
opiate
hallucinogen
designer drug
anabolic steroid

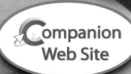

Companion Web Site

- **Print out the concept organizer at g-wlearning.com.**
- **Practice key terms with crossword puzzles, matching activities, and e-flash cards at g-wlearning.com.**

Objectives

After studying this chapter, you will be able to

- **explain** appropriate uses of drugs as medicine.
- **distinguish** between drug misuse and drug abuse.
- **identify** health risks associated with the abuse of stimulants, depressants, and hallucinogens.
- **summarize** the possible consequences of the use of drugs and dietary supplements to enhance physical performance.
- **suggest** ways to offer help for someone with a substance abuse problem.

Central Ideas

- The use of any drugs can have both positive and negative effects on total wellness.
- Misuse and abuse of drugs can cause damage to the body and possibly death.

More drugs, medicines, dietary supplements, and ergogenic aids are available today than ever before. A **drug** is any substance other than food or water that changes the way the body or mind operates. A **medicine** is a drug used to treat an ailment or improve a disabling condition. **Ergogenic aids** are any substances designed to enhance strength and endurance. They are promoted as performance enhancers that provide a competitive edge. Ergogenic aids can be a drug, dietary supplement, or piece of equipment.

Taking unnecessary drugs and high doses of dietary supplements or other performance aids often adds health risks, not health benefits. Misuse of drugs can have serious health consequences and cause harm, rather than enhance your chances for achieving physical power and strength.

This chapter will describe how various types of drugs and supplements can affect your health and physical performance. It will also discuss the physical, emotional, and social effects of the misuse and abuse of drugs.

Drugs Used as Medicine

Drugs used for medical reasons may be grouped according to their uses. New drugs are always being developed, and old ones are discontinued. Legal drugs are available to the consumer through prescription or as over-the-counter drugs.

Prescription Drugs

A **prescription drug** is a medicine that can only be obtained from a pharmacy with an order from a doctor, **19-1**. A physician has the training to decide which prescription drug best suits the needs of a patient.

When a doctor prescribes medicine for you, you need to be sure you know how to use it safely and effectively. A **side effect** is a reaction that differs from the drug's desired effect. However, it occurs alongside the desired effect. For instance, many drugs that relieve the sneezing and runny nose associated with colds and allergies also cause drowsiness. Most drugs produce some side effects in some people. For most people, however, the side effects are not even noticeable.

With each prescription, pharmacists often provide an information sheet explaining what the medicine is and how it should be used.

Over-the-Counter Drugs

Over-the-counter (OTC) drugs are the drugs sold legally that do not require a physician's prescription. OTC drugs are often called nonprescription drugs. They

---

Using Prescription Drugs Safely

- Ask the physician or the pharmacist about the medicine if you are not sure what it is and how it will help you. Ask whether the prescription can be refilled without a doctor's appointment.
- Read all the instructions and follow them carefully. Do not take more or less of the drug than the physician recommends.
- Take the medicine for the prescribed period of time even if you begin to feel better.
- While taking the drug, be sure to tell your physician about any unusual symptoms you experience.
- Use only one medicine at a time unless the physician indicates otherwise. Make sure the physician knows about all other drugs you are taking, even headache remedies, cold medicine, laxatives, or other nonprescription drugs.
- Never drink alcoholic beverages when taking medicine. Find out what other foods or medicines should be avoided.
- Never take someone else's prescribed medicine.
- Safely dispose of old medicines

19-1 Follow these guidelines to use prescription drugs safely.

are generally purchased off the shelves of supermarkets, drugstores, and convenience stores. When used as directed, OTC drugs are not as strong as prescription drugs. They also pose less potential risk than prescription drugs, even when self-administered.

The Food and Drug Administration (FDA) regulates the manufacture and sale of all drugs, including OTC drugs. A drug manufacturer must provide conclusive evidence to the FDA that a drug is safe and effective for the intended use. Only then is it approved for sale.

As a consumer, you decide which OTC drug to buy to treat a health problem or ailment. Read package labels carefully when choosing these products. Avoid buying OTC products designed to relieve symptoms you do not have.

When you have questions, ask your doctor or pharmacist. After choosing a product, be sure to read all information that comes with the drug. Heed all cautions and do not take more than the recommended dosage. Using the medication incorrectly could be dangerous and may damage your health.

Generic Versus Trade-Name Drugs

Most drugs have three names—chemical, generic, and trade or brand name. The chemical drug name describes the chemical composition of a drug. The *generic drug name* is the officially accepted name of the drug. A brand or trade name is the name a manufacturer uses to promote a drug product.

When the FDA approves a new drug for sale, the manufacturer has exclusive marketing rights to it for approximately 17 years. During this period, the drug is available only under the company's brand name, **19-2**. After this time, other manufacturers can sell

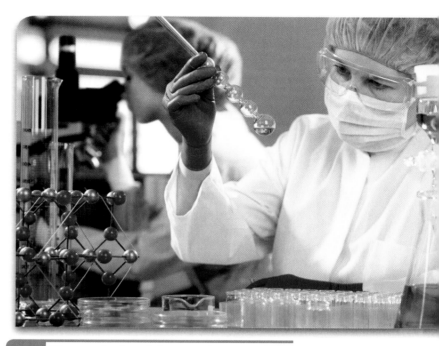

19-2 The exclusive right to a drug helps to pay for the company's enormous research and development costs.

the product under their own brand names and/or under the generic name. This is true for both prescription and OTC drugs.

A **generic drug** is a drug available under its generic name. For example, acetaminophen is the generic name for a common OTC drug. It relieves headache and pain in people sensitive to aspirin. You can buy it labeled *Tylenol*, *Anacin*, *Datril*, or any of the many other brand names currently used. You can also buy it labeled *acetaminophen*, which is the generic form of this product.

Many drug manufacturers produce a drug product in various forms, such as powder, liquid, tablets, caplets, and capsules. They often sell a product under a brand name while providing it under its generic name to pharmacies. Generic drugs contain the same active ingredients as comparable trade-name drugs. They are just as safe and effective as the brand-name products.

A company usually spends money to advertise its brand-name products. These costs are passed on to consumers. Therefore, brand-name drugs usually cost 20 to 70 percent more than generic drugs.

What the Body Does with Drugs

Like nutrients, drugs taken orally must be absorbed before they can have their intended effect on the body. Depending on the type of drug, absorption may take place in the mouth, stomach, or small intestine. As drugs are absorbed, they pass into the bloodstream. Then the blood carries them throughout the body.

The liver changes the structure of some drug chemicals to prepare them for use in the body. If the chemicals are toxic, the liver tries to convert them to less toxic substances. The liver also processes some chemicals for elimination, which usually occurs via the kidneys through the urine.

The body does not act on every chemical in the same way. Some chemicals may not be absorbed at all. Others may be absorbed, but not reduced to usable forms. The way the body uses the chemicals from drugs depends on many factors. These include the person's age, health status, use of other drugs, such as dietary supplements, and diet. The timing and content of meals also affect the body's use of drugs. Genetics play a role in drug utilization, too.

Food and Drug Interactions

Drugs, dietary supplements, and food can have physical and chemical effects on each other. These effects are called **food-drug interactions**. A food and a drug may affect the body differently when consumed together than when consumed separately. Supplements may also interact with drugs. Food-drug interactions may increase or decrease the effectiveness of a drug used for medical purposes. They may also have an effect on nutrients.

Interference with Appetite

Long-term use of some drugs can alter a person's nutritional status. One way drugs can do this is by interfering with appetite.

For instance, cancer treatment drugs often cause nausea, vomiting, diarrhea, and an altered sense of taste. Someone who is in a weakened state of health needs a full supply of nutrients to promote healing. This is why offering nutritious, appealing foods that stimulate a patient's appetite is an important aspect of health care.

Interference with Absorption

The most common interaction between foods and drugs is an interference with absorption. Pills and capsules need to dissolve before they release chemicals into the rest of the body. The amount and type of liquid consumed with drugs can affect how fast they dissolve and are absorbed.

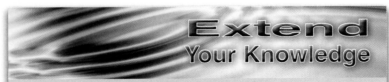

Extend Your Knowledge

Brand-Name Versus Generic Drugs

Interview a pharmacist to learn his or her opinion about the use of brand-name or generic drugs. When is one preferred over the other? What are the reasons? Who can make final decisions about which can be used? Report your findings to the class.

Soft drinks and fruit juices can increase the acidity levels of the mouth and stomach, **19-3**. This can block the absorption of some drugs. The calcium and protein in milk can also interfere with the absorption of some drugs. Unless otherwise directed by a physician or pharmacist, you should drink plenty of water when taking medicine. Water allows most drugs to dissolve and be absorbed efficiently.

Food in the stomach slows the absorption of many drugs. For some drugs, this is desirable because it allows the chemicals to reach the body more gradually. For other drugs, slowed absorption is undesirable because it reduces their effectiveness. This is why it is important to read and follow information about taking drugs with food.

Just as food can interfere with drug absorption, drugs can interfere with nutrient absorption. For instance, laxatives can reduce the absorption of fat-soluble vitamins. Antacids can hinder the absorption of iron. Long-term use of antibiotics can decrease the absorption of fats, amino acids, and a number of vitamins and minerals. When the body does not absorb enough nutrients, deficiency symptoms may begin to appear.

Interference with Metabolism

Taking drugs for a long time may gradually reduce the amounts of some nutrients in the body. For instance, bacteria in the intestinal tract make vitamin K. Antibiotics taken to kill the bacteria causing an infection can kill these helpful bacteria, too. This will reduce the amount of vitamin K available in the body.

Some drugs have a diuretic effect. They cause the body to increase urine production. When the body loses fluids, it also loses some minerals. These losses can lead to nutritional problems.

The labels provide warnings of potential food and drug interactions. You should consult your physician or pharmacist with any specific concerns you may have. Provide a list of all the drugs and supplements you are currently taking to let the physician decide which ones may interact negatively with each other.

Drug Misuse and Abuse

Drug misuse occurs when medicines are unintentionally used in a manner that could cause harm to the individual. Drug misuse occurs among people, especially older adults, who take several medicines daily. Sometimes they confuse *what* to take *when*. Common examples of drug misuse include the following:

- taking more or less medicine than the recommended dose

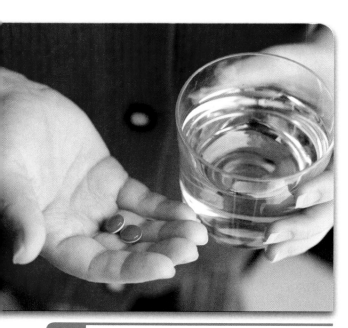

19-3 Juice and other beverages may prevent the absorption of some drugs. Drinking plenty of water is best.

- taking medicine more or less frequently per day or for longer or shorter periods than the directions state
- taking someone else's prescription medicine or sharing yours with others
- leaving medicine within children's reach, **19-4**

Misusing drugs presents a serious health risk because it may result in adverse drug reactions. Dangerous interactions can occur when various drugs are combined. One medication may increase or decrease the effectiveness of other medications. Therefore, drugs should not be taken in combination unless directed by a doctor.

Drugs should never be taken with alcohol because it alters the effects of drugs. Depending on the quantity consumed and the frequency of use, alcohol can dull or magnify a drug's

19-4 Special care must be taken to keep medicine away from children.

effects. Also, too much alcohol can damage the liver, making it less able to process certain drugs.

Drug abuse is the deliberate use of a drug or chemical substance for other than medical reasons and in such a way that the person's health or ability to function is threatened. Experimenting with drugs and their effects is one example of drug abuse.

Any type of drug can be abused. One form of serious drug abuse is teens who deliberately misuse prescription drugs. Much drug abuse occurs with the use of illegal drugs. **Illegal drugs**, also called "street drugs," are unlawful to buy or use. Many drugs fall in this category, some of which are legal when prescribed by a physician for treating patients. However, obtaining legal drugs through illegal means is against the law.

People who misuse or abuse drugs are likely to form addictions. An **addiction** is a psychological and/or physical dependence on a drug. When people stop taking an addictive drug, they are likely to go through **withdrawal**. Withdrawal symptoms vary from person to person. Symptoms also depend on how long and how much of the drug has been consumed. Withdrawal usually includes one or more symptoms such as irritability, nervousness, sleeplessness, nausea, vomiting, trembling, and cramps. To avoid forming dependencies, patients must carefully follow their doctors' directions when taking drugs that can be addictive.

The most commonly misused and abused drugs are psychoactive drugs. **Psychoactive drugs** affect the central nervous system. They interfere with normal brain activity and can affect moods and feelings. Psychoactive drugs can serve beneficial purposes when administered according to accepted medical use. However, a few psychoactive drugs have no known medical benefits or are too unsafe to use. Psychoactive drugs include stimulants, depressants, and hallucinogens.

Stimulants

Stimulants are a kind of psychoactive drug that speeds up the nervous system. They produce feelings of keen alertness and boundless energy. Stimulants have a number of effects on the body. They increase heart rate, blood pressure, and breathing rate. They can also affect appetite and cause headaches, dizziness, and insomnia. Many coffees, colas, and teas contain caffeine, a mild stimulant. Other well-known stimulants include amphetamines, cocaine, and nicotine.

Caffeine

Caffeine is a mild stimulant drug that occurs naturally in the leaves, seeds, or fruits of more than 60 plants. It is found in coffee, tea, cola drinks, and cocoa products. Caffeine is often used in OTC and prescription drugs. Be sure to check drug labels for caffeine in the list of active ingredients.

Many people in the United States consume caffeine on a daily basis. A morning mug of coffee may have 100 to 200 milligrams of caffeine, **19-5**. An after-school cola may contain approximately 50 milligrams. A cup of tea at bedtime contributes about 40 milligrams, whereas cocoa provides under 20. Some popular energy drinks can contain as much as 160 milligrams or more of caffeine.

Some individuals believe caffeine improves their performance. However, the effect of caffeine can vary greatly from person to person. Caffeine

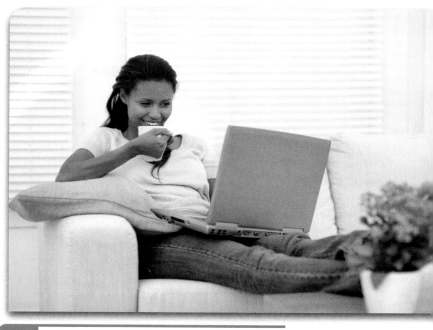

19-5 Coffee contains caffeine, a stimulant drug.

overload, or caffeine doping, is never advised as it may result in dizziness, headaches, and gastrointestinal distress. The reason caffeine is believed to improve physical performance is because it is a stimulant. The stimulant affects the central nervous system to improve mental alertness and increase focus on performance.

Caffeine affects the body in a number of ways. As with all stimulants, it increases breathing rate, heart rate, blood pressure, and the secretion of stress hormones. Too much caffeine may lead to irritability, lack of sleep, and an upset stomach. Caffeine causes diarrhea in some people. Caffeine has been the subject of much research. However, there is little proof linking caffeine to any specific diseases or health problems. As with other foods and drinks, it is wise to practice moderation with products containing caffeine. Many experts recommend limiting caffeine intake to no more than 300 milligrams per day.

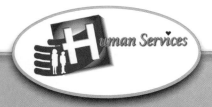

Substance Abuse Counselor

Substance abuse counselors help people who have problems with alcohol, drugs, gambling, and eating disorders. They counsel individuals to help them to identify behaviors and problems related to their addictions. Counselors are trained to assist in developing personalized recovery programs that help to establish healthy behaviors and provide coping strategies. Some counselors conduct programs and community outreach aimed at preventing addiction and educating the public.

Education: A master's degree usually is required to be licensed or certified as a counselor. Depending on the specialty, state licensure and certification requirements will vary. Fields of study for counselors may include substance abuse or addictions, rehabilitation, agency or community counseling, clinical mental health counseling, and related fields.

Job Outlook: Employment of substance abuse and behavioral disorder counselors is expected to grow much faster than the average for all occupations. As society becomes more knowledgeable about addiction, more people are seeking treatment.

To avoid the physical effects of caffeine, many people prefer to use caffeine-free products. Today, more choices of decaffeinated soft drinks, coffees, and teas are available than ever before. These products contain very little or no caffeine.

Caffeine is not an addictive drug, but it can be habit forming. People who suddenly stop drinking three or four cups of cola or coffee a day may experience withdrawal-like symptoms. These symptoms may include headaches, nausea, drowsiness, and irritability. A gradual withdrawal of caffeine will reduce these symptoms. To avoid feelings of fatigue from caffeine withdrawal, add daily exercise to your lifestyle.

Amphetamines

Amphetamines are commonly abused stimulant drugs. They are found in medicines used to treat certain sleep and attention disorders. They are also in some prescription medicines used to curb appetite for weight control.

Use of amphetamines to control weight is usually unsuccessful. The drugs only reduce appetite. They do not help dieters learn new eating behaviors. Once dieters stop using amphetamines, they usually regain weight rapidly. Also, dieters tend to build tolerance quickly to these drugs.

Amphetamines cause the same physical effects as other stimulants. They tend to increase physical performance, competitiveness, and aggression. However, side effects include sweating, poor sleep patterns, dizziness, and irregular cardiac rates. In addition, long-term use can result in malnutrition and various nutrient deficiency diseases. Amphetamine abusers sometimes report having strange visions and thoughts. Continued use can result in the development of **tolerance**. This is the ability of the body and mind to become less responsive to a drug.

When a user develops a drug tolerance, he or she must take ever larger doses to feel a drug's effects. Taking larger and more dangerous doses of a drug can lead to a drug **overdose**. This means taking an unsafe quantity of a drug. It can cause a slowdown in brain activity, coma, or even death. Use of stimulants, such as amphetamines, is banned by national and international sports associations.

Cocaine

Cocaine is a white powder made from the coca plant. The powder, often called "coke," is usually inhaled through the nose. When consumed, cocaine causes impulses that flood the brain within seconds. These chemical reactions affect appetite, sleep, and emotions. A feeling of high energy is often followed by an emotional letdown, anger, and irritability. Cocaine is illegal and highly addictive.

Crack cocaine is a newer, less expensive form of cocaine. Because crack cocaine is smoked, its effects are felt quickly, usually within seconds.

Cocaine can cause a number of nutritional and health problems related to weight loss and poor sleep patterns. Just one use can cause a heart attack or lung failure, resulting in death. Use of this stimulant is illegal.

Nicotine

Nicotine is a drug that occurs naturally in tobacco leaves. This highly addictive drug is found in cigarettes and all other tobacco products. It kills more people than all other drugs. According to the Surgeon General, more than 1,000 people in the United States die each day from smoking-related causes, **19-6**.

The Effects of Nicotine

What happens when smoke is inhaled? Nicotine first goes to the lungs and bloodstream. Within seconds, much of the nicotine has traveled through the bloodstream to the brain. Nicotine then begins to affect mood and alertness. More recent research indicates that adolescents who smoke have reduced memory and cognitive functions. This can affect school performance and sports performance. The younger the age of starting to smoke, the more of an impact there is on mental and physical performance.

Annual Deaths Attributable to Cigarette Smoking	
Cause	**Number of deaths**
Lung cancer	128,900
Other cancers	35,300
Ischemic Heart Disease	126,000
Chronic Obtrusive Pulmonary Disease	92,900
Stroke	15,900
Other diagnoses	44,000
Source: Centers for Disease Control	

19-6 Smoking is directly related to many fatal diseases.

Health Risks of Tobacco

According to estimates, each cigarette a person smokes shortens his or her life by about seven minutes. This means a person loses one day of the future for every ten packs of cigarettes he or she smokes. The main reasons for a smoker's reduced life expectancy are the effects of tobacco on the heart and lungs.

Math Link

Converting Percent to Milligrams

To qualify as decaffeinated, coffee must have at least 97% of its caffeine removed.

- If a cup of brewed coffee contains 160 mg of caffeine, what is the maximum amount of caffeine its decaffeinated version could contain? (Round answer to nearest whole milligram.)

Smoking is a major contributor to heart disease. Nicotine increases the heart rate. Carbon monoxide, a poisonous gas in cigarette smoke, decreases the amount of oxygen available in the blood. These two factors make the heart work harder. Smoking also causes blood clots to form more easily. This increases the risk of heart attack and stroke.

Tobacco smoke is the major cause of lung diseases, including lung cancer. When someone inhales smoke, irritating gases and particles slow the functioning of the lung's defense systems. Cigarette smoke can cause air passages to close up and make breathing more difficult. Cigarette smoke causes a sticky substance called *tar* to collect in the lungs. It can cause chronic swelling in the lungs, leading to coughs and bronchial infections. Lung tissue can be destroyed.

Smoking seems to increase the rate at which the body breaks down vitamin C. Nutrition researchers have found cigarette smokers need 35 milligrams more vitamin C each day than nonsmokers. Smokers must include extra sources of vitamin C in their diets to prevent deficiency.

A smoker is not the only one affected by his or her smoke. Other people inhale the smoke released into the air during smoking. This is called **secondhand smoke**. According to the American Lung Association, secondhand smoke can contain more cancer-causing compounds than the smoke inhaled by the smoker. The presence of smoke is especially harmful to infants and children. According to studies, babies of parents who smoke have a higher rate of respiratory problems than babies of nonsmokers.

Tobacco products that are not intended to be smoked, such as chewing tobacco or snuff, are called **smokeless tobacco**. These products also contain nicotine, making them addictive and harmful to health. Chewing tobacco is associated with cancer of the cheeks, gums, and throat. Some people's mouths begin to be affected within a few weeks after starting to use smokeless tobacco. Gums and lips can sting, crack, bleed, wrinkle, and develop sores and white patches.

Say No to Tobacco

Fortunately, information about the dangers of smoking has prompted many people to quit. The reasons to say no to smoking are many, **19-7**.

Anyone who smokes or uses other forms of tobacco knows that breaking the habit is not easy. Part of the dependence on nicotine is psychological. Some smokers associate smoking with relaxation, good food, and friends. Quitting smoking can be especially hard in a social network of friends who smoke.

Nicotine addiction is also physical. Common withdrawal symptoms include shakiness, anxiety, and grouchiness.

Reasons to Say No to Tobacco
• Healthier lungs, fewer colds, and less coughing and shortness of breath
• Decreased risk of blood clot formation
• Reduced cancer risk
• No nicotine addiction
• No risk of the shortened life span or premature aging of skin (especially the face) associated with smoking
• Fresher breath and whiter teeth
• Less debt (more spending money)
• No release of secondhand smoke
• Obedience to the law (regarding underage purchasers)

19-7 Can you name other reasons not to use tobacco?

Dizziness, headaches, difficulty sleeping, and changes in appetite are symptoms, too.

Some people claim they gain weight when they stop smoking. This may be partly because smoking elevates the body's basal metabolism about 10 percent. When a person quits smoking, his or her basal metabolism will drop back to normal. This accounts for a reduced energy need of about 100 calories a day. When a person is adjusting to not smoking, an extra walk or other physical activity will help control weight. Added activity will also help a smoker take his or her mind off smoking.

Making wellness a lifestyle means never starting to smoke, **19-8**. People who do smoke should quit. Programs are available to help people quit smoking. Doctors can prescribe medical aids to help the body adjust to nicotine withdrawal. Family members and friends can provide emotional support.

Former smokers must be patient and stay firm in their commitment to end the smoking habit. Withdrawal symptoms may last several months. Once a smoker has quit, it is vitally important never to

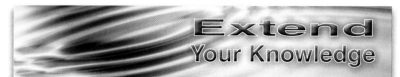

Extend Your Knowledge

Within 20 Minutes of Quitting...

Smoking causes damage to nearly every organ of the body. It causes disease and negatively impacts the health of not only smokers, but also the people in their lives. Fortunately, the human body is capable of reversing some of the negative effects of smoking. Visit the Centers for Disease Control and Prevention (CDC) Web site for *Smoking & Tobacco Use* for more information on tobacco addiction and quitting. Discover the series of changes to your body that begin "Within 20 Minutes of Quitting..."

have anything to do with tobacco again. The nicotine receptors in the brain will always be ready to respond to nicotine. Even a brief exposure to nicotine can stimulate the desire to smoke again. In time, a former smoker will realize the benefits of not smoking far outweigh any pleasures received from smoking. In addition, the financial rewards of not buying cigarettes can add up quickly.

Depressants

Depressants are drugs that decrease the activity of the central nervous system. They slow down certain body functions and reactions. Many drugs fall in this category. They can be grouped as barbiturates, tranquilizers, inhalants, and narcotics. Among the list of depressants, alcohol is the most often abused.

Alcohol

Alcohol, which is chemically called *ethanol*, is a drug. It is not a nutrient, although it supplies seven calories of energy per gram. Carbohydrates, fats,

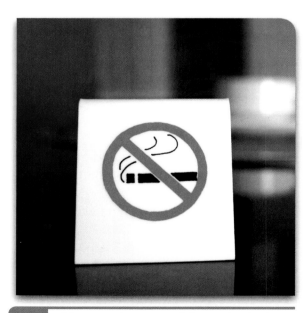

19-8   More and more public and private facilities are banning tobacco smoke.

and proteins must be digested before they are absorbed through the walls of the small intestine. Alcohol, by contrast, requires no digestion and can be absorbed through cells in the mouth and the walls of the stomach. This is what causes a person to feel the effects of alcohol so quickly. Food in the stomach helps slow the absorption of alcohol.

Alcohol in the Body

Once alcohol is absorbed, the bloodstream carries it to the liver. The liver is where alcohol metabolism occurs. The rate at which the liver can break down alcohol varies from person to person. Until alcohol is metabolized, it flows through the bloodstream, allowing it to reach and affect the brain.

In the brain, alcohol first suppresses the action of the area that controls judgment. Increased alcohol consumption affects the part of the brain that controls large muscle movements. This is why people who have consumed much alcohol begin to stagger when they walk. Loss of inhibitions, confusion, drowsiness, nausea, and vomiting are other symptoms. Further consumption affects the part of the brain that controls breathing and heartbeat.

The higher the level of blood alcohol, the greater is the risk to health and life. As blood alcohol content rises, more centers of the brain shut down. Many states declare a driver "drunk" when the blood alcohol level reaches 0.08 percent. However, a driver's judgment starts becoming impaired at a blood alcohol level of 0.05 percent. Use of poor judgment may result in serious accidents even at this blood alcohol level, **19-9**.

If a person passes out, it means the entire consciousness section of the brain has closed off. Meanwhile, the body continues to absorb the alcohol still in the stomach. This causes the blood alcohol levels to rise even though the person has stopped drinking.

The liver can metabolize alcohol only so fast. The higher the blood alcohol concentration, the longer it will take the liver to clear the body of the drug. The liver takes about six hours to break down the alcohol contained in four drinks. Drinking coffee, exercising, and using other techniques cannot speed up this process.

A person can feel sick the day after drinking large amounts of alcohol. This condition is called a *hangover*. A person with a hangover may experience

Effects of Alcohol on Behavior	
Percent of Blood Alcohol Concentration	**Behavioral Effect**
0.00–0.05%	Slight change in feeling; decreased alertness
0.05–0.10%	Reduced social inhibitions and motor coordination; slowed reaction time; legally drunk in many states
0.10–0.15%	Unsteadiness in standing and walking; loss of peripheral (side) vision
0.15–0.30%	Staggered walk and slurred speech; impaired pain receptors
0.30% and greater	Possible shutdown of heart and lungs; complete unconsciousness; death possible

19-9   As alcohol becomes more concentrated in the blood, health risks increase.

headache, nausea, vomiting, fatigue, thirst, and irritability. Alcohol consumption can also lower blood sugar levels and increase the heart rate.

Smoking seems to intensify the symptoms of a hangover. Drinking plenty of water will help prevent dehydration. Bland foods such as gelatin, puddings, and yogurt can help relieve stomach irritation. Complex carbohydrates such as whole-grain breads and cereals can counteract the low blood sugar. However, no remedy exists for curing a hangover. A person simply must wait until his or her body has time to recuperate.

Alcohol and Sports Performance

Alcohol use and athletes do not mix. As a depressant it is not useful to enhance performance. Much evidence shows that performance is reduced when alcohol is consumed. Several reasons are identified.

- *Alcohol acts as a diuretic in the body.* This means the body loses more water than is consumed. During physical activity, dehydration can occur even sooner. Dehydration upsets the balance of electrolytes in the body's fluids and cells. Athletes may experience some loss of strength, energy, and performance. The imbalance must be corrected with intake of water and foods to replace lost minerals and fluids.
- *Alcohol impairs mental and physical reaction times.* The effect may even be noticed days after the consumption. Because of impaired lactic acid breakdown, the person will likely feel more soreness after exercise.
- *Alcohol can reduce balance and coordination.* As a result, rough or uneven surfaces can be the source of unexpected injuries.

- *Alcohol impairs the body's ability to regulate temperature.* During endurance training, people are more prone to overheat in hot temperatures and experience danger of harming extremities in cold weather.
- *Alcohol is not utilized efficiently by the body for energy production.* It contains seven calories per gram as compared to carbohydrates and protein which has four calories per gram. The extra calories can add up to unwanted weight gain.
- *Alcohol consumption can negatively affect sleep patterns and ability to concentrate during the day.* This can be a problem for days to come after a drinking event.

Women athletes experience adverse effects sooner and with greater intensity. One reason is due to the smaller size of the female body and lower volume of blood. The effects of alcohol also put them at greater risk for traffic accidents and date rape or other forms of interpersonal violence, **19-10**.

Health Risks of Alcohol Abuse

One effect of long-term alcohol abuse is vitamin deficiencies. Many vitamins are affected, including vitamins A, C, D, K, and several B vitamins. Deficiencies may occur due to a couple of factors. If many calories in the diet come from alcohol, the diet may be poor in nutrients. Alcohol in the system also reduces the body's ability to absorb and use nutrients.

Alcohol abuse over time causes a fat buildup in the liver. Fat accumulation in the liver eventually chokes off the supply of blood to liver cells. Scar tissue forms. Eventually, liver cells begin to die. This is characteristic of a liver disease called **cirrhosis**. As cells die, the liver loses its ability to work. Without the function of this vital organ, a person will die. Seventy percent of deaths from cirrhosis are related to alcohol abuse.

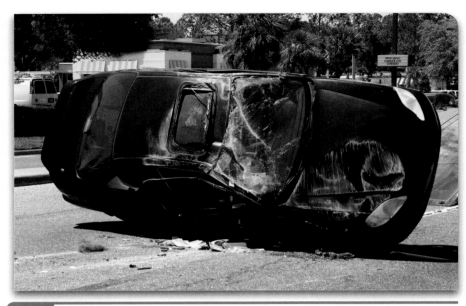

19-10 Alcohol is involved in nearly half of all vehicle accidents.

Other health risks of alcohol abuse include stomach problems, heart disease, and brain damage. Alcohol affects the immune system and the reproductive system, too. Great health risks also result from impaired judgment and slowed motor responses. These effects can lead to serious accidents.

Alcoholism

Alcoholism is an addiction to alcohol. It is fatal if left untreated. People who have this disease are called *alcoholics*. They cannot control the amount of alcohol they consume. Alcoholics do not always realize they have a disease. Many alcoholics find it hard to seek help. Close friends or family members can sometimes encourage an alcoholic to recognize he or she needs help to recover. However, few alcohol abusers seek help without facing a crisis.

One of the most successful resources for helping alcoholics recover is *Alcoholics Anonymous (AA)*. AA is a community-based program. It uses a self-help group format. This approach helps alcoholics learn to deal with its consequences and accept the fact they have a disease, **19-11**. Al-Anon and Alateen are support groups that help people who have alcoholic family members. Addresses and phone numbers for these groups can easily be found in the Yellow Pages or on the Internet.

Say No to Alcohol

Information about the dangers linked with alcohol has prompted many adults to use alcohol more responsibly. People who host parties make a point of offering nonalcoholic drinks. More people are avoiding driving if they have been drinking. Many people who drink alcohol limit their intake so they do not become drunk. They may alternate between alcohol and soft drinks. They also consume food along with alcohol to help slow alcohol's absorption.

Teens at Risk

From a wellness standpoint, the health hazards of consuming alcohol are greatest for someone who is still growing. The body is undergoing

Facts About Alcohol and Alcoholism
• Alcoholism is a disease, not a moral weakness. Alcoholism is treatable.
• More than two drinks a day doubles the chances of developing high blood pressure.
• Fifteen million Americans are allergic to the ingredients in alcoholic beverages.
• Teens and preteens are more vulnerable than adults to the toxic effects of alcohol.
• Many teenage suicides are directly related to alcohol and drug use.
• Approximately 45–60% of all fatal auto accidents are alcohol related.
• Over 50% of fire, drowning, and falling accidents are related to alcohol.

19-11 Alcohol abuse and addiction are linked to a number of health and safety risks.

many significant changes, such as hormonal alterations and brain development. Therefore, drinking alcohol is very hazardous for teens. In addition, drinking alcohol is illegal for teens. As teens begin to associate more with friends their own age and older, pressure to "fit in" with a group increases. Social acceptance is important. The effects of alcohol can quickly interfere with the ability to make correct or safe decisions. Rates of high-risk sex, sexual assault, suicide, and other dangerous behaviors increase when alcohol is consumed.

On a health level, researchers have found that exposing the brain to alcohol during the teen years may interrupt key processes of brain development. For some teens this can lead to mild cognitive difficulties and can become the source of worsening the drinking problems. There are many reasons that teens should say no to alcohol, **19-12**.

Reasons to Say No to Alcohol
• Less likely to have accidents
• Stay mentally alert
• Avoid dependency on alcohol to solve problems
• Reduce the risks of cancer
• Reduce the risk of nutritional and immune deficiencies
• Remain dependable for family and friends
• Avoid trouble with the law
• Maintain a healthy appearance
• Helps avoid liver disease
• Avoid dealing with hangovers
• Saves money

19-12 There are many reasons for saying no to alcohol. Can you think of others?

Barbiturates and Tranquilizers

Two groups of depressants are barbiturates and tranquilizers. *Barbiturates* create a feeling of drowsiness. Doctors may prescribe them for people who have trouble sleeping. *Tranquilizers* can calm emotions and relax muscles. Doctors may prescribe them for people who are feeling overly anxious or having muscle pain. Both of these groups of drugs can be addictive.

People who are taking barbiturates or tranquilizers must avoid drinking alcohol. The chemicals in the drugs and alcohol each intensify the effects of the other. The mixture can be deadly.

Inhalants

Inhalants are substances that are inhaled for their mind-numbing effects. Products used as inhalants include glue, spray paints, aerosols, and some petroleum products. People who abuse inhalants deeply breathe in their fumes. Inhalants can produce dizziness, confusion, and unconsciousness.

Abusing inhalants is very dangerous to health. Risks include a rapid increase in heart rate. Deeply breathing some substances can cause irreversible damage to lungs. Some inhalant abusers have also seen frightening visions and suffered permanent brain damage. Death from heart failure or suffocation is possible even with first-time inhalant use, **19-13**.

Narcotics

Narcotics are drugs that bring on sleep, relieve pain, and dull the senses. Some narcotics are made in the laboratory. Most, however, are made from the opium poppy and are called **opiates**. The opiates include codeine, morphine, opium, and heroin.

Some opiates are used medically to help people who are suffering from pain and discomfort. For example, codeine is used to control coughing. Cough medications are allowed to contain small amounts of this drug. Morphine, used to ease pain, is available only with a doctor's prescription. Doctors and pharmacists carefully monitor the availability and use of these drugs because they can cause addictions quickly.

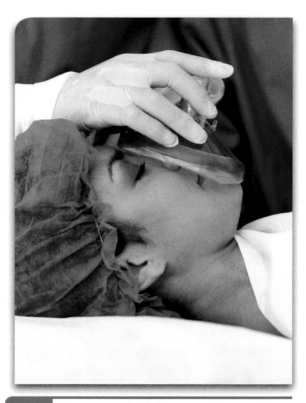

19-13 The powerful inhalant given to patients before surgery numbs all sense of pain. It is an example of a beneficial inhalant.

Heroin is the most addictive and dangerous narcotic known today. It is illegal in the United States, even for medical use. Heroin is illegal in most other countries, too.

Hallucinogens

Drugs that cause the mind to create images that do not really exist are called **hallucinogens**. The images the mind creates are called *hallucinations*. They may involve sounds and smells as well as visual images.

Users of hallucinogens cannot predict what effects the drugs will have from one time to the next. Some effects can be terrifying; some can be long lasting. Hallucinogens include marijuana, Ecstasy, LSD, PCP, and designer drugs. Use of street drugs is prohibited in sports.

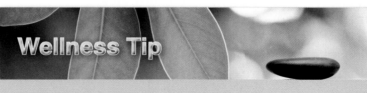

Wellness Tip

Ask a Pharmacist

Before taking any prescription drugs, ask your pharmacist for the package insert that addresses information on potential food-drug interactions. Ask whether you can take the medication with other drugs or whether you should avoid certain foods or beverages.

Marijuana

Large doses of marijuana can produce hallucinations. *Marijuana* is an illegal drug that comes from the cannabis plant. It is usually smoked and often referred to as "pot" or "grass." Marijuana contains over 400 chemicals. The effects of all these chemicals on the body are not fully known.

THC is the chief mood-altering ingredient in marijuana. It passes rapidly from the bloodstream into the brain. THC is fat-soluble and is attracted to the body's fatty tissues, where it can be stored for long periods. It takes about four weeks to rid the body of the THC from one marijuana cigarette.

Effects of Marijuana

Marijuana users cannot predict what the drug's effects will be. Purity levels of the drug may vary. Other substances may also be added to marijuana. These substances can alter the drug's effects.

Short-term effects of marijuana include apathy, mood swings, and a loss of concentration. Memory and coordination can also be affected. Someone who has used marijuana may feel its effects for only an hour or two. However, his or her judgment may be impaired for four or more hours.

Marijuana cigarettes release five times as much carbon monoxide into the lungs as tobacco cigarettes. They also release three times as much tar. These agents can damage the heart and lungs. Marijuana adversely affects the body's nervous and immune systems, too.

People who use marijuana can become psychologically dependent on it. It is common for marijuana users to experiment with more powerful drugs.

Ecstasy

Ecstasy, or MDMA (methylenedioxymethamphetamine), is produced in illegal laboratories around the world. This club drug causes both hallucinogenic and stimulant effects. Ecstasy is also known by a number of street names including "disco biscuits," "E," and "clarity."

Ecstasy is generally sold as a tablet. The tablets or capsules can be in various colors, shapes, and sizes. The drug is frequently imprinted with a design such as a butterfly, heart, star, or lightning bolt. Criminals with no education in drug manufacturing or chemistry are producing Ecstasy. The amounts and types of ingredients can vary greatly from pill to pill. Ecstasy is not a safe drug for human consumption.

Effects of Ecstasy

Ecstasy use can produce confusion, depression, sleep problems, drug craving, and severe anxiety. These problems may occur soon after taking the drug or days or weeks later. Chronic users have been identified as performing more poorly than nonusers on certain types of cognitive or memory tasks.

Using Ecstasy in combination with other drugs can increase the potential for harm to the brain. When combined with methamphetamine, the health consequences increase. Major concerns include the toxic effect on the brain and interference with the body's ability to regulate temperature. When Ecstasy is used with alcohol or other drugs, the chance of adverse health effects becomes even greater.

Ecstasy can be addictive for some people. Just under half of reported Ecstasy users meet the criteria for dependence on the drug. Withdrawal symptoms include fatigue, loss of appetite, depressed feelings, and trouble concentrating.

LSD and PCP

LSD (lysergic acid diethylamide) and *PCP* (phencyclidine) are two very powerful, illegal, and dangerous hallucinogens. They are made in illegal laboratories. LSD can cause *flashbacks*. These are hallucinations that occur long after the drug has been used. PCP has been known to produce confusion and violent behavior.

Users of both of these drugs can quickly develop tolerance. Even a single use of either drug can cause mental illness. While under the effects of these drugs, many people engage in bizarre or dangerous behaviors. A number of users have died as a result of these behaviors, **19-14**.

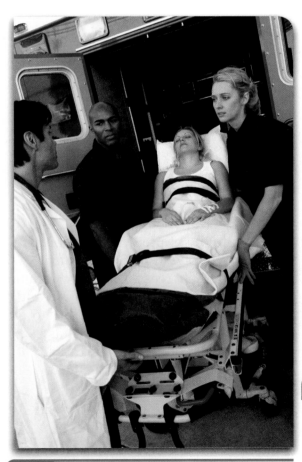

19-14 Believing that one can fly is a sensation associated with LSD use. Some users have walked off roofs and balconies under its influence.

Designer Drugs

Designer drugs are lab-created imitations of other street drugs. Most are much stronger than the drugs they are designed to imitate. When the drugs are being made in illegal laboratories, there is little concern for purity. They are never tested for contamination. These factors increase the already high risks of drug use.

Depending on the drug, effects may include confusion, depression, blurred vision, and nausea. Health risks include elevated blood pressure, rapid heart beat, seizures, and permanent brain damage.

Some designer drugs are hallucinogens. Others are classified as stimulants. Yet others are narcotics. The three categories of addictive drugs discussed in this chapter are summarized in **19-15**.

Psychoactive Drugs	
Stimulants	
Caffeine	Nicotine
Amphetamines	Designer drugs
Cocaine	
Depressants	
Alcohol	Inhalants
Barbiturates	Narcotics
Tranquilizers	Designer drugs
Hallucinogens	
Marijuana	PCP
Ecstasy	Designer drugs
LSD	

19-15 This chart lists the type of drugs that fall in the three main categories of psychoactive drugs.

Drugs, Supplements, and Athletes

Drug testing of athletes is occurring at all levels of sports. The athlete becomes disqualified for the event and may be asked to leave the team. The risk of fines and even serving jail time is possible. Of course, illegal drug use is always prohibited. However, most prescription stimulants and narcotics are banned from use, too. Also banned are diuretics and certain steroids. Most people agree sports should be a display of natural rather than chemically altered physical ability.

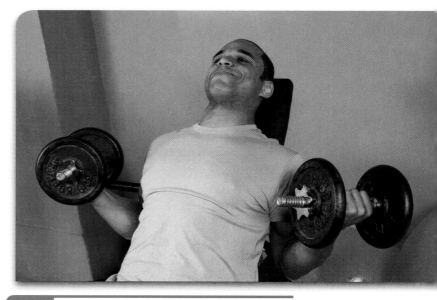

19-16 Exercise is a much better choice than anabolic steroids for building muscle.

Anabolic Steroids

Anabolic steroids are artificial hormones used to build a more muscular body. *Anabolic* means tissue-building. These steroids are a synthetic version of the male sex hormone testosterone. Both males and females have been known to use anabolic steroids to help build muscles, **19-16**. Some people use them simply to look better. Others are motivated to use the steroids because they believe the drugs will help them excel in sports.

Some anabolic steroids are prescribed by doctors for medical reasons. However, many of these steroids are made and sold illegally. Like designer drugs, steroids may be produced under unsafe conditions and contamination may occur. Some products sold as muscle-building steroids are bogus. They contain no ingredients that promote muscle growth.

As long as people want to look bigger, run faster, and be stronger, the temptation to use these ergogenic aids will exist. Before giving in to this temptation, athletes need to know the facts about the dangers of anabolic steroid use. Even brief use of the steroids can have harmful effects on a growing body, **19-17**. In people of both sexes, anabolic steroids can cause problems with acne, stunted growth, digestion, sleep, urination, weight gain, hair loss, mood swings, and unusual levels of aggression. Use of these steroids has also led to coronary artery disease, liver tumors, and death. With these dangers, it is easy to understand

Negative Effects of Using Anabolic Steroids	
For Females	**For Males**
• Deeper voice	• Greater risk of testicular or prostate cancer
• Growth of facial hair	• Enlarged breasts
• Reduced breast size	• Decreased testicle size
• Infertility	• Decreased sperm count

19-17 Some side effects from anabolic steroid use are permanent.

why so many professional athletes have spoken out strongly against anabolic steroid use.

Use of Performance Aids

How do you react to the following advertisement?

"Try the newly found secrets in **Master Muscle Builder**. *Two pills a day will enhance your muscle strength and endurance in just two weeks. The ingredients are all natural. Pay only $29.95 for a one-month supply! Buy it now to improve your looks and sports performance."*

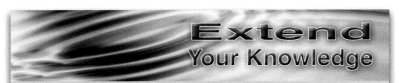

Ephedra Ban and Athletes

Once widely available in supermarkets and drugstores, the sale of supplements containing ephedra is now prohibited. Ephedra is also known as Ma huang. Historically, athletes used this drug to enhance strength, power, and endurance, and to prevent fatigue and feelings of pain. Although ephedra is a strong stimulant, evidence does not support the notion that athletic performance is enhanced. In addition, there are major safety concerns associated with the use of ephedra including resulting hypertension (high blood pressure), tachycardia, heart attack, and stroke. In 2004, the U. S. Food and Drug Administration (FDA) issued a rule prohibiting the sale of dietary supplements containing ephedrine alkaloids (ephedra). The supplements were identified as presenting an unreasonable risk of illness or injury.

The use of ephedra is banned in sports competition. Antihistamines may contain the substance and if the athlete is tested for drug use, he or she may be disqualified from the sporting event. Be sure to read the labels on antihistamines, cold, or cough medications. Research further to learn more about athletes and ephedra use. What were other reasons people used ephedra?

Does it sound too good to be true? Would you be willing to give it a try? Does the claim fit with what sports science professionals are saying? Perhaps if you really believed it worked, you would work out harder and then you would view the claim as true. The placebo effect may cause you to perform better because you believe you will. The supplement has nothing to do with the effect. There is nothing in the product that has caused the improvements, only your own determination to achieve.

Be aware of claims that sound too good to be true. Claims that rely on the testimonies of others to support an exaggerated expectation do not meet the rigors of scientific research.

A dietary supplement is an ingested product containing ingredients such as vitamins, minerals, amino acids, herbal aids, and/or other combinations of nutrients. Many sports enthusiasts call them ergogenic aids. These dietary supplements can be found in health food stores and frequently advertised in sports and fitness magazines. Some supermarkets sell these supplements.

Dietary supplements can be very expensive. In addition, these supplements do not require approval from the Food and Drug Administration (FDA) before they are sold. This differs from drugs which must be proven both safe and effective before they can be sold. If claims are made that a supplement is "unsafe," then the FDA may choose to investigate. You cannot assume that a supplement is safe simply because it is sold at the local supermarket or health store. Supplements can interact with medications. Supplement abuse may cause liver damage and even death. Most have little research to support the claims. Be sure to learn more about a dietary supplement before taking the advice of an enthusiastic coach or friend who is looking for short-cuts to "winning."

Drug testing in athletics is usually intended to check for substances that could either provide an unfair advantage over those who do not use them or contribute to problems in the individual's life. Common types of drug tests used in schools include tests for marijuana, cocaine, amphetamine/methamphetamine, opiates, PCP, and alcohol.

Getting Help for a Substance Abuse Problem

Drugs that lead to addiction create serious problems for the person who uses them. Families and friends are affected as well. Someone with a substance abuse problem needs to recognize a problem exists. A giant step toward recovery is the desire to seek help. The questions in **19-18** may help a person determine whether he or she has a problem.

Many forms of treatment are available for someone who has identified a substance abuse problem. Treatments range from inpatient therapy in treatment centers, to self-help groups. No one approach is right for everyone.

Therapy programs are offered through hospitals and clinics. If needed, clients receive medical treatment for the physical effects of substance abuse. Trained counselors help them understand the effects of substance abuse at a personal level.

For example, a drug problem for one family member creates stress for all other members. Therapy programs help clients develop the emotional tools they

Case Study: Winning at What Cost?

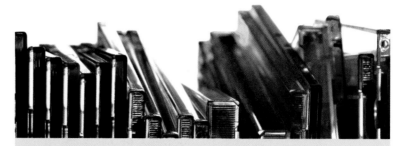

Competitive sports have a long history of tragedy and even death resulting from drug or supplement use. Some athletes are driven to win at all costs and resort to drugs or supplementation to gain an advantage over their competition. These athletes often pay a dear price for their choices. Consider the following incidents in competitive sports.

In the 1960 Olympics, cyclist Knud Jensen collapsed and died during a competitive team trial. His blood contained amphetamines and nicotinyl nitrate.

In the 1976 Olympic Games, the East German women's swim team dominated the pool. The women later discovered the "vitamins" the team doctors were giving them were actually anabolic steroids. Years later, the women and their children are suffering serious health side effects as a result.

In the 1996 Olympics, Irish swimmer Michelle Smith was excited as she won her gold medals. Later, her urine sample tested positive for whiskey, which was believed to be masking the presence of other substances. This, along with other factors, cast doubt on her success.

Track star Marion Jones won five medals in the 2000 Olympic Games. She later admitted to taking steroids and the medals were taken away.

In recent years, professional baseball has had a number of high-profile players testing positive for or admitting use of steroids or other performance-enhancing substances.

Case Review

1. Do you think performance-enhancing drugs should be allowed in the sports world?

2. Should there be a drug testing program for your school sports events?

Is There a Drug Problem?

- Do you miss school or work because of drinking or drugs?
- Does a drink or drugs help you build confidence?
- Do your friends comment about how much you drink or use drugs? Do you secretly feel angry at them?
- Do you drink or use drugs to break away from social, family, work, or school worries?
- Does a drink or other drug help you prepare for a date?
- Is finding enough money to buy alcohol or drugs a problem you are frequently facing?
- Do you choose to be friends with people who can get liquor or drugs easily?
- Do you eat very little or irregularly when you are drinking or getting high?
- Do you require more and more of the drug to get drunk or high?
- Have you ever been arrested for drunk driving or the illegal use of drugs?
- Do you get annoyed when friends or class discussions focus on the dangers of alcohol or drugs?
- Do you often think about alcohol or drugs?

19-18 Asking these questions might help a person determine if a drug problem exists.

need to stay drug free. Physicians and school counselors can refer people to therapy programs in their area.

Learning to control substance dependency can be a life-long process. Participation in self-help groups often follows other forms of treatment. These groups help people maintain drug-free lifestyles by attending regular meetings with supportive friends. Many self-help groups can be located by referring to the Yellow Pages or looking on the Internet.

Health and fitness means staying drug free and taking drugs only when needed, as directed by a health care provider, and for their intended purposes. Drug-free participation in sports protects your health and the integrity of the competition.

Reading Summary

Drug use has the potential for both positive and negative effects on wellness. When used appropriately, drugs can cure illness and save lives. However, drugs also have the potential to destroy health and even cause death. Drugs taken as medicine must be used as prescribed by a physician or as directed on the label. They contain chemicals that interact with the body in specific ways. As a consumer, you have a right to ask about the medicines you are taking.

Drugs should never be misused or abused. The most commonly misused and abused drugs are the psychoactive drugs. These include stimulants, depressants, and hallucinogens. The use of anabolic steroids by athletes is another example of drug abuse.

Body functioning and brain activity are affected in many ways by drugs. Mixing different drugs can compound the reactions. Prolonged drug use can lead to dependency and addiction. Impurities and contaminants present added dangers to illegal drugs. Some drugs are powerful enough to instantly cause brain damage, heart attack, coma, or death.

Drug testing is more common at all levels of sports. Various drugs and supplements used to enhance athletic performance can cause health problems, disqualification from competition, and worse.

Saying no to substances that may harm your health is a lifelong wellness choice. The risks to an individual's health and personal life from using these substances are enormous. People who decide to quit using them can turn to their physician or school counselor for help. The Yellow Pages or the Internet are other sources of information on drug treatment services.

Review Learning

1. Explain the difference between a drug and a medicine.
2. Why might a person choose a generic drug over a brand-name drug?
3. Explain the role of the liver in the body's use of drugs.
4. List the three basic ways in which food-drug interactions may interfere with a person's nutritional status.
5. State three examples of drug misuse.
6. True or false. Coffee and tobacco both contain stimulants.
7. What are the common health risks associated with smoking?
8. What effect can drinking alcohol have on a teen's brain?
9. How does the FDA approval process differ for dietary supplements and drugs?
10. To what sources of help may a person with a drug problem turn?

Critical Thinking

11. **Predict consequences.** Based on what you've read, predict the consequences of drugs on total wellness throughout the life span.
12. **Draw conclusions.** What conclusions can you draw about the impact of anabolic steroid use by professional athletes on teen athletes?

Applying Your Knowledge

13. **Guest speaker.** Invite a pharmacist or a representative from a pharmaceutical company to speak to the class. Ask the person to discuss how drugs are developed, approved, and marketed to the public.

14. **Supplement research.** Locate "muscle-enhancing" supplements in the health foods section of a store. Read the label to learn what claims the company makes about the product's benefits. What factors would help you decide if the claims are accurate?

15. **Poster displays.** Create poster campaign messages to inform teens about the effects of tobacco and alcohol on wellness. Request permission from your school administrator to hang the posters throughout the school.

16. **Newsletter article.** Develop a newsletter for the athletic department in your school. Inform readers about the dangers of using anabolic steroids to build muscles. Provide scientifically sound ideas for building body strength and endurance.

Technology Connections

17. **Electronic presentation.** Search the Internet to learn about the laws and procedures used by law enforcement and athletics governing bodies to prevent anabolic steroid use. Prepare an electronic presentation to share information with athletes and their coaches.

18. **Podcast review.** Search the *National Institutes of Health (NIH)* and the *Centers for Disease Control (CDC)* Web sites for podcasts related to effects of tobacco and/or alcohol on health. Listen to one or more podcasts and write a summary about what you learn. Share your findings with the class. If possible, have the class listen to the same podcast.

19. **Online video review.** Locate a video online depicting the effects of tobacco or alcohol on the brain, heart, liver, or other body systems from a reliable source. Get permission to show the video to the class.

Academic Connections

20. **Math.** Search the CDC Web site for statistics on tobacco use. Select data to compare that interests you. For example, you could compare percent of smokers by gender, by state, by year, or trends in smokeless tobacco use. Present your findings in a bar graph.

21. **Speech.** Debate the benefits and drawbacks of drug testing for high school athletics.

22. **Writing.** Write an opinion paper about whether the United States is a drug-dependent society.

23. **Social studies.** Research trends in substance abuse worldwide. Present your findings in class.

Workplace Applications

Acting Responsibly

Suppose you work in a manufacturing facility that utilizes heavy machinery. Safe actions are important to prevent employee injuries. In an effort to promote employee safety and health, the company strictly follows a random drug testing policy. One of your coworkers often bragged to you about his off-hours alcohol and drug use—the effects of which showed in his work performance. You question whether his actions were responsible, but go about your work without saying anything. After your coworker was not at work for three days, you asked your boss about him. All that your boss said was "he won't be back." You wonder if he failed his drug test. Then you begin to ask yourself, "Did I act responsibly in this situation by not talking to my boss about my coworker's behavior? Were my coworkers in danger because of these actions?" How should you handle situations such as this in the future?

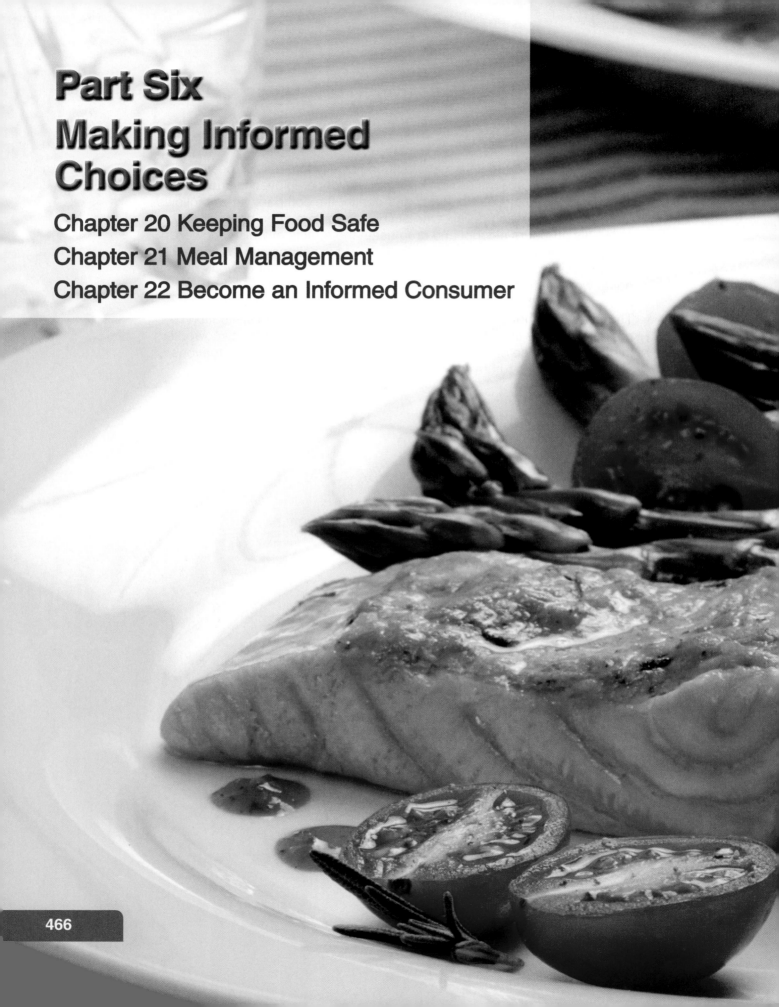

Part Six
Making Informed Choices

Poaching

Poaching is a food preparation method that uses gentle heat and liquid to cook food. This method is favored for delicate foods such as fish. The poaching liquid is often flavored to enhance the taste of the food being cooked. For example, a mixture of onions, carrots, and celery called *mirepoix* is often added. Other seasonings such as herbs, spices, vinegar, or lemon juice can be added to the poaching liquid as well. There are two ways to poach foods—shallow or deep poaching. Food is fully submerged in the liquid when using deep-poaching method. Shallow poaching uses only enough liquid to cover the food about halfway.

To poach properly, the temperature of the poaching liquid must be maintained between 160°F and 180°F. If you do not have a thermometer, use visual cues to maintain the appropriate temperature. Poaching liquid should barely move with small bubbles breaking the surface occasionally. If the poaching liquid becomes too hot, the food may disintegrate or become tough and rubbery. The fish is gently simmered until the flesh is opaque and flaky. The cooking liquid can be reduced and served as a sauce to accompany the fish.

Poaching is often used on foods such as fish, chicken, or eggs. It is a healthy cooking method because no fat is needed and the natural flavors and nutrients of the food are preserved.

Poached Salmon (6 servings)

Ingredients

- 1 tablespoon canola oil
- ⅓ cup onion, chopped
- ⅓ cup carrots, chopped
- ⅓ cup celery, chopped
- 4 cups water
- 1 lemon, sliced
- salt and pepper to taste
- 1½ pounds salmon fillets

Directions

1. In a large skillet, heat the oil and sauté the onions, carrots, and celery for 5 minutes. Add the water, lemon slices, and salt and pepper to the skillet. Let the mixture simmer for 5 additional minutes.
2. Place the salmon in liquid. Lower the heat and cook gently for about 15 minutes or until flesh is opaque and flaky. Cooking liquid should not be allowed to simmer or boil.
3. Remove salmon from the skillet carefully with a slotted spoon or spatula and serve hot.

Chapter 20

Keeping Food Safe

Concept Organizer

Use the T-chart diagram to identify the food safety responsibilities of those in the food supply chain.

Food Supply Chain Link	Safety Responsibilities
Producers	
Processors and Distributors	
Government Agencies	
Consumers	

Reading for Meaning

Use Internet resources to locate an article that relates to this chapter. Read the article and write four or more questions that you have about the article. Next, read the chapter. Based on what you read in the chapter, try to answer any of the questions you had about the article.

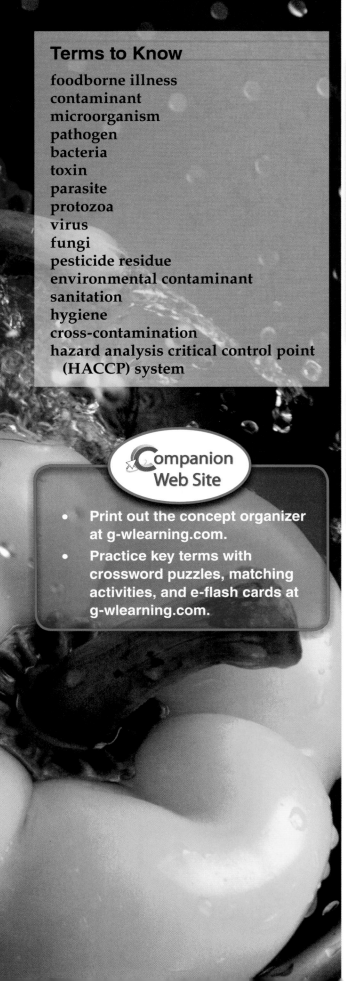

Terms to Know

foodborne illness
contaminant
microorganism
pathogen
bacteria
toxin
parasite
protozoa
virus
fungi
pesticide residue
environmental contaminant
sanitation
hygiene
cross-contamination
hazard analysis critical control point
   (HACCP) system

Companion Web Site

- **Print out the concept organizer at g-wlearning.com.**
- **Practice key terms with crossword puzzles, matching activities, and e-flash cards at g-wlearning.com.**

Objectives

After studying this chapter, you will be able to

- **identify** the common causes of food contamination.
- **practice** preventive measures when shopping for, storing, and preparing food to avoid foodborne illness.
- **identify** groups that are most at risk for foodborne illness.
- **recognize** symptoms and treatment of foodborne illnesses.
- **compare** the roles of food producers, food processors, government agencies, and consumers in protecting the safety of the food supply.

Central Ideas

- Keeping food safe to eat is the responsibility of all people involved in the food supply chain from producers to consumers.
- Ability to recognize symptoms of foodborne illness helps you to know what steps to take for treatment.

Food safety is of national importance. People rely on a safe food supply to stay healthy and productive in their work. However, the national headlines are sometimes a reminder that our food supply could be safer. In the past, food producers and food handlers have distributed contaminated foods and consumers have gotten sick. At home, foods can be handled and stored in a manner that causes food to spoil and illness results. **Foodborne illness**, also called *food poisoning*, is a disease transmitted by food. In the United States, millions of people are affected by food-borne illness each year. However, many cases go unreported because people mistake their symptoms for stomach flu.

Foodborne illness can be avoided. This chapter will help you learn how organisms that cause foodborne illness get into food. It will also help you apply guidelines to prevent the spread of these organisms. You will read about steps to take if foodborne illness occurs. You will study about agencies that are responsible for protecting the food supply, too.

Common Food Contaminants

Foodborne illness occurs when food is contaminated. A **contaminant** is an undesirable substance that unintentionally gets into food. The most common food contaminants are **microorganisms**. These are living beings so small you can see them only under a microscope. Organisms that cause foodborne illness are called **pathogens**. The types of pathogens that contaminate food are bacteria, parasites, viruses, and fungi. Although these organisms are tiny, the diseases they cause can have big impacts on people.

Harmful Bacteria

Much foodborne illness in the United States is caused by harmful **bacteria**. These single-celled microorganisms live in soil, water, and the bodies of plants and animals. Knowing how bacteria grow and multiply can help you prevent foodborne illnesses, **20-1**.

All foods contain bacteria, but not all bacteria are harmful. Certain types of bacteria are intentionally added to foods to produce desired effects. For instance, bacteria are used to make cultured milk products, such as buttermilk and yogurt.

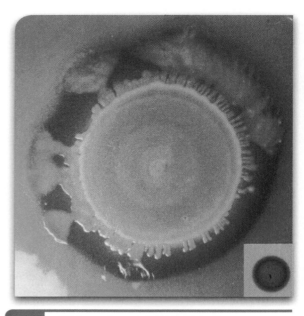

20-1   This colony of *Salmonella enteritidis* grew to just under 2½ inches in diameter in 16 hours. *(Photo by Jean Guard-Petter, ARS/USDA)*

One of the factors that causes foods to spoil is bacteria. However, foods that contain illness-causing bacteria often look, smell, and taste wholesome. Spoilage and contamination are not the same. *Spoiled* food has lost nutritional value and quality characteristics—such as flavor and texture—due to decay. *Contaminated* food has become unfit to eat due to the introduction of undesirable substances.

A number of bacteria are known to cause foodborne illness. Some bacteria cause sickness by irritating the lining of the intestines. Others produce **toxins**, or poisons, that cause illness, **20-2**.

Other Harmful Organisms

Other organisms that can cause foodborne illness include parasites, viruses, and fungi. A **parasite** is an organism that lives off another organism, called a *host*. *Trichinella* is a parasite sometimes found in raw or undercooked

Major Pathogens That Cause Foodborne Illness (Bacteria, Parasites, Viruses)

Pathogen	Methods of Transmission	Symptoms and Potential Impact
Anisakis simplex (parasite)	Raw and undercooked infected fish	Tingling in throat, coughing up worms
Campylobacter jejuni (bacteria)	Contaminated water Raw milk Raw or undercooked meat, poultry, or shellfish	Fever, headache, and muscle pain followed by diarrhea, abdominal pain, and nausea that appear 2 to 5 days after eating May spread to bloodstream and cause a serious life-threatening infection
Clostridium botulinum (bacteria)	Canned goods, improperly processed home-canned foods, luncheon meats	Bacteria produces toxin that causes double vision, inability to swallow, speech difficulty, progressive paralysis of the respiratory system that can lead to death Symptoms begin 12 to 36 hours after toxin enters the body
Clostridium perfringens (bacteria)	Food left for long periods on steam tables or at room temperature Meats, meat products, and gravy	Intense stomach cramps and diarrhea begin 8 to 22 hours after eating Complications and/or death are rare
Escherichia coli O157:H7 (One of several strains of E. coli bacterium that can cause human illness)	Undercooked beef, especially hamburger Unpasteurized milk and juice Contaminated raw fruits and vegetables, and water Person-to-person	Severe diarrhea that is often bloody; stomach cramps and vomiting; little or no fever; can begin 1 to 8 days after food is eaten Can cause acute kidney failure or even death, especially in the very young
Listeria monocytogenes (bacteria)	Contaminated hot dogs, luncheon meats, cold cuts, fermented or dry sausage, and other deli-style meat and poultry Soft cheeses and unpasteurized milk	Fever, chills, headache, stiff neck, backache, sometimes upset stomach, stomach pain and diarrhea; may take up to 3 weeks to become ill At-risk patients (including pregnant women) should seek medical advice
Noroviruses (and other caliciviruses)	Shellfish and fecally contaminated foods or water Ready-to-eat food touched by infected food workers, for example salads, sandwiches, ice, cookies, fruit	Nausea, vomiting, stomach pain, fever, muscle aches, and some headache usually appear within 1 to 2 days Diarrhea is more prevalent in adults, and vomiting is more prevalent in children

(Continued)

20-2   These pathogens can cause illnesses with symptoms of varying degrees.

20-2   *(Continued)*

Major Pathogens That Cause Foodborne Illness (Bacteria, Parasites, Viruses)		
Pathogen	**Methods of Transmission**	**Symptoms and Potential Impact**
Salmonella (over 2,300 types; bacteria)	Raw or undercooked eggs, poultry, and meat Raw milk or juice Cheese and seafood Contaminated fresh fruits and vegetables	Stomach pain, diarrhea, nausea, chills, fever, and headache usually appear 8 to 72 hours after eating A more severe illness may result if the infection spreads to the bloodstream
Staphylococcus aureus (bacteria)	Contaminated milk and cheeses Salty foods (such as ham), sliced meats Food made by hand that require no cooking; such as puddings, sandwiches Infected food workers	Nausea, vomiting, stomach cramps, and diarrhea usually occur within 30 minutes to 6 hours after eating contaminated food
Toxoplasma gondii (parasite)	Accidental ingestion of soil contaminated with cat feces on fruits and vegetables; raw or undercooked meat	Flu-like illness usually appears 5 to 23 days after eating—may last months; those with a weakened immune system may develop more serious illness Can cause problems with pregnancy, including miscarriage
Vibrio vulnificus (bacteria)	Undercooked or raw seafood, such as fish and shellfish	Diarrhea, stomach pain, and vomiting may appear within 1 to 7 days; may result in a blood infection; can result in death for those with a weakened immune system
Yersinia enterocolitica (bacteria)	Contaminated food-contact surfaces Raw milk, chitterlings (swine intestines), water, pork, other raw meats	Diarrhea, stomach pain, headache, fever, vomiting; can result in arthritis, meningitis, and inflammation of the skin for those with a weakened immune system

pork. It can cause a disease called *trichinosis*. Improved feeding conditions of hogs have made trichinosis rare in the United States today. Pork should be cooked to an internal temperature of at least 145°F (63°C) and allowed to rest for three minutes before eating. Parasites that are a more common cause of foodborne illness today are included in **Figure 20-2**.

Protozoa are single-celled animals. Some types of protozoa are parasites that can cause foodborne illness. *Entamoeba histolytica* and *Giardia lamblia* are two such protozoa. They are both found in water polluted with animal or human feces. Safe drinking water is tested and treated to destroy these and other harmful microorganisms.

A **virus** is a disease-causing agent that is the smallest type of life-form. Viruses are the chief cause of foodborne illness. A few viruses, such as *hepatitis A* and *Norwalk virus*, can be transmitted by foods. These viruses are commonly spread through ready-to-eat foods prepared by infected foodworkers. People can also contract these viruses by eating raw or under-cooked shellfish, such as oysters, clams, and mussels. Although most shellfish are safe, those taken from polluted waters may be contaminated.

Fungi are organisms that vary greatly in size and structure, and are classified as plants. Mold and yeast are two types of fungi. Molds are mainly associated with food spoilage, but can cause illness. Molds often form on foods that have been stored for extended periods after opening. Some molds produce toxins. When mold forms on liquids or soft foods, such as jelly, soft cheese, or shredded cheese, you should discard the whole food. The mold cannot be safely removed.

With hard cheese, you can cut away the moldy part and eat the rest of the cheese. Keep the knife out of the mold itself so that it doesn't touch other parts of the cheese. Cut off at least one inch around and below the moldy spot. Discard the moldy portion.

Yeasts can spoil foods quickly. Food that smells or tastes like alcohol is an indication of yeast and should be thrown away. Yeast can also cause discoloration or slime on foods.

Natural Toxins

Many plants produce substances to defend themselves against insects, birds, and animals. These substances are called *natural toxins*. Although many of these substances are not toxic to humans, others are. For instance, eating

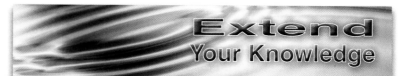

Nanotechnology and Food Safety

Nanotechnology is the understanding and control of extremely small matter that measures between 1 and 100 nanometers. A nanometer is one-billionth of a meter. One gold atom is approximately one-third nanometer in diameter.

Nanotechnology is a very young technology that many believe holds potential benefits for the food industry. Food packaging is one aspect of the food industry that might benefit with improved safety, quality, strength, and stability. Smart, or active, packaging is an example of nanotechnology's role in food quality and safety. For example, a nanolayer of aluminum is used to line many snack food packages. In the future, nanosensors may be used in packaging to detect and signal the presence of contaminants such as chemicals, bacteria, viruses, toxins, or allergens in foods. Research further to learn about the potential challenges and concerns regarding nanotechnology.

some varieties of wild berries and mushrooms can cause illness. Avoid foods that do not come from reputable food sellers.

Some types of fish, such as tuna and blue marlin, also produce a natural toxin when they begin to spoil. This toxin, *scombroid toxin*, is not destroyed by cooking. People who eat fish containing this toxin may develop symptoms of foodborne illness immediately. These symptoms last less than 24 hours.

Chemicals

Chemicals that come in contact with the food supply can be another source of foodborne illness. Some chemicals are purposely used to produce and process foods. Such chemicals include pesticides and food additives. A pesticide is a substance used to repel or destroy insects, weeds, or fungi on plant crops. Pesticides are also used to protect foods during transportation. Food additives are chemicals added to food during processing.

Pesticide residues are chemical pesticide particles left on food after it is prepared for consumption. Some consumers are concerned about the effects long-term exposure to these residues may have. Farmers must follow strict guidelines when applying pesticides. They must keep residues within legal limits. These limits are set by state and federal agencies to protect public health. Government agencies also check the food supply to be sure foods are safe.

Some chemicals unintentionally come in contact with the food supply. **Environmental contaminants** are substances released into the air or water by industrial plants. These substances eventually make their way into foods. They can build up in the body over time until they reach toxic levels.

Environmental contaminants can accumulate in fish that live in waters polluted by industrial wastes. The larger the fish, the more time it had to store toxins. Eating lean fish may help you avoid chemical toxins, which tend to be stored in fishes' fatty tissues. Some health experts caution people to eat freshwater fish no more than once a week. This helps you avoid the potential buildup of toxins, just in case contamination exists.

Helpful Microorganisms

Some microorganisms are used to change foods to create positive effects on food taste and texture. For instance, special molds are used to age some cheeses. Lactic acid bacteria are used to give yogurt its tangy taste and thick, creamy texture. One type of yeast is used as a *leavening agent*. A leavening agent is a substance used to produce a gas that causes batter or dough to rise, **20-3**.

Outwitting the Food Contaminators

Most foodborne illness is due to improper food handling. You need to use care when buying, storing, and preparing food. You must correct conditions that allow bacteria to spread and multiply. This will help you protect yourself and your family from foodborne illnesses.

Shopping with Safety in Mind

Fortunately, the food supply in the United States is one of the safest in the world. However, you still need to be on guard for possible sources of contamination.

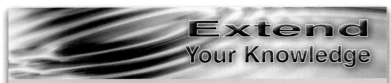

Extend Your Knowledge

What About BPA?

Bisphenol A (BPA) is a chemical that has been used in many hard plastic bottles and food and beverage cans. In recent years, concerns about its safety have been raised. The Food and Drug Administration (FDA) has supported studies to learn more about the risks of human exposure to BPA. In addition, the FDA has issued recommendations regarding BPA. Research the FDA Web site to learn what those recommendations are. What population is most likely to be affected by BPA? How can you tell if a product has BPA in it? How are manufacturers responding? Evaluate research on the topic and form an opinion. Share your findings with the class.

Bringing safe foods into your home is your first step toward outwitting the food contaminators. Begin by shopping at stores known for food safety and sanitation. **Sanitation** involves keeping everything that comes in contact with food clean to help prevent disease. Check to see if store refrigerators, shelves, and floors are clean. Poor sanitation in these areas may indicate low standards for food handling overall.

Bacteria grow most rapidly in the temperature range between 40°F and 140°F (4°C–60°C). This temperature range is called the "Danger Zone" because bacteria thrive in this range. The number of bacteria can double in as little as 20 minutes in these temperatures. For this reason, time and temperature are two important factors for keeping food safe. When shopping, care must be taken that food is transported carefully and not out of refrigeration for more than two hours. If the outside temperature is 90°F (32°C) or higher, food should be refrigerated within one hour. Frozen food quality can be maintained by transporting items in coolers or thermal bags.

Protecting yourself and others from foodborne illness begins with following a few simple tips when selecting and transporting food purchases, **20-4**.

How Does Yeast Make Bread Rise?

1. Liquid ingredients used to make bread dough are heated to a temperature that helps activate the yeast.

2. Bread is kneaded, or folded and pushed with the hands. This action helps develop an elastic protein in the dough called *gluten*.

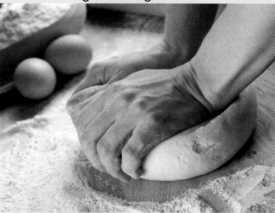

3. After kneading, the dough is allowed to rise in a warm environment, which promotes a process called *fermentation*. During this process, the yeast causes a chemical reaction that produces carbon dioxide gas.

4. After time, the carbon dioxide causes the dough to rise.

5. Physical changes to the size and shape of the dough result in a high-quality bread product that is flavorful and light in texture.

20-3 Yeast is a helpful microorganism that is used as a leavening agent to make bread rise.

Math Link

Exponential Growth of Bacteria

Lena took a piece of leftover chicken from the refrigerator to eat for her lunch. Before she could eat, Josie called needing a ride. Lena ran out the door to pick up Josie, leaving the chicken on the counter. Lena returned home two hours and forty minutes later. She knows bacteria can double in 20 minutes and wonders if the chicken was still safe to eat.

- If there were 12 bacteria on the chicken when Lena removed it from the refrigerator, how many bacteria are on the chicken now?

Tips for Buying Safe Foods

- Select foods that appear fresh and wholesome.
- Check dates on the package. Choose the freshest foods with the most time available before having to use the food.
- Do not buy food in cans that are swollen, rusted, or deeply dented.
- Check package for leaking which could be a source of contamination.
- Buy from stores that practice safe food handling.
- Research door-to-door food companies for safety and reliability before buying their food products.
- Ensure labels on meat and poultry products display the USDA inspection stamp.
- Select meats, fish, and poultry that smell fresh and have good color. Avoid any that smell of ammonia.
- Place meats, poultry, and fish in separate plastic bags to avoid cross-contamination.
- Shop for refrigerated and frozen foods last to avoid prolonged time at room temperature.
- Avoid frozen products that are covered with heavy layer of frost or have indications of thawing and refreezing.
- Take food home promptly and store properly.

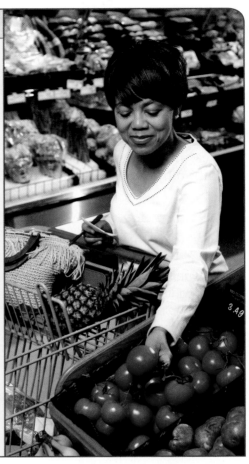

20-4   An important tip for buying safe food is to shop at food stores that appear clean and sanitary.

Storing Foods Safely

When you come home from the grocery store, put away your perishable foods first. The temperature in the refrigerator should be 40°F (4°C) or below. The freezer should be 0°F (-18°C) or lower. These cold temperatures do not kill bacteria. However, they do slow bacterial growth. Consider keeping refrigerator/freezer thermometers in your refrigerator and freezer. This can help you make sure your appliances are maintaining the correct temperatures.

Store eggs in the cartons in which you purchased them. These cartons help reduce the evaporation of moisture from the egg through the porous eggshell. Place eggs on an interior shelf of the refrigerator. The refrigerator door is not as cold as the interior.

Wrap or cover all foods for refrigerator or freezer storage. This keeps bacteria from settling on foods. It also keeps foods from dripping onto one another. Plastic or glass lids are good covers because they can be reused. However, plastic wrap and aluminum foil make fine food covers, too. They cannot be reused because they cannot easily be sanitized.

The sooner foods are chilled, the less chance there will be for bacteria to grow to unsafe numbers. Store foods in shallow containers to promote quick cooling. Arrange foods in the refrigerator in a manner that allows air to circulate freely around the containers.

Put dates on leftovers. This will help you remember how soon you must use the food, **20-5**.

Store foods that do not need refrigeration, such as dry beans, pasta, and canned goods, in a cool, dry place. Store foods away from cleaning supplies, which are likely to be toxic. Also avoid storing foods in damp areas, such as under the sink. Dampness encourages

Cold Storage Chart		
Product	**Refrigerator (40°F, 4°C)**	**Freezer (0°F, -18°C)**
Eggs		
Fresh in shell	3 weeks	Do not freeze
Hard cooked	1 week	Do not freeze well
Salads		
Egg, chicken, ham, tuna, and macaroni salads	3 to 5 days	Do not freeze well
Hot Dogs		
Opened package	1 week	1 to 2 months
Unopened package	2 weeks	1 to 2 months
Luncheon Meat		
Opened package or deli meat	3 to 5 days	1 to 2 months
Unopened package	2 weeks	1 to 2 months
Bacon and Sausage		
Bacon	7 days	1 month
Sausage, raw (chicken, turkey, pork, beef)	1 to 2 days	1 to 2 months
Hamburger and Other Ground Meats		
Hamburger, ground beef, turkey, veal, pork, lamb, and mixtures	1 to 2 days	3 to 4 months
Fresh Beef, Veal, Lamb, and Pork		
Steaks	3 to 5 days	6 to 12 months
Chops	3 to 5 days	4 to 6 months
Roasts	3 to 5 days	4 to 12 months
Fresh Poultry		
Chicken or turkey, whole	1 to 2 days	1 year
Chicken or turkey, pieces	1 to 2 days	9 months
Soups and Stews		
Vegetable or meat added	3 to 4 days	2 to 3 months
Leftovers		
Cooked meat or poultry	3 to 4 days	2 to 6 months
Chicken nuggets or patties	3 to 4 days	1 to 3 months
Pizza	3 to 4 days	1 to 2 months

Source: USDA Kitchen Companion: Your Safe Food Handbook

20-5   Temperature can have an effect on the growth of bacteria.

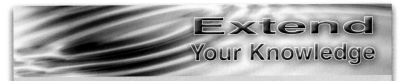

Food Safety During an Emergency

Emergencies such as power outages, flooding, or fire can place your food supply at risk. Select one of the emergencies listed and prepare guidelines for maintaining a safe supply of food and water. Check out food safety on the Homeland Security department's *Ready America* Web site. Share your guidelines with your family.

bacterial growth. Check to be sure boxes and bottles are tightly closed and plastic bags are completely sealed.

Keeping Clean in the Kitchen

Many people are unaware of basic safe food handling techniques. When working with food, one of the most important points to remember is to use good personal hygiene. **Hygiene** refers to practices that promote good health. It involves making a conscientious effort to keep dirt and germs from getting into food.

Always wash your hands with soap and warm running water for 20 seconds before beginning to work with food. Try singing "Happy Birthday" twice while you wash your hands to be sure you are spending a full 20 seconds. You need this much time to get hands thoroughly clean. Be sure to clean under your nails and around cuticles, too. Use paper towels or clean cloth towels to dry hands.

If you have any kind of cut or infection on your hand, wear gloves when preparing foods. Bacteria grow in open wounds and may contaminate the food you are preparing. Gloves should be changed whenever you move from one task to another or the gloves become contaminated. For example, if you answer the phone with your glove on, you must get a new glove before returning to food preparation.

Be sure to wash your hands when moving from one food preparation task to the next. Rewash your hands every time you touch another object such as a pet, money, refrigerator door, or unwashed utensils. Wash hands after coughing, sneezing, touching your hair, and using the bathroom, too.

Wear clean clothes or a clean apron when working with food. If you have long hair, pull it back to keep loose strands from falling into food.

You need to keep your work area clean when preparing foods. **Cross-contamination** occurs when harmful bacteria from one food are transferred to another food. This can happen when one food drips on or touches another. Cross-contamination can also happen when an object that touches a contaminated food later touches another food. For instance, suppose a knife used to

Wellness Tip

Removing Pesticide Residues

To avoid potential exposure to pesticide residues, use the following tips:

- Thoroughly wash and dry fruits and vegetables with clear water. Do not use soaps and detergents to wash food—these products leave residues, too!
- Remove outer leaves of vegetables such as cabbage and lettuce.
- Eat a moderate, nutritious diet with plenty of variety to reduce the risk of toxicity from any one food source.
- Trim fat from meat and poultry. Discard the fats and oils from broth and pan drippings since some residues from animal feed concentrate in the fatty tissue.
- Eat kidneys, liver, and other organ meats sparingly. Chemical residues from animal feeds may also be stored in these organs.

cut raw poultry is then used to cut fresh vegetables. Bacteria from the poultry can get on the knife and then be transferred to the vegetables, **20-6**.

To prevent cross-contamination, be sure to wash all utensils and surfaces thoroughly after each use. Using a bleach solution of three-fourths teaspoon bleach to a quart of water will help eliminate bacteria. Choose tools and cutting boards that are easy to clean. Plastic materials are good choices. Wooden surfaces are porous and more difficult to keep clean. Allow cutting boards to air dry rather than drying them with cloth towels, which can transmit bacteria.

Keep shelves and drawers clean. Bacteria from these surfaces can be transferred to foods by utensils and dishes. Carefully cleaning appliances is another way to avoid contamination. For example, cleaning the cutting edge of a can opener keeps it from transferring bacteria when it touches food.

Allow dishcloths and sponges to dry thoroughly. Damp cloths and sponges are breeding grounds for bacteria. Wash dishcloths and sponges often in the hot cycle of the washing machine. Replace used dishcloths and sponges frequently. They can be washed in a bleach solution or microwave wet sponges for 30 seconds to kill bacteria. To guard against fire, be sure the sponge is completely wet and place in a microwave-safe dish. Use caution when removing the sponge from the microwave as it may still be very hot.

Preparing Foods Safely

Following safety guidelines when preparing and serving food is another major part of food safety. The time food spends in the temperature "Danger Zone" is also important during food preparation and serving.

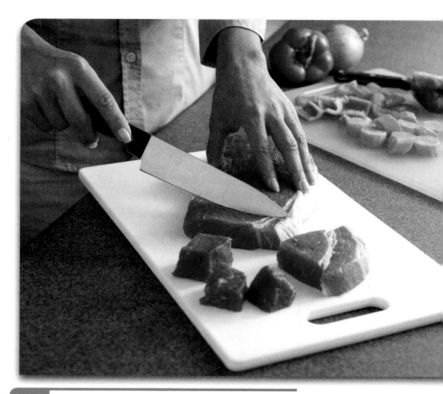

20-6   To avoid cross-contamination, use one cutting board for fresh produce and a different board for raw meat, poultry, and seafood. *(USDA/FSIS)*

Never thaw frozen meat at room temperature. Bacteria in the portions of the meat that reach room temperature will reproduce rapidly. The safest way to thaw all foods is to defrost them in the refrigerator. Another acceptable thawing technique is to place foods under cold running water. You can also use a microwave oven for quick, safe defrosting just before cooking. Follow the directions of the microwave manufacturer.

Do not eat or taste raw or partially cooked meat or poultry. Cook foods to appropriate safe minimum internal temperatures, **20-7**. Appearance alone is not a good indication of doneness. Use a thermometer to check the internal temperature. When checking temperature of meats, insert the tip of the thermometer into the thickest part of the meat, avoiding fat and bone.

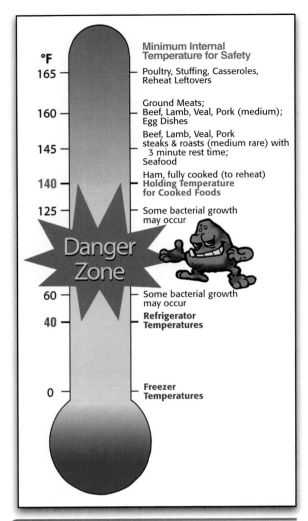

°F

Minimum Internal
Temperature for Safety

165 — Poultry, Stuffing, Casseroles, Reheat Leftovers

160 — Ground Meats; Beef, Lamb, Veal, Pork (medium); Egg Dishes

145 — Beef, Lamb, Veal, Pork steaks & roasts (medium rare) with 3 minute rest time; Seafood

140 — Ham, fully cooked (to reheat) **Holding Temperature for Cooked Foods**

125 — Some bacterial growth may occur

Danger Zone

60 — Some bacterial growth may occur

40 — **Refrigerator Temperatures**

0 — **Freezer Temperatures**

20-7   Use a thermometer to ensure foods are cooked to safe temperatures. *(USDA/FSIS)*

Eggs may be contaminated with salmonella bacteria. Therefore, avoid eating raw or undercooked eggs. Cooking eggs until whites are completely set and yolks are solid helps destroy salmonella bacteria.

Do not place cooked meat on the same plate that held uncooked meat. Bacteria from the uncooked meat can remain on the plate and contaminate the cooked meat. Brush sauces only on cooked surfaces of meat and poultry. This prevents bacteria on the surface of raw meat and poultry from getting on the basting brush and contaminating the sauce. If you want to use a marinade as a sauce for cooked meat, reserve a portion before adding raw meat.

When cooking foods in a microwave oven, be sure to follow instructions on product labels. Keep in mind microwave ovens vary in power and operating efficiency. Also remember microwave ovens often do not cook foods evenly. Some parts of a food may not reach a high enough temperature to destroy harmful microorganisms. Incidents of food poisoning have occurred because people were not cooking frozen chicken dinners to recommended temperatures. To promote uniform cooking, arrange foods evenly in covered containers. Stir or rotate foods several times during the cooking period. (Many microwave ovens come with turntables for this purpose.) Use a temperature probe or thermometer to make sure food has reached a safe internal temperature.

When serving foods, remember to limit the time the foods are held at room temperature to no more than two hours to limit bacterial growth. If possible, it is best to hold cold foods at or below 40°F (4°C) and hot foods above 140°F (60°C) during service. Refrigerate leftover foods as soon as possible.

Packing Food to Go

Some members of your family may pack lunches to take to work or school. You might need to transport a casserole to a relative's home for a holiday celebration. Perhaps you are going on a picnic with some friends. Whatever the situation, you need to take special steps to keep food safe when carrying it away from home.

When packing food to go, place all perishable items in an insulated bag or cooler, **20-8**. Be sure cold foods are frozen or well chilled before packing. For instance, you might freeze sandwiches for lunches the night before. The next day they will stay cold longer. (Freezing sandwiches with mayonnaise or fresh lettuce on them is not a good idea. Mayonnaise tends to separate and lettuce wilts during freezer storage.) Use ice packs to keep cold foods cold and safe for several hours. Try to keep foods out of the direct sun and avoid storage in a hot car. If possible, refrigerate packed food until you are ready to eat it.

You can store hot foods in a wide-mouth thermal container to keep them at safe temperatures for several hours. Rinse the container with hot water before adding the food. Food should be hot to the touch at serving time. Throw away any perishable food that does not get eaten.

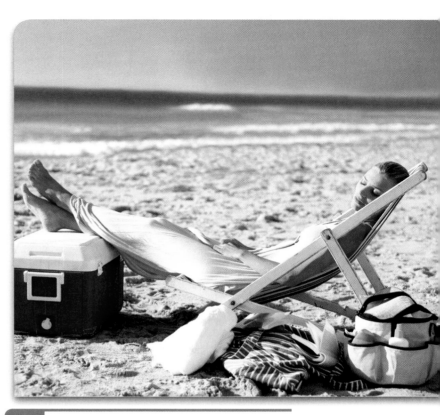

20-8   The beach can be fun and safe if cold foods are kept cold and hot foods are kept hot.

When Foodborne Illness Happens

Foodborne illnesses can affect people differently. A contaminated food eaten by two people may cause different symptoms to appear in each person. One person may become sick and the other may not. Genetic makeup may play a role in the way your body reacts to certain contaminants. Your age and state of health may also affect how you will react to foodborne contaminants.

Who Is Most at Risk?

Foodborne illness can be more serious for some groups of people than others. Infants, young children, pregnant women, older adults, substance abusers, and people with immune disorders are at the greatest

risk, **20-9**. Infants' and children's immune systems are not mature enough to easily fight a virus or buildup of harmful bacteria. A given amount of toxin poses more danger to their small bodies than to the larger bodies of adults. Pregnant women need to avoid any type of illness due to potential danger to their fetuses. Older people have lost some of their ability to fight off dangerous bacteria. Immune systems weaken as people age. In addition, stomach acid also decreases with age. Stomach acid plays an important role in reducing the number of bacteria in our intestinal tracts.

Contaminants from foods place added stress on the bodies of people who are already in poor health. People who are HIV positive or have AIDS are at a greater risk of problems from foodborne illness. People who have

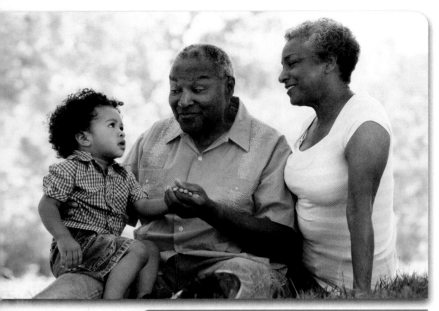

20-9 Older adults and young children are at greater risk for foodborne illness.

cancer, diabetes, or liver disease are also in more danger when foodborne illness occurs.

Recognizing the Symptoms

Foodborne illnesses produce an array of symptoms that range in severity. The most common symptoms are vomiting, stomach cramps, and diarrhea. The type and amount of bacteria in a food affects how sick a person becomes. The symptoms of most foodborne illnesses appear within a day or two after eating tainted food. However, some illnesses take up to 30 days to develop.

The symptoms of most foodborne illnesses last only a few days. A small percentage of cases lead to other illnesses. Spontaneous abortions (miscarriages), kidney failure, and arthritis have all been linked to foodborne illness. Complications caused by foodborne illnesses result in thousands of deaths each year.

Treating the Symptoms

Prevention is the best approach to foodborne illness. Do not eat any food you suspect might be contaminated. If in doubt about a food, throw it out! Dispose of it safely away from other humans and animals.

If foodborne illness does occur, you may be able to provide treatment at home. Self-treatment is appropriate when symptoms are mild and the person affected is not in a high-risk group. Replace the fluids lost through diarrhea and vomiting by drinking plenty of water. This will help prevent dehydration. Get a lot of rest. If symptoms continue for more than two or three days, call a physician.

If symptoms are severe, you should not wait to call a doctor. Severe symptoms include a high fever (101.5°F), blood in your stools, and dehydration (noticed by dizziness while standing). Diarrhea or vomiting lasting more than a few hours should be viewed as a severe symptom, too. You should also seek immediate medical advice when someone in a high-risk group presents symptoms of foodborne illness. Infants, young children, pregnant women, older adults, and chronically ill people need prompt medical care. If symptoms include double vision, inability to swallow, or difficulty speaking, you should go directly to a hospital. These symptoms suggest botulism, which is a type of foodborne illness that can be fatal without immediate treatment.

Reporting Foodborne Illness

Determining the source of foodborne illness can be hard. Symptoms may not appear until a day or two after eating contaminated food. However, if you suspect the contaminated food came from a public source, you should call your local health department. If you ate the food at a restaurant or large gathering, such as a party, you should file a report. You should also report commercial products suspected of causing illness, such as canned goods, prepared salads, or precooked meats. Information you will need to present to the local health department when you phone in your report is presented in **20-10**.

If you still have some of the suspected food, wrap it in a plastic bag. Clearly mark the bag to warn people not to eat the food. Store the bag in the refrigerator. Health officials may want to examine the food to see if a product *recall* is necessary. This means removing the product from stores and warehouses and announcing a consumer alert to the public.

People and Public Food Safety

The food supply chain includes food producers, food processors and distributors, government agencies, and consumers. A weak link at any

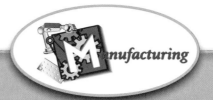

Food Inspector

Food inspectors work to ensure that your food will not make you sick. These workers monitor or audit quality standards for foods. Inspectors work to guarantee the quality of the goods their firms produce. Some jobs involve only a quick visual inspection; others require a longer, detailed one. Some firms have completely automated inspection with the help of advanced vision inspection systems using machinery installed at one or several points in the production process. Inspectors in these firms monitor the equipment, review output, and perform random product checks.

Education: Training requirements vary with the responsibilities of the inspector. For workers who perform simple "pass/fail" tests of products, a high school diploma generally is sufficient, together with limited in-house training. Training for new inspectors may cover the use of special meters, gauges, computers, and other instruments. There are some postsecondary training programs, but many employers prefer to train inspectors on the job. USDA food inspectors must have at least a bachelor's degree in food science.

Job Outlook: Employment is expected to decline slowly primarily because of the growing use of automated inspection.

Information to Report When Foodborne Illness Is Suspected
• Your name, address, and phone number
• Description of what happened: where the food was purchased, how many people ate the food, when the food was eaten
• If food is a commercial product, the manufacturer's name and address listed on the container
• On meat and poultry products, the USDA inspection stamp number for the identification of the processing plant or establishment number
• Lot or batch number, which will indicate on what day and factory shift the item was produced.

20-10 If foodborne illness is suspected and a number of people may be affected, health officials may request the above information.

point in the chain may mean the difference between safety and illness. Poorly maintained farms and unclean processing plants can introduce microorganisms into the food supply. A careless inspection or improper handling at home can also allow tainted food to reach the dining table. Everyone in the chain has a role to play in keeping food safe.

A hazard analysis critical control point (HACCP) system is used to protect the wholesomeness of the food supply. A **hazard analysis critical control point (HACCP) system** identifies the steps at which a food product, as it moves through an operation, is at risk of biological, chemical, or physical contamination. Once the steps are identified, a plan is created to minimize or eliminate the risk. A seven-step process is used to develop a HACCP plan, **20-11**. HACCP plans are used by various links in the food supply chain.

Developing a HACCP Plan

1. Analyze how foods move through the operation.
2. Identify the points (critical control points) in the process where risks to the food can be reduced or avoided.
3. Establish the limits that must be met at each step to achieve safety.
4. Establish a procedure to monitor the limits at each step.
5. Identify a corrective action to take when limits are not met.
6. Evaluate the plan regularly to make sure it works.
7. Establish a system for record keeping and documentation.

20-11   HACCP plans are used to control risk as food moves through the food supply chain.

Food Producers

Farmers who raise plants and animals for food have a duty to use chemicals carefully. They must use pesticides according to label directions. They might also explore alternatives to chemical pesticides as part of a crop management system. Farmers need to follow regulations when treating animals with medications. They must also be sure medications have cleared the animal's system before selling the animal for meat.

Food Processors and Distributors

From the farm to the grocery store, the responsibility for safe foods lies with food processors and distributors. Reputable companies know safe food is good business. To compete in the food industry, they must provide wholesome foods. Processors should not accept farm products they suspect of being tainted. They need to keep their facilities clean. Distributors must be sure food is kept at safe temperatures during shipping.

To ensure food safety, some processing companies set guidelines that exceed government standards for handling food. They may have their own inspectors in addition to government inspectors. These steps help guarantee the quality of products placed on grocery store shelves.

People who handle foods at supermarkets and restaurants also have a duty to protect public health. They must follow proper procedures to keep food wholesome.

Government Agencies

A number of federal and state agencies look after the food supply. Each agency plays a role in maintaining food safety.

U.S. Food and Drug Administration (FDA)

The FDA is in charge of ensuring the safety of all foods sold except meat, poultry, and eggs. The FDA monitors pesticide residues left on farm products. FDA inspectors check farms, food processing plants, and imported food products. They also oversee recalls of foods that have been found to be unsafe.

U.S. Department of Agriculture (USDA) and Food Safety and Inspection Service (FSIS)

The USDA and FSIS work together to monitor the safety and quality of poultry, egg, and meat products. USDA inspectors place a stamp of approval on food products that meet their standards for wholesomeness. They also check to be sure food handlers are practicing good sanitation.

Food processors may choose to have USDA inspectors judge the quality of products. A grade shield is placed on products to indicate their level of quality.

A large part of the USDA's and FSIS's efforts are geared to educating the public. They developed a safe food handling label to help consumers prepare and store foods with safety in mind, **20-12**. The USDA also maintains the Meat and Poultry Hotline to answer consumers' food safety questions.

Case Study: Contaminated Peanut Butter

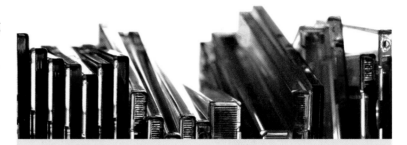

Blaine is listening to the news and hears a story about peanut butter being linked to incidents of foodborne illness across the country. ACME Peanut Butter Company sells peanut butter to food manufacturers. The news report states this company is responsible for a nationwide salmonella outbreak. Five hundred cases of illness due to salmonella have been reported. This company ships peanut butter to many manufacturers who make products with peanut butter, such as cookies, crackers, and ice cream.

Blaine is interested in learning more about the outbreak and decides to research further online. He finds out the company had received multiple citations for food safety violations from inspectors in recent years. A company manager was quoted anonymously as "having concerns about the safety of the peanut butter, but was afraid to say anything for fear of losing his job." The more Blaine reads about the situation, the angrier he gets.

Case Review

1. Which link(s) in the food supply chain failed to protect the consumers in this situation? Explain.

2. What factors might contribute to lapses in the safety of the food supply chain?

National Marine Fisheries Service (NMFS)

The NMFS has a voluntary inspection program for fish products. Fish processors can choose to have their products inspected for quality. A quality seal can be placed on the labels of fish that meet quality standards.

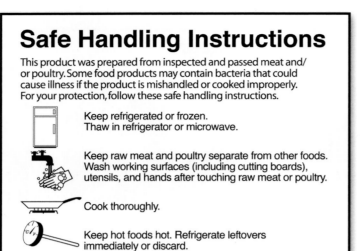

Safe Handling Instructions

This product was prepared from inspected and passed meat and/or poultry. Some food products may contain bacteria that could cause illness if the product is mishandled or cooked improperly. For your protection, follow these safe handling instructions.

Keep refrigerated or frozen. Thaw in refrigerator or microwave.

Keep raw meat and poultry separate from other foods. Wash working surfaces (including cutting boards), utensils, and hands after touching raw meat or poultry.

Cook thoroughly.

Keep hot foods hot. Refrigerate leftovers immediately or discard.

20-12 This label, which is required on raw and partially cooked meat and poultry products, helps educate consumers about safe food handling. *(USDA/FSIS)*

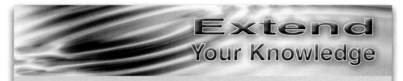

Extend Your Knowledge

Protecting the Food Supply

In 2004, Homeland Security Presidential Directive 9 established a national policy to defend the U.S. agriculture and food system against terrorist attacks, major disasters, and other emergencies. This policy charges the Secretary of Homeland Security with coordinating efforts of the USDA, FDA, EPA, Federal Bureau of Investigation (FBI), state governments, and private industry to protect the country's essential infrastructure and resources. The directive identifies responsibilities for the following:

- monitoring and surveillance systems to detect, track, and diagnose disease, pest, or poisoning agents
- collection and analysis of information regarding threats to the system
- creation of a new biological threat awareness role that incorporates and analyzes information from national as well as international sources

In 2005, an initial assessment to identify and assess weaknesses in the existing system was performed. This assessment, called the *Strategic Partnership Program Agroterrorism (SPPA) Initiative*, is required to be updated every two years.

U.S. Environmental Protection Agency (EPA)

The EPA plays a role in food safety by regulating pesticides. The EPA evaluates the safety of new pesticides and publishes directions for their safe use. It sets limits for pesticide residues and prosecutes growers who exceed these limits, too. The EPA also sets standards for water quality.

Federal Trade Commission (FTC)

The FTC's Bureau of Consumer Protection regulates food advertisements. Advertising claims must be truthful. They cannot mislead consumers about the contents or nutritional value of a product. The FTC handles complaints about a company, organization, or business practice.

State and Local Agencies

Federal agencies cannot keep the food supply safe without support. State and local government agencies help ensure the safety of food produced in their regions. State departments of agriculture set standards and inspect farms. Local health departments check food handling in grocery stores. They also inspect food service operations, such as schools, nursing homes, and restaurants.

Food Consumers

As a consumer, you are the last link in the food supply chain. The responsibility for choosing wholesome food and handling it properly ultimately lies with you. You must select foods carefully to minimize food-related risks. You must practice safe food-handling techniques to prevent foodborne illnesses. If illness occurs, you need to report it to the appropriate agencies.

Reading Summary

Foodborne illness is common in the United States. Many foodborne illnesses are caused by harmful bacteria. Parasites, viruses, and fungi in foods can cause illness, too. Natural toxins and chemicals can also contaminate foods.

You can take steps to help prevent foodborne illness. These steps begin with careful shopping to select only foods that appear wholesome. Then you need to store foods at safe temperatures. Prepare foods using safe food-handling standards in a clean kitchen environment. When packing food to eat away from home, you need to take special precautions to keep it at safe temperatures.

Despite your best efforts, members of your family may still experience foodborne illness at some point. Knowing who is most at risk and recognizing the symptoms will help you know what steps to take. You can often treat mild symptoms at home. Severe symptoms and people in high-risk groups require treatment from a physician. If you suspect the cause of foodborne illness came from a public source, you should contact local health authorities.

Many people play a role in helping keep the food supply safe. Food producers, processors, and distributors each have a duty to maintain the wholesomeness of food before it reaches consumers. Government agencies set and enforce guidelines for food safety. The final burden for preventing foodborne illness lies with you, the consumer, through safe food handling practices.

Review Learning

1. Describe the differences between bacteria that are harmful and those that are helpful.
2. What causes food to spoil?
3. How are foodborne illnesses caused by viruses commonly spread?
4. What are three steps a person can take to limit his or her intake of pesticide residues?
5. Why is the temperature range 40°F to 140°F called the "Danger Zone?"
6. When should you wash your hands during food preparation?
7. List three ways to thaw foods safely.
8. What six groups of people are most at risk when foodborne illness occurs?
9. What are the most common symptoms of foodborne illness?
10. Describe the treatment of mild symptoms of foodborne illness for someone who is not in a high-risk group.
11. What is the role of food distributors in keeping food safe?
12. How does government help ensure the consumer of a safe food supply?

Critical Thinking

13. **Identify evidence.** Read an article about a recent recall on a food product. Follow the chain of evidence in the article. Who identified the problem? What was the source of the problem? When and where did the problem initially occur? How was the problem resolved?

14. **Draw conclusions.** Suppose you and a friend went out for dinner. Your friend had a chicken sandwich and green salad and you had a well-done burger and fries. Two days later, your friend has a fever, severe headache, abdominal pain, and diarrhea but you are fine. What conclusions can you draw about your friend's symptoms?

Applying Your Knowledge

15. **Food safety posters.** Research sources for food safety information and prepare posters to place around the school cafeteria. Your target audience is both the school cafeteria staff and students who bring lunches from home.

16. **Kitchen inspection.** Find out what a health inspector looks for when he or she is making an on-site inspection of a foodservice facility. Use these points to inspect your home kitchen or the kitchen in your school foods lab.

17. **Identify food recalls.** Locate the FDA Web site where food recalls are posted. Check your kitchen for any recalled food products.

Technology Connections

18. **Web site review.** Select two Web sites that serve as food safety resources for consumers. Write a one-page review comparing each for their ease of use and quality of information.

19. **Food safety inquiry.** Prepare a food safety question. Locate the USDA automated response system called "Ask Karen." Key in your question. Share your question and the response with the class.

20. **Video PSA.** As a class, prepare a 10-question survey to measure knowledge about basic food safety. Questions should focus on guidelines for selecting, storing, preparing, and transporting food. Each student should ask one adult and one student outside the class to complete the survey. Compile your survey findings. Then video-record a public service announcement (PSA) to educate people about the food safety question that was most often answered incorrectly.

Academic Connections

21. **Science.** Use a food science text or lab manual to learn how to grow bacterial cultures. Follow the procedure to transfer bacteria from at least three kitchen surfaces to a growth medium. Observe the bacterial growth over a three-day period. Use a microscope to view the organisms. Record your observations and write a paper detailing your conclusions.

22. **Speech.** Prepare and perform a humorous skit that portrays the use of improper food safety behaviors during the preparation of a meal. Have classmates identify each unsafe behavior they observed and how it could be corrected.

23. **Science.** Traveler's diarrhea (TD) is the most common illness affecting international travelers. Research the symptoms, causes, and preventive measures for TD. Prepare an electronic presentation to share your findings with the social sciences classes or a geography club.

Workplace Applications

Using Ethical Behavior

Presume you work on the wait staff of a very busy, up-and-coming trendy restaurant. One of your customers has complained that he ordered his steak to be cooked to medium doneness but the steak he received is well-done. You return the steak to the kitchen, and pick up an appropriately cooked one for your customer. As you turn to go to the dining area, you notice the chef re-plating the well-done steak for another customer instead of throwing it away as dictated by the health department. The code states that once food has been served to someone, it cannot be served to someone else. What is the ethical way to handle this situation? Write your explanation.

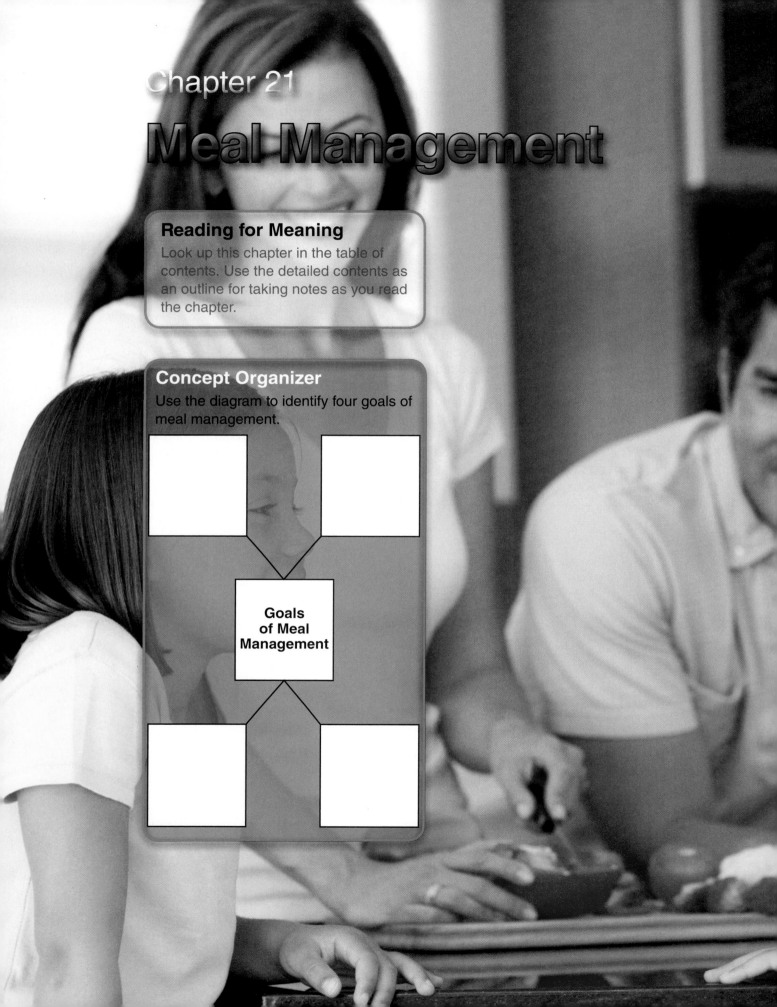

Chapter 21
Meal Management

Reading for Meaning

Look up this chapter in the table of contents. Use the detailed contents as an outline for taking notes as you read the chapter.

Concept Organizer

Use the diagram to identify four goals of meal management.

Goals
of Meal
Management

Terms to Know

meal management
reduction
budget
congregate meal
convenience food

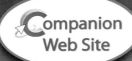

Companion Web Site

- **Print out the concept organizer at g-wlearning.com.**
- **Practice key terms with crossword puzzles, matching activities, and e-flash cards at g-wlearning.com.**

Objectives

After studying this chapter, you will be able to
- **plan** menus that include a variety of food flavors, colors, textures, shapes, sizes, and temperatures.
- **recognize** how life-cycle stage can influence food preferences.
- **plan** healthy meals to address special needs of household members.
- **identify** resources to use for planning healthy menus.
- **select** healthy ingredients and cooking methods when preparing meals.
- **implement** techniques for controlling food spending to stay within the household food budget.
- **identify** methods for saving time when preparing foods.
- **explain** how to meet meal-management goals when eating meals away from home.

Central Ideas

- Meal management involves planning meals ahead, preparing healthful meals, and saving time and money.
- Household member food preferences, factors that affect appealing meals, and the life cycle all influence effective meal management.

At mealtime, have you ever just opened the refrigerator and grabbed what was handy? Meals thrown together without planning often lack balanced nutrition and taste appeal. Meal management can help you avoid haphazard meals.

Meal management involves using resources to meet nutritional needs through food selection and preparation. As individuals and households progress through stages of the life cycle, their needs and resources change. The resources a meal manager uses include knowledge of nutrition and food safety. Food preparation skills, time, and money are meal management resources, too, **21-1**.

Lifestyle, income, health, and other factors influence nutritional needs as well as food selection and preparation during a lifetime. In this chapter, you will learn how to plan healthy meals that make wise use of the varied types of available resources. By developing meal management skills, you will begin to focus on addressing food preferences and nutritional needs. You will also discover how to stay within a spending plan while preparing meals that suit your lifestyle. You will even pick up some pointers about managing your resources and healthy options when eating meals away from home.

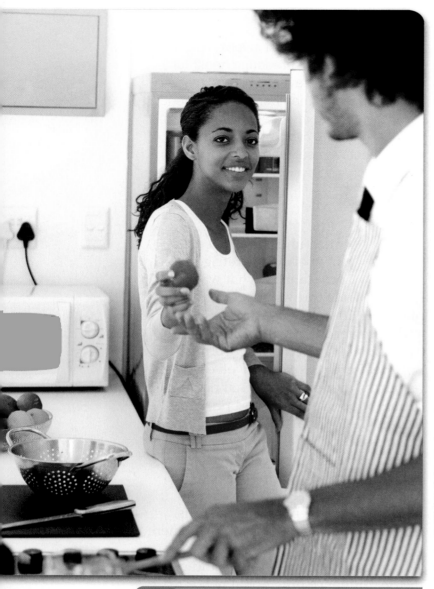

21-1 Today's lifestyles are hectic. The meal-planning process includes knowing how to prepare simple menus.

Planning for Appeal

Meal managers have found many advantages of planning meals. One advantage is being able to serve meals household members enjoy eating. A meal will not meet nutritional needs if no one will eat it. Considering individuals' likes and dislikes will help you plan a meal they will find appealing.

Besides individual preferences, you can use variety to make meals more appealing. Variety adds interest to each meal served. It also adds interest to weekly menus because the same foods are not served repeatedly. You can add variety to meals with different flavors, colors, textures, shapes and sizes, and temperatures. Keep in mind that an individual's life-cycle stage may influence his or her preference for flavors, textures, or other factors.

Flavor

You may be tempted to always include favorite foods in your meal plans. This assures you that household members will find the meals appealing. For variety, however, consider introducing new foods from time to time. Ethnic foods offer a broad range of interesting new flavors household members might enjoy. For example, you might want to try a Brazilian black bean soup or an Asian stir-fry recipe.

Keep in mind that eating habits change slowly. Household members may not like every new dish you try. Do not be discouraged. Continue to prepare tasty and attractive new foods now and then. Soon you will learn which flavor combinations generally meet with approval and which ones are usually disliked.

Flavor gives food a distinctive taste. Use a variety of flavors in your meal planning. This means more than serving different dishes throughout the week. You need to include a variety of flavors in every meal. Think about a meal with tomato juice as an appetizer, tomatoes on the salad, and tomato sauce on the pasta. So much tomato flavor would make the meal seem rather boring. Substituting marinated peppers for the appetizer and toasted almonds on the salad would introduce variety.

Make a point of balancing strongly flavored foods with those that are more subtle. For instance, you could complement a spicy burrito with some mild pinto beans. You might balance a dish of tart apple slices with a drizzle of sweet caramel topping.

When experimenting with flavor, consider the age of those who will be eating the dish. Children are often more sensitive to tastes than adults and may prefer milder flavors. Older adults or people with certain health conditions may have lost some of their sense of taste or smell. For these people, more highly seasoned foods may act to stimulate their appetites.

Color

Color appeals to the eye and stimulates appetite at all stages of the life cycle. Picture a meal of poached fish, scalloped potatoes, and steamed cabbage. These foods are all pale. Now envision how the plate would look if you top the fish with a mango and jalapeño salsa. Sprinkle the scalloped potatoes with bright red paprika. Replace the cabbage with deep green broccoli. By making a few changes, a bland-looking meal has become quite colorful, **21-2**.

Texture

Food texture refers to the properties of food that are sensed by the mouth. Texture variety makes meals more enjoyable to eat. How appealing would you find a meal of creamed turkey, mashed sweet potatoes, and applesauce? These foods all have a smooth, creamy texture. A meal that includes crunchy and chewy textures as well as soft would be more appetizing. You

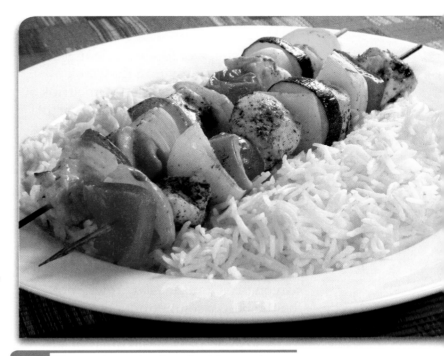

21-2 The variety of colors in this meal adds interest and makes the meal more attractive.

could introduce some different textures by changing the menu to roast turkey with mashed sweet potatoes. Then replace the applesauce with a salad of crisp apple wedges on a bed of fresh spinach.

Texture should not present a challenge to the person eating the food. Remember that children and older adults may have difficulty with certain textures. Young children may be in the process of losing baby teeth and gaining permanent teeth. Loose or missing teeth can present challenges when eating. Older individuals are more likely to have dental issues which make chewing difficult as well. They may not be able to safely eat regular textures. Softer, cut up, ground, or minced foods may be necessary. Enhancing the flavor and appearance of the texture modified foods will help improve food enjoyment.

Shape and Size

The shape of foods on your plate can affect how inviting they look. Think about a plate filled with strips of pepper steak, French fries, and carrot sticks. These foods are all in long, skinny pieces. The plate would be more appealing if you served a baked potato and sliced carrots with the pepper steak. Creating food in fun shapes is particularly appealing to children.

Also try to vary the size of food pieces. For instance, a tuna and rice casserole is made up of little pieces. Green peas and coleslaw might not be the best accompaniments for this casserole. They too are made up of little pieces. Snow peas and a salad of sliced tomatoes might complement the casserole better.

Temperature

Most people enjoy a balance of hot and cold foods in their meals. Consider a breakfast of scrambled eggs, toast, warm fruit compote, and hot chocolate. These foods are all hot. Changing the fruit compote to a chilled fruit salad and the hot chocolate to cold chocolate milk adds temperature variety.

Whatever foods are on your menu, be sure to serve them at the proper temperature. Few people enjoy lukewarm soup or milk that is barely cool. They prefer their soup to be piping hot and their milk to be icy cold, **21-3**. Besides being more appealing, foods are safer when they are served at the correct temperatures. Keep hot foods hot, above 140°F (60°C), and cold foods cold, below 40°F (5°C). This will help prevent growth of bacteria and other pathogens that can cause foodborne illness.

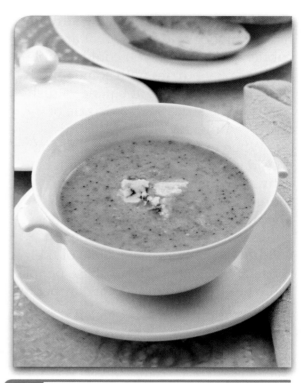

21-3 Soups such as this broccoli soup are more appealing when they are served hot.

Planning Healthy Meals

A second advantage of meal planning is that it helps meal managers provide for their household members' nutritional and health needs. Remember that no single food can provide all the needed nutrients. Serving a variety of foods is the best way to be sure household members are getting a variety of nutrients.

However, simply providing meals featuring a variety of foods does not guarantee the meals are healthy. Some household members may have special nutritional needs which make meal planning more complex. Meal planners may benefit from resources to help them in their planning. Learning to recognize healthy ingredients and cooking methods will also help them plan healthy meals.

Addressing Special Needs

You have learned everyone needs the same set of nutrients. However, the amounts of nutrients each person needs may vary. For instance, children need smaller amounts of nutrients, but they have greater proportional needs than adults. The age, sex, body size, and activity level of an individual affects his or her nutrient needs. Meal managers do not need to plan a separate menu to meet each person's needs. All household members can usually enjoy the same meal in different portion sizes.

Older adults who are living on their own may experience problems with nutrition and meal planning. This group is more likely to be at nutritional risk due to health issues. Social isolation, poor mobility, or lack of income can contribute to problems with meal planning. A few simple tips can be used to improve meal planning for older adults, **21-4**.

Factors other than age can impact an individual's nutritional needs. Sometimes one or more members of a household follow a special diet due to a health condition. A household member with high blood pressure may follow a low-sodium diet. Individuals with food allergies need to avoid certain foods. A vegetarian chooses not to include eggs or meat products in his or her diet.

Adapting meals to the special needs of individuals helps them continue to enjoy good nutrition. Meal managers must consider each of these needs when planning menus. Special resources may be needed to help meal managers with this task.

Meal Planning Tips for Older Adults
• Grocery shop with a friend and divide quantities that are too big for one person. For example, share a bunch of broccoli, bag of potatoes, or a melon.
• Cook extra and freeze to have healthy, easy meals on days when cooking is difficult.
• Keep frozen or canned vegetables, beans, and fruits on hand for quick, healthy additions to meals.
• Rinse canned vegetables under cold running water to lower their salt content. If fruit is canned in heavy syrup, drain the juice unless added calories are needed.
• Perk up bland-tasting foods with herbs, spices, and lemon juice rather than relying solely on salt or sugar.
• Set the table with a cheerful, clean cloth and flowers to make mealtime enjoyable.
• Eat regularly with someone whose company you enjoy.
• Learn about community programs in the area that serve or deliver meals to older adults.

21-4 A few tips may help older adults with meal planning.

Resources for Planning Healthy Meals

Meal managers can use a number of resources to help them meet nutritional needs of household members. The USDA nutrition Web site provides links to many excellent resources including the MyPlate food guidance system and the *Dietary Guidelines for Americans*. A meal manager may also choose to seek the advice of a registered dietitian about meeting the special needs of individuals when planning meals.

Following MyPlate can help you plan meals that provide recommended amounts of nutrients for household members. Each day's menus should provide household members with the suggested amounts from the five major food groups. As you choose foods from each group, remember to keep the *Dietary Guidelines for Americans* in mind. Following the *Guidelines* will help you control the fats, sugar, and sodium in your family's diet. At the same time, you will be selecting foods that are rich sources of vitamins, minerals, and fiber.

MyPlate "Food Planner" is a tool you can use when menu planning. It helps you make healthy food choices and compares your choices to your MyPlate food plan. You can add other household members to the "Food Planner" as well, **21-5**.

Many meal managers plan for household members to meet nutrient needs by eating three meals a day. Breakfast generally supplies about one-fourth of the day's nutrient and calorie needs. Lunch and dinner each furnish one-third of the day's needs. Healthful snacks chosen from the five food groups can provide the remaining needs. Some meal managers plan lighter meals and heartier snacks. You can choose the meal schedule that is most convenient for members of your household. The important point is they receive their full allowance of nutrients throughout the day.

Preparing Healthy Meals

Healthy meals result when healthy ingredients are prepared using healthy cooking methods. Once a meal planner can recognize healthy ingredients and cooking methods, he or she will be able to make adjustments to recipes, meals, and menus to create healthier versions.

Healthy Ingredients

To prepare a healthy meal, you must start with healthy ingredients. Luckily, healthy ingredients can be found in all the food groups and oils.

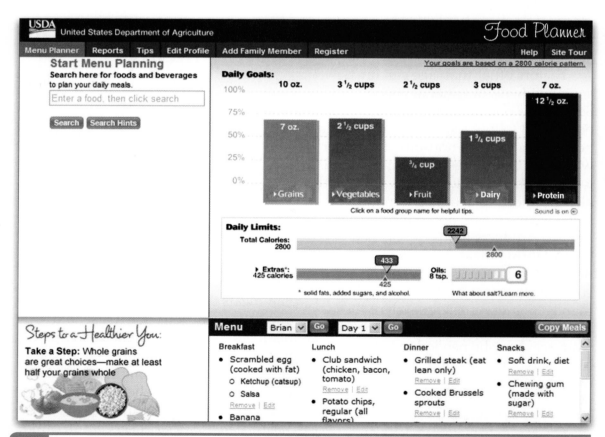

21-5 The MyPlate "Food Planner" (formerly MyPyramid "Menu Planner") is a useful tool for planning healthy meals.

The *Dietary Guidelines* recommend making at least half of the grains you eat be whole grains. Incorporating whole-grain ingredients into recipes and meals will result in a healthier meal. Substitute whole-grain flour for a portion of the refined flour in baked goods. Use whole-grain pastas for salads and casseroles. Mix brown rice in with white rice. Over time, gradually increase the proportion of brown rice to white as individuals adjust to the change in texture and flavor.

Use low-fat dairy products in place of full fat products. For example, try substituting fat-free milk when a recipe calls for whole milk. Some cheeses are naturally lower in fat than others. Parmesan cheese contains about 25 percent less fat than cheddar cheese. Feta cheese contains approximately two-thirds the amount of fat found in cheddar cheese.

Use healthier protein ingredients for meals. Try leaner cuts of meat. Cuts of red meat that include "round" or "loin" in the name are considered lean. Look for ground meats or poultry with less than five percent fat content. Trim visible fat off meat before cooking. Nuts, seeds, dried beans and peas are good alternate sources of protein. Top salads with garbanzo beans or add walnuts to oatmeal. Combining these foods with whole grains will provide your body with all the indispensable amino acids. For example, peanut butter on whole-wheat bread, red beans and rice, or pinto beans in a corn tortilla will provide the needed amino acids.

Whole, unpeeled fruits and vegetables generally retain more of their nutrients. Therefore, if you have the time to wash and trim produce yourself, avoid buying precut produce. Use a variety of fruits and vegetables in meals to benefit from the different nutrients each supplies. Make vegetables a bigger portion of the meal or recipe.

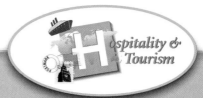

Personal Chef

Personal chefs work for individuals. They plan and prepare meals in private homes according to the client's tastes or dietary needs. They order groceries and supplies, clean the kitchen, and wash dishes and utensils. They also may serve meals. Personal chefs usually prepare a week's worth of meals in the client's home for the client to heat and serve according to directions. These chefs typically work full-time for one client, such as corporate executives, university presidents, or diplomats, who regularly entertain as a part of their official duties.

Education: Most personal chefs have some postsecondary training. Formal training may take place at a community college, technical school, culinary arts school, or a college with a degree in hospitality. A growing number of chefs participate in training programs sponsored by independent cooking schools, professional culinary institutes, or in the armed forces.

Job Outlook: Job openings for personal chefs are expected to be good. However, competition should be keen.

Few ingredients or foods need to be completely avoided. However, some ingredients should be used sparingly or less often. Fat, sugar, and salt are three ingredients that should be reduced or replaced when cooking healthy meals.

Select healthier fats. Use more oils which contain less saturated and *trans* fats than solid fats such as butter, lard, and shortening.

Americans often consume too much salt and sugar. Gradually decrease the use of salt and sugar. Fill the flavor void with herbs, spices, lemon juice, or flavored vinegars. Marinades and rubs can be used on meats before cooking to enhance flavor.

Healthy Cooking Methods

The cooking methods you use affect the flavor and nutrient content of your food. Healthy cooking methods enable you to prepare flavorful foods while retaining nutrients and avoiding the use of too much fat or salt.

To prepare healthier foods, use cooking methods such as roasting, baking, grilling, broiling, poaching, sautéing, braising, steaming, and stir-frying, **21-6**. Rather than panfrying fish, try poaching it in flavorful liquid. Instead of deep-fat frying, try marinating chicken and then grilling it. To remove fat remaining in cooking liquid after braising or stewing food, place in refrigerator. As the food cools, the fat will rise to the surface and harden. This can be easily skimmed off before reheating.

Make healthier sauces using reduction. **Reduction** is the process of cooking a liquid with the intent of losing volume through evaporation. This technique concentrates the flavors and thickens the liquid without the use of fat or starches.

When cooking fruits and vegetables, keep them in larger pieces and avoid peeling, if possible. This reduces the amount of exposed surface area and helps to reduce the amount of nutrients that leach into the cooking liquid. Use the smallest amount of cooking liquid possible to help preserve water-soluble nutrients. Protect heat-sensitive nutrients, such as folate and vitamin C, by cooking foods for the shortest time possible.

Your choice of kitchen equipment can affect the nutrients in foods and your food preparation options. Choose cookware that provides even heat distribution. You want to avoid cookware that creates hotspots, which scorch foods. Scorching causes an unappealing taste and damage to some nutrients.

A microwave oven can be a wise choice in kitchen equipment that helps protect the nutrients in foods. High heat and long cooking periods can result in vitamin losses. A microwave oven cooks foods quickly, minimizing such losses. Microwave cooking also requires less water than conventional cooking methods. Therefore, fewer nutrients leach into the cooking liquid.

A deep fryer is a less healthful option in kitchen equipment. Frying adds fat and calories to foods. In addition, high frying temperatures can destroy heat-sensitive vitamins.

Healthy Cooking Methods	
Method	**Description**
Baking	Food is cooked in the oven surrounded by hot air. Can be covered or uncovered. Typically used to cook foods with a certain amount of added moisture.
Braising	Food is first browned in a pan on the stovetop. Liquid is added and the food is covered and simmered until tender.
Broiling	Food is placed on a grate or pan and then placed below the heat source. This method uses high temperatures.
Grilling	Similar to broiling, but food is located above the heat source. Fat drips away from food as it cooks.
Poaching	Foods are placed in liquid and gently cooked at a low temperature. The cooking liquid is often flavored.
Roasting	Similar to baking, but food is uncovered so moisture evaporates. Food is often placed on a rack allowing fats to drip away and air to circulate for even cooking.
Sautéing	Food is cooked in a small amount of fat over high heat. Just enough fat is used to cover the bottom of pan. Both the pan and fat should be hot before food is added.
Steaming	Food is placed on a rack over boiling liquid and covered. The steam from the boiling liquid surrounds and cooks the food.
Stir-frying	Similar to sautéing, but food is cut into small, uniform pieces. A piece of cookware called a *wok* is often used for this method.

21-6 Healthy cooking methods add little or no fat to the food.

Slow cookers can help you save time and energy as you prepare nutritious foods. You can put the ingredients for a one-dish dinner in a slow cooker in the morning. In the evening, your dinner will be ready with a minimal amount of preparation time. Slow cookers use low heat for long periods. Nutrients destroyed by high temperatures can be preserved. The cooking liquid is often eaten with one-dish meals prepared in slow cookers. Therefore, you will not lose the benefit of any nutrients that have escaped into the cooking liquid.

Healthy Recipes

How do you know if a recipe is healthy? A very basic way is to simply look at the list of ingredients and the cooking method. Knowing which ingredients and cooking methods are healthy helps you select healthy recipes. You can also use this knowledge to make recipes healthier. For example, substitute unsaturated for saturated fats when cooking with fat. If the recipe says to panfry the chicken in butter, you could sauté it in a small amount of olive oil instead, **21-7**. Add a vegetable ingredient to a recipe that lacks vegetables. Adding broccoli to a chicken rice casserole recipe improves color appeal and adds nutrients to the dish. In baked goods recipes, experiment with replacing half the fat with unsweetened applesauce or prune purée. Rather than basting a turkey with fatty drippings or butter, use fat-free broth.

Many recipes include a nutritional analysis. To determine if the recipe meets your health needs, you could compare the nutritional analysis against specific recommendations. For example, compare the fat per serving against the recommendations of the American Heart Association or *Dietary Guidelines*.

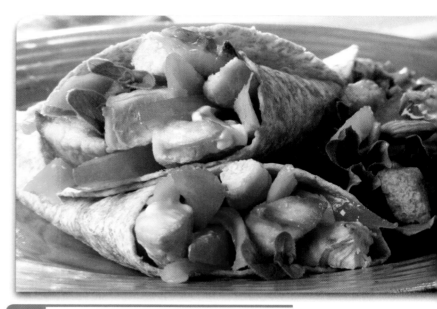

21-7 Make a wrap recipe healthier by using whole-grain tortillas.

Controlling Food Costs

A third advantage of meal planning is being able to manage how much money your household spends on food. Food can be very expensive. When people have limited incomes, food expenses become difficult. During an economic crisis, the situation only gets worse. Be assured, you can use a few techniques to help you control food costs without giving up appetite appeal or nutrients.

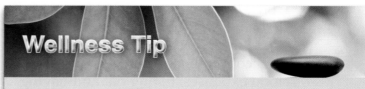

Wellness Tip

Healthful Quick Cooking

When planning meals for a busy week, choose healthful quick-cooking methods such as steaming, microwaving, and stir-frying to retain more nutrients. Use high-temperature cooking methods, such as deep frying, less often because they result in greater nutrient loss.

Use a Spending Plan

To plan meals that stay within your household's financial limits, you first need to decide what those limits are. Preparing a **budget**, or a spending plan, will help you make this decision. A budget helps you plan how to use your sources of income to meet your various expenses. Many expenses occur on a monthly basis. Therefore, many people find it convenient to set up a monthly budget.

It is not a good idea to spend more money than you receive. The amount of money you budget for food must fit in with all your other expenses. These include *fixed expenses*, such as rent and car payments, which are the same each month. You also have *flexible expenses*, such as clothing purchases and utility bills, which vary from month to month. The food category of a budget is generally considered a flexible expense.

As the meal manager, you are responsible for staying within the established food budget. Saving all your food receipts for a few weeks will help you see if you are meeting this goal. If you find you are spending too much, you must make some adjustments. Consider all the resources available to you as you plan for your food needs and look for ways to lower costs. Take advantage of coupon Web sites to save on food. You may also consider planting a vegetable garden to help lower food costs. Keep in mind that buying meats, gourmet foods, and convenience products adds to food expenses. Eating out and having frequent dinner guests increases your food spending, too. You may need to cut back on these types of food purchases if you are not staying within your budget, **21-8**.

Food Budget		
Month: *January*		
Food Eaten at Home		
	Money Planned	**Money Spent**
Week one	$150	$130
Week two	150	165
Week three	150	180
Week four	150	115
Total	$600	$590
Restaurants/Takeout		
	Money Planned	**Money Spent**
Week one	$30	$40
Week two	30	38
Week three	30	42
Week four	30	50
Total	$120	$170
Total Food Expenses	$720	$760

21-8 If you are not meeting your monthly food budget, you may have to make adjustments in spending.

Cost-Cutting Menu Plans

Most people are concerned about food costs. When incomes are limited, food budgets must also be limited. One way to keep food spending under control is to build menus around low-cost foods in each food group. For instance, brown rice and fresh pasta are both in the grain group. You could use either as the basis of a tasty, nutritious casserole. However, fresh pasta costs about three times more than the brown rice.

When planning menus, plan to use less costly foods from all the food groups. From the fruit and vegetable groups, choose fresh produce that is in season. Frozen and canned plain fruits and vegetables are usually good buys, too. Those that come with extras, such as sauces, are more costly. In the dairy group, you can save money by using nonfat dry milk in your menu plans. Dry legumes and peanut butter are the best buys in the protein foods group. You can use them to create high-fiber, low-fat meatless main dishes.

Plan menus that take advantage of advertised store specials. If broccoli is on sale, you might plan to serve it for several meals. You could use it in a salad one day and in a side dish another day.

Control the cost of your menu by planning the appropriate amounts of foods. Base the amount of food on individuals' nutrient needs—do not prepare more food than is needed. If you have an active teen male in the household, the menu plan will include more food than if you are feeding a toddler. Consider planning leftovers into the menu. Rather than throwing away leftovers, plan ahead for their use in your menu. If roast chicken is on the menu for Sunday, plan chicken casserole for later in the week. Make the casserole with leftover chicken and any leftover vegetables from the week.

Careful shopping can also help you save money when buying food, **21-9**.

Food Assistance Resources

People need to know what resources exist to help them when they have food needs. The following programs are available through the United States Department of Agriculture (USDA). Some of these programs are funded jointly by the states. These programs provide resources for eligible individuals at various life-cycle stages.

Supplemental Nutrition Assistance Program (SNAP)

The Supplemental Nutrition Assistance Program was formerly called the Federal Food Stamp Program. The focus is on nutrition and making healthy food accessible to low income households. Some states use a different name for the program. You apply for benefits by completing a state application form.

Tips for Saving on Food Shopping

- Prepare a shopping list from your menu and stick to it
- Avoid shopping when tired or hungry
- Buy good quality store and generic brands when possible
- Shop at stores which have the low-priced, good quality foods
- Buy only the amount of food needed or that can be safely stored
- Look for marked down foods that are day old or close to their expiration dates—be sure to use before expiration to avoid food losses
- Avoid the snack aisles, instead purchase healthier fruits and vegetables
- Avoid individual packs which are usually more costly than buying in bulk and repackaging for lunches and traveling
- Use nonfat dry milk instead of fluid milk for puddings, sauces, and desserts
- Buy blocks of cheese and grate or slice it yourself
- Leave soda, sweetened juices, and bottled waters off your shopping list—drink tap water instead
- Select lean cuts of meat, poultry, and fish on sale
- Consider loss due to bones and fat when comparing price per pound for various meats

---

21-9 You can cut costs in food spending and still purchase foods you need for a nutritious diet.

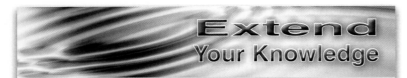

Resource Conservation in the Kitchen

Meal managers should establish practices to conserve resources related to food preparation. The entire household should participate in conservation of resources on a daily basis. The Environmental Protection Agency (EPA) suggests individuals reduce, reuse, and recycle waste to conserve resources.

Households can reduce the amount of trash thrown away by
- reusing containers
- composting food scraps and yard trimmings
- recycling waste when possible and buying products made with recycled materials
- purchasing products with as little packaging as possible
- using cloth napkins rather than disposable

Households can reduce energy and water use by
- turning off lights when not in use
- running dishwasher only when full
- allowing dishes to air dry and skipping dishwasher's dry cycle
- using the appropriate-size burner for the pot or pan
- cleaning and maintaining refrigerators and freezers
- using as little water as possible when cooking
- scraping dishes (not rinsing) before placing in dishwasher
- keeping drinking water in the refrigerator rather than running faucet water until it is cool
- defrosting foods in refrigerator overnight rather than in running water

Learn more about composting and other conservation practices at the EPA Web site.

add money to their SNAP allotment to meet their nutritional needs.

National School Programs

The National School Lunch program provides nutritious lunches at reduced or no cost to eligible children. The lunches must meet the *Dietary Guidelines'* recommendations for the age group being served. Additional programs offered through schools include the Afterschool Snack, Fresh Fruit and Vegetable, Seamless Summer, School Breakfast, and Special Milk programs.

Special Supplemental Nutrition Program for Women, Infants, and Children (WIC)

The Special Supplemental Nutrition Program for Women, Infants, and Children (WIC) is intended to help children get a healthy start in life. It focuses on children up to age five and pregnant and lactating (breast-feeding) women. The program is designed to help low-income mothers and children who are at nutritional risk. WIC services provide vouchers for the purchase of specific nutritious foods. These foods supply nutrients to meet the nutritional needs of the WIC clients. The program also provides nutrition education as well as referrals to other health and social services.

Elderly Nutrition Program

The Elderly Nutrition Program provides funding to support nutrition services to older adults throughout the United States. The nutrition services include congregate and home-delivered meals. The meals must provide at least one-third of estimated required nutrients.

Congregate meals are designed to meet both the social and nutritional needs of people age 50 and older. A **congregate meal** is a group meal.

Benefits are provided on an electronic card that is used like an ATM card. The card is accepted at most grocery stores as well as some food cooperatives and farmers' markets. Through educational training programs, SNAP helps clients learn to make healthy eating and active lifestyle choices.

This assistance program supplements food needs for a family, it is not enough to purchase a complete nutritionally adequate diet. Families must

Group meals are provided at local places of worship, community centers, or other facilities one or more days a week.

Home-delivered meals are delivered by volunteers to the homes of individuals who cannot leave their homes and are unable to prepare their own meals.

Commodity Supplemental Food Program

The Commodity Supplemental Food Program (CSFP) gives commodity food to low-income pregnant and breastfeeding women, new mothers, infants, children up to age six, and elderly people 60 years and older. A commodity food is a common, mass-produced item. Instant dry milk, flour, sugar, and cornmeal are often given out through this program. Perishable foods, such as butter, cheese, fruits, and vegetables, may also be issued. Unlike some of the other food programs, CSFP distributes the food directly to individuals. Many of the individuals who qualify for SNAP and WIC will qualify for this program as well. Resources through this program may shrink as farm policies change and food costs continue to rise.

Expanded Food and Nutrition Education Program (EFNEP)

The Expanded Food and Nutrition Education Program (EFNEP) does not distribute food supplies. Instead, this program provides individuals with limited resources with the knowledge and skills needed to make healthy food choices. Participants attend a series of classes on food preparation, storage, and safety and sanitation. They will learn how to manage their food budgets effectively. The EFNEP also offers youth programs with topics including nutrition, health, and food preparation.

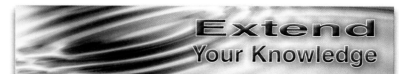

Food Banks and Soup Kitchens

Food banks, or pantries, are nonprofit organizations which distribute nonperishable goods and perishable food items to nonprofit agencies involved in local emergency food programs. Food banks raise money to purchase food. Much of the food they receive comes from for-profit companies. These companies donate food they cannot sell or serve. The food bank ensures the food is healthy and safe before distributing it. The food is sorted, packed, and taken to community pantries. Mobile food pantries distribute food throughout a region.

Soup kitchens are locations that provide prepared meals to those in need. Many of these programs are run by religious or other charitable organizations. Some programs encourage individual gardeners to plant additional produce in their gardens and donate the surplus to local food banks or soup kitchens.

Learn what types of programs exist in your community.

Saving Time

Saving time and effort is a fourth advantage of meal planning. Efficient use of time is important to people with busy schedules. Some people skip meals if they cannot prepare foods quickly and easily. For them, fast and simple meal preparations are essential to good nutrition.

A number of tools can help you make the best use of your time in the kitchen. You can use organizational skills and timesaving appliances. You can also use recipes and food products designed to speed your food preparation tasks.

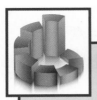

Math Link

Unit Cost Comparison

Selena plans to bake blueberry muffins for the choir potluck. She needs 2 cups of berries for her recipe. Fresh blueberries are on sale for $3.99 a pint. Frozen blueberries are $4.79 for a 1-quart bag.

- Calculate which blueberries cost less. Show your work. Round answers up to 2 decimals. (Hint: 2 cups in a pint, 2 pints in a quart)

Organize Work Space and Equipment

A first step for saving time in food preparation is organizing your work space and equipment. Store kitchen utensils close to where you are likely to use them. For instance, you might store a pancake turner close to the range and a vegetable peeler close to the sink. Keeping cupboards and drawers neat makes it easier to find the items that are stored in them. Store appliances in handy locations. If appliances are difficult to get out and put away, you are less likely to use them.

Ingredients need to be on hand when you are ready to use them. Keeping a shopping list handy will help you remember to jot down items as you discover you need them. This will allow you to avoid running to the store at the last minute to pick up missing ingredients.

Use Timesaving Appliances

Many small appliances can save preparation and cooking time. Food processors can save time when chopping, grating, or mixing large portions of fruits, vegetables, or other ingredients. Pressure cookers reduce cooking time. Slow cookers and bread machines allow you to prepare foods in the morning and have them ready to eat at dinnertime, **21-10**.

Microwave ovens are useful for reducing time when cooking and reheating leftovers. Using a microwave oven can also save serving and cleanup time. This is because many foods can be cooked, served, and stored in the same container.

Select Quick and Easy Menu Items

With planning, you can prepare many meals in 30 minutes or less. These meals can be as tasty and healthful as those that take more time and trouble to prepare.

Quick and easy meals begin with quick and easy recipes. Most simple recipes require only a few ingredients. Ingredients are generally foods that most people have on hand. These recipes have a small number of preparation steps and require only a few utensils.

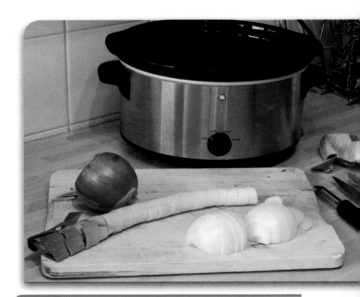

21-10 Slow cookers are timesaving appliances used in many households.

They usually rely on fast cooking techniques, such as microwaving and stir-frying.

Keep a file of simple recipes household members enjoy. Organize them into categories, such as main dishes, salads, and desserts. You might also want to keep a file of quick menu ideas for various types of meals. This will make it easy for you to prepare complete meals when you are in a hurry.

Another way to prepare quick and easy meals is through the planned use of leftovers. When you have time to cook, double recipes and store half in the refrigerator or freezer. In the time it takes to cook or reheat the stored portion, you can prepare accompanying menu items. In a matter of minutes you will be able to serve a complete meal. Meat loaf, soups, and casseroles work especially well for this type of meal planning.

Consider Convenience Foods

Nearly all meal managers use some convenience foods to help them save time in the kitchen. **Convenience foods** are food items that are purchased partially or completely prepared. Cake mixes, canned soups, and frozen entrées are typical convenience foods, **21-11**.

Convenience foods are popular for several reasons other than time savings. Meal managers who have limited cooking skills like convenience foods because the instructions are simple to follow. Many people enjoy the taste of convenience foods. Creative cooks appreciate recipes found on many convenience food packages calling for the convenience products as ingredients.

Convenience foods often cost more than foods made from scratch. You must decide whether the time savings,

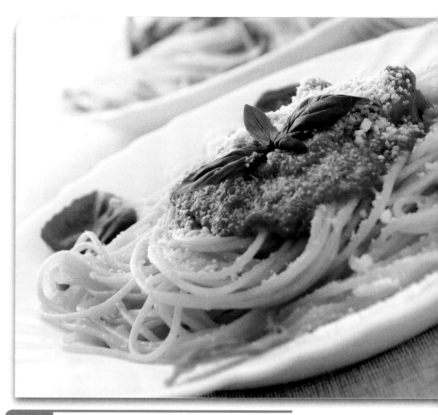

21-11 Heating ready-made spaghetti sauce and cooking the noodles for this dish could be done easily in a short time.

taste, and nutritional contributions of convenience products are worth the cost. Be sure to read nutrition labels when choosing convenience products. Many are higher in sodium and fat than foods you would prepare yourself.

Healthy Meals Away from Home

Meal managers are responsible for making sure household members' nutrient needs are met and the food budget is maintained. This is true even when individuals eat meals away from home. Managing nutrition and food costs is not difficult when meals are prepared at home and packed to go. These management tasks are more challenging when meals are prepared elsewhere.

Case Study: Latrell's Lunch Makeover

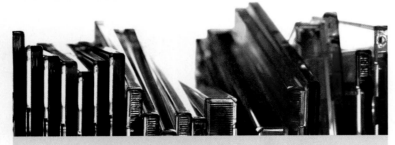

Jada was on the phone with her brother Latrell one day. Latrell had recently moved into his own apartment closer to his new job in the city. He is trying to save money on food by packing his own lunch for work. He complains to Jada that he is bored with his lunch and feels sluggish and tired many days. Jada asks what he usually packs for lunch. Latrell says "I pack the same lunch every day—a bag of potato chips, can of soda, and bologna and mayonnaise on white bread." Jada starts laughing and says "No wonder you don't feel well! Your lunch needs a makeover."

Case Review

1. What do you think Jada means when she says Latrell's lunch needs a makeover?

2. What suggestions would you make for improving Latrell's lunch?

Packing a Lunch

Many students and working household members carry meals from home to eat at school or the workplace. These meals are most often lunches.

Carrying a lunch from home has many advantages over purchasing food from a restaurant or vending machine. When you pack a lunch, you can include your favorite foods. You can use ingredients that meet the *Dietary Guidelines.* You will save money, too.

Packing a lunch can also have a down side. Creatively choosing what to put into a lunch is not always easy. Finding the time to pack it requires planning.

Sandwiches are frequently the main course in a packed lunch. Look for new recipes if you like variety. You can add interest to sandwiches by using different kinds of breads and rolls and preparing various fillings.

When packing lunches, try to include a variety of foods from the five food groups. Limit snack foods, cookies, and cakes that are high in fats, sugar, and sodium. Choose some foods that are high in dietary fiber, such as whole-grain breads and fresh fruits and vegetables.

Packing a lunch need not take much time. Many people pack lunches the night before and keep them in the refrigerator. When clearing the dinner table, store leftovers in serving-sized containers. Put them directly into lunch bags and refrigerate. Try setting up an assembly line to make sandwiches for the entire household. You can quickly complete each meal by adding a piece of fresh fruit. Packing a thermos of milk or a frozen box of juice will provide a cool drink with lunch.

Keep food safety in mind when packing lunches. Use food containers that will keep foods at the proper temperatures until they will be eaten.

Choosing from a Menu

Eating out often serves as a solution to time problems for busy meal managers and their household members. In the United States, many food dollars are spent on foods prepared away from home. This includes foods purchased from concession stands, vending machines, take-out counters, and all types of restaurants.

You have less control over the appeal, nutrient content, and cost of foods when eating out. However, your choice of restaurant will affect the type of foods available and how much you will spend.

Many restaurants offer a variety of choices for their health-conscious customers. Sometimes healthful options are marked by a special symbol on the menu. In addition, menu terms can help you identify foods that may be high in fat and sodium, **21-12**.

You may find healthful eating a bit more challenging when eating at fast-food restaurants. This is because many fast foods are high in sodium, fat, and calories. One large burger, French fries, and a milk shake can supply half a day's calorie needs for many teens. This meal is low in fiber and vitamins A and C. It contains approximately 1,400 milligrams of sodium, and over 50 percent of the calories come from fat. On the positive side, fast-food meals are usually excellent sources of protein and iron.

You do not have to avoid fast-food meals. Registered dietitians suggest selecting foods wisely and adjusting other meals throughout the day to balance calorie and nutrient intake.

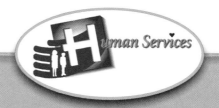

Food Bank Director

Food bank directors are responsible for the acquisition of food and its storage and distribution. This includes the evaluation of inventory and processing orders for each distribution site in the community. The director is responsible for regular training workshops for staff and volunteers. The food bank director also develops eligibility guidelines and oversees the eligibility of recipients. Many food bank directors promote awareness of hunger throughout the community through public presentations, press conferences and interviews.

Education: A bachelor's degree in community services or a related field is preferred.

Job Outlook: The job outlook is expected to be good due to poor economic conditions in most areas.

Menu Clues	
Terms Suggesting Higher Fat Content	
Au gratin or in cheese sauce	Hollandaise
Breaded	In its own gravy, with gravy, pan gravy
Buttered or buttery	Pastry
Creamed, creamy, or in cream sauce	Rich
Fried, French-fried, deep-fried, batter-fried, panfried	Scalloped
Terms Suggesting Higher Sodium Content	
Barbecued	Mustard sauce
Creole sauce	Parmesan
In a tomato base	Pickled
In broth	Smoked
In cocktail sauce	Soy sauce
Marinated	Teriyaki

21-12 Be aware of menu items described using these words. The food will be higher in fat and sodium.

The following tips can help you meet your goals for good nutrition when eating out:

- Resist the temptation to order double burgers, large fries, and supersized drinks. Stick with regular-sized menu items.
- Order half-size, appetizer, or children's portions or consider sharing an entrée with a friend.
- Limit high-fat creamy and oily salads, such as potato salad, tuna salad, and marinated pasta and vegetable salads.
- Go easy on toppings such as cheese and bacon. Request that gravies, sauces, and salad dressings be served on the side.
- Use low-calorie condiments, such as reduced-fat dressings on salads and lemon juice on fish instead of tartar sauce.
- Avoid adding salt at the table.
- Trim fat from meat, skin from chicken, and breading from fish. Blot the oil on pizza with a napkin, **21-13**.
- Choose fruit or nonfat frozen yogurt for dessert.
- Order fruit juice instead of soda. Choose low-fat milk instead of a milk shake. Ask for water to drink with your meal along with or instead of other beverages.
- Get some exercise after eating out. Walk home from the restaurant or plan other light activities to help burn a few calories.

Through planning, you can enjoy eating out. As people have become more nutrition conscious, restaurants have increased their offerings of healthful menu items. Many restaurants post the nutrition information for their menu items on their Web site and on their menus. This allows meals eaten away from home to better meet all the goals of meal management.

Healthful Menu Choices			
Chicken Menu Choices	**Calories**	**Fat (g)**	**Sodium (mg)**
3 oz. cooked skinless chicken breast	140	3	65
3 oz. cooked chicken breast (meat and skin)	165	7	60
3 oz. fried chicken breast (meat, skin, and breading)	220	11	235

21-13 When eating out, evaluate the choices available to you.

Reading Summary

Meal management involves using resources to plan and prepare meals. One of the goals of meal management is to make meals appealing. Planning meals that include foods with a variety of flavors, colors, textures, shapes, sizes, and temperatures will meet this goal.

A second goal of meal management is to plan healthy meals that meet nutritional needs. Different needs of each household member must be considered. The *Dietary Guidelines for Americans* and MyPlate food guidance system are resources for meeting this goal. Preparing healthy meals requires the ability to recognize healthy ingredients, cooking methods, and recipes.

A third meal management goal is to control food costs. A meal manager can prepare a budget. This will allow him or her to determine how much money is available to spend on food. A number of cost-cutting techniques can help a meal manager stay within his or her budget. Food assistance resources are available for individuals at various life-cycle stages.

Saving time is a fourth goal for most meal managers. Keeping the kitchen and equipment organized and using timesaving appliances will help keep meal preparations moving. Choosing quick and easy recipes and taking advantage of convenience products will save time, too.

A meal manager must try to meet these four basic goals even when household members eat meals away from home. These goals are not difficult to achieve when packing meals to eat at school or the workplace. Meal management is more of a challenge when meals are purchased from sources such as restaurants. Meal managers can help household members learn to make nutritious choices that are within food spending limits.

Review Learning

1. What are two tips for adding flavor appeal to meals?
2. Which characteristic of an appealing meal is not met by a menu of cranberry juice, cabbage slaw, and spaghetti with tomato sauce?
   A. Flavor.
   B. Color.
   C. Texture.
   D. Shape and size.
3. Besides making foods more appealing, why is it important to serve them at proper temperatures?
4. Which of the following is a good resource for planning healthy meals?
   A. American Medical Association
   B. *Physical Activity Guidelines for Americans*
   C. MyPlate food guidance system
5. True or false. Cuts of red meat that include "round" or "loin" are considered high fat.
6. List three healthy ways to enhance the flavor of a food.
7. What is the difference between fixed expenses and flexible expenses?
8. Give one example of a low-cost food in each of three food groups from MyPlate.

9. Give two examples of how appliances can help save time in the kitchen.
10. What are three characteristics of a quick and easy recipe?
11. What is one advantage and one disadvantage of using convenience foods?
12. What are two tips for saving time when packing lunches?
13. What are five tips for meeting the goal of good nutrition when eating out?

Critical Thinking

14. **Predict outcomes.** Think about the goals of meal management. Predict several outcomes of using these principles effectively.
15. **Draw conclusions.** What are your food choices like when you go out to eat with friends? Do you choose healthful options or go along with the crowd? Draw conclusions about ways that you can improve your food choices when you eat away from home.

Applying Your Knowledge

16. **Meal appeal evaluation.** Cut a picture of a plated meal from a magazine. (You may choose to use pictures to prepare your own plated meal.) Attach your pictured meal to a written evaluation of the meal's flavors, colors, textures, shapes, sizes, and temperatures.
17. **Menu planning.** Write a one-day menu for your household. Use resources discussed in the chapter to help you. Make note of healthy ingredients, cooking methods, and recipes you use to write the menu.
18. **Evaluate restaurant menus.** Collect menus from various local restaurants. Evaluate them based on the recommendations from the *Dietary Guidelines for Americans*. Highlight these menu choices. Explain why they are health promoting choices.

Technology Connections

19. **Meal analysis.** Conduct a meal analysis of the school's cafeteria meals for one week. Prepare a rubric to evaluate the menus using the various factors that contribute to the appeal and health of a meal. Use ChooseMyPlate.gov to evaluate nutritional content of the menus.
20. **Ingredient substitutions.** Select a family favorite recipe. Substitute healthier ingredients or cooking methods or both to create a healthier version of the recipe. Perform a nutrient analysis for each version using the USDA National Nutrient Database found online.
21. **Life-cycle menu planning.** Use MyPlate "Food Planner" to create a menu for yourself. Add two or more "household members" at different stages of the life cycle. For example, you could add a mother who is pregnant and a three-year-old brother. Be sure the menus meet each individual's daily nutritional needs. Print out the menu plans. For an additional challenge, assume one of the household members has a special nutritional need such as vegetarianism or lactose intolerance. Make adjustments to the menu to meet the entire household's needs.

22. **Interactive meal activity.** Find the interactive activity "Analyze My Plate" on the CDC's Fruits & Veggies Matter Web site. Complete the activity to learn how to create a healthy plate.

Academic Connections

23. **History.** Learn about what was involved in meal planning in the 1930s. Prepare a presentation comparing it to meal planning today.

24. **Science.** Plan and conduct a small taste test to evaluate the effect of flavor, color, texture, shape, size, or temperature on food choices. Divide a batch of mashed potatoes in half. Color one half blue and leave the other half unaltered. Ask people to taste both potatoes and tell you which they prefer and why. Next, have the same people wear blindfolds and sample the potatoes again. Note their responses. Perform the taste test comparing cheese at room temperature to the same cheese served cold. Summarize your findings and write a conclusion about factors that affect food appeal.

25. **Writing.** Research the international slow foods movement. Based on your findings, write a persuasive paper either in favor of or against the movement.

26. **Math.** Create a list of 10 food items which your household often purchases. Visit three different food stores and record the prices for the 10 food items at each location. Prepare a report that includes the purchase price, pack size, and unit price for each item on the list organized by store. Determine which stores in your community have lower food prices. Note: A variety of food items may need to be compared to get an accurate comparison.

Workplace Applications

Teaching Skills to Others

The director of the food pantry at which you volunteer overheard you explaining the directions for cooking a low-cost chicken dish to a client. The director has asked you to demonstrate your dish to a group of clients at the monthly nutrition and cooking class. She said the food pantry will supply your ingredients. You will need to supply the recipe and prepare a cost list—showing the total cost and cost-per-portion. Your chicken dish is a one-dish meal that uses chicken, broccoli, whole-grain noodles, and grated cheese topping and makes eight portions. Think about the following as you prepare your demonstration:
- thrifty substitutions that can be made that are equally nutritious and utilize foods from every food group
- ways to save time during preparation
- methods for keeping food safe
- ways to utilize leftovers

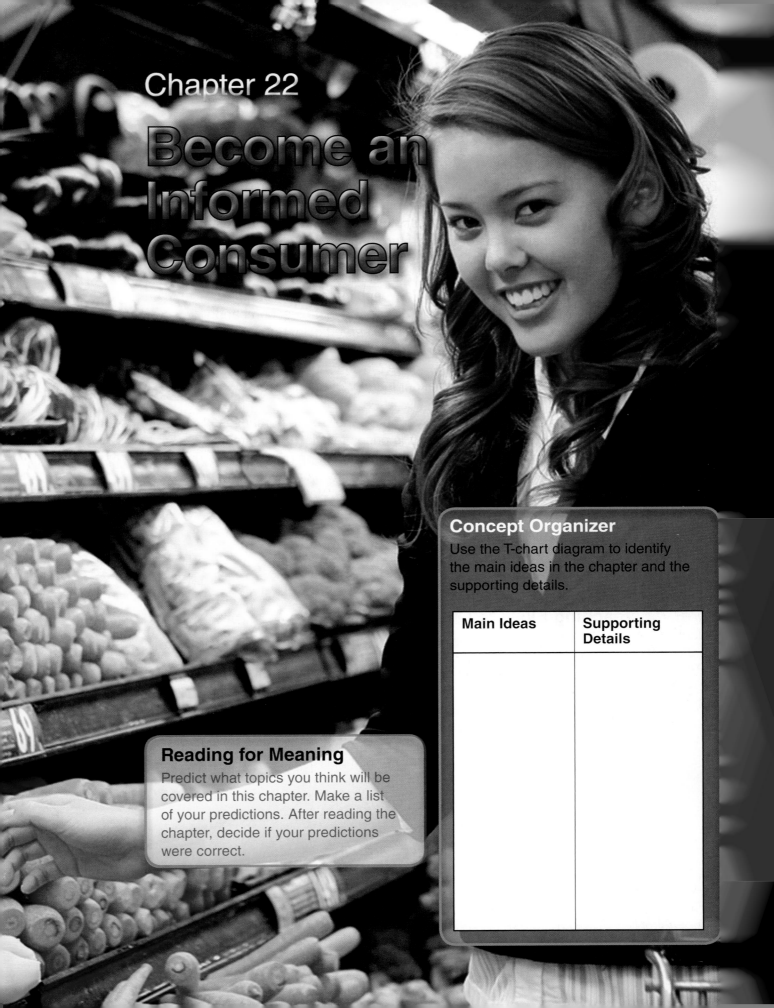

Chapter 22

Become an Informed Consumer

Concept Organizer

Use the T-chart diagram to identify the main ideas in the chapter and the supporting details.

Main Ideas	Supporting Details

Reading for Meaning

Predict what topics you think will be covered in this chapter. Make a list of your predictions. After reading the chapter, decide if your predictions were correct.

Terms to Know

consumer
food processing
food irradiation
food additive
generally recognized as safe (GRAS)
  list
organic foods
comparison shopping
unit price
national brand
store brand
generic product
impulse buying
serving size

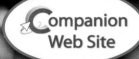

Companion Web Site

- **Print out the concept organizer at g-wlearning.com.**
- **Practice key terms with crossword puzzles, matching activities, and e-flash cards at g-wlearning.com.**

Objectives

After studying this chapter, you will be able to
- **compare** various places people shop for food.
- **recognize** food shopping trends.
- **explain** factors that can affect consumer choices.
- **use** information on food labels to make healthful food choices.
- **evaluate** the quality of fitness products and services.
- **identify** your consumer rights and responsibilities.

Central Ideas

- Understanding shopping trends and where and how to shop can help you make wise purchasing decisions.
- Utilizing nutrition labels, understanding labeling regulations, seeking reliable information about fitness products and services, and knowing consumer rights help consumers get the most out of the purchasing dollars.

How do you decide which food and fitness items to buy? Are your decisions swayed by advertising? Do you base your food choices on the way products taste, their nutritional value, or their package appeal? Do you buy fitness equipment because it is the latest fad or because you are truly interested in an activity? How much does cost affect what you buy? Perhaps you buy certain products out of habit. These and many other factors influence your market decisions.

You are a consumer. A **consumer** is someone who buys and uses products and services. You purchase food, sports equipment, clothing, movie tickets, and hundreds of other items. You pay people to serve you meals, lead your fitness classes, and dry-clean your clothes.

This chapter will help you develop skills as a consumer. You will consider your options for where to buy foods and fitness products and services. You will become aware of the impact advertising can have on you. You will determine what quality standards are important to you when choosing nutritious foods and quality fitness equipment. You will learn to read and interpret information on food and product labels. This chapter will also help you practice shopping skills to control spending. You will form a plan of action to take when you have problems in the marketplace, too.

Where to Shop for Food

How do you decide where to buy the foods you need? If you are like most people, one of the factors that affects your choice of stores is food prices. However, you will probably not want price to be your only consideration. If you drive from store to store to get the lowest price, you may not end up saving money. This shopping strategy takes time and adds to your transportation costs.

You may find it more practical to do most of your shopping in one or two stores. Choose stores that give you the best overall price and quality. Look for stores that are conveniently located. You are likely to want stores that offer cleanliness, customer services, and variety, too. As you become familiar with favorite stores, you will learn where to quickly find the items on your shopping list.

A great variety of stores sell food products. These include supermarkets, warehouse stores and clubs, convenience stores, outlet stores, specialty stores, health food stores food cooperatives, roadside stands and farmers' markets, and on-line shopping. Conveniences, type of service, quality of food, products available, and cost are primary reasons for choosing one store over another. Each alternative offers particular advantages and disadvantages.

Supermarkets

Supermarkets offer a wide range of products. Besides foods, they carry household items, health and beauty products, and pet supplies. Many stores have bakery, deli, and meat departments. Some have pharmacies, bank branches, and cafeterias. Supermarkets offer consumers selection and convenience, **22-1**. However, some shoppers have trouble finding the products they need in such large stores.

Warehouse Stores and Clubs

Warehouse stores and clubs offer a variety of products other than foods. Selections and variety may be limited. Many items are sold in large containers and multiunit packages. This can be a convenience for shoppers who like to stock up on food items. Prices at warehouse stores can be lower than supermarket prices. Some warehouses clubs charge membership fees and may not accept coupons. These factors make warehouse prices less of a bargain.

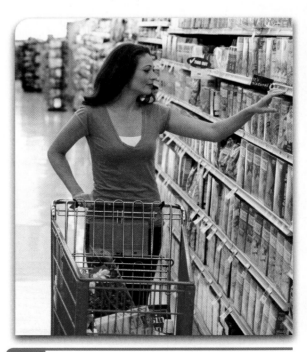

22-1 Supermarkets offer shoppers many brands and choices.

Convenience Stores

These stores usually have longer business hours than other food stores. Many stay open around the clock. They stock a limited variety of food items and household essentials. They often sell a variety of sports drinks, snacks, and ready-to-eat foods, such as sandwiches and pizza. These stores are in locations that make it easy to quickly stop and pick up a few needed items. Prices at convenience stores are often higher than supermarket prices.

Outlet Stores

Outlet stores usually sell products made by one food manufacturer and are sometimes located in outlet malls. Although these items are wholesome, some of them may not have met the manufacturer's standards for quality. For instance, bagels may be slightly misshapen or the frosting on a cake may be smudged. Products at outlet stores are usually sold at substantial discounts over retail prices. However, the consumer has no opportunity to compare and select competing brands.

Specialty Stores

Specialty stores include ethnic markets, dairies, bakeries, and meat or fish markets. These stores specialize in selling one type of product. Their products are usually high quality and very fresh. Most specialty stores charge premium prices, **22-2.**

Health Food Stores

Health food stores often emphasize natural foods, whole foods, organic foods, herbal supplements, and may specialize in sports supplements and energy drinks. In the last 15 years,

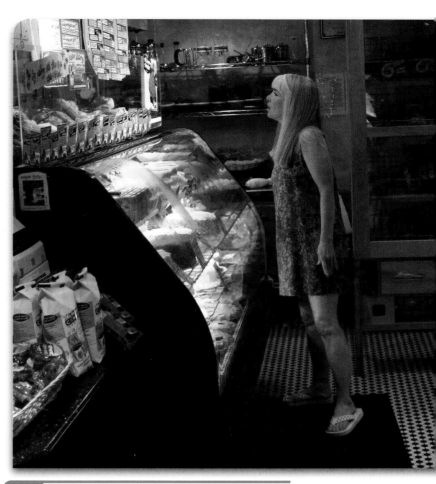

22-2 Specialty stores such as bakeries often offer products you cannot find at other stores.

these stores grew at a tremendous rate. The variety of choices is great but the dollar cost may be higher than in supermarkets. You may find food choices not found in other stores. Claims regarding the benefit of using health promoting foods or food supplements are often not supported by scientific research.

Food Cooperatives

Most food cooperatives, or co-ops, are not open to the public. They are owned and run by a group of consumers. Only members of the group may take advantage of the discounted food prices. Food prices are low because the group buys foods in bulk and adds no charge for profit. Co-ops also save labor costs by requiring members to volunteer at the co-op for a few hours each month. Members may also need to pay an annual fee.

Roadside Stands and Farmers' Markets

Roadside stands and farmers' markets offer consumers the chance to buy fruits and vegetables fresh from the field. Roadside stands are operated by individual produce growers during the growing season. Farmers' markets sell produce from a number of farmers, often in a city location. Roadside stands and farmers' markets usually have

limited hours. However, their produce is fresher, usually grown locally, and priced comparably or lower than supermarket produce, **22-3**

Shopping On-Line

Shopping on-line eliminates the need for consumers to travel to a store. Food stores that provide on-line shopping allow customers to order food using their home computer. On-line shoppers can choose from a wide range of food and nonfood items. Specified brands, amounts, and sizes can be selected. The shopper can even view product labels on the computer screen. After a consumer completes a shopping list, he or she submits it to the on-line service provider. Professional shoppers then fill the customer's order and deliver it to his or her home. Electronic payment for services is usually completed before the delivery occurs.

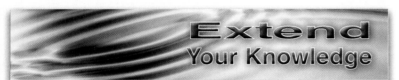

Shopping for Locally Grown Food

A growing number of people are interested in participating in sustainable living practices. Eating locally grown foods is an example of a sustainable living practice. People choose to shop for locally grown foods for many social and environmental reasons. How far food travels from farm to plate is called *food miles*. Some people believe food miles are the way to judge the food's impact on the climate. However, some studies have shown that transporting food accounts for only 11 percent of greenhouse gases related to food consumption. The majority of these gases result from the practices used to grow and harvest the foods. For example, it may be more efficient to transport lettuce from a warmer growing climate than to heat a greenhouse to grow lettuce locally.

The sustainable food movement also emphasizes use of agricultural methods that value respect for workers, provide fair wages to farmers, and support farming communities. Humane treatment of animals is emphasized. Investigate to learn more about the sustainable food movement.

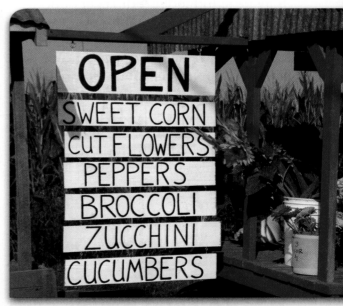

22-3 Freshly picked fruits and vegetables are offered at roadside stands and farmers' markets.

Food Shopping Trends

Changes are taking place in food stores to meet the emerging needs of consumers. Supermarkets are becoming larger and are focusing more on convenience. Other food stores want to emphasize natural, whole foods, or foods for easy living. The larger stores offer pharmacies, eye glass care, financial services, and ready-to-eat meals. They are adding more nonfood departments. New supermarket departments may include floral arranging, DVD rentals, and postal services. This trend allows consumers to do much of their shopping at one store. There may be separate entrances to specialty sections of the store, such as the deli and bakery departments.

Some large supermarkets are adding educational centers. These are classrooms in which stores offer cooking and wellness classes for their customers.

Stores increasingly rely on *demographic data*. Demographic data provides information about people in the communities in which the stores are located. This trend helps stores tailor the items they carry to the needs of their customers. For instance, a store might expand its ethnic food line to meet the needs of local consumers.

New marketing methods are being introduced in the supermarket. Look for food demonstrations or cooking contests as ways to advertise products. Video screens mounted on shopping carts may promote products as you walk up and down the store aisles. Monitors in specific store departments may show videotapes about how to prepare foods sold in those departments. Electronic coupons or automated discounts may be used to promote

items. These forms of savings will be automatically deducted from your bill at the checkout. Stores are using electronic communications to deliver "savings" messages through social networks and cell phones.

Stores are introducing services that reduce the amount of time needed to shop. Self-service scanners are being used in some stores to speed checkout. Some supermarkets are allowing consumers to call in grocery orders for pickup.

Many stores are also showing more concern for the environment. They may have facilities for recycling store bags and bottle returns. Stores may encourage you to bring your own bags for carrying food out of the store. Offering bulk foods reduces the use of packaging.

Factors That Affect Consumer Food Choices

A number of factors affect the choices you make when you are shopping for nutritious and wholesome food. You may want to try products you learn about through advertising. You may think about how a food is processed and the types of additives it contains, **22-4**. You might evaluate the pros and cons of buying organic foods or locally grown foods. You may be drawn to some products by their packaging.

Food Advertising

Food advertising can influence your buying behavior. Manufacturers spend billions of dollars each year promoting products. Their intent is nutrients. This type of information can help you decide how products might fit into your meal planning. Special nutrients found in the product may be highlighted. *Persuasive advertising* appeals to your human needs and desires for love, beauty, physical power, social approval, and happiness. Often, food is advertised for its impact on your life rather than for its nutritional value. For instance, an advertisement may imply you will be more popular if you serve your friends a certain soft drink.

Be aware of how advertising is affecting your shopping decisions. Some ads are helpful, but others may cause you to overspend or buy items you do not need or want.

Food Processing

The degree to which foods are processed may influence some of your consumer decisions. **Food processing** refers to any procedure performed on food to prepare it for consumers. Food processing offers consumers many advantages. Canning green beans preserves them for long-term storage. Pasteurizing milk kills harmful bacteria and makes the milk safer to drink. Washing, cutting, and boning chicken save consumers preparation time. Fortifying margarine makes it more nutritious. Some chemical and physical changes occur during processing, **22-5**. As you may realize from these examples, preparing meals without some processed foods would be nearly impossible in today's society.

Food processing also has some disadvantages for consumers. Processing adds to the cost of foods. The more processed a food is, the higher its price tends to be. Some processing methods cause a loss of essential nutrients in foods. For

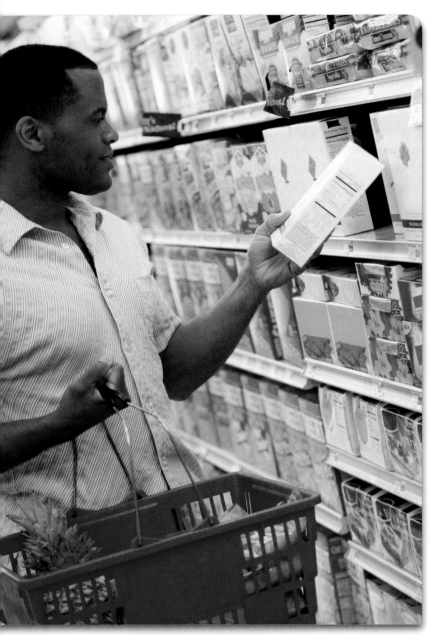

22-4 Evaluating the additives and price of a product will help you decide whether or not to purchase it.

to sway how you spend your food dollars. They want to convince you one product is different from or better than a competing product.

Advertisers use a number of methods to encourage consumers to buy products. *Informational advertising* tends to focus on facts, such as ingredients, prices, and

Effects of Food Processing

Processing Technique	Chemical and Physical Effects on Foods
Canning	Canning involves heating foods in sealed containers to destroy organisms that can cause disease or produce toxins. Heat causes changes in texture, color, and nutritive value of food products. Canned foods maintain quality for 1 to 2 years.
Aseptic canning	This processing method may use temperatures as high as 302°F (150°C) to sterilize food in as little as one second. This short time minimizes changes to the food product. Sterilized food is then placed in sterilized packages within a sterile environment.
Dehydration	Dehydration preserves food by lowering its water content. This stops microbe growth and inactivates enzymes. As food loses water, its weight and size are reduced. Its texture may become leathery or brittle. Flavors often become more concentrated. Treatments used to prevent enzymatic browning may destroy some vitamins in the food.
Fermentation	Microbes are added to cause specific enzymatic changes in some food products. As enzymes break down components in the food product, by-products such as carbon dioxide, acidic and lactic acids, and ethanol may be released. These by-products can change the texture, flavor, and keeping quality of foods such as bread, cheeses, and pickles.
Freezing	Freezing increases shelf life of food by slowing the growth of microbes and the chemical reaction rate of enzymes. Most frozen foods maintain their quality for three to nine months. Rapid freezing right after harvesting is best for preserving food texture and nutrients. Treatment of fruits and vegetables before freezing helps prevent darkening.
Irradiation	Irradiation exposes approved foods to radiant energy which kills bacteria and parasites in the food. This improves food safety and increases shelf life. Irradiation does not change food's nutritional value or flavor.
Pasteurization	Pasteurization involves heating a food product to 161°F (72°C) for 15 seconds to reduce enzyme activity and destroy pathogens and some spoilage bacteria. This improves food safety and increases shelf life. Pasteurization can affect food flavors and destroy heat-sensitive nutrients, which may be replaced through fortification.
Ultrapasteurization	Ultrapasteurization heats a food product to a higher temperature (280°F, 138°C) for a shorter time (2 seconds) than pasteurization. This process also affects food flavors and destroys heat-sensitive nutrients, which may be replaced through fortification. Foods treated with this process can be stored at room temperature until opened.

22-5 Food processing may affect the chemical and physical characteristics of food products.

instance, refining grains removes parts of the grain kernels that are rich in vitamins, minerals, protein, and fiber. Most refined grain products are enriched to add back some of the lost nutrients. However, enriched products still do not match the nutrient levels of whole-grain products.

Your shopping task is not easy. There is a lot to consider in the new marketing age—convenience, cost, potential environmental impact from processing or packaging, and nutritional value of the food. Think about what has been added to the food during the processing, for example increased amounts of salt, sugar, and fats. Think about what has been removed from the processed foods, such as fiber, vitamins, minerals, and phytochemicals. Weighing all these factors can help you decide which foods you want to put in your shopping cart.

Food Irradiation

In 1963, the FDA determined food irradiation to be a safe process. **Food irradiation** is the treatment of approved foods with ionizing energy. Ionizing energy creates positive and negative charges. Irradiation of foods is a useful method for

- food preservation
- food sterilization
- control of sprouting, ripening, and insect damage
- control of foodborne illness

Irradiation improves food safety and extends shelf life by killing or inactivating organisms that cause food spoilage and decomposition. It kills harmful bacteria and parasites (not viruses) that can cause foodborne illness. Irradiation does not change the food itself in any way. It does not make the food radioactive. It is impossible to detect if food has been exposed to irradiation.

The first food approved for irradiation by the FDA was for U.S. space program astronauts. If you have eaten any spices, you probably already sampled irradiated food. Spices are the most commonly irradiated food in the world. The other foods approved by the FDA for irradiation include fruits, vegetables, lettuce, spinach, wheat flour, potatoes, fresh shell eggs, pork, poultry, and red meat. The FDA requires a special symbol on the labels of irradiated food, **22-6**.

During irradiation, foods go through some slight chemical and nutritional changes. Electromagnetic waves strike molecules in the food product. The force breaks molecular bonds, and new compounds are produced, such as carbon dioxide, formic acid, and glucose. These substances are commonly found in all types of foods. No substances produced have been found to be harmful. Keeping food temperatures and oxygen levels in check during irradiation limits damage to nutrients. It causes little change in flavor, texture, or color of most foods.

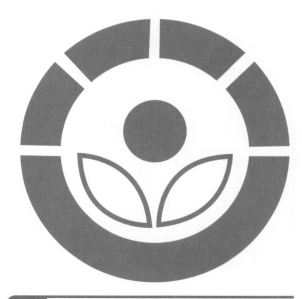

22-6 The international symbol named *radura* is used to identify irradiated foods.

Irradiation is a safe, effective, and thoroughly tested method for preserving food. Food irradiation does not protect against future contamination because no residue remains in the food. Consumers are still expected to wash and refrigerate irradiated foods for safe use.

Many consumers are confused about the processes used for irradiation and what is required to keep foods safe in the kitchen. Consumers who receive education about the process are far more likely to purchase irradiated foods.

Food Additives

Food additives are substances added to food products to cause desired changes in the products. Substances added to foods during processing may affect some of your consumer choices. The Food and Drug Administration (FDA) regulates the use of food additives. The FDA places food additives that have proven to be safe on the **generally recognized as safe (GRAS) list**. The GRAS list includes sugar, salt, and hundreds of other substances. GRAS list substances are also called *ingredients* of processed foods. The FDA has reviewed substances on the GRAS list and removed those whose safety is suspect. Manufacturers can freely use any of the substances on the GRAS list.

Manufacturers must seek FDA approval to use any food additives other than those on the GRAS list. The FDA will not approve the use of any substance found to cause cancer in humans or animals. Aspartame, nitrites, and synthetic food colorings are among the hundreds of additives used in foods.

Most packaged foods contain additives to perform one or more of the following functions:

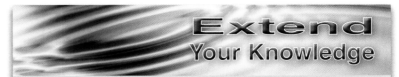

The Delaney Clause

The Delaney Clause was included in the Food Additives Amendment of 1958 and the Color Additives Amendment of 1960. This clause stated that no food or color additives could be approved for use in foods if they were shown to cause cancer in humans or animals.

The intent of the clause was good, but it created some problems. Experts questioned whether results of experiments in which lab animals were fed extremely high levels of a substance over a lifetime were relevant to humans eating much smaller amounts. In addition, advances in technology made the zero-cancer-risk standard established by this clause impractical.

In 1996, U.S. foods safety laws were reformed. As a result, a new safety standard was established limiting quantities of these substances in foods to levels that ensured reasonable certainty of no harm to consumers.

- preserve food (For example, additives that control the growth of bacteria, yeast, or molds improve keeping quality of foods. Additives that prevent damage due to oxidation keep fats from becoming rancid and fruits from turning brown.)
- enhance colors, flavors, or textures
- maintain or improve nutritional quality
- aid processing

Food manufacturers must limit additive use to the smallest amount needed to produce a desired effect. Even so, some people have adverse reactions to certain food additives. Others want to limit their intake of food additives. Reading ingredient labels on food products will help people avoid specific additives if desired. As a wise consumer, you must weigh the costs and benefits of buying foods that contain additives.

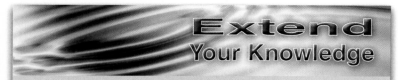

Extend Your Knowledge

Organic Labeling

When shopping for organic foods, look for the USDA organic seal. You will find the seal on fresh or processed products that contain organic ingredients. Be familiar with the different levels of organic labeling:

- If the product is labeled "100 Percent Organic," the product must contain only organic ingredients, not including water and salt.
- Products labeled "Organic" must contain at least 95 percent organic products, not including water and salt.
- Foods labeled "Made with Organic Ingredients or Foods" must contain 70 percent or more organic ingredients, not including water and salt. These labels cannot display the USDA Organic Seal.
- Products containing less than 70 percent organic ingredients can list organic ingredients in the ingredients statement, but cannot display the USDA Organic Seal.

Organically Grown

Like the chemicals used to process foods, the chemicals used to grow foods may concern you as a consumer. If so, you may want to shop for organic foods. **Organic foods** are produced without the use of synthetic fertilizers, pesticides, antibiotics, herbicides, or growth hormones. Materials and farming methods are used that are designed to be in ecological balance. Organic farmers often use manure or compost to enrich the soil. They may hoe to control weeds and use natural pesticides to control insects.

The United States Department of Agriculture (USDA) established standards and a certification program for organic products sold in this country. The USDA organic seal on a product means the ingredients and production methods have been verified by a certifying agency as meeting or exceeding USDA standards for organic production, **22-7**. This seal assures consumers they are buying a product that is uniform and consistent with federal standards.

The organics food industry is growing. Sales of organic foods are expected to continue to increase. The average cost of organic foods is usually higher than similar nonorganic foods. Many organic farms are small although larger food manufacturers are interested in a share of the organic food sales, too. Small organic farms cannot produce and ship foods as economically as large farming operations. Covering their production costs raises food prices.

Some health-conscious consumers prefer organic produce, eggs, milk, meats, and other products. They may think these foods are more nutritious. However, research has not found this to be the case. Many consumers who choose organics are also concerned about the pesticide residues on nonorganic fruits and vegetables. However, many residues can be removed from

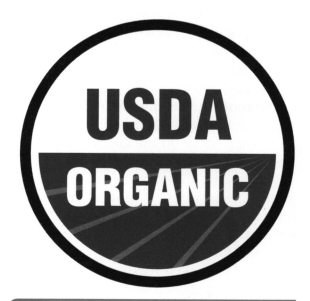

22-7 Look for this seal when buying organic foods to be sure they have been produced according to USDA standards.

nonorganics by washing them in running water. Washing is an important step when preparing organic produce to remove soil and insects.

Food Prices

Perhaps the price of products is one of the biggest factors that will affect your decisions when shopping for food. Most people have a certain amount of money available to spend on food. Comparison shopping will help you avoid overspending. **Comparison shopping** is assessing prices and quality of similar products. It enables you to choose those that best meet your needs and fit your price range.

Use Unit Prices

Unit pricing makes it easy to comparison shop. A **unit price** is a product's cost per standard unit of weight or volume. For instance, the unit price for breakfast cereal would tell you the cost in cents per ounce. The unit price for milk might be in cents per quart. Unit prices for products such as eggs and paper napkins are based on count, such as cents per dozen.

Unit prices are usually on tags attached to the shelves on which products are sitting. You can use unit pricing to compare different forms, sizes, or brands of products to find the best buy.

Compare Brands

You need to compare more than price when comparing brands. You also need to compare product quality. **National brand** products are distributed and advertised throughout the country by major food companies. These products are generally considered to be high quality. To cover the costs of nationwide advertising, the prices of these products are usually high.

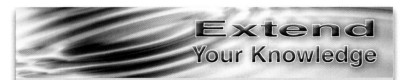

Shopping for Fair Trade?

Are there ethical considerations when shopping for food? Some food products include a Fair Trade logo on their label. Fair Trade is still a relatively new concept. There are a number of different organizations that certify, label, and market Fair Trade products. Research to learn more about Fair Trade. What types of food stores sell Fair Trade foods? Form an opinion on the concept of Fair Trade. Next time you are shopping, see if you can find foods with a Fair Trade logo.

Store brand products are sold only in specific chains of food stores. These products are often of similar quality to national brand products. However, because they are not widely advertised, their prices are usually lower than national brands.

Generic products are unbranded and have no trade name. You can identify them by their plain, simple packaging. You may find generic products to be of somewhat lower quality. For instance, the size of generic green beans may not be uniform.

Math Link

Calculating Unit Cost

Lena wants to compare the unit price of frozen peas to canned peas. A 10-ounce box of frozen peas has 2½ servings and costs 79 cents. A 15-ounce can of peas has 3½ servings and costs 99 cents.
- Calculate the price per ounce for both the frozen and canned peas. Which has the lower unit cost?

However, the nutritional value of generic products is comparable to other products. They are usually less expensive than national or store brands.

Consider how you intend to use a food when choosing among national brands, store brands, and generic products. For example, suppose you are going to cut up canned peaches for a salad. Irregular shapes and sizes will not be noticeable in this type of dish. Therefore, you do not need to pay a high price for the top-quality national brand. Consider buying store brand or generic peaches instead. The nutritional quality will remain the same, and you will save money.

Use a Shopping List

One of the best ways to control food spending is to prepare a shopping list, **22-8**. A shopping list can help you avoid **impulse buying**, or making unplanned purchases. Impulse buying can cause you to spend money you had not planned to spend on items you do not need. A shopping list can also help you save the time required to return to the store for forgotten items.

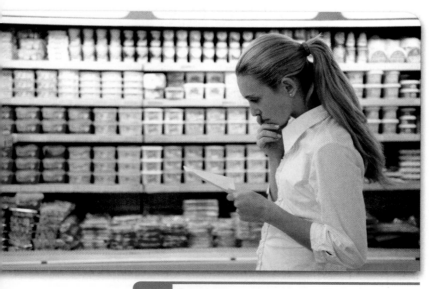

22-8 Food buyers can save time and money by using a shopping list set up according to store layout.

To prepare your list, begin by reviewing the menus and recipes you plan to use. Write all the ingredients you do not have on hand on your shopping list. Keep the shopping list handy and add needed food items as supplies run low.

Organize your shopping list according to the way foods are grouped in the store. This will save you time and keep you from missing items you need. Your list might include such headings as *produce*; *canned foods*; *rice, beans*, and *pasta*; *baking needs*; *cereals*; and *breads*. Place the headings *meats, dairy products*, and *frozen foods* at the bottom of the list. You should pick up perishable foods in these categories last to reduce the chance of spoilage.

Control Food Spending

The following shopping pointers may help you get more food value for your dollar:

- Plan meals around advertised specials.
- Try to avoid shopping when you are tired, hungry, or rushed. You are more likely to make unplanned purchases under these conditions.
- Buy foods in season. When foods are plentiful, they are usually a good buy, **22-9**.
- If you have the storage space, stock up on sale items that will stay fresh in your home. Canned and frozen foods may be bought in larger quantities if properly stored. Pay attention to expiration dates.
- Avoid overbuying foods that spoil if not eaten right away. Fresh produce spoils more quickly than canned, dried, or frozen fruits and vegetables.
- Avoid foods that are packaged in individual servings. Extra packaging usually adds to the costs of products. Packaging also places a strain on the environment.

Preventing food spoilage helps you get the most from the money you spend. You can maintain wholesome quality of the foods you buy by storing them properly. Go directly home from the store. As soon as you get home, remember to refrigerate all perishable foods. Rewrap meats and other bulk items for the freezer in meal-sized portions. Place flour, mixes, and other dry foods in tightly covered containers to avoid insect problems. Store dry and canned foods in cool, dry places.

Using Food Labels

As an informed consumer, you will want to use food labels to guide your buying decisions. Food labeling is regulated by the FDA, but the USDA governs labels on meat and poultry products. Labels are your main source of information about food products.

A few food products are exempt from labeling laws. Foods prepared by small businesses do not need to display label information. For example, the local baker does not need to label fresh baked goods. Restaurant and deli foods intended to be eaten right away do not need to supply label information. However, restaurant and vending machine chains of a certain size are required to provide nutritional information for their menu items, **22-10**. Custom processed fish and meats, donated foods, and individual foods from multiunit packages are exempt from labeling laws. Foods in small packages, such as chewing gum, do not need nutrition labeling. However, manufacturers must include a phone number or address for consumers to call or write if they have questions. Foods of limited nutritional value, such

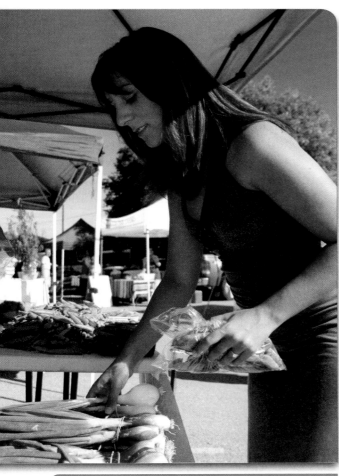

22-9 The best prices can be found when foods are in their growing season.

- Compare prices of uncut and precut items, such as chunk and shredded cheeses or whole fruit and fruit salad. Precut items tend to cost more. They may also spoil more quickly.
- Use coupons to buy items you need or use regularly. Before you use a coupon, however, compare quality and prices of similar products. Even with coupons, some foods are not cheaper than other brands.
- Be aware of methods stores use to entice you to make impulse purchases. Store displays may tempt you to buy items not on your shopping list. For example, a display of toppings with the frozen desserts may encourage you to make an unplanned purchase.

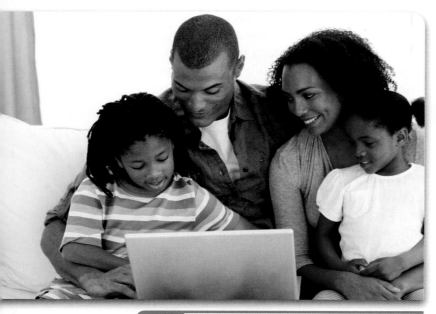

22-10 Many restaurants provide nutritional information for their menu items on their Web site.

as tea and coffee, are not required to have nutrition labeling, either. Companies may choose voluntary labeling to provide nutrition information, even if not required by law.

Basic Information

Federal laws require certain information on the label of every processed, packaged food product. This information includes the name and form of the food, such as French cut green beans. The label must also state the amount of food in the package in both U.S. and metric units of measure. The name and address of the manufacturer, packer, or distributor must appear, too. A list of ingredients and a Nutrition Facts panel are also required on almost all foods.

Ingredient Labeling

The law requires all the ingredients in a food product to be listed on the label. Manufacturers must list ingredients in descending order by weight. Flavorings,

color additives, and some spices must be listed by their common names.

A complete list of ingredients helps consumers know what is in the foods they buy. People are interested in this information for various reasons. They may want to buy the canned beef stew that contains more beef than any other ingredient. Others want to avoid certain ingredients for religious or cultural reasons. For instance, a vegetarian would want to know that a can of vegetable soup contains beef broth.

Some consumers want to avoid substances to which they may be allergic or sensitive. Eight foods or food groups are responsible for 90 percent of food allergies. The eight major food allergens include milk, egg, fish, crustacean shellfish, tree nuts, wheat, peanuts, and soybeans. Food manufacturers are required by law to include a list of any ingredients that are major food allergens, **22-11**.

Nutrition Labeling

The Nutrition Labeling and Education Act (NLEA) requires most foods to include nutrition labeling. When purchasing a food item, take time to look at the Nutrition Facts panel on the product label. The information listed there can help you decide how the food will contribute to your day's total diet. It can help you meet special dietary needs, too. For instance, this information can help you select foods that are lower in fats or higher in fiber. The Nutrition Facts panel can also help you quickly compare the nutritional value of similar foods.

Serving Sizes

On all labels, serving size of food products must be stated in common household terms and metric measures. For example, a serving of milk or yogurt is one cup (240 mL). **Serving size** is based on the amount of a food most people eat at one time. Labels must be read carefully. On snack foods, what often appears to be one serving may be listed as two or more on the package label. Daily nutrients and calories may be more than expected when serving sizes are doubled. A listed serving size is the same for all foods in the same general category. This allows you to compare the nutrient content of similar products. For example, you can easily compare vitamin C per serving of grape drink and grape juice. Both products will list nutrients based on the same serving size.

Compare the serving sizes listed on product labels with the sizes of portions you consume. Suppose a serving of cereal is one cup. However, you may pour one and a half cups into your bowl. This means you are consuming one and a half times the calories and nutrients listed on the cereal package. Knowing this will help you more accurately calculate your daily calorie and nutrient intakes.

Below the serving size on the Nutrition Facts panel is the number of servings per container. You can divide the total cost of the product by the number of servings to figure the cost per serving. This can help you compare food prices when shopping. For instance, suppose a 12-ounce can of frozen orange juice concentrate costs $1.49 and makes six servings. A 64-ounce carton of orange juice costs $1.89 and contains eight servings. (In this case, the unit price is not helpful. The concentrated weight of the frozen juice is not comparable to the fluid volume of the reconstituted juice.) You can figure the frozen juice costs nearly $0.248 per serving whereas juice from the carton costs $0.236 per serving. Costs per serving are nearly the same. Personal taste preference and storage consideration will be the deciding factors.

Calories and Nutrients

The Nutrition Facts panel lists information about food products on a per serving basis. You will find the number of calories a serving of the product provides. The number of calories from fat is also stated. This information can help you limit your fat intake to no more than 30 percent of your total calories.

The next section of the Nutrition Facts panel contains the amounts of nutrients per serving. Amounts of total fat, saturated fat, *trans* fat, cholesterol, sodium, total carbohydrates, dietary

Nutrition Facts
Serving Size 2 bars (42g)
Servings Per Container 6

Amount Per Serving	2 bars		1 bar	
Calories	190		90	
Calories from Fat	60		30	
		%DV*		%DV*
Total Fat	7g	**10%**	3.5g	**5%**
Saturated Fat	1g	**4%**	0.5g	**2%**
Trans Fat	0g		0g	
Cholesterol	0mg	**0%**	0mg	**0%**
Sodium	180mg	**7%**	90mg	**4%**
Total Carbohydrate	28g	**9%**	14g	**5%**
Dietary Fiber	2g	**8%**	1g	**4%**
Sugars	11g		16g	
Protein	5g		2g	
Iron		4%		2%

Not a significant source of vitamin A, vitamin C and calcium.

*Percent Daily Values (DV) are based on a 2,000 calorie diet. Your daily values may be higher or lower depending on your calorie needs:

	Calories	2,000	2,500
Total Fat	Less Than	65g	80g
Sat Fat	Less Than	20g	25g
Cholesterol	Less Than	300mg	300mg
Sodium	Less Than	2,400mg	2,400mg
Total Carbohydrates		300g	375g
Dietary Fiber		25g	30g

Ingredients: Whole Grain Oats, Sugar, Canola Oil, Peanut Butter (peanuts, salt), Yellow Corn Flour, Brown Sugar Syrup, Soy Flour, Salt, Soy Lecithin, Baking Soda.

CONTAINS PEANUT, SOY; MAY CONTAIN ALMOND AND PECAN INGREDIENTS.

22-11 According to law, ingredients that are major allergens must be clearly listed on food labels.

fiber, sugars, and protein are listed. The nutrient amounts are listed in grams or milligrams.

To the right of the nutrient amounts on the Nutrition Facts panel, you will see percent *Daily Values* (%DV). *Daily Values* are recommended nutrient intakes used as references on food labels, though there is no Daily Value for *trans* fat. The percent Daily Values are based on daily calorie needs on a 2,000-calorie diet. If you need more or less than 2,000 calories daily, you will need to adjust your Daily Values accordingly, **22-12**.

Percent Daily Values for vitamins A and C, calcium, and iron are also required on the nutrition panel. Manufacturers may choose to list information about other nutrients, such as the B vitamins. They must provide information about all nutrients that are added to the food.

The percent Daily Values serve as general guidelines. They can help you know how a food serving fits into your daily nutrient needs. A high percent Daily Value (20 percent or more) for a given nutrient means a food provides a lot of that nutrient. A low percentage (5 percent or less) means the food provides a small amount of the nutrient.

The bottom of the Nutrition Facts panel provides some reference information. Daily Values are listed for several nutrients for a 2,000- and a 2,500-calorie diet. You can use these numbers to estimate your daily limits for fat, saturated fat, cholesterol, and sodium. You can also estimate your recommended intakes of carbohydrate and dietary fiber. A conversion guide reminds you how many calories a gram of fat, carbohydrate, or protein provides.

Modified Labels

You will find modified nutrition labels on some foods. For instance, no recommended fat intake levels are given on foods intended for children under two years of age. This is because restricting fat in the diets of young children may be harmful to health.

Another label modification you may notice is on boxed mixes for products like muffins and pudding. Two columns of nutrient amounts may appear on these products. Manufacturers must list nutrient amounts per serving of mix as packaged. However, manufacturers may also list nutrition information for the products as prepared.

You may find a simplified label on products like candy, which do not provide significant amounts of some nutrients. Also, smaller food items, such as canned tuna, may use simpler labels that fit more easily on their packages.

Sample label for Macaroni & Cheese

① **Start Here** ➡

Nutrition Facts
Serving Size 1 cup (228g)
Servings Per Container 2

Amount Per Serving

② **Check Calories**   **Calories** 250   Calories from Fat 110

	% Daily Value*
Total Fat 12g	18%
Saturated Fat 3g	15%
Trans Fat 3g	
Cholesterol 30mg	10%
Sodium 470mg	20%
Total Carbohydrate 31g	10%
Dietary Fiber 0g	0%
Sugars 5g	
Protein 5g	
Vitamin A	4%
Vitamin C	2%
Calcium	20%
Iron	4%

③ **Limit these Nutrients**

⑥ **Quick Guide to % DV**

• **5% or less is Low**

• **20% or more is High**

④ **Get Enough of these Nutrients**

* Percent Daily Values are based on a 2,000 calorie diet. Your Daily Values may be higher or lower depending on your calorie needs.

	Calories:	2,000	2,500
Total Fat	Less than	65g	80g
Sat Fat	Less than	20g	25g
Cholesterol	Less than	300mg	300mg
Sodium	Less than	2,400mg	2,400mg
Total Carbohydrate		300g	375g
Dietary Fiber		25g	30g

⑤ **Footnote**

22-12 The nutrition label can help consumers choose the most healthful foods.

Fresh fruits, vegetables, meats, poultry, and fish may not have labels. However, most stores have posters, notebooks, or pamphlets with nutrition information about these foods. The produce department should offer information about the 20 most popular raw fruits and vegetables. The fish department should provide nutrition details about the 20 most common fish sold raw. The meat department has nutrient data on the 45 best-selling cuts of raw meat and poultry, **22-13**.

Using Label Information to Meet Your Needs

Suppose you are reading the label on a can of baked beans. It tells you one serving provides 5 grams of total fat, or 8 percent of the Daily Value. You know this percentage is based on a 2,000-calorie diet. How can you use this information if you need 2,800 calories per day?

Recommendations for daily total fat intake are based on 30 percent of daily calorie needs. If you need 2,800 calories per day, no more than 840 of those calories should come from fat (2,800 calories x 0.30 = 840 calories). Fat provides 9 calories per gram. This means you should limit daily fat intake to no more than 93 grams (840 calories ÷ 9 calories/gram = 93 grams). Therefore, 5 grams of total fat from a serving of the baked beans equals 5 percent of your Daily Value (5 grams ÷ 93 grams = 0.05 x 100 = 5%).

What if you need only 1,600 calories per day? The same series of calculations would tell you your daily limit for total fat is 53 grams. This means a serving of baked beans would provide 9 percent of your Daily Value for total fat.

Check the Nutrition Facts panel to compare similar types of foods. Serving sizes are generally similar. This will help you identify heart-healthy foods. For example, you can combine the grams of saturated fat and *trans* fat

Seafood Nutrition Facts

Cooked (by moist or dry heat with no added ingredients), edible weight portion. Percent Daily Values (%DV) are based on a 2,000 calorie diet.

Seafood, Serving Size (84 g/3 oz)	Calories	Calories from Fat	Total Fat g	%DV	Saturated Fat g	%DV	Cholesterol mg	%DV	Sodium mg	%DV	Potassium mg	%DV	Total Carbohydrate g	%DV	Protein g	Vitamin A %DV	Vitamin C %DV	Calcium %DV	Iron %DV
Blue Crab	100	10	1	2	0	0	95	32	330	14	300	9	0	0	20g	0%	4%	10%	4%
Catfish	130	60	6	9	2	10	50	17	40	2	230	7	0	0	17g	0%	0%	0%	0%
Clams, about 12 small	110	15	1.5	2	0	0	80	27	95	4	470	13	6	2	17g	10%	0%	8%	30%
Cod	90	5	1	2	0	0	50	17	65	3	460	13	0	0	20g	0%	2%	2%	2%
Flounder/Sole	100	15	1.5	2	0	0	55	18	100	4	390	11	0	0	19g	0%	0%	2%	0%
Haddock	100	10	1	2	0	0	70	23	85	4	340	10	0	0	21g	2%	0%	2%	6%
Halibut	120	15	2	3	0	0	40	13	60	3	500	14	0	0	23g	4%	0%	2%	6%
Lobster	80	0	0.5	1	0	0	60	20	320	13	300	9	1	0	17g	2%	0%	6%	2%
Ocean Perch	110	20	2	3	0.5	3	45	15	95	4	290	8	0	0	21g	0%	2%	10%	4%
Orange Roughy	80	5	1	2	0	0	20	7	70	3	340	10	0	0	16g	2%	0%	4%	2%
Oysters, about 12 medium	100	35	4	6	1	5	80	27	300	13	220	6	6	2	10g	0%	6%	6%	45%
Pollock	90	10	1	2	0	0	80	27	110	5	370	11	0	0	20g	2%	0%	0%	2%
Rainbow Trout	140	50	6	9	2	10	55	18	35	1	370	11	0	0	20g	4%	4%	8%	2%
Rockfish	110	15	2	3	0	0	40	13	70	3	440	13	0	0	21g	4%	0%	2%	2%
Salmon, Atlantic/Coho/Sockeye/Chinook	200	90	10	15	2	10	70	23	55	2	430	12	0	0	24g	4%	4%	2%	2%
Salmon, Chum/Pink	130	40	4	6	1	5	70	23	65	3	420	12	0	0	22g	2%	0%	2%	4%
Scallops, about 6 large or 14 small	140	10	1	2	0	0	65	22	310	13	430	12	5	2	27g	2%	0%	4%	14%
Shrimp	100	10	1.5	2	0	0	170	57	240	10	220	6	0	0	21g	4%	4%	6%	10%
Swordfish	120	50	6	9	1.5	8	40	13	100	4	310	9	0	0	16g	2%	2%	0%	6%
Tilapia	110	20	2.5	4	1	5	75	25	30	1	360	10	0	0	22g	0%	2%	0%	2%
Tuna	130	15	1.5	2	0	0	50	17	40	2	480	14	0	0	26g	2%	2%	2%	4%

Seafood provides negligible amounts of *trans* fat, dietary fiber, and sugars.

U.S. Food and Drug Administration
(January 1, 2008)

22-13 Stores may use posters to present nutrition information for items such as seafood.

and look for the lowest total. Also, look for the lowest percent Daily Value for cholesterol. Check all three nutrients to make the best choice for a healthful diet. Similarly, compare foods to seek lower Daily Values of sodium and sugar and higher Daily Values for fiber, vitamins, and minerals.

Claims

In addition to nutrition labeling, the NLEA requires any food labels that make nutrient content claims or health claims meet specific requirements. There are four types of claims used on food labels—nutrient content claims, health claims, qualified health claims, and structure/function claims.

Nutrient Content Claims

You may be swayed by words used on food packaging to make products sound healthful. Manufacturers use claims on their labels to convince you to buy their product. A nutrient content claim either directly states or implies a level of nutrient in a food. For example, a cereal label that reads "Low-fat granola" is stating the cereal contains a low level of the nutrient fat.

Terms may be used that can be confusing. For instance, lite whipped topping sounds more healthful than regular whipped topping. However, you need to know what the term *lite* means. Then you can decide if eating lite foods will improve the quality of your diet. Products must meet specific definitions for manufacturers to use terms such as *light, low sodium*, and *fat free* on labels, **22-14**.

Nutrient Content Claims	
Claim	**Definition (per serving)**
Calorie free	Fewer than 5 calories
Low calorie	40 calories or fewer
Reduced or fewer calories	At least 25% fewer calories
Light or lite	One-third fewer calories or 50% less fat
Sugar free	Fewer than 0.5 grams sugars
Reduced sugar or less sugar	At least 25% less sugars
No added sugar	No sugars added during processing or packing, including ingredients that contain sugars, such as juice or dry fruit
Fat free	Fewer than 0.5 grams fat
Low fat	3 grams or fewer of fat
Reduced or less fat	At least 25% less fat
Saturated fat free	Fewer than 0.5 grams saturated fat and less than 0.5 grams *trans* fatty acids
Low saturated fat	1 gram or less and 15% less calories from saturated fat
Reduced/less saturated fat	At least 25% less saturated fat
Cholesterol free	Fewer than 2 milligrams cholesterol and 2 grams or fewer of saturated fat
Low cholesterol	20 milligrams or fewer cholesterol and 2 grams or fewer of saturated fat
Reduced or less cholesterol	At least 25% less cholesterol and 2 grams or fewer saturated fat
Sodium free	Fewer than 5 milligrams sodium
Very low sodium	35 milligrams or fewer sodium
Low sodium	140 milligrams or fewer sodium
Reduced or less sodium	At least 25% less sodium
Light in sodium	At least 50% less sodium

22-14 Foods labeled with a nutrient content claim must meet the appropriate criteria.

Health Claims

Besides claims about nutrient content, manufacturers may put certain health claims on product labels. These claims are based on research showing solid evidence of links between foods or nutrients and diseases. For instance, a yogurt container might have a claim about the link between calcium and a reduced risk of osteoporosis. Claims cannot state a certain food prevents or causes a disease, only that risk for the disease may be reduced.

Health claims must be reviewed and evaluated by the FDA before they can be used on labels. FDA approves a health claim only if it finds "significant scientific agreement (SSA)" to support the claim, **22-15**.

Health Claims on Food Product Labels	
Approved Claim	**Model Claim Statement**
Calcium and osteoporosis	Regular exercise and a healthy diet with enough calcium helps teens and young adult white and Asian women maintain good bone health and may reduce their high risk of osteoporosis later in life.
Dietary fat and cancer	Development of cancer depends on many factors. A diet low in total fat may reduce the risk of some cancers.
Dietary saturated fat and cholesterol and coronary heart disease	While many factors affect heart disease, diets low in saturated fat and cholesterol may reduce the risk of this disease.
Fiber-containing grain products, fruits, and vegetables and cancer	Low-fat diets rich in fiber-containing grain products, fruits, and vegetables may reduce the risk of this disease.
Fruits, vegetables, and grain products that contain fiber, particularly soluble fiber, and risk of coronary heart disease	Diets low in saturated fat and cholesterol and rich in fruits, vegetables, and grain products that contain some types of dietary fiber, particularly soluble fiber, may reduce the risk of heart disease, a disease associated with many factors.
Sodium and hypertension (high blood pressure)	Diets low in sodium may reduce the risk of high blood pressure, a disease associated with many factors.
Fruits and vegetables and cancer	Low-fat diets rich in fruits and vegetables (foods that are low in fat and may contain dietary fiber, vitamin A, or vitamin C) may reduce the risk of some types of cancer, a disease associated with many factors. Broccoli is high in vitamins A and C, and is a good source of dietary fiber.
Folate and neural tube birth defects	Healthful diets with adequate folate may reduce a woman's risk of having a child with a brain or spinal cord defect.
Dietary noncariogenic carbohydrate sweeteners and dental caries	Frequent between-meal consumption of foods high in sugars and starches promotes tooth decay. The sugar alcohols in [name of food] do not promote tooth decay.

(Continued)

22-15   Health claims continue to be submitted to the FDA for review and addition to this list.

22-15   *(Continued)*

Health Claims on Food Product Labels *(Continued)*

Approved Claim	Model Claim Statement
Soluble fiber from certain foods and risk of coronary heart disease	Soluble fiber from foods such as [name of soluble fiber source and food product] as part of a diet low in saturated fat and cholesterol, may reduce the risk of heart disease. A serving of [name of food product] supplies _____ grams of the soluble fiber from [name of soluble fiber source] necessary per day to have this effect.
Soy protein and risk of coronary heart disease	(1) 25 grams of soy protein a day, as part of a diet low in saturated fat and cholesterol, may reduce the risk of heart disease. A serving of [name of food] supplies _____ grams of soy protein. (2) Diets low in saturated fat and cholesterol that include 25 grams of soy protein a day may reduce the risk of heart disease. One serving of [name of food] supplies _____ grams of soy protein.
Plant sterol/stanol esters and risk of coronary heart disease	(1) Foods containing at least 0.65 gram per reference amount of vegetable oil sterol esters, eaten twice a day with meals for a daily total intake of at least 1.3 grams, as part of a diet low in saturated fat and cholesterol, may reduce the risk of heart disease. A serving of [name of food] supplies _____ grams of vegetable oil sterol esters. (2) Diets low in saturated fat and cholesterol that include two servings of foods that provide a daily total of at least 3.4 grams of plant stanol esters in two meals may reduce the risk of heart disease. A serving of [name of food] supplies _____ grams of plant stanol esters.
Whole-grain foods and risk of heart disease and certain cancers	Diets rich in whole-grain foods and other plant foods and low in total fat, saturated fat, and cholesterol may reduce the risk of heart disease and some cancers.
Potassium and the risk of high blood pressure and stroke	Diets containing foods that are a good source of potassium and that are low in sodium may reduce the risk of high blood pressure and stroke.
Fluoridated water and reduced risk of dental caries	Drinking fluoridated water may reduce the risk of dental caries or tooth decay.
Saturated fat, cholesterol, and *trans* fat, and reduced risk of heart disease	Diets low in saturated fat and cholesterol, and as low as possible in *trans* fat, may reduce the risk of heart disease.

Qualified Health Claims

Similar to health claims, qualified health claims suggest a link between a food or nutrient and its ability to reduce risk for a disease or health condition. However, qualified health claims do not require the scientific support to be as strong as for a health claim.

Sometimes you may see dietary guidance statements on food labels. These statements cannot include both a reference to a specific food or nutrient and to a disease or health condition as health and qualified health claims do. Dietary guidance statements include only one of these elements. For example, the statement "Calcium is good for you" contains a reference to a specific nutrient, but not to a disease or health condition. Truthful dietary guidance statements that are not deceiving do not require review and approval from the FDA before being used on a label. However, if the FDA decides the statement is misleading, its use may be disallowed.

Structure/Function Claims

A fourth type of claim found on food labels is a structure/function claim. A structure/function claim describes the effect that a food or nutrient has on the structure or function of the body. This claim differs from health and qualified health claims because there is no reference to a disease or health condition in the claim. An example of a structure/function claim would be "Calcium (the nutrient) builds strong bones (the body structure)."

Product Dating

Take note of dates on food product labels. Under federal regulations, all infant formula, baby food, and over the counter drugs sold in the United States are required to have product dating, Food manufacturers voluntarily use several types of dates. There are three basic types of open dates:

- "Use-by" date is the last date recommended for consumer use of the product while at peak quality. The date is determined by the packer of the product.
- "Sell-by" date identifies to the store management how long a product should be displayed for sale.
- "Best if used by (or before)" date is useful to the consumer to predict for best flavor or quality, although it is technically not a "sell-by" or safety date.

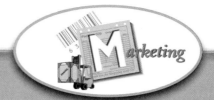

Food Purchasing Agent

Food purchasing agents buy a vast array of food products for companies and institutions. They attempt to get the best deal for their companies—the highest quality at the lowest possible cost. These agents accomplish this by studying sales records and inventory levels of current stock and identifying foreign and domestic suppliers. Food purchasing agents also keep abreast of changes affecting both the supply of and demand for needed products.

Education: Requirements tend to vary with the size of the organization. Large stores and distributors prefer applicants who have a bachelor's degree with an emphasis in business. Many manufacturing firms put an even greater emphasis on formal training, preferring applicants with a bachelor's or master's degree in engineering, business, economics, or one of the applied sciences.

Job Outlook: Employment for purchasing agents is expected to increase. Job growth and opportunities, however, will differ among different occupations in this category.

If foods have been stored properly, they should still be wholesome after the dates have expired. For maximum eating and keeping quality, however, avoid buying products with expired dates.

Country-of-Origin Labeling (COOL)

Much of the food supply in the United States comes from other countries. Grapes may come from Chile, avocados from Mexico, and apples from Canada. The *country-of-origin labeling (COOL)* law requires that full-line food stores provide consumers with information at the point of

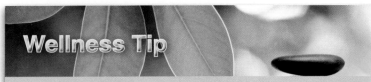

Wellness Tip

Wash Reusable Grocery Bags

Although reusable grocery bags are good for the environment, they can be bad for your health without proper care. Without regular washing, these reusable bags can be a breeding ground for food-borne bacteria. To keep your reusable grocery bags safe, clean them after every use. Wash fabric bags in your washing machine. Clean bags made of plastic-like materials in a sink filled with soapy water and a ¼ cup of distilled vinegar.

purchase about the sources of certain foods. Not all foods are covered by this law, **22-16**. Processed foods such as canned tuna, roasted peanuts, or fruit medley are examples of foods not covered by COOL.

Businesses such as butchers and fish markets do not have to provide COOL information because they do not sell fruits and vegetables. Restaurants, cafeterias, food stands, salad bars, and delicatessens are also not covered by this law.

The COOL information may appear on a food label, sign, twist tie, band, or other display, but it must be easy to

Foods Covered by Country-of-Origin Labeling Law
• Muscle cuts of beef, veal, lamb, pork, goat, and chicken
• Ground beef, veal, lamb, pork, goat, and chicken
• Fish and shellfish (wild and farm raised)
• Fresh and frozen fruits and vegetables
• Peanuts
• Pecans and macadamia nuts
• Ginseng

22-16 Certain foods must display country-of-origin labeling.

read. The label must list the country (or countries) where the food was grown, or born, raised, and slaughtered. In some cases, an animal may have been born and raised in Canada, but slaughtered in the United States. The label for this food would include both Canada and the United States.

Being a Consumer of Fitness Products and Services

The basic items required for taking part in physical activity are sturdy, comfortable shoes and nonbinding clothes. If you choose to buy more specialized fitness products and services, you need to know where to shop. You must also learn to use product information and evaluate quality.

Shopping for Apparel

Some people prefer the comfort and appearance of fitness apparel that is tailored to specific activities. Sports clothing is designed to meet the needs of people who will be performing a certain set of motions. For instance, bicycle shorts are often made with padding in the seat to provide cushioning on a long ride. Tennis shorts are made with large pockets to hold spare tennis balls.

Fitness apparel is available at discount, department, and sporting goods stores. You can also buy it through catalogs and Internet shopping services. Some companies charge premium prices for their high-tech garments. You must decide if you want multipurpose clothing or items designed for specific activities. You will need to think about what garment features are most important to you.

One of the most important clothing items for fitness activities is shoes. You need to choose shoes that provide support for your feet. The shoes need to be flexible and lightweight to provide comfort as you move. They should not create any sore spots on your feet. The soles should be designed to give you an adequate amount of traction. You may also look for cushioning that absorbs shock and reduces jarring to the body. Absorbent socks will also help cushion and pull perspiration away from the feet, **22-17**.

Your choices of other fitness clothing will depend on the activities you plan to do. For some activities, you may prefer garments made from stretchy fabrics that hug the body. For other activities, loose-fitting clothes may be a better choice. Whatever the fit, you are likely to sweat when you exercise. Therefore, you will be more comfortable in garments made from fabrics that carry perspiration away from your body.

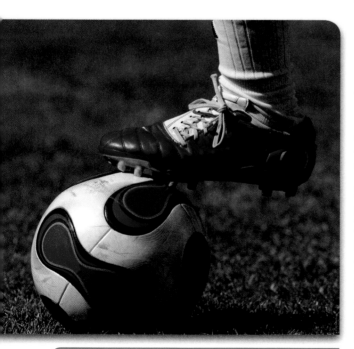

22-17 Shoes are specifically designed for different sports activities to provide the kind of support each activity requires.

Shopping for Equipment

Many sports and exercise activities require special equipment. From golf clubs to free weights to treadmills, you need to know what to look for when shopping for fitness products.

Safety gear is one of the most important fitness purchases you can make. Even the most skilled athletes can have accidents when participating in physical activities. Equipment such as bicycle helmets and wrist guards for in-line skating can protect you from injury. Choose sturdy items that are designed to withstand the forces placed on them by a particular activity.

Having gym equipment at home may make it more convenient for you to exercise. Factors such as bad weather and lack of transportation will not hinder your ability to work out. For most people, less than $200 will set up a basic home gym. This includes a jump rope, a floor mat, stretch bands, and some hand weights. However, some people choose to purchase more complex fitness equipment. Popular items often include rowing machines, treadmills, elliptical machines, exercise bikes, and home gyms, **22-18**.

Many brands and models of fitness equipment are available. To compare various pieces of equipment, you might begin by reading consumer product reviews. When you go to the store, study the features listed on product labels. You can also talk to salespeople. Sometimes talking to several salespeople is helpful because you can get more than one person's opinion about a product. Whenever possible, rent or borrow equipment to try it out before buying.

Watch out for expensive gadgets that do not enhance fitness. Avoid passive devices driven by electric belts,

Popular Fitness Equipment	
Equipment	**Pros and Cons**
Elliptical trainer	Exercises upper body as you work to move the poles and lower body as you pedal. The impact is low on knees. Machine should be comfortable to match your stride.
Rowing machine	Strengthens back, arms, thighs, hips, calves as you pull. Good training for swimmers. Requires care to avoid excess strain on the back.
Stair climber	Provides a good workout for hips, buttocks, and legs. Exercise is low impact and weight bearing. Good training for hikers and skiers. Not a good choice for individuals with knee problems.
Stationary bicycle	Works lower body. Less stress is placed on knees and feet. Not useful for upper body exercise.
Treadmill	Exercises lower body. Incline and speed can be adjusted for greater or lesser intensity. Provides weight-bearing exercise. Older adults or beginners with balance problems can hold handrails until balance improves. No upper body workout.

22-18 Select fitness equipment that helps you fulfill your training goals.

shakers, or rollers. These machines cannot massage the inches away or reduce fat by jarring, squeezing, or rubbing it off, **22-19**.

Evaluating Fitness Equipment

- How often will I use this equipment?
- Can I afford this equipment?
- What safety features does this equipment have?
- Are clear instructions given for proper use?
- Will I get an effective workout with this equipment?
- Can I vary the intensity of exercise easily?
- Will the equipment fit on the available floor space? Is the ceiling high enough to accommodate a person on the equipment?
- How sturdy is the equipment?
- Will the equipment run smoothly?
- Will the machine fit my body size?
- Is the noise level acceptable?

22-19 Answering these questions will help you when selecting fitness equipment.

Choosing Exercise Digital Media

Exercise DVD's, TV exercise programs, and some video-gaming systems offer fitness opportunities at home. They provide some instruction and give you a sense of companionship. Some of these options are far less costly than hiring a trainer or joining a club.

The programs vary by the type and intensity of exercise they include. Some are aerobic for heart health; others are geared toward muscle conditioning for strength and toning. Stretching activities enhance flexibility. Some programs combine all three types of exercise. Some workouts are for beginners, whereas others are intended for advanced exercisers.

Before you buy a DVD or gaming system, consider renting it or borrowing it from the library. This will help you see if you like the music, activity, or style of the leader. It will also allow you to evaluate whether the intensity of exercise is suited to your fitness level.

Watch out for programs that support the use of dangerous techniques. Injuries can happen if complicated twists, turns, and jumps are used. A safe workout should include a warm-up period and a cool-down period. The workout should encourage viewers to work at their own pace.

When doing a home program workout, be sure to wear shoes that offer appropriate support. Work out on an exercise mat or carpet. Check your pulse to be sure you are staying within your safe target heart rate zone, **22-20**.

Hiring a Personal Trainer

Personal trainers offer one-on-one coaching to help you reach your physical fitness goals. A good trainer should be able to design a safe program suited to your needs.

To find a trainer, search the Internet for certified trainers in your area. Call a fitness center, dance studio, or physical education department at a local college. Ask for the names of people who offer individualized fitness instruction.

When you interview a trainer, ask about his or her credentials. Certification and registration programs are offered by a number of sports and fitness organizations. Certifications from National Commission for Certifying Agencies (NCCA)-accredited programs are recommended. You might want to contact the organization through which a trainer received his or her credentials. Ask what qualifications this organization requires to bestow its credential. Decide whether these qualifications meet your standards for a personal trainer. Regardless of other credentials, a trainer should be certified in cardiopulmonary resuscitation (CPR). A trainer with CPR certification can assist a client who is experiencing an exercise-related emergency.

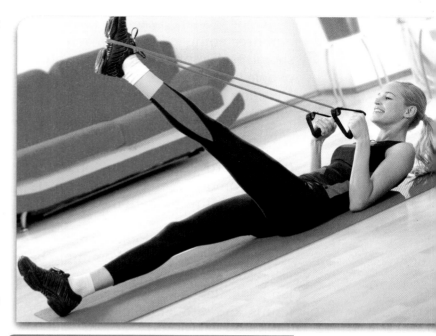

22-20 Sturdy shoes and an exercise mat will provide support and cushioning when working out with an exercise video.

Before hiring a trainer, ask for the names of people who have used his or her services. Call a few of these references to see if they were pleased with the trainer's work.

You may pay $40 to over $100 per hour for personalized fitness services at health clubs or at private business locations. Ask about rates before signing a contract.

Selecting a Health or Fitness Club

You may feel joining a health or fitness club will help you meet your exercise goals. Health facilities range from high-cost clubs with deluxe equipment and many services to inexpensive, no-frills gyms. When deciding what type of facility would meet your needs, examine all the options in your community. These may include spas, Ys, colleges, schools, and community centers. Weigh the costs and conveniences.

Choose a facility with a pleasant, nonthreatening atmosphere. You should feel comfortable with the other people who go there. You should also feel comfortable with the instructors. Ask about their training and experience. The International Health, Racquet and Sportsclub Association (IHRSA) provides accreditation for clubs promoting safety for consumers and works directly with the personal trainers, **22-21**.

Evaluate the equipment and services a facility offers. You might be interested in a running track and a lap pool. Maybe you want basketball, tennis, and racquetball courts. Perhaps an aerobics class and a weight room are important to you. Look at the cleanliness of locker rooms, saunas, and hot tubs. You must decide if the features available fit your needs.

The cost of membership is part of your consumer decision. The costs should reflect the quality of the equipment and services offered by the facility. Many clubs have specials and package deals. Be sure

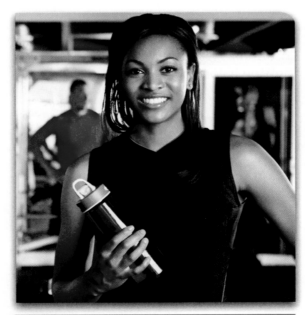

22-21 Trying out the equipment and services at a health club before joining will help you make a good consumer decision.

to ask about any extra charges. Some clubs charge for court time and fitness classes in addition to basic membership fees. Comparison shop with other facilities. No matter what you pay, you must exercise regularly to get the full value of your membership dollar.

Choose a club that is conveniently located. Make sure the hours are convenient, too. You are more likely to go to a facility that is not out of your way. You will also be more inclined to use your membership if you can avoid waiting in line for equipment.

Work out at a facility several times before deciding to buy a membership. Choose a fitness club that is right for you and your budget.

Consumer Rights

As a consumer, you have power. People who produce and sell goods and services want to keep you happy. They want you to keep spending your money on the items they offer.

Consumers have specific rights, some of which are protected by federal laws. Consumers also have responsibilities. You must use your consumer power in appropriate ways when you have problems in the marketplace. The following points give some brief examples of your consumer rights and responsibilities when buying products:

- *You have the right to safety.* The foods you buy should be wholesome. Fitness products should list safety precautions. In turn, you have the responsibility to handle foods and fitness equipment correctly to avoid problems with use.
- *You have the right to be informed.* Labeling on food and other products should be complete and accurate. You have a responsibility to use package information to choose foods that do not contain

ingredients you want to avoid. Read Nutrition Facts panels to select products that will meet your nutritional needs. You also have a responsibility to heed cautions on fitness equipment.

- *You have the right to choose.* You should be able to select from a variety of brands, forms, and sizes of products. You have a responsibility to choose carefully by comparing the cost, convenience, and value of items.
- *You have the right to be heard.* You should be able to expect a satisfactory response when you express your concern about a product. You have a responsibility to be truthful when making a complaint.
- *You have the right to redress.* You should be able to expect a company or product mistake to be corrected. You have a responsibility to receive compensation when errors are made or products are not acceptable.
- *You have the right to education.* You should be able to access information through media, printed material, or organized programs that will help you make the best decision possible. Your responsibility is to seek out information before making a consumer decision.
- *You have the right to a healthy environment.* You should be able to live and carry out consumer activities without danger to health. Your responsibility is to be environmentally aware of your choices on personal and public health.
- *You have the right to have basic needs met.* You should be able to have adequate access to food, drinkable water, and shelter. Your responsibility is to use resources carefully to ensure future availability.

Case Study: A Fit Decision

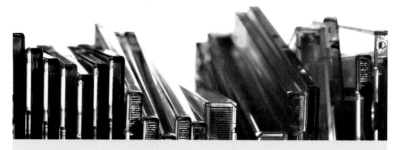

Abby was lying on the couch watching TV as she does most evenings. A commercial came on for a fitness club. The advertisement showed young, attractive individuals performing many types of fitness activities. The people in the commercial appeared very happy and physically fit. Abby knows she needs to be more active. Her parents bought a treadmill last year, but she has only used it once. She is sure if she joins the fitness club in the advertisement, she will go every day.

Abby had been considering joining a fitness club for some time. None of Abby's friends belong to the fitness club and she wasn't comfortable going alone. She was aware many of the athletes from her school had memberships at this club. Abby doesn't socialize with this group much, but thought this might be a way to make new friends. The club even had indoor tennis courts—maybe she would take up tennis. Abby decides to join the next day!

Case Review

1. What kind of advertising is the fitness club using in the commercial?

2. Do you believe Abby will utilize the fitness club? Why?

3. What advice would you give Abby about signing up for the fitness club membership?

Making a Consumer Complaint

For one reason or another, you may find the need to make a consumer complaint. Perhaps you bought a package of cheese that was moldy when you opened it. Maybe a piece of fitness equipment did not operate as advertised. For these and other reasons, a complaint may be in order.

To receive a satisfactory response to your complaint, you need to complain to the right party. If the product you bought came from a local store, your first step is to return the item. Bring your receipt to document when and where you bought the item. State your complaint to the manager. The manager may simply return your money or offer you a replacement product.

Sometimes it may be more appropriate to contact the manufacturer of a product. Look for a toll-free number, Web site, or e-mail address on the product package. You can use these resources to contact a consumer service representative. Clearly explain your problem. Have the product package handy to answer manufacturer queries regarding package code numbers and other identification information.

If a store or manufacturer cannot resolve your problem, you may want to contact an appropriate government office. State, county, and city government consumer protection offices can settle complaints and conduct investigations. The FDA can help you with problems with food products. The U.S. Consumer Product Safety Commission (CPSC) can help solve problems related to other types of products. These agencies are listed under *government offices* in the telephone directory.

When you call, ask to speak to a consumer affairs officer. Again, clearly explain your problem. The officer may be able to take action on your behalf to find an acceptable solution.

Reading Summary

Becoming familiar with some consumer skills and resources will help you make wise choices in the marketplace. One of the decisions you must make as a consumer is where to shop for food. You can choose from many types of food stores; each has advantages and disadvantages. The latest supermarket trends are geared toward making food shopping more convenient for consumers.

A number of factors affect your choices when shopping for food. You may be swayed by advertising. The degree to which foods are processed and the additives they contain may influence some of your food purchases. The availability of organic foods may attract your attention in the store. Food prices are likely to affect many of your choices, too. You can learn how to use unit prices, compare brands, and use a shopping list to control food spending.

Food labels provide much information that can help you as a consumer. Ingredient labeling allows you to identify what is in food products. Claims on packages may encourage you to choose some food products for health reasons. Nutrition labeling can help you analyze how a food will fit into your diet. Product dating can assist you in choosing foods that are fresh and wholesome. The food's country of origin may influence your choice.

You may be a consumer of fitness products and services as well as a consumer of foods. Look for apparel that meets your needs for comfort, appearance, and design features. Choose equipment that meets standards for safety and fits your budget and desired level of quality. When choosing exercise digital media, look for one that is intended for your fitness level. When hiring a personal trainer, or selecting a health club, analyze the important details before signing any contracts.

As a consumer, you have a number of rights, which are protected by law. You must be aware these rights carry the weight of certain responsibilities. Going through proper channels to make a complaint can help you address problems in the marketplace.

Review Learning

1. List five places people shop for food and give one advantage and one disadvantage of each.
2. Describe three supermarket trends that are intended to make shopping more convenient for consumers.
3. Compare the differences between informational advertising and persuasive advertising.
4. True or false. Irradiated foods are protected from future contamination.
5. What are the four main functions of food additives?
6. Why do organic foods tend to cost more than nonorganic food?
7. Products sold only in specific chains of food stores are _____.
    A.   generic products
    B.   local brand products
    C.   national brand products
    D.   store brand products
8. Give five tips for controlling food spending.

9. In what order are ingredients listed on a food product label?
10. True or false. A product labeled "light in sodium" contains 35 milligrams or fewer sodium.
11. On what type of diet are the percent Daily Values on food labels based?
12. True or false. Health claims on food labels must have "significant scientific agreement" to support the claim.
13. List five foods that must be labeled with their country of origin.
14. What are five questions you might ask yourself when evaluating fitness equipment?
15. What type of program certification is recommended for personal trainers?
16. True or false. The first step in filing a consumer complaint is to speak with the appropriate government agency.

Critical Thinking

17. **Compare and contrast.** Examine an organically grown food product and its traditionally grown counterpart. Use the labels to compare and contrast the nutrient content and cost. What are the advantages and disadvantages of each?
18. **Draw conclusions.** How do you think food advertising impacts consumer purchases? Draw conclusions about whether food advertising influences consumers to purchase less-healthful food choices.

Applying Your Knowledge

19. **Price comparison.** List five specific food products. For each product on the list, record the prices charged at two types of food stores discussed in this chapter. Calculate an equivalent unit price comparison for each product and report your findings in class. Which types of stores seem to have the lowest prices?
20. **Nutrition summary.** Read the Nutrition Facts panel from your favorite cereal. Find a similar cereal that is healthier based on a comparison of the Nutrition Facts panel with that from your favorite cereal. Write a paragraph of your findings. Would you consider switching cereals?
21. **Facility evaluation.** Visit a health or fitness club and write a one-page evaluation of the facility. List the criteria you chose for your evaluation.

Technology Connections

22. **Coupon research.** Research current ways—such as wireless electronic coupons—food marketers are using technology to distribute coupons to consumers.
23. **Food label PSA.** Prepare and video-record a public service announcement to teach consumers how to read and understand food labels.
24. **Consumer alert.** Visit the Better Business Bureau (BBB) Web site for your area to learn about current consumer alerts or to check out a business from which you are considering purchasing a product or service. Use presentation software to share your findings with the class.

Academic Connections

25. **Math.** Select one food that is also processed and sold in a variety of forms. For example, a potato is processed and sold as French fries, potato chips, and dehydrated mashed potatoes. Visit the supermarket and record the price per serving for each product. Rank the products by their price per serving. Write a brief paragraph explaining the cost variations.

26. **Speech.** In small groups, debate the following topic: "Food irradiation should be used on more foods to improve the safety of the food supply." Each team should conduct research to support its arguments.

27. **Social studies.** Visit a supermarket. List 10 foods that were imported from another country. List the name of the food and the country of origin. Write a short survey to learn people's attitudes about the foods on your list. Would they buy the foods? What is their opinion about imported foods? How do they decide which food products to buy? Give the survey to five adults who are responsible for purchasing food for their household. Share the survey results with the class.

28. **Speech.** Start a campaign to serve healthier foods in the schools. Develop a 10-minute personal testimony to be given to an authoritative body. Be creative. Ask them to support increased availability of healthy food information and choices. Prepare your arguments.

Workplace Applications

Using Writing and Computer Skills

Imagine that you are a nutrition educator for a national supermarket chain. Your job responsibilities include giving supermarket tours focused on healthful eating, demonstrating recipes to customers, and writing articles for the supermarket's information center. This month you will write an article about how to choose the best quality, low-cost fresh foods. Focus especially on in-season produce, low-fat cuts of meat and poultry, quality fish, and low-fat dairy foods. Be sure to include a healthful recipe or two that use six or fewer ingredients.

Appendix A

Career Planning

Making a Career Choice

Can you picture yourself working in the nutrition and wellness field? What type of occupations interest you most? One way to narrow the long list of career possibilities is to examine your interests, aptitudes, values, and goals. Then you can focus on the career options that best suit you.

Know Your Interests

Everyone has a unique set of interests, and no one knows yours better than you. One person's interests are not better than another's. Interests simply help define an individual. Knowing your interests is important to choosing a satisfying career. Career interests can be classified into three broad categories.

- *Interest in people.* Do you prefer to be with a group or on your own? Do you like projects that involve teamwork or those you accomplish yourself? If you enjoy being around others, you are probably suited for a career that focuses on interacting with people. Counseling hospital patients and working with youth are examples of people-oriented careers.
- *Interest in information.* Do you like to keep track of facts and details? Do you regularly check information sources, such as magazines, newspapers, TV, or the Internet? Do you enjoy making discoveries? If you like to gather facts and share what you know, you are probably

suited for a career that focuses on information. Researching nutrition theories and reporting discoveries appeal to people interested in information.

- *Interest in material items.* Do you like to work with your hands? Perhaps you enjoy assembling objects or taking items apart to find out how they operate. If you do, a career that focuses on tools and material items could be ideal for you. Related nutrition and fitness jobs range from developing new sports equipment to artistic presentation of food on a plate.

Many careers involve all three interest areas to varying degrees. If you have trouble narrowing your interests, however, using an interest assessment can help. Consider taking the *O*NET Interest Profiler*—a self-assessment tool to discover work activities you might find exciting. You can find this tool on the O*NET Web site. Your school guidance counselor can help you with other interest-assessment options.

Identify Aptitudes and Abilities

When choosing a career, it is very important to consider your *aptitudes* and *abilities.* An aptitude is a natural talent. Most people have several aptitudes. These are areas in which you excel, develop your greatest skills, and generally find satisfaction. For example, people with an aptitude for singing do it well even without practice. Because they enjoy singing, they also enjoy practicing. With more practice, their singing improves.

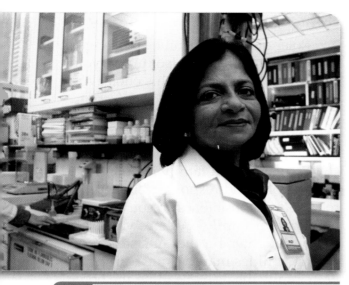

A-1   Working as a research dietitian is just one career option related to nutrition and wellness. *Used with permission by the American Dietetic Association*

A person without an aptitude for singing may still be able to develop singing ability. An ability is a skill a person learns through practice. Someone who practices frequently may be able to achieve some singing success. However, that person is unlikely to achieve as much success as a person with natural singing aptitude.

The same is true in the world of employment. People who perform a job using a natural talent often do it better and quicker than others. For example, a person with little talent for math can develop math ability through practice. However, if that person takes a job requiring math ability, the job is likely to be a struggle. A person with a natural math aptitude, on the other hand, will find the job easy and fun.

When you match yourself against your peers, in what areas do you excel? The activities you most enjoy are probably those you do best. Your school counselor can help you recognize your natural talents through aptitude and ability assessments. This information can help you identify possible career paths that match your interests. One such tool is the *O*NET Ability Profiler*.

Know Your Career Goals

Most people can improve their lives by setting goals. Goals are the aims you strive to reach. Without goals, you will not know what direction to take when faced with choices.

Short-term career goals relate to work you want to achieve within the next few months. Each short-term goal is a springboard to a long-term goal. *Long-term* career goals are the specific job or career destinations you plan to reach in a year or more. For example, passing a class is a short-term career goal. It is one step in the path to a long-term career goal, such as getting a college degree in foodservice management. All goals have deadlines. Some long-term career goals take many years to reach. Working toward short-term goals now will help you reach long-term goals in the future. Effective goals are

- *Achievable.* Carefully consider whether a goal is or is not reachable. Talk to your parents and listen to your friends. If the goal seems achievable to you, then go for it. You may be able to accomplish what others thought was impossible.
- *Personal.* Avoid copying someone else's goals. You must feel your future plans are right for you.
- *Positive.* You will find it easier to meet your goals if you state them positively. For instance, suppose you have a problem with tardiness. A positive way to state your goal is "I will be on time every day."
- *Specific.* A specific goal gives more direction about the actions to take to reach your target. For example, saying "I will do better this semester" is too general. Saying "I will get at least a B in every class this semester" is more defined.

Understand Your Values

Your family, friends, and life experiences shape your *values*, or beliefs that are important to you. What you value will determine the career you choose and shape the way you live your life. People who value independence, for example, desire flexibility in their work hours. People who value education want a job that pays for job-related degrees they earn while employed. A person who values family life avoids employment options that require constant travel. Carefully considering your values will point you to the job that best suits you.

By considering your interests and aptitudes, you can usually narrow the wide list of career options to a select few. Then use your values to guide which of these selections will bring you the most joy.

Think About Lifestyle

The career you choose affects your lifestyle in many ways. It affects your income, which in turn impacts how much you can spend on housing, clothing, food, and other items you need and want. Your career choice, as mentioned earlier, may also impact where you live. If you want to live away from a large city, choose a career that is available in other areas.

Your career choice may also affect your friendships. Although you will likely become friends with some work associates, it is also likely you will live a distance from lifelong friends. The work hours and vacation policies at your job will also affect your available leisure time. For example, you will want to avoid job options that require overtime, early and late shifts, or weekend work if you desire normal business hours.

Balancing Work and Family

Roles and responsibilities that relate to your home life will also impact your career choice. Likewise, this choice also influences job success and satisfaction with your personal and family life. Maintaining a balance between work and home helps bring satisfaction to both.

Belonging to a family includes certain roles and responsibilities. What roles and responsibilities do you currently hold in your family? Perhaps you are a son or daughter, brother or sister. Your responsibilities may include helping with family meals or cleaning the home. Adding a part-time job into the mix complicates matters. This will require you to manage time more carefully.

The multiple roles of spouse, parent, homemaker, and employee are demanding, and at times conflicting. In order to fully meet the requirements of these roles, you will need to find ways to balance them.

Parents may need to adjust work responsibilities to spend more time with their families. Some may participate in *flextime*—a program that allows employees greater flexibility in setting their work hours. Others may have the option to telecommute, work less overtime, or start a home-based business. In *dual-career families*, parents must also provide substitute care for their children.

Researching Careers

In your lifetime, you will likely have several occupations that relate by a common skill, purpose, or interest. An *occupation* is paid employment involving one or more jobs or tasks. In contrast, a *career* is a series of related occupations that show your progression

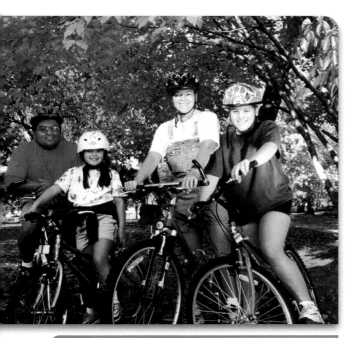

A-2   Taking time for a family outing helps build relationships and bring balance to busy daily schedules.

in a field of work. As you move from one occupation to the next, you will continue gaining new skills and knowledge.

The Career Clusters

The *career clusters* are 16 groups of occupations or career specialties that are similar to or related to one another. The occupations within a cluster demand a set of common knowledge and skills—or *essential knowledge and skills*—for career success. Career clusters relating to nutrition and wellness include

- Agriculture, Food & Natural Resources
- Education & Training
- Health Science
- Hospitality & Tourism
- Human Services
- Manufacturing
- Marketing
- Science, Technology, Engineering & Mathematics

If one or two jobs in a career cluster appeal to you, it is likely that others will, too. This is because occupations within a cluster share certain similarities. To help narrow your options, each career cluster is broken further into *career pathways*. These career subgroups often require additional or more specialized knowledge and skills.

Programs of Study

Because occupations in a career pathway require similar knowledge and skill, they also require similar *programs of study*. A program of study is a sequence of courses or instruction that prepares you for occupations within a certain career pathway. A program generally includes classroom instruction along with service-learning and workplace experiences. You may also want to become involved with student chapters of related professional organizations.

Customizing your program of study results in a *personal plan of study*. This plan will help prepare you for your career direction of choice. Your plan of study will involve appropriate high school classes and participation in related organizations. With this foundation, you can select programs that address your career goals. Some of your high school courses may also count toward college credit. Check with your high school counselor about this option. Be sure to update your plan at least yearly, but more often if your goals change.

Career Information Sources

One of the best ways to find employment is to use the Internet. You can search for open positions in your area or across the country. Many of these Web sites also provide tips for job hunting. You can start by using the U.S. Department of Labor Web site.

Online Career Resources	
Source	**Internet Address**
Career Guide to Industries, U.S. Department of Labor	www.bls.gov/oco/cg/
CareerOneStop	www.careeronestop.org/
Occupational Outlook Handbook, U.S. Department of Labor	www.bls.gov/oco/
Occupational Outlook Quarterly, U.S. Department of Labor	www.bls.gov/ooq/home.htm
O*NET, The Occupational Information Network	www.onetcenter.org/
U.S. Department of Labor Employment and Training Administration	www.doleta.gov/
USAJOBS, the official job site of the U.S. Federal Government	www.usajobs.gov/

Consider Education and Training

Some employment opportunities in nutrition and wellness careers require little training beyond high school. Some require occupational training and others require college and advanced degrees. When planning your career, you will need to determine how much education you need and want. There are a number of ways to acquire the education and training you need.

Work-Based Learning Programs

Work-based learning programs offer students an opportunity for job placement while still taking classes. A program coordinator works with students and the work sites to make these work experiences successful. Participating in such work-based learning programs can help ease the transition from school to career. Here are some program options to explore.

- *Cooperative programs (co-ops).* High school work-based learning programs are often called *cooperative programs.* The program coordinators place students in part-time positions.

Students generally attend school for at least half the day and then work the remainder of the day. The program coordinators and workplace supervisors evaluate student performance on the job, giving students a realistic view of job realities and responsibilities.

- *Internships.* Work-based learning opportunities at the postsecondary or college level are called *internships.* Such internships offer paid or unpaid supervised practical work experience. Students enroll in internship programs much like they enroll in courses. They may work several days per week with a reduced class load, or work during the summer. Students generally receive college credit for internships while gaining valuable work skills.

Occupational Training

Occupational training can help you prepare for a career in a specific field. This type of training is available through apprenticeship programs, technical schools, and trade schools.

Apprenticeship programs offer students the opportunity to learn a trade or skill on-the-job under the direction and supervision of a skilled worker. Apprenticeships may last several months or many years. Requirements for entering apprenticeship programs will vary from state to state and one trade to another.

Technical schools offer job training at both secondary and postsecondary levels. Students who attend classes at technical schools during high school often receive a certificate for a specific job skill with their high school diplomas. Postsecondary programs at technical schools may offer a two-year degree or a certificate.

Trade schools provide job-specific training at the postsecondary level. Programs at trade schools may take one, two, or three years to complete. Successful completion of these programs may result in a certificate or possibly an associate's degree.

Colleges and Universities

Careers that require a high level of skills or creativity and have great potential for advancement are highly competitive. Obtaining higher education at a college or university is generally needed for acquiring such positions. You can obtain degrees from community or junior colleges and four-year colleges or universities.

Attending a community or junior (two-year) college leads to earning an *associate's degree*. Completing a program at a four-year college or university results in a *bachelor's degree*. For careers that require a higher level of education, students can take additional courses which result in a *master's degree*. It usually takes another one to two years of study to obtain a master's. Other professional occupations, such as research scientists, require a *doctorate*, or *Ph.D.* Doctoral degrees often require three to six years of additional study beyond a master's degree, especially if the student works part-time while attending classes.

To find out about schools that offer the education and training you desire in nutrition and wellness, begin by talking with your school guidance counselor. You may also want to explore schools of interest on the Internet. These Web sites generally describe curriculum programs along with school size and costs. In addition, such Web sites address student life on campus, housing options, and financial aid programs. You will also find contact information for each school's admissions office.

Certification and Licensing

People who work in jobs that deal with people's lives, health, or safety must often have certification or a license. Doctors, dentists, and teachers are examples of such professions. Many people in the nutrition and fitness field have these requirements, too.

Meeting certification and licensing requirements means a person has a clear grasp of the science involved. It also means the person has proven ability to apply scientific principles correctly with each client or patient. This helps keep unqualified people from holding important jobs. It also helps prevent any physical harm that may result from bad advice.

Certification is a special standing within a profession as a result of meeting specific requirements of a certifying organization. A *license* is a work requirement set by a government agency. Licensing requirements are similar or identical to the certification requirements. The one main difference is license requirements carry the force of law. The government controls the performance standards of licensed professionals.

Education and Careers

Education Levels	Possible Careers
High School Diploma*	Baker, Cook, Diet clerk, Foodservice worker, Food and nutrition tech, Food inspector, Home health aid, Restaurant server
Associate's (2 years)*	Dietetic technician, Food meal supervisor, Food and drug inspector, Group exercise instructor, Lactation consultant, Occupational health and safety inspector, Personal chef, Registered nurse
Bachelor's (4+ years)*	Athletic trainer, Biochemist, Clinical dietitian, Exercise physiologist, USDA Extension Specialist, Fitness trainer, Food and drug inspector, Food bank director, Food writer/editor, Food purchasing agent, Food scientist, Food technologist, Health and safety sanitarian, Hydrologist, Journalist, Media spokesperson, Registered dietitian, Soil scientist, School counselor, Sports nutrition consultant
Master's (Bachelor's+)*	Clinical psychologist, Hydrologist, Research dietitian, Research food scientist, Research soil scientist, School counselor, Substance abuse counselor
Doctorate (Master's+)*	Clinical psychologist, Research biochemist, Research dietitian, Research food scientist

May require a combination of apprenticeship, internship, licensing, and/or certification.

Certification and licensing usually require the following:

- completion of an acceptable program of study
- minimum level of education or degree(s)
- completion of an internship and/or on-the-job experience
- minimum grade or score on a national exam
- continuing education

Those who meet the requirements receive a certificate or license. Many professionals choose to display these documents at their workplaces. This allows clients to know they are dealing with qualified professionals.

Certificates and licenses usually have expiration dates. If the person takes the suggested courses and/or attends a required number of approved meetings, renewal is granted. Having regular renewal requirements helps ensure professionals keep their knowledge and skills up-to-date.

The use of certain initials after a person's name often indicates certification. The following includes a list of some of the certifying organizations for nutrition and wellness careers:

- *American Dietetic Association (ADA).* A certified dietitian is called a *registered dietitian*. He or she uses the initials *RD*. Some RDs also hold special board certifications in such areas as sports, gerontology, pediatrics, or renal care.
- *American College of Sports Medicine (ACSM).* A certified fitness director uses the initials *ACSM*.
- *National Commission of Health Education Credentialing.* A certified health education specialist uses the initials *CHES*.

- *National Athletic Trainers Association (NATA).* Certified athletic trainers use the initials *AT.*

Regardless of other credentials, people employed in nutrition and wellness careers should have cardiopulmonary resuscitation (CPR) certification. This will enable the employee to offer help if a client has a health-related emergency.

When a license is a job requirement, the government controls the use of related titles and initials. For example, a person who uses the initials *LD* or the title *Licensed Dietitian* must have the qualifications to do so. If not, fines or penalties may result.

Many states have licensing require-ments for dietitians. Some have them for anyone using the term *nutritionist.* The licensing process for nutrition and fitness professionals in general is expanding due to increasing consumers complaints. Consumers are concerned about deceitful people who give harmful nutrition or exercise advice. Such frauds lack proper training and are primarily interested in selling a product or service.

Professional associations are also expanding their certification efforts to cover more job categories. Jobs that direct, counsel, or treat people are their main focus. Their goal is to keep unqualified people from spreading wrong information.

Evaluate Employment Outlook

Knowing the future of careers that interest you is important to your career research. For example, in the next 10 years will the demand for certain occupations increase, stay the same, or decrease compared to average employment trends? If the job outlook is poor, fewer oppor-tunities will exist. For more employment opportunities, focus on career areas that are growing.

Weighing Other Factors

When planning your career, there are other factors to consider. Some or all of these factors may be important to you.
- *Rewards.* People have different ideas about what embodies a "reward." For some, frequent travel is a reward, while others find it an interruption to their lifestyle. Remember that each occupation presents certain conditions that involve personal preferences.
- *Employer location.* What workplaces employ people with your expertise? Are these employers in a convenient location? Will certain employers require you to move to a new location?
- *Workplace conditions.* Is the work environment quiet or noisy? Is it near public transportation, or will you need a car? How long is the daily commute? Think carefully about your preferences.

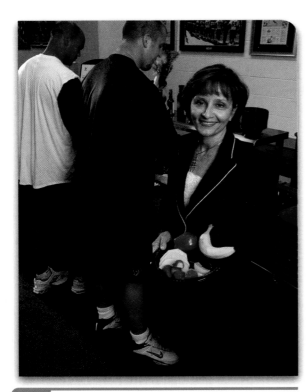

A-3   This dietitian works with sport teams to help them meet their nutritional needs.
Using with permission by the American Dietetic Association

Finding Meaningful Employment

To acquire employment that meets your needs and provides satisfaction, you must take the appropriate steps. These include locating job sources, preparing a résumé, creating a portfolio, and writing letters of application. In addition, you will need to complete job applications, have one or more interviews, and evaluate job offers.

Locate Jobs

Knowing how and where to find work is a valuable skill. When looking for a job, consider as many sources of information as possible. Your teachers, school counselors, and parents may know some job openings for you to pursue.

Friends and relatives are often your most fruitful resources. The process of connecting with the people you know is networking. *Networking* means to alert a wide circle of people about your interest in a job. By networking, you simply reach out for assistance. You will find that most people are happy to help you.

Finding meaningful employment will probably require a time-consuming search. Those who find success say networking and hard work are the two key ingredients to a successful job search.

While you are networking, check other information sources about job openings.

Resources for Locating Jobs	
Resource	**Description**
Internet	Hundreds of data banks from companies, unions, trade associations, government agencies, and universities announce job openings. Many employers use the Internet exclusively to post their positions.
Job Boards	Check Internet job boards and bulletin boards for job announcements. Start with those in your school's career center. Community organizations may also post job announcements in public buildings or on a community Web site.
Career Fairs	At these events, many employers have booths to promote available jobs and careers. You can talk with employer representatives and learn more about the companies. Stay alert to TV, radio, and newspaper promotions announcing career events.
Print Resources	Read the job listings in the classified ads in local newspapers and in state and national publications. Most advertised job openings appear in these classified ads. If you qualify, apply for positions by carefully following the directions the publication provides.
Employment Services	*Public employment services* are free services existing solely to inform job-seekers of job openings in the state and beyond. *Private employment agencies* are businesses that receive job listings from employers who pay them a fee to fill the openings. Private agencies may specialize in specific types or levels of jobs. Some may charge a fee for their service.

Join Professional Organizations

Professional organizations can help you explore career options. They also connect you with members who can help you establish your career. While still in school, you can join student chapters of various professional organizations, such as the American Dietetics Association and American College of Sports Medicine. Membership in such organizations can help you land your ideal job. Membership shows employers that you are serious about a career in a particular area. Many professional organizations also provide career-search help to their members.

Prepare a Résumé

A *résumé* outlines on paper a person's job qualifications. It is a quick reference for the employer to determine if a person meets specific job qualifications. When you apply for a job, attach a copy of your résumé to your letter of application. More and more job applications are received through the Internet. You may be asked to give an extra copy of your résumé to the interviewer during a job interview.

Carefully prepare your résumé and print it on fine-quality paper. Computer programs and high-quality printers create résumés that look professionally prepared. The appearance of a résumé may be as important as the information in it. A well-prepared résumé can make you stand out from the crowd of many applicants.

The information in your résumé should show all the key facts about you and your accomplishments. A résumé includes the following categories:

- *Identifying information*—your name, address, and telephone number or e-mail address by which employers can reach you
- *Career objective*—state your objective in clear, simple language

- *Work experience*—list both volunteer and paid employment (including company names, addresses, service dates, and job titles)
- *Education information*—include the school's name and address, the program of study, special courses completed relative to job success, grade average or grade point, and the graduation date
- *Awards and activities*—list any honors, awards, or recognition you receive through school or other organizations
- *Interests and hobbies*—although these items are optional, include them if they directly relate to the job you seek

Provide references upon request. A *reference* is a person who will speak highly of your skills and abilities. Have at least three references ready to give to employers. The list should include the names, titles, work addresses, phone numbers, fax numbers, and e-mail addresses of your references. Be sure to acquire each person's permission before adding his or her name to your list.

For your references, select people who know you well and are respected in the community. Teachers, counselors, employers, and religious leaders are ideal choices. Never name family members or personal friends since their opinions may be viewed as biased.

Omit information about your race, ethnic background, religion, gender, marital status, or disabilities from your résumé. This information is personal and has no bearing on your qualifications for the job. Also, equal opportunity laws prohibit employers from considering these facts in deciding whom to hire.

Create a Portfolio

A *portfolio* is an organized collection of your best and most creative work. It should give a balanced view of who you are as a potential employee. A portfolio

Laws Providing Employee Protection

Americans with Disabilities Act—Prohibits discrimination against people with disabilities within the United States. This legislation opens up employment and service opportunities to citizens with disabilities. The act requires employers to give reasonable accommodations to persons with disabilities during the hiring process. Employers must also make reasonable accommodations—such as physical changes to workspace, time off for treatment, and so forth—to allow a person with a disability to successfully perform job duties.

Equal Employment Opportunity Act—Prohibits employers from discriminating against any employee or job applicant because of race, color, religion, national origin, sex, physical or mental disability, or age.

Equal Pay Act—Requires that men and women be paid the same amount for doing the same jobs under the same conditions.

Fair Labor Standards Act—Sets the national minimum wage and overtime pay practices.

provides a visible way to demonstrate your skills and achievements to those who might want to hire you.

Contents of the portfolio will vary, but should always include a copy of your résumé and any letters of recommendation. Keep your portfolio up-to-date by adding new items and replacing others to make the portfolio relate to the requirements of the job you are seeking. If you use a binder or folder, you can easily add or remove items. Carefully label and date everything you include.

Display the items in your portfolio neatly and simply to showcase your skills. During job interviews, offer the employer an opportunity to review your portfolio. Be prepared to discuss any item included, highlighting only the main points. Always take your portfolio with you when you leave an interview.

Your Personal Portfolio

What skills would each of the following examples illustrate to a potential employer?

- Transcript of completed courses
- National and state test results
- Recognitions and documented accomplishments
- Career/technical training records
- Evidence of involvement in extracurricular activities
- Samples of school papers and projects
- Samples of graphs, charts, computer-assisted designs (CAD), brochures produced using a computer
- Letters of recommendations from teachers or former employers
- Photos, newspaper clippings, Web pages created, videos produced, and other documentation of completed projects
- List of positions held in career-related organizations, with a brief description of what was learned and/or accomplished in each

Write a Letter of Application

Your first contact with a potential employer will likely be a *letter of application*. It can make a lasting impression. Make sure your letter is neat and follows a standard business-letter format. Use a standard font and be sure to check the spelling and punctuation. Consider having several people proofread your letter and offer advice for improvements. Print your letter on high-quality paper that is neutral in color (ivory or white). Make sure it is free of smudges and mistakes. Always mail your résumé with a letter of application.

The letter should be brief, positive, and to the point. Send the letter only to places at which you are truly interested in working. When responding to newspaper or online ads, be sure to follow the specific instructions given. Review the following table for items to include in your letter of application.

Complete a Job Application

An employer will generally have you complete a job application before an interview. An *application form* requests your personal, academic, and employment information. Although some questions may duplicate your résumé, the employer may still require you to complete an application. Remember the following guidelines when completing an application:

- Read the entire application before filling it out.
- Follow the directions exactly.
- Fill out the form neatly.
- Omit your social security number to protect your identity. Instead, write *will provide if hired*.
- Give complete responses. If an item does not apply to you, write *N/A* or *does not apply*.
- Ask for clarification on items you do not understand.
- Refer to an extra copy of your résumé for employment history dates and other information the form requires. Remember to include part-time jobs, too.
- Review your application before submitting it to the employer. If you need to make changes, neatly draw a line through incorrect information and write the correct information.

Items to Include in a Letter of Application

When writing your letter of application, use the following guidelines:

- *Heading and salutation.* List the date, your name, and contact information. If possible, address the letter to a specific person or title, such as the Human Resources Director or Hiring Manager.
- *Opening paragraph.* Explain who you are and the title of the position you are seeking. Note how you heard about the position.
- *Middle paragraph(s).* Be sure to target the letter to the employer and the industry or profession. Identify your specific strengths, skills, and abilities, describing how you think they benefit the employer.
- *Closing paragraph and signature.* In your closing paragraph, thank the reader for his or her time. Politely request an interview and state when you can begin working. Identify when you will recontact the reader. Then sign the letter. Use blue ink for your signature because it best shows the letter is original and not a photocopy.

The Interview

The *job interview* is a discussion between the job applicant and the person doing the hiring. The purpose of the interview is to give you and the employer a chance to seek information and ask questions. The interviewer will want to know more about your work skills, likes and dislikes, and future goals. You will probably want to know more details about the position available.

For a successful job interview, you must first do your homework. This means preparing for the interview in much the same way as you prepare for school assignments. Interview readiness requires you to do the following:

- Learn as much as possible about the employer and the business.
- Prepare a résumé and a portfolio—highlighting the qualifications that relate to the job you are considering.
- Prepare, if possible, for any testing that is part of the interview.
- Make a list of questions to ask the employer about the job and opportunities for advancement.
- Plan what you will to wear for the interview—look neat, clean, and dressed in business attire one step above what your future coworkers may wear. Polish your shoes, neatly groom your hair and fingernails, and—if you wear makeup or jewelry—make sure it is subtle.
- Gather the materials you plan to take to the interview.
- Practice your responses to possible interview questions with a friend or family member. Make sure you maintain eye contact and your composure when answering questions. Practice will help you answer with better accuracy and appropriate enthusiasm.
- Verify the interview location and plan to arrive at least 10 minutes early.

After completing a job interview, send a follow-up letter right away using

---

Common Interview Questions

The interviewer will probably begin by saying, "Tell me about yourself." Then expect the following questions:

- What do you know about this job and organization?
- How does your education or work experience relate to this position?
- What are your most (or least) favorite subjects in school? Why?
- Describe your computer skills.
- What school or club team projects involved you? Be specific about your contributions.
- What did you like, or dislike, about working on team projects?
- What types of work do you dislike doing?
- Tell me about a time when you made a serious mistake. What did you do?
- How would others describe your strengths and weaknesses?
- Why would you like to work here?
- What would you like to be doing five years from now?
- What does success mean to you?
- What hours are you willing to work?
- What would you do if . . . ? (This could involve any ethical dilemma or problem-solving situation related to the work.)

standard business-letter format. Thank the interviewer for his or her time and express your continuing interest in the position. This also is your chance to clarify any points about your qualifications.

If you do not get the job, try not to be discouraged. Often there are many applicants competing for the same job. Learn from this experience by evaluating what went well in the interview and what you would do differently. Then continue your job search. Try to be positive and think about all the other employment opportunities that may be better than the job you did not get.

Evaluate Job Offers

As you consider a job offer or compare two or more positions, you will need to examine the items that follow. Remember, you will need to use considerable diplomacy when approaching these topics.

- *Physical workplace.* Is the workplace location convenient? Is the atmosphere conducive to your working style? Is public transportation conveniently located, or will you need a car?
- *Work schedule.* Do the work days and work hours blend with your lifestyle? Is occasional overtime a work requirement?
- *Income and benefits.* Is the salary or wage proposal fair? Will you receive benefits that are just as valuable as extra income? Carefully examine policies for sick leave, vacation leave, and medical and life insurance. Will the employer pay for college tuition for additional courses or programs related to the job? Is there a cafeteria with foodservice provided or refrigerated storage if you bring your lunch?
- *Job obligations.* Will you be required to join a union or other professional organization? If so, what are the costs? Is there reimbursement for these costs? Will meetings occur after work hours?
- *Potential for advancement.* Is there opportunity for advancement? How soon after demonstrating good performance can you pursue additional responsibilities? Does advancement require additional degrees or certifications? What training program does the employer offer?

Succeeding in the Workplace

Workplace success results from hard work, high motivation, and diverse skills. Whatever career path you choose, you will need to give it your best effort. Employees who are successful display energy, cooperation, and enthusiasm for their work. They follow instructions, take constructive criticism well, and finish tasks in a timely manner. Maintaining confidentiality is also an important workplace responsibility. Willingness to do more than what is expected and respecting the work of others are traits employers value.

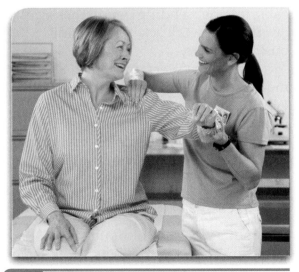

A-4 A physical therapist plays an important role in this woman's wellness team.

Work Habits

Employers want employees who are reliable, punctual, and responsible. They want their employees to be capable of taking initiative—working both independently and with team members. Employees to who have high *self-esteem* have a deep sense of their worth and are able to work hard with a positive attitude.

As a member of the workforce, your employer will expect you to be prompt and on time. You should arrive at work on time, and return promptly from breaks and lunches. Dependable employees keep their word and meet deadlines. It is important to call your supervisor right away when illness or other emergencies prevent you from coming to work. Then make alternative arrangements with your employer for making up work. Many people lose jobs because of failure to check in with a supervisor about time off.

Time Management

Successful employees prioritize their work assignments, complete them on time, and avoid wasting time. Time-wasting behaviors include talking with coworkers, making personal phone calls, texting, sending e-mail messages, or other nonwork activities during business hours.

Ability to determine which assignments are most important is a key skill. When uncertain, ask your supervisor. It is important to avoid putting excessive effort into minor assignments when something crucial demands attention.

Attitude on the Job

Your *attitude* is your outlook on life. Your response to events and people around you reflects your attitude.

Cheerfulness, cooperation, and courteous behavior help pave the way to successful working relationships.

Enthusiasm spreads quickly from one person to another. When you are enthusiastic about your work, it is a sign that you enjoy what you do. This leads to pride in your accomplishments and a desire to achieve greater goals.

Ethical Workplace Behavior

As a member of the workforce, you may face problems daily for which solutions are not always clear. The decisions you make in these situations can affect your ability to maintain your job. You will need to apply professional ethics. *Ethics* are standards, guidelines, and codes that guide behaviors. Ethics should rule over every aspect of your job—every decision you make and every action you take.

What do you need to consider when applying ethics to a particular decision? Ask yourself the following questions:

- Are my actions aimed at improving the quality of life for others?
- Would the people I respect agree with my decision?
- Do my actions show I respect others regardless of their ethnic background, race, religion, sex, or age?
- Will my actions cause other people to have their freedoms denied?
- Do my actions show I respect the privacy and confidentiality of others and my employer?
- Do my actions reflect truthfulness and open communication?

Always allow ethics to guide your actions. In addition, make a point of associating with other professionals who display high standards of ethics to the public.

Decision Making and Problem Solving

Ability to make responsible decisions and use problem-solving skills applies to the workplace and all other aspects of life. Using these skills well shows your employer that you can handle additional work responsibilities. Effective use of these skills can also help strengthen team efforts and help all employees take pride in their work.

Your problem-solving skills can help you answer tough questions and resolve difficult situations. Often, problem solving involves adapting to a new way of doing things. Employers highly value employees who can solve problems effectively. The problem-solving steps include

1. Clearly identify the real problem.
2. List alternative courses of action.
3. Evaluate the consequences of each course of action.
4. Choose an alternative and take action.
5. Assess the outcome for reference when facing future problems.

Interpersonal Skills

Interpersonal skills are those skills you use to relate to others. They involve communicating, teamwork, and leadership.

Effective Communication

Good communication is central to the smooth operation of any business. Through communication, you and your coworkers exchange ideas, thoughts, and information. The primary forms of communication are verbal and nonverbal.

- *Verbal communication* involves sending and receiving messages through speaking, listening, and writing.
- *Nonverbal communication* includes sending and receiving messages without using words. It involves body language, such as your facial expressions and your body posture.

Listening and feedback are key to effective workplace communication. If you do not understand what a coworker or supervisor has said (or if body language and verbal communication send mixed signals), be sure to ask questions. Remember, maintaining eye contact tells the other person you are paying attention to what he or she is saying. Clear communication helps avoid costly mistakes and wasted time in the workplace.

Skillful communication also applies to telephone and written communications. Answering a telephone promptly, with a positive tone of voice and pleasant attitude conveys a positive message about your employer. Likewise, using written communication—especially letters and e-mail—requires your special attention. Carefully craft your messages to say precisely what you mean. Think about how others will interpret the message without hearing or seeing body language. Then check your spelling, grammar, and punctuation. Periodically give yourself a communications checkup. Ask your supervisor to suggest areas in which you can improve.

Teamwork

Employers seek employees who can effectively serve as good team members. A *team* is a small group of people with similar skills who share a common purpose. Effective team members focus on the goals of the group. Creative ideas and solutions often develop from building on the shared ideas of others. With a team, all members help carry out tasks to meet team goals. Cooperation and effective communication among team members allows each person to express ideas fully and honestly. All team members use problem-solving skills to help build consensus on ways

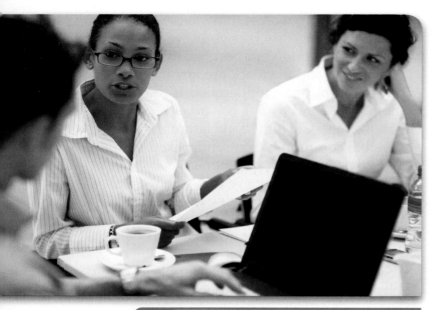

A-5 Effective teamwork requires cooperation and good communication.

to meet group goals. Team membership involves striking a balance between group productivity and personal satisfaction.

Leadership

Employers want to know how you function as a team leader. If you have ever made a decision that helped others achieve a goal, you have used leadership skills. Leadership skills go hand in hand with problem-solving skills. Although a number of leadership styles exist, a democratic style of leadership is often favored. It encourages all group members to take initiative, help carry out goals, and assume responsibility for group accomplishments in a timely manner. In general, traits of effective leaders include the ability to

- help individual team members resolve problems and differences of opinion
- guide the team to overcome hurdles in reaching the team goals
- work with the team to make change happen
- take responsibility for their actions and the actions of the team
- be inspiring, flexible, and creative

Making Job Changes

Whatever the reasons for leaving a job, you can grow from analyzing the pros and cons of a work experience. A positive attitude and a willingness to learn from mistakes can make your next job more productive and satisfying. A new job can offer a chance to begin again and put your experience to work.

When you leave a job, it is important to behave professionally. Most employers request at least a two-week notice that you will be leaving. This gives your employer time to find someone else to take over your responsibilities. You should give this notice in writing. Briefly explain that you are leaving and give the date of your last day on the job. Some people also choose to state why they are resigning and mention where they will be working next. Convey this type of information in a positive tone.

You do not want to anger an employer you may need to list as a reference someday. Therefore, avoid focusing on what you do not like about the job you are leaving. Instead, you might describe the challenges that attracted you to your new position. Remember that even unpleasant work experiences can provide chances to learn and grow as a professional. Be sure to thank your employer for the opportunities your present position offered.

Becoming an Entrepreneur

Would you like to start a business of your own someday? People who start, own, and operate their own businesses are called *entrepreneurs*. Many opportunities exist for entrepreneurs in the area

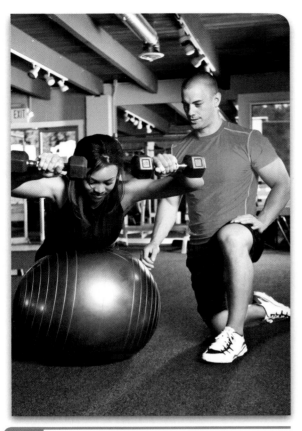

A-6   Many entrepreneurs in nutrition and wellness serve as personal consultants.

entrepreneurs are people who stick with their dreams. They know what needs to be done and they do it.

Entrepreneurs get their business ideas by doing market research. Many start with observing consumer needs. Then they search for ways to meet those needs with new products or services.

Advances in technology also create new opportunities for entrepreneurs. Through technology, new research findings can be revealed and new products and services can be developed. For instance, technology might lead to the development of a testing device. This device could be used in a laboratory study to reveal new benefits of a certain phytochemical. This research could prompt an ambitious dietitian to develop and sell a line of drinks made from plants rich in this phytochemical. Technology comes into play again to invent the machine that will extract the plant juices used in the drinks.

of nutrition and fitness. For example, a dietitian may develop a program on drug-free muscle building to present to athletes at area schools. A fitness specialist may create an exercise program to help factory workers avoid repetitive-motion injuries.

Successful entrepreneurs have three key traits. They are

- *Innovative.* Entrepreneurs have creativity to take old or new ideas and market them effectively to their target audience.
- *Risk takers.* Entrepreneurs take reasonable risks. They are willing to invest their time and resources to put their business plan into action.
- *Persistent.* Willingness to repeatedly adapt a product or service until it fully meets the needs of the target market is true to the persistent nature of entrepreneurs. Most

Appendix B

Eating Well with Canada's Food Guide

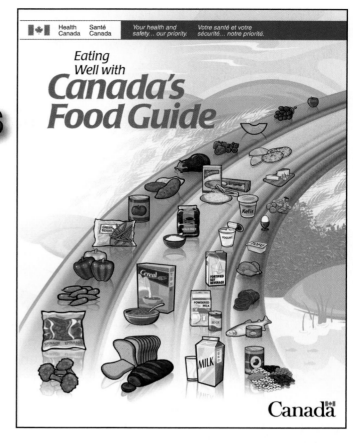

Health Canada / Santé Canada — Your health and safety... our priority. / Votre santé et votre sécurité... notre priorité.

Eating Well with Canada's Food Guide

Canada

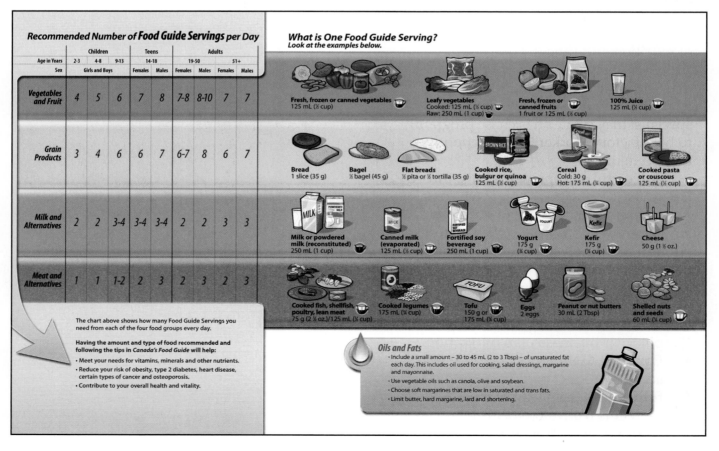

Recommended Number of Food Guide Servings per Day

	Children			Teens		Adults			
Age in Years	2-3	4-8	9-13	14-18		19-50		51+	
Sex	Girls and Boys			Females	Males	Females	Males	Females	Males
Vegetables and Fruit	4	5	6	7	8	7-8	8-10	7	7
Grain Products	3	4	6	6	7	6-7	8	6	7
Milk and Alternatives	2	2	3-4	3-4	3-4	2	2	3	3
Meat and Alternatives	1	1	1-2	2	3	2	3	2	3

The chart above shows how many Food Guide Servings you need from each of the four food groups every day.

Having the amount and type of food recommended and following the tips in *Canada's Food Guide* will help:

- Meet your needs for vitamins, minerals and other nutrients.
- Reduce your risk of obesity, type 2 diabetes, heart disease, certain types of cancer and osteoporosis.
- Contribute to your overall health and vitality.

What is One Food Guide Serving?
Look at the examples below.

Fresh, frozen or canned vegetables 125 mL (½ cup)

Leafy vegetables Cooked: 125 mL (½ cup) Raw: 250 mL (1 cup)

Fresh, frozen or canned fruits 1 fruit or 125 mL (½ cup)

100% Juice 125 mL (½ cup)

Bread 1 slice (35 g)

Bagel ½ bagel (45 g)

Flat breads ½ pita or ½ tortilla (35 g)

Cooked rice, bulgur or quinoa 125 mL (½ cup)

Cereal Cold: 30 g Hot: 175 mL (¾ cup)

Cooked pasta or couscous 125 mL (½ cup)

Milk or powdered milk (reconstituted) 250 mL (1 cup)

Canned milk (evaporated) 125 mL (½ cup)

Fortified soy beverage 250 mL (1 cup)

Yogurt 175 g (¾ cup)

Kefir 175 g (¾ cup)

Cheese 50 g (1 ½ oz.)

Cooked fish, shellfish, poultry, lean meat 75 g (2 ½ oz.)/125 mL (½ cup)

Cooked legumes 175 mL (¾ cup)

Tofu 150 g or 175 mL (¾ cup)

Eggs 2 eggs

Peanut or nut butters 30 mL (2 Tbsp)

Shelled nuts and seeds 60 mL (¼ cup)

Oils and Fats
- Include a small amount – 30 to 45 mL (2 to 3 Tbsp) – of unsaturated fat each day. This includes oil used for cooking, salad dressings, margarine and mayonnaise.
- Use vegetable oils such as canola, olive and soybean.
- Choose soft margarines that are low in saturated and trans fats.
- Limit butter, hard margarine, lard and shortening.

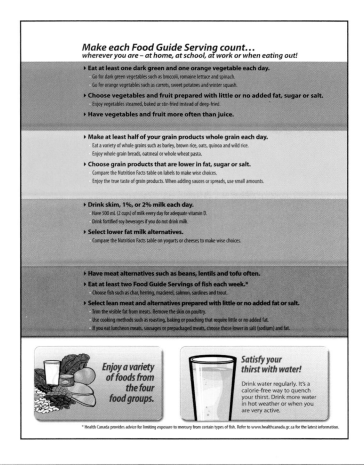

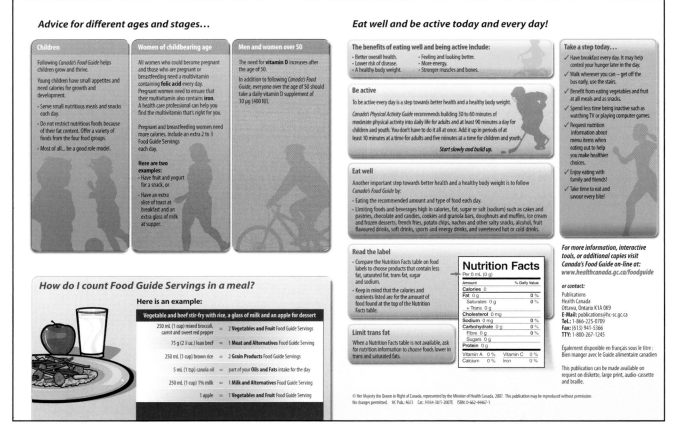

Appendix C
Dietary Reference Intakes

Dietary Reference Intakes (DRIs): Recommended Dietary Allowances and Adequate Intakes, Vitamins
Food and Nutrition Board, Institute of Medicine, National Academies

Life Stage Group	Vitamin A (µg/d)[a]	Vitamin C (mg/d)	Vitamin D (µg/d)[b,c]	Vitamin E (mg/d)[d]	Vitamin K (µg/d)	Thiamin (mg/d)	Riboflavin (mg/d)	Niacin (mg/d)	Vitamin B$_6$ (mg/d)[e]	Folate (µg/d)[f]	Vitamin B$_{12}$ (µg/d)	Pantothenic Acid (mg/d)	Biotin (µg/d)	Choline (mg/d)[g]
Infants														
0 to 6 mo	400*	40*	15	4*	2.0*	0.2*	0.3*	2*	0.1*	65*	0.4*	1.7*	5*	125*
6 to 12 mo	500*	50*	15	5*	2.5*	0.3*	0.4*	4*	0.3*	80*	0.5*	1.8*	6*	150*
Children														
1–3 y	300	15	15	6	30*	0.5	0.5	6	0.5	150	0.9	2*	8*	200*
4–8 y	400	25	15	7	55*	0.6	0.6	8	0.6	200	1.2	3*	12*	250*
Males														
9–13 y	600	45	15	11	60*	0.9	0.9	12	1.0	300	1.8	4*	20*	375*
14–18 y	900	75	15	15	75*	1.2	1.3	16	1.3	400	2.4	5*	25*	550*
19–30 y	900	90	15	15	120*	1.2	1.3	16	1.3	400	2.4	5*	30*	550*
31–50 y	900	90	15	15	120*	1.2	1.3	16	1.3	400	2.4	5*	30*	550*
51–70 y	900	90	15	15	120*	1.2	1.3	16	1.7	400	2.4[h]	5*	30*	550*
> 70 y	900	90	20	15	120*	1.2	1.3	16	1.7	400	2.4[h]	5*	30*	550*
Females														
9–13 y	600	45	15	11	60*	0.9	0.9	12	1.0	300	1.8	4*	20*	375*
14–18 y	700	65	15	15	75*	1.0	1.0	14	1.2	400[i]	2.4	5*	25*	400*
19–30 y	700	75	15	15	90*	1.1	1.1	14	1.3	400[i]	2.4	5*	30*	425*
31–50 y	700	75	15	15	90*	1.1	1.1	14	1.3	400[i]	2.4	5*	30*	425*
51–70 y	700	75	15	15	90*	1.1	1.1	14	1.5	400	2.4[h]	5*	30*	425*
> 70 y	700	75	20	15	90*	1.1	1.1	14	1.5	400	2.4[h]	5*	30*	425*
Pregnancy														
14–18 y	750	80	15	15	75*	1.4	1.4	18	1.9	600[j]	2.6	6*	30*	450*
19–30 y	770	85	15	15	90*	1.4	1.4	18	1.9	600[j]	2.6	6*	30*	450*
31–50 y	770	85	15	15	90*	1.4	1.4	18	1.9	600[j]	2.6	6*	30*	450*
Lactation														
14–18 y	1,200	115	15	19	75*	1.4	1.6	17	2.0	500	2.8	7*	35*	550*
19–30 y	1,300	120	15	19	90*	1.4	1.6	17	2.0	500	2.8	7*	35*	550*
31–50 y	1,300	120	15	19	90*	1.4	1.6	17	2.0	500	2.8	7*	35*	550*

NOTE: This table (taken from the DRI reports, see www.nap.edu) presents Recommended Dietary Allowances (RDAs) in **bold type** and Adequate Intakes (AIs) in ordinary type followed by an asterisk (*). An RDA is the average daily dietary intake level; sufficient to meet the nutrient requirements of nearly all (97-98 percent) healthy individuals in a group. It is calculated from an Estimated Average Requirement (EAR). If sufficient scientific evidence is not available to establish an EAR, and thus calculate an RDA, an AI is usually developed. For healthy breastfed infants, an AI is the mean intake. The AI for other life stage and gender groups is believed to cover the needs of all healthy individuals in the groups, but lack of data or uncertainty in the data prevent being able to specify with confidence the percentage of individuals covered by this intake.

[a] As retinol activity equivalents (RAEs). 1 RAE = 1 µg retinol, 12 µg β-carotene, 24 µg α-carotene, or 24 µg β-cryptoxanthin. The RAE for dietary provitamin A carotenoids is two-fold greater than retinol equivalents (RE), whereas the RAE for preformed vitamin A is the same as RE.[b] As cholecalciferol. 1 µg cholecalciferol = 40 IU vitamin D.

[c] Under the assumption of minimal sunlight.

[d] As α-tocopherol. α-Tocopherol includes *RRR*-α-tocopherol, the only form of α-tocopherol that occurs naturally in foods, and the *2R*-stereoisomeric forms of α-tocopherol (*RRR*-, *RSR*-, *RRS*-, and *RSS*-α-tocopherol) that occur in fortified foods and supplements. It does not include the *2S*-stereoisomeric forms of α-tocopherol (*SRR*-, *SSR*-, *SRS*-, and *SSS*-α-tocopherol), also found in fortified foods and supplements.

[e] As niacin equivalents (NE). 1 mg of niacin = 60 mg of tryptophan; 0–6 months = preformed niacin (not NE).

[f] As dietary folate equivalents (DFE). 1 DFE = 1 µg food folate = 0.6 µg of folic acid from fortified food or as a supplement consumed with food = 0.5 µg of a supplement taken on an empty stomach.

[g] Although AIs have been set for choline, there are few data to assess whether a dietary supply of choline is needed at all stages of the life cycle, and it may be that the choline requirement can be met by endogenous synthesis at some of these stages.

[h] Because 10 to 30 percent of older people may malabsorb food-bound B$_{12}$, it is advisable for those older than 50 years to meet their RDA mainly by consuming foods fortified with B$_{12}$ or a supplement containing B$_{12}$.

[i] In view of evidence linking folate intake with neural tube defects in the fetus, it is recommended that all women capable of becoming pregnant consume 400 µg from supplements or fortified foods in addition to intake of food folate from a varied diet.

[j] It is assumed that women will continue consuming 400 µg from supplements or fortified food until their pregnancy is confirmed and they enter prenatal care, which ordinarily occurs after the end of the periconceptional period—the critical time for formation of the neural tube.

SOURCES: *Dietary Reference Intakes for Calcium, Phosphorous, Magnesium, Vitamin D, and Fluoride* (1997); *Dietary Reference Intakes for Thiamin, Riboflavin, Niacin, Vitamin B$_6$, Folate, Vitamin B$_{12}$, Pantothenic Acid, Biotin, and Choline* (1998); *Dietary Reference Intakes for Vitamin C, Vitamin E, Selenium, and Carotenoids* (2000); *Dietary Reference Intakes for Vitamin A, Vitamin K, Arsenic, Boron, Chromium, Copper, Iodine, Iron, Manganese, Molybdenum, Nickel, Silicon, Vanadium, and Zinc* (2001); *Dietary Reference Intakes for Water, Potassium, Sodium, Chloride, and Sulfate* (2005); and *Dietary Reference Intakes for Calcium and Vitamin D* (2011). These reports may be accessed via www.nap.edu. Reprinted with permission from the National Academies Press, National Academy of Sciences.

Dietary Reference Intakes (DRIs): Tolerable Upper Intake Levels, Vitamins
Food and Nutrition Board, Institute of Medicine, National Academies

Life Stage Group	Vitamin A (µg/d)[a]	Vitamin C (mg/d)	Vitamin D (µg/d)	Vitamin E (mg/d)[b,c]	Vitamin K	Thia-min	Ribo-flavin	Niacin (mg/d)[c]	Vitamin B6 (mg/d)	Folate (µg/d)[c]	Vitamin B12	Panto-thenic Acid	Bio-tin	Cho-line (g/d)	Carote-noids[d]
Infants															
0 to 6 mo	600	ND[e]	25	ND	ND	ND	ND	ND	ND	ND	ND	ND	ND	ND	ND
6 to 12 mo	600	ND	38	ND	ND	ND	ND	ND	ND	ND	ND	ND	ND	ND	ND
Children															
1–3 y	600	400	63	200	ND	ND	ND	10	30	300	ND	ND	ND	1.0	ND
4–8 y	900	650	75	300	ND	ND	ND	15	40	400	ND	ND	ND	1.0	ND
Males															
9–13 y	1,700	1,200	100	600	ND	ND	ND	20	60	600	ND	ND	ND	2.0	ND
14–18 y	2,800	1,800	100	800	ND	ND	ND	30	80	800	ND	ND	ND	3.0	ND
19–30 y	3,000	2,000	100	1,000	ND	ND	ND	35	100	1,000	ND	ND	ND	3.5	ND
31–50 y	3,000	2,000	100	1,000	ND	ND	ND	35	100	1,000	ND	ND	ND	3.5	ND
51–70 y	3,000	2,000	100	1,000	ND	ND	ND	35	100	1,000	ND	ND	ND	3.5	ND
> 70 y	3,000	2,000	100	1,000	ND	ND	ND	35	100	1,000	ND	ND	ND	3.5	ND
Females															
9–13 y	1,700	1,200	100	600	ND	ND	ND	20	60	600	ND	ND	ND	2.0	ND
14–18 y	2,800	1,800	100	800	ND	ND	ND	30	80	800	ND	ND	ND	3.0	ND
19–30 y	3,000	2,000	100	1,000	ND	ND	ND	35	100	1,000	ND	ND	ND	3.5	ND
31–50 y	3,000	2,000	100	1,000	ND	ND	ND	35	100	1,000	ND	ND	ND	3.5	ND
51–70 y	3,000	2,000	100	1,000	ND	ND	ND	35	100	1,000	ND	ND	ND	3.5	ND
> 70 y	3,000	2,000	100	1,000	ND	ND	ND	35	100	1,000	ND	ND	ND	3.5	ND
Pregnancy															
14–18 y	2,800	1,800	100	800	ND	ND	ND	30	80	800	ND	ND	ND	3.0	ND
19–30 y	3,000	2,000	100	1,000	ND	ND	ND	35	100	1,000	ND	ND	ND	3.5	ND
31–50 y	3,000	2,000	100	1,000	ND	ND	ND	35	100	1,000	ND	ND	ND	3.5	ND
Lactation															
14–18 y	2,800	1,800	100	800	ND	ND	ND	30	80	800	ND	ND	ND	3.0	ND
19–30 y	3,000	2,000	100	1,000	ND	ND	ND	35	100	1,000	ND	ND	ND	3.5	ND
31–50 y	3,000	2,000	100	1,000	ND	ND	ND	35	100	1,000	ND	ND	ND	3.5	ND

NOTE: A Tolerable Upper Intake Level (UL) is the highest level of daily nutrient intake that is likely to pose no risk of adverse health effects to almost all individuals in the general population. Unless otherwise specified, the UL represents total intake from food, water, and supplements. Due to a lack of suitable data, ULs could not be established for vitamin K, thiamin, riboflavin, vitamin B12, pantothenic acid, biotin, and carotenoids. In the absence of a UL, extra caution may be warranted in consuming levels above recommended intakes. Members of the general population should be advised not to routinely exceed the UL. The UL is not meant to apply to individuals who are treated with the nutrient under medical supervision or to individuals with predisposing conditions that modify their sensitivity to the nutrient.

[a] As preformed vitamin A only.
[b] As α-tocopherol; applies to any form of supplemental α-tocopherol.
[c] The ULs for vitamin E, niacin, and folate apply to synthetic forms obtained from supplements, fortified foods, or a combination of the two.
[d] β-Carotene supplements are advised only to serve as a provitamin A source for individuals at risk of vitamin A deficiency.
[e] ND = Not determinable due to lack of data of adverse effects in this age group and concern with regard to lack of ability to handle excess amounts. Source of intake should be from food only to prevent high levels of intake.

SOURCES: *Dietary Reference Intakes for Calcium, Phosphorous, Magnesium, Vitamin D, and Fluoride* (1997); *Dietary Reference Intakes for Thiamin, Riboflavin, Niacin, Vitamin B6, Folate, Vitamin B12, Pantothenic Acid, Biotin, and Choline* (1998); *Dietary Reference Intakes for Vitamin C, Vitamine E, Selenium, and Carotenoids* (2000); *Dietary Reference Intakes for Vitamin A, Vitamin K, Arsenic, Boron, Chromium, Copper, Iodine, Iron, Manganese, Molybdenum, Nickel, Silicon, Vanadium, and Zinc* (2001); and *Dietary Reference Intakes for Calcium and Vitamin D* (2011). These reports may be accessed via www.nap.edu. Reprinted with permission from the National Academies Press, National Academy of Sciences.

Dietary Reference Intakes (DRIs): Recommended Dietary Allowances and Adequate Intakes, Elements
Food and Nutrition Board, Institute of Medicine, National Academies

Life Stage Group	Calcium (mg/d)	Chromium (µg/d)	Copper (µg/d)	Fluoride (mg/d)	Iodine (µg/d)	Iron (mg/d)	Magnesium (mg/d)	Manganese (mg/d)	Molybdenum (µg/d)	Phosphorus (mg/d)	Selenium (µg/d)	Zinc (mg/d)	Potassium (g/d)	Sodium (g/d)	Chloride (g/d)
Infants															
0 to 6 mo	200*	0.2*	200*	0.01*	110*	0.27*	30*	0.003*	2*	100*	15*	2*	0.4*	0.12*	0.18*
6 to 12 mo	260*	5.5*	220*	0.5*	130*	11	75*	0.6*	3*	275*	20*	3	0.7*	0.37*	0.57*
Children															
1–3 y	700	11*	340	0.7*	90	7	80	1.2*	17	460	20	3	3.0*	1.0*	1.5*
4–8 y	1,000	15*	440	1*	90	10	130	1.5*	22	500	30	5	3.8*	1.2*	1.9*
Males															
9–13 y	1,300	25*	700	2*	120	8	240	1.9*	34	1,250	40	8	4.5*	1.5*	2.3*
14–18 y	1,300	35*	890	3*	150	11	410	2.2*	43	1,250	55	11	4.7*	1.5*	2.3*
19–30 y	1,000	35*	900	4*	150	8	400	2.3*	45	700	55	11	4.7*	1.5*	2.3*
31–50 y	1,000	35*	900	4*	150	8	420	2.3*	45	700	55	11	4.7*	1.5*	2.3*
51–70 y	1,000	30*	900	4*	150	8	420	2.3*	45	700	55	11	4.7*	1.3*	2.0*
> 70 y	1,200	30*	900	4*	150	8	420	2.3*	45	700	55	11	4.7*	1.2*	1.8*
Females															
9–13 y	1,300	21*	700	2*	120	8	240	1.6*	34	1,250	40	8	4.5*	1.5*	2.3*
14–18 y	1,300	24*	890	3*	150	15	360	1.6*	43	1,250	55	9	4.7*	1.5*	2.3*
19–30 y	1,000	25*	900	3*	150	18	310	1.8*	45	700	55	8	4.7*	1.5*	2.3*
31–50 y	1,000	25*	900	3*	150	18	320	1.8*	45	700	55	8	4.7*	1.5*	2.3*
51–70 y	1,200	20*	900	3*	150	8	320	1.8*	45	700	55	8	4.7*	1.3*	2.0*
> 70 y	1,200	20*	900	3*	150	8	320	1.8*	45	700	55	8	4.7*	1.2*	1.8*
Pregnancy															
14–18 y	1,300	29*	1,000	3*	220	27	400	2.0*	50	1,250	60	12	4.7*	1.5*	2.3*
19–30 y	1,000	30*	1,000	3*	220	27	350	2.0*	50	700	60	11	4.7*	1.5*	2.3*
31–50 y	1,000	30*	1,000	3*	220	27	360	2.0*	50	700	60	11	4.7*	1.5*	2.3*
Lactation															
14–18 y	1,300	44*	1,300	3*	290	10	360	2.6*	50	1,250	70	13	5.1*	1.5*	2.3*
19–30 y	1,000	45*	1,300	3*	290	9	310	2.6*	50	700	70	12	5.1*	1.5*	2.3*
31–50 y	1,000	45*	1,300	3*	290	9	320	2.6*	50	700	70	12	5.1*	1.5*	2.3*

NOTE: This table (taken from the DRI reports, see www.nap.edu) presents Recommended Dietary Allowances (RDAs) in **bold type** and Adequate Intakes (AIs) in ordinary type followed by an asterisk (*). An RDA is the average daily dietary intake level; sufficient to meet the nutrient requirements of nearly all (97-98 percent) healthy individuals in a group. It is calculated from an Estimated Average Requirement (EAR). If sufficient scientific evidence is not available to establish an EAR, and thus calculate an RDA, an AI is usually developed. For healthy breastfed infants, an AI is the mean intake. The AI for other life stage and gender groups is believed to cover the needs of all healthy individuals in the groups, but lack of data or uncertainty in the data prevent being able to specify with confidence the percentage of individuals covered by this intake.

Dietary Reference Intakes (DRIs): Tolerable Upper Intake Levels, Elements
Food and Nutrition Board, Institute of Medicine, National Academies

Life Stage Group	Arsenic[a]	Boron (mg/d)	Calcium (mg/d)	Chromium	Copper (µg/d)	Fluoride (mg/d)	Iodine (µg/d)	Iron (mg/d)	Magnesium (mg/d)[b]	Manganese (mg/d)	Molybdenum (µg/d)	Nickel (mg/d)	Phosphorus (g/d)	Selenium (µg/d)	Silicon[c]	Vanadium (mg/d)[d]	Zinc (mg/d)	Sodium (g/d)	Chloride (g/d)
Infants																			
0 to 6 mo	ND[e]	ND	1,000	ND	ND	0.7	ND	40	ND	ND	ND	ND	ND	45	ND	ND	4	ND	ND
6 to 12 mo	ND	ND	1,000	ND	ND	0.9	ND	40	ND	ND	ND	ND	ND	60	ND	ND	5	ND	ND
Children																			
1–3 y	ND	3	2,500	ND	1,000	1.3	200	40	65	2	300	0.2	3	90	ND	ND	7	1.5	2.3
4–8 y	ND	6	2,500	ND	3,000	2.2	300	40	110	3	600	0.3	3	150	ND	ND	12	1.9	2.9
Males																			
9–13 y	ND	11	3,000	ND	5,000	10	600	40	350	6	1,100	0.6	4	280	ND	ND	23	2.2	3.4
14–18 y	ND	17	3,000	ND	8,000	10	900	45	350	9	1,700	1.0	4	400	ND	ND	34	2.3	3.6
19–30 y	ND	20	2,500	ND	10,000	10	1,100	45	350	11	2,000	1.0	4	400	ND	1.8	40	2.3	3.6
31–50 y	ND	20	2,500	ND	10,000	10	1,100	45	350	11	2,000	1.0	4	400	ND	1.8	40	2.3	3.6
51-70 y	ND	20	2,000	ND	10,000	10	1,100	45	350	11	2,000	1.0	4	400	ND	1.8	40	2.3	3.6
> 70 y	ND	20	2,000	ND	10,000	10	1,100	45	350	11	2,000	1.0	3	400	ND	1.8	40	2.3	3.6
Females																			
9–13 y	ND	11	3,000	ND	5,000	10	600	40	350	6	1,100	0.6	4	280	ND	ND	23	2.2	3.4
14–18 y	ND	17	3,000	ND	8,000	10	900	45	350	9	1,700	1.0	4	400	ND	ND	34	2.3	3.6
19–30 y	ND	20	2,500	ND	10,000	10	1,100	45	350	11	2,000	1.0	4	400	ND	1.8	40	2.3	3.6
31–50 y	ND	20	2,500	ND	10,000	10	1,100	45	350	11	2,000	1.0	4	400	ND	1.8	40	2.3	3.6
51-70 y	ND	20	2,000	ND	10,000	10	1,100	45	350	11	2,000	1.0	4	400	ND	1.8	40	2.3	3.6
> 70 y	ND	20	2,000	ND	10,000	10	1,100	45	350	11	2,000	1.0	3	400	ND	1.8	40	2.3	3.6
Pregnancy																			
14–18 y	ND	17	3,000	ND	8,000	10	900	45	350	9	1,700	1.0	3.5	400	ND	ND	34	2.3	3.6
19–30 y	ND	20	2,500	ND	10,000	10	1,100	45	350	11	2,000	1.0	3.5	400	ND	ND	40	2.3	3.6
61–50 y	ND	20	2,500	ND	10,000	10	1,100	45	350	11	2,000	1.0	3.5	400	ND	ND	40	2.3	3.6
Lactation																			
14–18 y	ND	17	3,000	ND	8,000	10	900	45	350	9	1,700	1.0	4	400	ND	ND	34	2.3	3.6
19–30 y	ND	20	2,500	ND	10,000	10	1,100	45	350	11	2,000	1.0	4	400	ND	ND	40	2.3	3.6
31–50 y	ND	20	2,500	ND	10,000	10	1,100	45	350	11	2,000	1.0	4	400	ND	ND	40	2.3	3.6

NOTE: A Tolerable Upper Intake Level (UL) is the highest level of daily nutrient intake that is likely to pose no risk of adverse health effects to almost all individuals in the general population. Unless otherwise specified, the UL represents total intake from food, water, and supplements. Due to a lack of suitable data, ULs could not be established for vitamin K, thiamin, riboflavin, vitamin B_{12}, pantothenic acid, biotin, and carotenoids. In the absence of a UL, extra caution may be warranted in consuming levels above recommended intakes. Members of the general population should be advised not to routinely exceed the UL. The UL is not meant to apply to individuals who are treated with the nutrient under medical supervision or to individuals with predisposing conditions that modify their sensitivity to the nutrient.

[a] Although the UL was not determined for arsenic, there is no justification for adding arsenic to food or supplements.
[b] The ULs for magnesium represent intake from a pharmacological agent only and do not include intake from food and water.
[c] Although silicon has not been shown to cause adverse effects in humans, there is no justification for adding silicon to supplements.
[d] Although vanadium in food has not been shown to cause adverse effects in humans, there is no justification for adding vanadium to food and vanadium supplements should be used with caution. The UL is based on adverse effects in laboratory animals and this data could be used to set a UL for adults but not children and adolescents.
[e] ND = Not determinable due to lack of data of adverse effects in this age group and concern with regard to lack of ability to handle excess amounts. Source of intake should be from food only to prevent high levels of intake.

SOURCES: *Dietary Reference Intakes for Calcium, Phosphorous, Magnesium, Vitamin D, and Fluoride* (1997); *Dietary Reference Intakes for Thiamin, Riboflavin, Niacin, Vitamin B_6, Folate, Vitamin B_{12}, Pantothenic Acid, Biotin, and Choline* (1998); *Dietary Reference Intakes for Vitamin C, Vitamine E, Selenium, and Carotenoids* (2000); *Dietary Reference Intakes for Vitamin A, Vitamin K, Arsenic, Boron, Chromium, Copper, Iodine, Iron, Manganese, Molybdenum, Nickel, Silicon, Vanadium, and Zinc* (2001); *Dietary Reference Intakes for Water, Potassium, Sodium, Chloride, and Sulfate* (2005); and *Dietary Reference Intakes for Calcium and Vitamin D* (2011). These reports may be accessed via www.nap.edu. Reprinted with permission from the National Academies Press, National Academy of Sciences.

Estimated Energy Requirements (EER)

Estimated amount of calories[a] needed to maintain calorie balance for various gender and age groups at three different levels of physical activity. The estimates are rounded to the nearest 200 calories. An individual's calorie needs may be higher or lower than these average estimates.

Gender/ Activity level[b]	Male/ Sedentary	Male/ Moderately Active	Male/ Active	Female[c]/ Sedentary	Female[c]/ Moderately Active	Female[c]/ Active
Age (years)						
2	1,000	1,000	1,000	1,000	1,000	1,000
3	1,200	1,400	1,400	1,000	1,200	1,400
4	1,200	1,400	1,600	1,200	1,400	1,400
5	1,200	1,400	1,600	1,200	1,400	1,600
6	1,400	1,600	1,800	1,200	1,400	1,600
7	1,400	1,600	1,800	1,200	1,600	1,800
8	1,400	1,600	2,000	1,400	1,600	1,800
9	1,600	1,800	2,000	1,400	1,600	1,800
10	1,600	1,800	2,200	1,400	1,800	2,000
11	1,800	2,000	2,200	1,600	1,800	2,000
12	1,800	2,200	2,400	1,600	2,000	2,200
13	2,000	2,200	2,600	1,600	2,000	2,200
14	2,000	2,400	2,800	1,800	2,000	2,400
15	2,200	2,600	3,000	1,800	2,000	2,400
16	2,400	2,800	3,200	1,800	2,000	2,400
17	2,400	2,800	3,200	1,800	2,000	2,400
18	2,400	2,800	3,200	1,800	2,000	2,400
19–20	2,600	2,800	3,000	2,000	2,200	2,400
21–25	2,400	2,800	3,000	2,000	2,200	2,400
26–30	2,400	2,600	3,000	1,800	2,000	2,400
31–35	2,400	2,600	3,000	1,800	2,000	2,200
36–40	2,400	2,600	2,800	1,800	2,000	2,200
41–45	2,200	2,600	2,800	1,800	2,000	2,200
46–50	2,200	2,400	2,800	1,800	2,000	2,200
51–55	2,200	2,400	2,800	1,600	1,800	2,200
56–60	2,200	2,400	2,600	1,600	1,800	2,200
61–65	2,000	2,400	2,600	1,600	1,800	2,000
66–70	2,000	2,200	2,600	1,600	1,800	2,000
71–75	2,000	2,200	2,600	1,600	1,800	2,000
76+	2,000	2,200	2,400	1,600	1,800	2,000

a: Based on Estimated Energy Requirements (EER) equations, using reference heights (average) and reference weights (healthy) for each age-gender group. For children and adolescents, reference height and weight vary. For adults, the reference man is 5 feet 10 inches tall and weighs 154 pounds. The reference woman is 5 feet 4 inches tall and weighs 126 pounds. EER equations are from the Institute of Medicine. Dietary Reference Intakes for Energy, Carbohydrate, Fiber, Fat, Fatty Acids, Cholesterol, Protein, and Amino Acids. Washington (DC): The National Academies Press; 2002.

b: Sedentary means a lifestyle that includes only the light physical activity associated with typical day-to-day life. Moderately active means a lifestyle that includes physical activity equivalent to walking about 1.5 to 3 miles per day at 3 to 4 miles per hour, in addition to the light physical activity associated with typical day-to-day life. Active means a lifestyle that includes physical activity equivalent to walking more than 3 miles per day at 3 to 4 miles per hour, in addition to the light physical activity associated with typical day-to-day life.

c: Estimates for females do not include women who are pregnant or breastfeeding.

Source: *Dietary Guidelines for Americans, 2010*. 7th Edition.

Appendix D

Nutritive Value of Foods

(Tr indicates nutrient present in trace amount.)

Item No. (A)	Foods, approximate measures, units, and weight (edible portion only) (B)		Water (C) Per-cent	Food energy (D) Cal-ories	Pro-tein (E) Grams	Fat (F) Grams	Satur-ated fat (G) Grams	Cho-lesterol (H) Milligrams	Carbo-hydrate (I) Grams	Dietary fiber (J) Grams	Calcium (K) Milligrams	Iron (L) Milligrams	Potas-sium (M) Milligrams	Sodium (N) Milligrams	Vitamin A (O) Micrograms	Thiamin (P) Milligrams	Ribo-flavin (Q) Milligrams	Niacin (R) Milligrams	Vitamin C (S) Milligrams
		Grams																	
Beverages																			
Carbonated:[2]																			
Club soda	12 fl. oz.	355	100	0	0	0	0.0	0	0	0	18	Tr	0	78	0	0.00	0.00	0.0	0
Cola type:																			
Regular	12 fl. oz.	369	89	160	0	0	0.0	0	41	0	11	0.2	7	18	0	0.00	0.00	0.0	0
Diet, artificially sweetened	12 fl. oz.	355	100	Tr	0	0	0.0	0	Tr	0	14	0.2	7	32	0	0.00	0.00	0.0	0
Ginger ale	12 fl. oz.	366	91	125	0	0	0.0	0	32	0	11	0.1	4	29	0	0.00	0.00	0.0	0
Grape	12 fl. oz.	372	88	180	0	0	0.0	0	46	0	15	0.4	4	48	0	0.00	0.00	0.0	0
Lemon-lime	12 fl. oz	372	89	155	0	0	0.0	0	39	0	7	0.4	4	33	0	0.00	0.00	0.0	0
Orange	12 fl. oz.	372	88	180	0	0	0.0	0	46	0	15	0.3	7	52	0	0.00	0.00	0.0	0
Pepper type	12 fl. oz.	369	89	160	0	0	Tr	0	41	0	11	0.1	5	37	0	0.00	0.00	0.0	0
Root beer	12 fl. oz.	370	89	165	0	0	0.0	0	42	0	15	0.2	4	48	0	0.00	0.00	0.0	0
Cocoa and chocolate-flavored beverages. See Dairy Products																			
Coffee:																			
Brewed	6 fl. oz.	180	100	Tr	Tr	Tr	0.0	0	Tr	0	4	Tr	124	2	0	0.00	0.02	0.4	0
Instant, prepared (2 tsp. powder plus 6 fl. oz. water)	6 fl. oz.	182	99	Tr	Tr	Tr	0.0	0	1	0	2	0.1	71	Tr	0	0.00	0.03	0.6	0
Fruit drinks, noncarbonated:																			
Canned:																			
Fruit punch drink	6 fl. oz.	190	88	85	Tr	0	0.0	0	22	0	15	0.4	48	15	2	0.03	0.04	Tr	[4]61
Grape drink	6 fl. oz.	187	86	100	Tr	0	0.0	0	26	Tr	2	0.3	9	11	Tr	0.01	0.01	Tr	[4]64
Pineapple-grapefruit juice drink	6 fl. oz.	187	87	90	Tr	Tr	Tr	0	23	Tr	13	0.9	97	24	6	0.06	0.04	0.5	[4]110
Frozen:																			
Lemonade concentrate:																			
Undiluted	6-fl.-oz. can	219	49	425	Tr	Tr	Tr	0	112	1	9	0.4	153	4	4	0.04	0.07	0.7	66
Diluted with 4 1/3 parts water by volume	6 fl. oz.	185	89	80	Tr	Tr	Tr	0	21	Tr	2	0.1	30	1	1	0.01	0.02	0.2	13
Limeade concentrate:																			
Undiluted	6-fl.-oz. can	218	50	410	Tr	Tr	Tr	0	108	1	11	0.2	129	Tr	Tr	0.02	0.02	0.2	26
Diluted with 4-1/3 parts water by volume	6 fl. oz	185	89	75	Tr	Tr	0.0	0	20	Tr	2	Tr	24	Tr	Tr	Tr	Tr	Tr	4
Fruit juices. See type under Fruits and Fruit Juices.																			
Milk beverages. See Dairy Products.																			
Tea:																			
Brewed	8 fl. oz.	240	100	Tr	Tr	Tr	0.0	0	Tr	0	0	Tr	36	1	0	0.00	0.03	Tr	0
Instant, powder, prepared:																			
Unsweetened (1 tsp. powder plus 8 fl. oz. water)	8 fl. oz.	241	100	Tr	Tr	Tr	0.0	0	1	0	1	Tr	61	1	0	0.00	0.02	0.1	0
Sweetened (3 tsp. powder plus 8 fl. oz. water)	8 fl. oz.	262	91	85	Tr	Tr	Tr	0	22	0	1	Tr	49	Tr	0	0.00	0.04	0.1	0
Dairy Products																			
Butter. See Fats and Oils																			
Cheese:																			
Cheddar:																			
Cut pieces	1 oz.	28	37	115	7	9	0.6	30	Tr	0	204	0.2	28	176	86	0.01	0.11	Tr	0
	1 in.³	17	37	70	4	6	3.6	18	Tr	0	123	0.1	17	105	52	Tr	0.06	Tr	0
Shredded	1 cup	113	37	455	28	37	23.8	119	1	0	815	0.8	111	701	342	0.03	0.42	0.1	0
Cottage (curd not pressed down):																			
Creamed (cottage cheese, 4% fat):																			
Large curd	1 cup	225	79	235	28	10	6.4	34	6	0	135	0.3	190	911	108	0.05	0.37	0.3	Tr
Small curd	1 cup	210	79	215	26	9	6.0	31	6	0	126	0.3	177	850	101	0.04	0.34	0.3	Tr
Lowfat (2%)	1 cup	226	79	205	31	4	2.8	19	8	0	155	0.4	217	918	45	0.05	0.42	0.3	Tr

(A)	(B)	(C)	(D)	(E)	(F)	(G)	(H)	(I)	(J)	(K)	(L)	(M)	(N)	(O)	(P)	(Q)	(R)	(S)
Uncreamed (cottage cheese dry curd, less than 1/2% fat)	1 cup	145	125	25	1	1.4	10	3	0	46	0.3	47	19	12	0.04	0.21	0.2	0
Cream	1 oz.	28	100	2	10	6.2	31	1	0	23	0.3	34	84	124	Tr	0.06	Tr	0
Mozzarella, made with:																		
Whole milk	1 oz.	28	80	6	6	3.7	22	1	0	147	0.1	19	106	68	Tr	0.07	Tr	0
Part skim milk (low moisture)	1 oz.	28	80	8	5	3.1	15	1	0	207	0.1	27	150	54	0.01	0.10	Tr	0
Parmesan, grated:																		
Tablespoon	1 tbsp.	5	25	2	2	1.0	4	Tr	0	69	Tr	5	93	9	Tr	0.02	Tr	0
Ounce	1 oz.	28	130	12	9	5.4	22	1	0	390	0.3	30	528	49	0.01	0.11	0.1	0
Swiss	1 oz.	28	105	8	8	5.0	26	1	0	272	Tr	31	74	72	0.01	0.10	Tr	0
Pasteurized process cheese:																		
American	1 oz.	28	105	6	9	5.6	27	Tr	0	174	0.1	46	406	82	0.01	0.10	Tr	0
Swiss	1 oz.	28	95	7	7	4.6	24	1	0	219	0.2	61	388	65	Tr	0.08	Tr	0
Pasteurized process cheese:																		
food, American	1 oz.	28	95	6	7	4.4	18	2	0	163	0.2	79	337	62	0.01	0.13	Tr	0
spread, American	1 oz.	28	80	5	6	3.8	16	2	0	159	0.1	69	381	54	0.01	0.12	Tr	0
Cream, sweet:																		
Half-and-half (cream and milk)	1 cup	242	315	7	28	17.3	89	10	0	254	0.2	314	98	259	0.08	0.36	0.2	2
	1 tbsp.	15	20	Tr	2	1.1	6	1	0	16	Tr	19	6	16	Tr	0.02	Tr	Tr
Light, coffee, or table	1 cup	240	470	6	46	28.8	159	9	0	231	0.1	292	95	437	0.08	0.36	0.1	2
	1 tbsp.	15	30	Tr	3	1.8	10	1	0	14	Tr	18	6	27	Tr	0.02	Tr	Tr
Whipping, unwhipped (volume about double when whipped):																		
Light	1 cup	239	700	5	74	46.1	265	7	0	166	0.1	231	82	705	0.06	0.30	0.1	1
	1 tbsp.	15	45	Tr	5	2.9	17	Tr	0	10	Tr	15	5	44	Tr	0.02	Tr	Tr
Heavy	1 cup	238	820	5	88	54.7	326	7	0	154	0.1	179	89	1,002	0.05	0.26	0.1	1
	1 tbsp.	15	50	Tr	6	3.4	21	Tr	0	10	Tr	11	6	63	Tr	0.02	Tr	Tr
Whipped topping, (pressurized)	1 cup	60	155	2	13	8.3	46	7	0	61	Tr	88	78	124	0.02	0.04	Tr	Tr
	1 tbsp.	3	10	Tr	1	0.6	2	Tr	0	3	Tr	4	4	6	Tr	Tr	Tr	0
Cream, sour	1 cup	230	495	7	48	29.9	102	10	0	268	0.1	331	123	448	0.08	0.34	0.2	2
	1 tbsp.	12	25	Tr	3	1.8	5	1	0	14	Tr	17	6	23	Tr	0.02	Tr	Tr
Cream products, imitation (made with vegetable fat):																		
Whipped topping:																		
Frozen	1 cup	75	240	1	19	16.4	0	17	0	5	0.1	14	19	565	0.00	0.00	0.0	0
	1 tbsp.	4	15	Tr	1	1.1	0	1	0	Tr	Tr	1	1	53	0.00	0.00	0.0	0
Pressurized	1 cup	70	185	1	16	13.2	0	11	0	4	Tr	13	43	533	0.00	0.00	0.0	0
	1 tbsp.	4	10	Tr	1	0.8	0	1	0	Tr	Tr	1	2	52	0.00	0.00	0.0	0
Ice cream. See Milk desserts, frozen.																		
Ice milk. See Milk desserts, frozen.																		
Milk:																		
Fluid:																		
Whole (3.3% fat)	1 cup	244	150	8	8	5.1	33	11	0	291	0.1	370	120	76	0.09	0.40	0.2	2
Lowfat (2%):																		
No milk solids added	1 cup	244	120	8	5	2.9	18	12	0	297	0.1	377	122	139	0.10	0.40	0.2	2
Milk solids added, label claim less than 10 g of protein per cup	1 cup	245	125	9	5	2.9	18	12	0	313	0.1	397	128	140	0.10	0.42	0.2	2
Lowfat (1%):																		
No milk solids added	1 cup	244	100	8	3	1.6	10	12	0	300	0.1	381	123	144	0.10	0.41	0.2	2
Milk solids added, label claim less than 10 g of protein per cup	1 cup	245	105	9	2	1.5	10	12	0	313	0.1	397	128	145	0.10	0.42	0.2	2
Nonfat (skim):																		
No milk solids added	1 cup	245	85	8	Tr	0.3	4	12	0	302	0.1	406	126	149	0.09	0.34	0.2	2
Milk solids added, label claim less than 10 g of protein per cup	1 cup	245	90	9	1	0.4	5	12	0	316	0.1	418	130	149	0.10	0.43	0.2	2
Buttermilk	1 cup	245	100	8	2	1.3	9	12	0	285	0.1	371	257	20	0.08	0.38	0.1	2
Canned:																		
Condensed, sweetened	1 cup	306	980	24	27	16.8	104	166	0	868	0.6	1,136	389	248	0.28	1.27	0.6	8
Evaporated:																		
Whole milk	1 cup	252	340	17	19	11.6	74	25	0	657	0.5	764	267	136	0.12	0.80	0.5	5
Nonfat milk	1 cup	255	200	19	1	0.3	9	29	0	738	0.7	845	293	298	0.11	0.79	0.4	3
Dried:																		
Nonfat, instantized:																		
Envelope, 3.2 oz., net wt.[6]	1 envelope	91	325	32	1	0.4	17	47	0	1,120	0.3	1,552	499	7,646	0.38	1.59	0.8	5

Nutritive Value of Foods – Continued
(Tr indicates nutrient present in trace amount.)

Nutrients in Indicated Quantity

Item No. (A)	Foods, approximate measures, units, and weight (weight of edible portion only) (B)		Water (C)	Food energy (D)	Protein (E)	Fat (F)	Saturated fat (G)	Cholesterol (H)	Carbohydrate (I)	Dietary fiber (J)	Calcium (K)	Iron (L)	Potassium (M)	Sodium (N)	Vitamin A (O)	Thiamin (P)	Riboflavin (Q)	Niacin (R)	Vitamin C (S)
		Grams	Percent	Calories	Grams	Grams	Grams	Milligrams	Grams	Grams	Milligrams	Milligrams	Milligrams	Milligrams	Micrograms	Milligrams	Milligrams	Milligrams	Milligrams
Milk beverages:																			
Chocolate milk (commercial):																			
Regular	1 cup	250	82	210	8	8	5.2	31	26	3	280	0.6	417	149	73	0.09	0.41	0.3	2
Lowfat (2%)	1 cup	250	84	180	8	5	3.1	17	26	3	284	0.6	422	151	143	0.09	0.41	0.3	2
Lowfat (1%)	1 cup	250	85	160	8	3	1.5	7	26	3	287	0.6	425	152	148	0.10	0.42	0.3	2
Cocoa and chocolate-flavored beverages:																			
Powder containing nonfat dry milk	1 oz.	28	1	100	3	1	0.7	1	22	Tr	90	0.3	223	139	Tr	0.03	0.17	0.2	Tr
Powder without nonfat dry milk	3/4 oz.	21	1	75	1	1	0.4	0	19	1	7	0.7	136	56	Tr	Tr	0.03	0.1	Tr
Eggnog (commercial)	1 cup	254	74	340	10	19	11.3	149	34	0	330	0.5	420	138	203	0.09	0.48	0.3	4
Malted milk:																			
Chocolate:																			
Powder	3/4 oz.	21	2	85	1	1	0.5	1	18	Tr	13	0.4	130	49	5	0.04	0.04	0.4	0
Shakes, thick:																			
Chocolate	10-oz. container	283	72	335	9	8	6.5	30	60	Tr	374	0.9	634	314	59	0.13	0.63	0.4	0
Vanilla	10-oz. container	283	74	315	11	9	5.3	33	50	Tr	413	0.3	517	270	79	0.08	0.55	0.4	0
Milk desserts, frozen:																			
Ice cream, vanilla:																			
Regular (about 11% fat):																			
Hardened	1/2 gal.	1,064	61	2,155	38	115	72.4	476	254	1	1,406	1.0	2,052	929	1,064	0.42	2.63	1.1	6
	1 cup	133	61	270	5	14	9.0	59	32	Tr	176	0.1	257	116	133	0.05	0.33	0.1	1
Soft serve (frozen custard)	1 cup	173	60	375	7	23	12.9	153	38	Tr	236	0.4	338	153	199	0.08	0.45	0.2	1
Ice milk, vanilla:																			
Hardened (about 4% fat)	1/2 gal.	1,048	69	1,470	41	45	27.7	146	232	1	1,409	1.5	2,117	836	419	0.61	2.78	0.9	6
	1 cup	131	69	185	5	6	3.5	18	29	Tr	176	0.2	265	105	52	0.08	0.35	0.1	1
Soft serve (about 3% fat)	1 cup	175	70	225	8	5	2.8	13	38	Tr	274	0.3	412	163	44	0.12	0.54	0.2	1
Sherbet (about 2% fat)	1/2 gal.	1,542	66	2,160	17	31	17.9	113	469	0	827	2.5	1,585	706	308	0.26	0.71	1.0	31
	1 cup	193	66	270	2	4	2.2	14	59	0	103	0.3	198	88	39	0.03	0.09	0.1	4
Yogurt:																			
With added milk solids:																			
Made with lowfat milk:																			
Fruit-flavored[8]	8-oz. container	227	74	230	10	2	1.6	10	43	1	345	0.2	442	133	25	0.08	0.40	0.2	1
Plain	8-oz. container	227	85	145	12	4	2.3	14	16	0	415	0.2	531	159	36	0.10	0.49	0.3	2
Made with nonfat milk	8-oz. container	227	85	125	13	Tr	0.3	4	17	0	452	0.2	579	174	5	0.11	0.53	0.3	2
Eggs																			
Eggs, large (24 oz. per dozen):																			
Raw:																			
Whole, without shell	1 egg	50	75	80	6	6	1.6	274	1	0	28	1.0	65	69	78	0.04	0.15	Tr	0
White	1 white	33	88	15	3	Tr	0.0	0	Tr	0	4	Tr	45	50	0	Tr	0.09	Tr	0
Yolk	1 yolk	17	49	65	3	6	1.6	272	Tr	0	26	0.9	15	8	94	0.04	0.07	Tr	0
Cooked:																			
Fried in butter	1 egg	46	68	95	6	7	1.9	278	1	0	29	1.1	66	162	94	0.04	0.14	Tr	0
Hard-cooked, shell removed	1 egg	50	75	80	6	6	1.6	274	1	0	28	1.0	65	69	78	0.04	0.14	Tr	0
Poached	1 egg	50	74	80	6	6	1.6	273	1	0	28	1.0	65	146	78	0.03	0.13	Tr	0
Scrambled (milk added) in butter. Also omelet	1 egg	64	73	110	7	8	2.2	282	2	0	54	1.0	97	176	102	0.04	0.18	Tr	Tr
Fats and Oils																			
Butter (4 sticks per lb.):																			
Tablespoon (1/8 stick)	1 tbsp.	14	16	100	Tr	11	7.1	31	Tr	0	3	Tr	4	[9]116	[10]106	Tr	Tr	Tr	0
Pat (1 in. square, 1/3 in. high; 90 per lb.)	1 pat	5	16	35	Tr	4	2.5	11	Tr	0	1	Tr	1	[9]41	[10]38	Tr	Tr	Tr	0
Fats, cooking (vegetable shortenings)	1 cup	205	0	1,810	0	205	51.5	0	0	0	0	0.0	0	0	0	0.00	0.00	0.0	0
	1 tbsp.	13	0	115	0	13	3.3	0	0	0	0	0.0	0	0	0	0.00	0.00	0.0	0

(A)	(B)	(g)	(C)	(D)	(E)	(F)	(G)	(H)	(I)	(J)	(K)	(L)	(M)	(N)	(O)	(P)	(Q)	(R)	(S)
Margarine:																			
Imitation (about 40% fat), soft	8-oz. container	227	58	785	1	88	14.5	0	1	0	40	0.0	[11]57	2,178	[12]2,254	0.01	0.05	Tr	Tr
	1 tbsp.	14	58	50	Tr	5	0.9	0	Tr	0	2	0.0	4	[11]134	[12]139	Tr	Tr	Tr	Tr
Regular (about 80% fat):																			
Hard (4 sticks per lb.):																			
Tablespoon (1/8 stick)	1 tbsp.	14	16	100	Tr	11	1.8	0	Tr	0	4	Tr	6	[11]132	[12]139	Tr	Tr	Tr	Tr
Pat (1 in. square, 1/3 in. high; 90 per lb.)	1 pat	5	16	35	Tr	4	0.8	0	Tr	0	1	Tr	2	147	150	Tr	Tr	Tr	Tr
Soft	8-oz. container	227	16	1,625	2	183	30.7	0	1	0	60	0.0	[11]86	2,449	[12]2,254	0.02	0.07	Tr	Tr
	1 tbsp.	14	16	100	Tr	11	1.9	0	Tr	0	4	0.0	5	[11]151	[12]139	Tr	Tr	Tr	Tr
Spread (about 60% fat):																			
Hard (4 sticks per lb.):																			
Tablespoon (1/8 stick)	1 tbsp.	14	37	75	Tr	9	2.0	0	0	0	3	0.0	4	[11]139	[12]139	Tr	Tr	0.0	0
Pat (1 in. square, 1/3 in. high; 90 per lb.)	1 pat	5	37	25	Tr	3	0.7	0	0	0	1	0.0	1	150	150	Tr	Tr	0.0	0
Soft	8-oz. container	227	37	1,225	1	138	29.1	0	0	0	47	0.0	[11]68	2,256	[12]2,254	0.02	0.06	0.0	0
	1 tbsp.	14	37	75	Tr	9	1.8	0	0	0	3	0.0	4	[11]139	[12]139	Tr	Tr	0.0	0
Oils, salad or cooking:																			
Corn	1 cup	218	0	1,925	0	218	29.4	0	0	0	0	0.0	0	0	0	0.00	0.00	0.0	0
	1 tbsp.	14	0	125	0	14	1.8	0	0	0	0	0.0	0	0	0	0.00	0.00	0.0	0
Safflower	1 cup	218	0	1,925	0	218	19.8	0	0	0	0	0.0	0	0	0	0.00	0.00	0.0	0
	1 tbsp.	14	0	125	0	14	1.3	0	0	0	0	0.0	0	0	0	0.00	0.00	0.0	0
Soybean oil, hydrogenated (partially hardened)	1 cup	218	0	1,925	0	218	31.4	0	0	0	0	0.0	0	0	0	0.00	0.00	0.0	0
	1 tbsp.	14	0	125	0	14	2.0	0	0	0	0	0.0	0	0	0	0.00	0.00	0.0	0
Sunflower	1 cup	218	0	1,925	0	218	25.0	0	0	0	0	0.0	0	0	0	0.00	0.00	0.0	0
	1 tbsp.	14	0	125	0	14	1.5	0	0	0	0	0.0	0	0	0	0.00	0.00	0.0	0
Salad dressings:																			
Commercial:																			
Blue cheese	1 tbsp.	15	32	75	1	8	1.5	3	1	Tr	12	Tr	6	164	10	Tr	0.02	Tr	Tr
French:																			
Regular	1 tbsp.	16	35	85	Tr	9	1.5	0	1	Tr	2	Tr	2	188	Tr	Tr	Tr	Tr	Tr
Low calorie	1 tbsp.	16	75	25	Tr	2	0.1	0	2	Tr	6	Tr	3	306	Tr	Tr	Tr	Tr	Tr
Italian:																			
Regular	1 tbsp.	15	34	80	Tr	9	1.0	0	1	Tr	1	Tr	5	162	3	Tr	Tr	Tr	Tr
Low calorie	1 tbsp.	15	86	5	Tr	Tr	0.2	0	2	Tr	1	Tr	4	136	Tr	Tr	Tr	Tr	Tr
Mayonnaise:																			
Regular	1 tbsp.	14	15	100	Tr	11	1.6	8	Tr	0	3	0.1	5	80	12	0.00	0.00	Tr	0
Imitation	1 tbsp.	15	63	35	Tr	3	0.5	4	2	0	Tr	0.0	2	75	0	0.00	0.00	0.0	0
Tartar sauce	1 tbsp.	14	34	75	Tr	8	1.5	4	1	Tr	3	0.1	11	182	9	Tr	Tr	Tr	Tr
Thousand Island:																			
Regular	1 tbsp.	16	46	60	Tr	6	1.0	4	2	Tr	2	0.1	18	112	15	Tr	Tr	Tr	0
Low calorie	1 tbsp.	15	69	25	Tr	2	0.2	2	2	Tr	2	0.1	17	150	14	Tr	Tr	Tr	0
Prepared from home recipe:																			
Cooked type	1 tbsp.	16	69	25	1	2	0.5	9	2	Tr	13	0.1	19	117	20	0.01	0.02	Tr	Tr
Vinegar and oil	1 tbsp.	16	47	70	0	8	1.5	0	Tr	0	0	0.0	1	Tr	0	0.00	0.00	0.0	0

Fish and Shellfish

(A)	(B)	(g)	(C)	(D)	(E)	(F)	(G)	(H)	(I)	(J)	(K)	(L)	(M)	(N)	(O)	(P)	(Q)	(R)	(S)
Clams:																			
Raw, meat only	3 oz.	85	82	65	11	1	0.1	43	2	0	59	2.6	154	102	26	0.09	0.15	1.1	9
Crabmeat, canned	1 cup	135	77	135	23	3	0.3	135	1	0	61	1.1	149	1,350	14	0.11	0.11	2.6	0
Fish sticks, frozen, reheated, (stick, 4 by 1 by 1/2 in.)	1 fish stick	28	52	70	6	3	0.9	26	4	Tr	11	0.3	94	53	5	0.03	0.05	0.6	0
Haddock, breaded, fried[14]	3 oz.	85	61	175	17	9	3.2	75	7	1	34	1.0	270	123	20	0.06	0.10	2.9	0
Halibut, broiled, with butter and lemon juice	3 oz.	85	67	140	20	6	0.5	62	Tr	0	14	0.7	441	103	174	0.06	0.07	7.7	1
Salmon:																			
Canned (pink), solids and liquid	3 oz.	85	71	120	17	5	1.7	34	Tr	0	[15]167	0.7	307	443	18	0.03	0.15	6.8	0
Sardines, Atlantic, canned in oil, drained solids	3 oz.	85	62	175	20	9	1.7	85	2	0	[15]371	2.6	349	425	56	0.03	0.17	4.6	0
Scallops, breaded, frozen, reheated	6 scallops	90	59	195	15	10	2.5	70	1	Tr	39	2.0	369	298	21	0.11	0.11	1.6	0
Shrimp:																			
Canned, drained solids	3 oz.	85	70	100	21	1	0.2	128	1	0	98	1.4	1	1,955	15	0.01	0.03	1.5	0
French fried (7 medium)[16]	3 oz.	85	55	200	16	10	3.8	168	11	Tr	61	2.0	189	384	26	0.06	0.09	2.8	0
Tuna, canned, drained solids:																			
Oil pack, chunk light	3 oz.	85	61	165	24	7	1.3	55	0	0	7	1.6	298	303	20	0.04	0.09	10.1	0
Water pack, solid white	3 oz.	85	63	135	30	1	0.2	48	0	0	17	0.6	255	468	32	0.03	0.10	13.4	0

Nutritive Value of Foods – Continued
(Tr indicates nutrient present in trace amount.)

Nutrients in Indicated Quantity

Item No. / Foods (A)	Measure, units, weight (B)	Grams	Water, Percent (C)	Food energy, Calories (D)	Protein, Grams (E)	Fat, Grams (F)	Saturated fat, Grams (G)	Cholesterol, mg (H)	Carbohydrate, Grams (I)	Dietary fiber, Grams (J)	Calcium, mg (K)	Iron, mg (L)	Potassium, mg (M)	Sodium, mg (N)	Vitamin A, Micrograms (O)	Thiamin, mg (P)	Riboflavin, mg (Q)	Niacin, mg (R)	Vitamin C, mg (S)
Fruits and Fruit Juices																			
Apples:																			
Raw:																			
Unpeeled, without cores:																			
2-3/4-in. diam. (about 3 per lb. with cores)	1 apple	138	84	80	Tr	Tr	0.1	0	21	3	10	0.2	159	Tr	7	0.02	0.02	0.1	8
Peeled, sliced	1 cup	110	84	65	Tr	Tr	0.1	0	16	2	4	0.1	124	Tr	5	0.02	0.01	0.1	4
Dried, sulfured	10 rings	64	32	155	1	Tr	Tr	0	42	6	9	0.9	288	56[18]	0	0.00	0.10	0.6	2[20]
Apple juice, bottled or canned[19]	1 cup	248	88	115	Tr	Tr	Tr	0	29	Tr	17	0.9	295	7	Tr	0.05	0.04	0.2	2[20]
Applesauce, canned:																			
Sweetened	1 cup	255	80	195	Tr	Tr	Tr	0	51	3	10	0.9	156	8	3	0.03	0.07	0.5	4[20]
Unsweetened	1 cup	244	88	105	Tr	Tr	Tr	0	28	3	7	0.3	183	5	7	0.03	0.06	0.5	3[20]
Apricots:																			
Raw, without pits (about 12 per lb. with pits)	3 apricots	106	86	50	1	Tr	Tr	0	12	2	15	0.6	314	1	277	0.03	0.04	0.6	11
Canned (fruit and liquid):																			
Heavy syrup pack	1 cup	258	78	215	1	Tr	Tr	0	55	3	23	0.8	361	10	317	0.05	0.06	1.0	8
Juice pack	1 cup	248	87	120	2	Tr	Tr	0	31	3	30	0.7	409	10	419	0.04	0.05	0.9	12
Dried:																			
Uncooked (28 large or 37 medium halves per cup)	1 cup	130	31	310	5	1	Tr	0	80	6	59	6.1	1,791	13	941	0.01	0.20	3.9	3[20]
Apricot nectar, canned	1 cup	251	85	140	1	Tr	Tr	0	36	2	18	1.0	286	8	330	0.02	0.04	0.7	2[20]
Avocados, raw, whole, without skin and seed:																			
California (about 2 per lb. with skin and seed)	1 avocado	173	73	305	4	30	4.5	0	12	6	19	2.0	1,097	21	106	0.19	0.21	3.3	14
Bananas, raw, without peel:																			
Whole (about 2-1/2 per lb. with peel)	1 banana	114	74	105	1	1	0.2	0	27	2	7	0.4	451	1	9	0.05	0.11	0.6	10
Blackberries, raw	1 cup	144	86	75	1	1	0.3	0	18	6	46	0.8	282	Tr	24	0.04	0.06	0.6	30
Blueberries:																			
Raw	1 cup	145	85	80	1	1	Tr	0	20	4	9	0.2	129	9	15	0.07	0.07	0.5	19
Frozen, sweetened	10-oz. container	284	77	230	1	Tr	0.1	0	62	6	17	1.1	170	3	12	0.06	0.15	0.7	3
Cantaloupe. See Melons																			
Cherries:																			
Sour, red, pitted, canned, water pack	1 cup	244	90	90	2	Tr	0.1	0	22	2	27	3.3	239	17	184	0.04	0.10	0.4	5
Sweet, raw, without pits and stems	10 cherries	68	81	50	1	1	0.1	0	11	Tr	10	0.3	152	Tr	15	0.03	0.04	0.3	5
Cranberry juice cocktail, bottled, sweetened	1 cup	253	85	145	Tr	Tr	0.1	0	38	Tr	8	0.4	61	10	1	0.01	0.04	0.1	108[21]
Cranberry sauce, sweetened, canned, strained	1 cup	277	61	420	1	Tr	Tr	0	108	3	11	0.6	72	80	6	0.04	0.06	0.3	6
Dates:																			
Whole, without pits	10 dates	83	23	230	2	Tr	0.2	0	61	6	27	1.0	541	2	4	0.07	0.08	1.8	0
Fruit cocktail, canned, fruit and liquid:																			
Heavy syrup pack	1 cup	255	80	185	1	Tr	Tr	0	48	3	15	0.7	224	15	52	0.05	0.05	1.0	5
Juice pack	1 cup	248	87	115	1	Tr	Tr	0	29	3	20	0.5	236	10	76	0.03	0.04	1.0	7
Grapefruit:																			
Raw, without peel, membrane and seeds (3-3/4 in. diam., 1 lb. 1 oz., whole, with refuse)	1/2 grapefruit	120	91	40	1	Tr	Tr	0	10	1	14	0.1	167	Tr	1[22]	0.04	0.02	0.3	41
Grapefruit juice:																			
Canned:																			
Unsweetened	1 cup	247	90	95	1	Tr	Tr	0	22	Tr	17	0.5	378	2	2	0.10	0.05	0.6	72
Sweetened	1 cup	250	87	115	1	Tr	Tr	0	28	Tr	20	0.9	405	5	2	0.10	0.06	0.8	67
Frozen concentrate, unsweetened																			
Diluted with 3 parts water by volume	1 cup	247	89	100	1	Tr	0.1	0	24	Tr	20	0.3	336	2	2	0.10	0.05	0.5	83
Grapes, European type (adherent skin); raw:																			
Thompson seedless	10 grapes	50	81	35	Tr	Tr	0.1	0	9	Tr	6	0.1	93	1	4	0.05	0.03	0.2	5
Grape juice:																			
Canned or bottled	1 cup	253	84	155	1	Tr	0.1	0	38	2	23	0.6	334	8	2	0.07	0.09	0.7	Tr[20]
Frozen concentrate, sweetened:																			
Diluted with 3 parts water by volume	1 cup	250	87	125	Tr	Tr	0.1	0	32	Tr	10	0.3	53	5	2	0.04	0.07	0.3	160[2]
Lemons, raw, without peel and seeds (about 4 per lb. with peel and seeds)	1 lemon	58	89	15	1	Tr	Tr	0	5	2	15	0.3	80	1	2	0.02	0.01	0.1	31

(A)	(B)	(C)	(D)	(E)	(F)	(G)	(H)	(I)	(J)	(K)	(L)	(M)	(N)	(O)	(P)	(Q)	(R)	(S)
Lemon juice:																		
Canned or bottled, unsweetened	1 cup	92	50	1	1	0.1	0	16	1	27	0.3	249	2³51	4	0.10	0.02	0.5	61
Frozen, single-strength, unsweetened	6 fl. oz. can	244 92	55	1	1	0.1	0	16	1	20	0.3	217	2	3	0.14	0.03	0.3	77
Lime juice:																		
Canned, unsweetened	1 cup	246	93	50	1	1	0.1	0	16	1	30	0.6	185	2³39	4	0.08	0.01	0.4	16
Melons, raw, without rind and cavity contents:																		
Cantaloupe, orange-fleshed																		
(5 in. diam., 2-1/3 lb., whole, with rind and cavity contents)	1/2 melon	267	90	95	2	1	0.1	0	22	2	29	0.6	825	24	861	0.10	0.06	1.5	113
Honeydew (6-1/2 in. diam., 5-1/4 lb., whole, with rind and cavity contents)	1/10 melon	129	90	45	1	Tr	Tr	0	12	1	8	0.1	350	13	5	0.10	0.02	0.8	32
Nectarines, raw, without pits (about 3 per lb. with pits)1 nectarine	1 nectarine	136	86	65	1	1	0.1	0	16	2	7	0.2	288	Tr	100	0.02	0.06	1.3	7
Oranges, raw:																		
Whole, without peel and seeds (2-5/8 in. diam., about 2-1/2 per lb., with peel and seeds)	1 orange	131	87	60	1	Tr	Tr	0	15	3	52	0.1	237	Tr	27	0.11	0.05	0.4	70
Orange juice:																		
Raw, all varieties	1 cup	248	88	110	2	Tr	Tr	0	26	Tr	27	0.5	496	2	50	0.22	0.07	1.0	124
Canned, unsweetened	1 cup	249	89	105	1	Tr	Tr	0	25	Tr	20	1.1	436	5	44	0.15	0.07	0.8	86
Frozen concentrate:																		
Diluted with 3 parts water by volume	1 cup	249	88	110	2	Tr	Tr	0	27	Tr	22	0.2	473	2	19	0.20	0.04	0.5	97
Orange and grapefruit juice, canned	1 cup	247	89	105	1	Tr	Tr	0	25	Tr	20	1.1	390	7	29	0.14	0.07	0.8	72
Peaches:																		
Raw:																		
Whole, 2-1/2 in. diam., peeled, pitted (about 4 per lb. with peels and pits)	1 peach	87	88	35	1	Tr	Tr	0	10	2	4	0.1	171	Tr	47	0.01	0.04	0.9	6
Canned, fruit and liquid:																		
Heavy syrup pack	1 cup	256	79	190	1	Tr	Tr	0	51	3	8	0.7	236	15	85	0.03	0.06	1.6	7
Juice pack	1 cup	248	87	110	2	Tr	Tr	0	29	4	15	0.7	317	10	94	0.02	0.04	1.4	9
Dried:																		
Uncooked	1 cup	160	32	380	6	1	0.1	0	98	12	45	6.5	1,594	11	346	Tr	0.34	7.0	8
Frozen, sliced, sweetened 10 oz. container	10-oz container	284	75	265	2	Tr	Tr	0	68	4	9	1.1	369	17	81	0.04	0.10	1.9	2¹268
	1 cup	250	75	235	2	Tr	Tr	0	60	4	8	0.9	325	15	71	0.03	0.09	1.6	2¹236
Pears:																		
Raw, with skin, cored:																		
Bartlett, 2-1/2 in. diam. (about 2-1/2 per lb. with cores and stems)	1 pear	166	84	100	1	1	Tr	0	25	4	18	0.4	208	Tr	3	0.03	0.07	0.2	7
Bosc, 2-1/2 in. diam. (about 3 per lb. with cores and stems)	1 pear	141	84	85	1	1	Tr	0	21	3	16	0.4	176	Tr	3	0.03	0.06	0.1	6
Canned, fruit and liquid:																		
Heavy syrup pack	1 cup	255	80	190	1	Tr	Tr	0	49	5	13	0.6	166	13	1	0.03	0.06	0.6	3
Juice pack	1 cup	248	86	125	1	Tr	Tr	0	32	5	22	0.7	238	10	1	0.03	0.03	0.5	4
Pineapple:																		
Raw, diced	1 cup	155	87	75	1	1	Tr	0	19	2	11	0.6	175	2	4	0.14	0.06	0.7	24
Canned, fruit and liquid:																		
Heavy syrup pack:																		
Crushed, chunks, tidbits	1 cup	255	79	200	1	Tr	Tr	0	52	1	36	1.0	265	3	4	0.23	0.06	0.7	19
Juice pack:																		
Chunks or tidbits	1 cup	250	84	150	1	Tr	Tr	0	39	2	35	0.7	305	3	10	0.24	0.05	0.7	24
Pineapple juice, unsweetened, canned	1 cup	250	86	140	1	Tr	Tr	0	34	Tr	43	0.7	335	3	1	0.14	0.06	0.6	27
Plums, without pits:																		
Raw:																		
2-1/8 in. diam. (about 6-1/2 per lb. with pits)	1 plum	66	85	35	1	Tr	Tr	0	9	1	3	0.1	114	Tr	21	0.03	0.06	0.3	6
Canned, purple, fruit and liquid:																		
Heavy syrup pack:	1 cup	258	76	230	1	Tr	Tr	0	60	3	23	2.2	235	49	67	0.04	0.10	0.8	1
Juice pack:	1 cup	252	84	145	1	Tr	Tr	0	38	3	25	0.9	388	3	254	0.06	0.15	1.2	7
Prunes, dried:																		
Uncooked	4 extra large or 5 large prunes	49	32	115	1	Tr	Tr	0	31	4	25	1.2	365	2	97	0.04	0.08	1.0	2
Cooked, unsweetened, fruit and liquid	1 cup	212	70	225	2	Tr	Tr	0	60	14	49	2.4	708	4	65	0.05	0.21	1.5	6
Prune juice, canned or bottled	1 cup	256	81	180	2	Tr	Tr	0	45	3	31	3.0	707	10	1	0.04	0.18	2.0	10
Raisins, seedless:																		
Cup, not pressed down	1 cup	145	15	435	5	1	0.2	0	115	5	71	3.0	1,089	17	1	0.23	0.13	1.2	5

Nutritive Value of Foods – Continued
(Tr indicates nutrient present in trace amount.)

Item No. (A)	Foods, approximate measures, units, and weight (weight of edible portion only) (B)	Grams	Water Percent (C)	Food energy Calories (D)	Protein Grams (E)	Fat Grams (F)	Saturated fat Grams (G)	Cholesterol Milligrams (H)	Carbohydrate Grams (I)	Dietary fiber Grams (J)	Calcium Milligrams (K)	Iron Milligrams (L)	Potassium Milligrams (M)	Sodium Milligrams (N)	Vitamin A Micrograms (O)	Thiamin Milligrams (P)	Riboflavin Milligrams (Q)	Niacin Milligrams (R)	Vitamin C Milligrams (S)
Raspberries:																			
Raw	1 cup	123	87	60	1	1	Tr	0	14	5	27	0.7	187	Tr	16	0.04	0.11	1.1	31
Frozen, sweetened	10-oz. container	284	73	295	2	Tr	Tr	0	74	5	43	1.8	324	3	17	0.05	0.13	0.7	47
Rhubarb, cooked, added sugar	1 cup	240	68	280	1	Tr	Tr	0	75	5	348	0.5	230	2	17	0.04	0.06	0.5	8
Strawberries:																			
Raw, capped, whole	1 cup	149	92	45	1	1	Tr	0	10	2	21	0.6	247	1	4	0.03	0.10	0.3	84
Tangerines:																			
Raw, without peel and seeds (2-3/8 in. diam., about 4 per lb., with peel and seeds)	1 tangerine	84	88	35	1	Tr	Tr	0	9	1	12	0.1	132	1	77	0.09	0.02	0.1	26
Watermelon, raw, without rind and seeds:																			
Piece (4 by 8 in wedge with rind and seeds; 1/16 of 32-2/3 lb. melon, 10 by 16 in.)	1 piece	482	92	155	3	2	0.6	0	35	1	39	0.8	559	10	176	0.39	0.10	1.0	46
Grain Products																			
Bagels, plain or water, enriched, 3-1/2 in. diam.[24]	1 bagel	68	29	200	7	2	0.1	0	38	2	29	1.8	50	245	0	0.26	0.20	2.4	0
Biscuits, baking powder, 2 in. diam. (enriched flour, vegetable shortening):																			
From home recipe	1 biscuit	28	28	100	2	5	1.2	Tr	13	Tr	47	0.7	32	195	3	0.08	0.08	0.8	Tr
From mix	1 biscuit	28	29	95	2	3	0.8	Tr	14	1	58	0.7	56	262	4	0.12	0.11	0.8	Tr
From refrigerated dough	1 biscuit	20	30	65	1	2	2.0	1	10	Tr	4	0.5	18	249	0	0.08	0.05	0.7	0
Breads:																			
Cracked-wheat bread (3/4 enriched wheat flour, 1/4 cracked wheat flour):[25]																			
Slice (18 per loaf)	1 slice	25	35	65	2	1	0.2	0	12	2	16	0.7	34	106	Tr	0.10	0.09	0.8	Tr
French or Vienna bread, enriched:[25]																			
Slice:																			
French, 5 by 2-1/2 by 1 in.	1 slice	35	34	100	3	1	0.2	0	18	1	39	1.1	32	203	Tr	0.16	0.12	1.4	Tr
Vienna, 4-3/4 by 4 by 1/2 in.	1 slice	25	34	70	2	1	0.2	0	13	1	28	0.8	23	145	Tr	0.12	0.09	1.0	Tr
Italian bread, enriched:[25]																			
Slice, 4-1/2 by 3-1/4 by 3/4 in.	1 slice	30	32	85	3	Tr	0.3	0	17	1	5	0.8	22	176	0	0.12	0.07	1.0	0
Pita bread, enriched, white, 6-1/2 in. diam.	1 pita	60	31	165	6	1	0.1	0	33	1	49	1.4	71	339	0	0.27	0.12	2.2	0
Pumpernickel (2/3 rye flour, 1/3 enriched wheat flour):[25]																			
Slice, 5 by 4 by 3/8 in.	1 slice	32	37	80	3	1	0.1	0	16	1	23	0.9	141	177	0	0.11	0.17	1.1	0
Raisin bread, enriched:[25]																			
Slice (18 per loaf)	1 slice	25	33	65	2	1	0.3	0	13	1	25	0.8	59	92	Tr	0.08	0.15	1.0	Tr
Rye bread, light (2/3 enriched wheat flour, 1/3 rye flour):[25]																			
Slice, 4-3/4 by 3-3/4 by 7/16 in.	1 slice	25	37	65	2	1	0.2	0	12	2	20	0.7	51	175	0	0.10	0.08	0.8	0
Wheat bread, enriched:[25]																			
Slice (18 per loaf)	1 slice	25	37	65	2	1	0.2	0	12	1	32	0.9	35	138	Tr	0.12	0.08	1.2	Tr
White bread, enriched:[25]																			
Slice (18 per loaf)	1 slice	25	37	65	2	1	0.2	0	12	1	32	0.7	28	129	Tr	0.12	0.08	0.9	Tr
Slice (22 per loaf)	1 slice	20	37	55	2	1	0.2	0	10	1	25	0.6	22	101	Tr	0.09	0.06	0.7	Tr
Cubes	1 cup	30	37	80	2	1	0.2	0	15	1	38	0.9	34	154	Tr	0.14	0.09	1.1	Tr
Crumbs, soft	1 cup	45	37	120	4	2	0.3	0	22	1	57	1.3	50	231	Tr	0.21	0.14	1.7	Tr
Whole-wheat bread:[25]																			
Slice (16 per loaf)	1 slice	28	38	70	3	1	0.3	0	13	2	20	1.0	50	180	Tr	0.10	0.06	1.1	Tr
Bread stuffing (from enriched bread), prepared from mix:																			
Dry type	1 cup	140	33	500	9	31	2.4	0	50	4	92	2.2	126	1,254	273	0.17	0.20	2.5	0

(A)	(B)	(C)	(D)	(E)	(F)	(G)	(H)	(I)	(J)	(K)	(L)	(M)	(N)	(O)	(P)	(Q)	(R)	(S)
Moist type	1 cup	203	61	9	26	3.0	67	40	4	81	2.0	118	1,023	256	0.10	0.18	1.6	0
Breakfast cereals:																		
Hot type, cooked:																		
Corn (hominy) grits:																		
Regular and quick, enriched	1 cup	242	85	145	3	0.1	0	31	5	0	[27]1.5	53	[28]0	[29]0	[27]0.24	[27]0.15	[27]2.0	0
Instant, plain	1 pkt.	137	85	80	2	Tr	0	18	Tr	7	[27]1.0	29	343	0	[27]0.18	[27]0.08	[27]1.3	0
Cream of Wheat®:																		
Regular, quick, instant	1 cup	244	86	140	4	0.1	0	29	1	[30]54	[30]10.9	46	[31]325	0	[30]0.24	[30]0.07	[30]1.5	0
Mix'n Eat, plain	1 pkt.	142	82	100	3	Tr	0	21	Tr	[30]20	[30]8.1	38	241	[30]376	[30]0.43	[30]0.28	[30]5.0	0
Malt-O-Meal®	1 cup	240	88	120	4	Tr	0	26	1	5	[30]9.6	31	[32]2	0	[30]0.48	[30]0.24	[30]5.8	0
Oatmeal or rolled oats:																		
Regular, quick, instant, nonfortified	1 cup	234	85	145	6	0.4	0	25	4	19	1.6	131	342	4	0.26	0.05	0.3	0
Instant, fortified:																		
Plain	1 pkt.	177	86	105	4	0.3	0	18	3	[27]163	[27]6.3	99	[27]285	[27]453	[27]0.53	[27]0.28	[27]5.5	0
Ready-to-eat:																		
All-Bran® (about 1/3 cup)	1 oz.	28	3	70	4	0.1	0	21	10	23	[30]4.5	350	320	[30]375	[30]0.37	[30]0.43	[30]5.0	[30]15
Cap'n Crunch® (about 3/4 cup)	1 oz.	28	3	120	1	2.2	0	23	1	5	[27]7.5	37	213	4	[27]0.50	[27]0.55	[27]6.6	[30]15
Cheerios® (about 1-1/4 cup)	1 oz.	28	5	110	4	0.3	0	20	2	48	[30]4.5	101	307	[30]375	[30]0.37	[30]0.43	[30]5.0	[30]15
Corn Flakes (about 1-1/4 cup):																		
Toasties®	1 oz.	28	3	110	2	Tr	0	24	1	1	[27]0.7	33	297	[30]375	[30]0.37	[30]0.43	[30]5.0	0
40% Bran Flakes:																		
Kellogg's® (about 3/4 cup)	1 oz.	28	3	90	4	0.1	0	22	6	14	[30]8.1	180	264	[30]375	[30]0.37	[30]0.43	[30]5.0	[30]15
Froot Loops® (about 1 cup)	1 oz.	28	3	110	2	0.2	0	25	1	3	[30]4.5	26	145	[30]375	[30]0.37	[30]0.43	[30]5.0	[30]15
Golden Grahams® (about 3/4 cup)	1 oz.	28	2	110	2	2.9	Tr	24	1	17	[30]4.5	63	346	[30]375	[30]0.37	[30]0.43	[30]5.0	[30]15
Grape-Nuts® (about 1/4 cup)	1 oz.	28	3	100	3	Tr	0	23	3	11	1.2	95	197	[30]375	[30]0.37	[30]0.43	[30]5.0	0
Honey Nut Cheerios® (about 3/4 cup)	1 oz.	28	3	105	3	0.1	0	23	1	20	[30]4.5	99	257	[30]375	[30]0.37	[30]0.43	[30]5.0	[30]15
Nature Valley® Granola (about 1/3 cup)	1 oz.	28	4	125	3	5.0	0	19	2	18	0.9	98	58	2	0.10	0.05	0.2	0
Product 19® (about 3/4 cup)	1 oz.	28	3	110	3	Tr	0	24	1	3	[30]18.0	44	325	[30]1,501	[30]1.50	[30]1.70	[30]20.0	[30]60
Raisin Bran:																		
Kellogg's® (about 3/4 cup)	1 oz.	28	8	90	3	0.2	0	21	5	10	[30]3.5	147	207	[30]288	[30]0.28	[30]0.34	[30]3.9	0
Rice Krispies® (about 1 cup)	1 oz.	28	2	110	2	Tr	0	25	Tr	4	[30]1.8	29	340	[30]375	[30]0.37	[30]0.43	[30]5.0	[30]15
Shredded Wheat (about 2/3 cup)	1 oz.	28	5	100	3	0.2	0	23	4	11	1.2	102	3	0	0.07	0.08	1.5	0
Special K® (about 1-1/3 cup)	1 oz.	28	2	110	6	Tr	Tr	21	Tr	8	[30]4.5	49	265	[30]375	[30]0.37	[30]0.43	[30]5.0	[30]15
Frosted Flakes,																		
Kellogg's® (about 3/4 cup)	1 oz.	28	3	110	1	Tr	0	26	1	1	[30]1.8	18	230	[30]375	[30]0.37	[30]0.43	[30]5.0	[30]15
Golden Crisps® (about 3/4 cup)	1 oz.	28	3	105	2	Tr	0	25	1	3	[30]1.8	42	75	[30]375	[30]0.37	[30]0.43	[30]5.0	[30]15
Total® (about 1 cup)	1 oz.	28	4	100	3	0.1	0	22	4	48	[30]18.0	106	352	[30]1,501	[30]1.50	[30]1.70	[30]20.0	[30]60
Wheaties® (about 1 cup)	1 oz.	28	5	100	3	0.1	0	23	3	43	[30]4.5	106	354	[30]375	[30]0.37	[30]0.43	[30]5.0	[30]15
Buckwheat flour, light, sifted	1 cup	98	12	340	6	0.2	0	78	6	11	1.0	314	2	0	0.08	0.04	0.4	0
Cakes prepared from cake mixes with enriched flour:[35]																		
Angel food:																		
Piece, 1/12 of cake	1 piece	53	38	125	3	0.1	0	29	1	44	0.2	71	269	0	0.03	0.11	0.1	0
Coffeecake, crumb:																		
Piece, 1/6 of cake	1 piece	72	30	230	5	1.3	47	38	1	44	1.2	78	310	32	0.14	0.15	1.3	Tr
Devil's food with chocolate frosting:																		
Piece, 1/16 of cake	1 piece	69	24	235	3	3.2	37	40	2	41	1.4	90	181	31	0.07	0.10	0.6	Tr
Cupcake, 2-1/2 in. diam.	1 cupcake	35	24	120	2	1.9	19	20	1	21	0.7	46	92	16	0.04	0.05	0.3	Tr
Gingerbread:																		
Piece, 1/9 of cake	1 piece	63	37	175	2	1.6	1	32	2	57	1.2	173	192	0	0.09	0.11	0.8	Tr
Yellow with chocolate frosting:																		
Piece, 1/16 of cake	1 piece	69	26	235	3	3.3	36	40	1	63	1.0	75	157	29	0.08	0.10	0.7	Tr
Cakes prepared from home recipes using enriched flour:																		
Carrot, with cream cheese frosting:[36]																		
Piece, 1/16 of cake	1 piece	96	23	385	4	5.5	74	48	1	44	1.3	108	279	15	0.11	0.12	0.9	1
Fruitcake, dark:[36]																		
Piece, 1/32 of cake, 2/3 in. arc	1 piece	43	18	165	2	0.5	20	25	2	41	1.2	194	67	13	0.08	0.08	0.5	16
Plain sheet cake:[37]																		
Without frosting:																		
Piece, 1/9 of cake	1 piece	86	25	315	4	3.3	61	48	Tr	55	1.3	68	258	41	0.14	0.15	1.1	Tr
With uncooked white frosting:																		
Piece, 1/9 of cake	1 piece	121	21	445	4	2.9	70	77	1	61	1.2	74	275	71	0.13	0.16	1.1	Tr

Nutritive Value of Foods – Continued
(Tr indicates nutrient present in trace amount.)

Nutrients in Indicated Quantity

Item No. Foods, approximate measures, units, and weight (weight of edible portion only) (A)	(B) Grams	Water (C) Percent	Food energy (D) Calories	Protein (E) Grams	Fat (F) Grams	Saturated fat (G) Grams	Cholesterol (H) Milligrams	Carbohydrate (I) Grams	Dietary fiber (J) Grams	Calcium (K) Milligrams	Iron (L) Milligrams	Potassium (M) Milligrams	Sodium (N) Milligrams	Vitamin A (O) Micrograms	Thiamin (P) Milligrams	Riboflavin (Q) Milligrams	Niacin (R) Milligrams	Vitamin C (S) Milligrams
Pound:38																		
Slice, 1/17 of loaf	30	22	120	2	5	0.3	32	15	Tr	20	0.5	28	96	60	0.05	0.06	0.5	Tr
Cakes, commercial, made with enriched flour:																		
Pound:																		
Slice, 1/17 of loaf	29	24	110	2	5	3.2	64	15	Tr	8	0.5	26	108	41	0.06	0.06	0.5	0
Snack cakes:																		
Devil's food with creme filling (2 small cakes per pkg.) 1 small cake	28	20	105	1	4	0.9	15	17	Tr	21	1.0	34	105	4	0.06	0.09	0.7	0
Sponge with creme filling (2 small cakes per pkg.) 1 small cake	42	19	155	1	5	0.5	7	27	Tr	14	0.6	37	155	9	0.07	0.06	0.6	0
White with white frosting:																		
Piece, 1/16 of cake	71	24	260	3	9	2.8	3	42	1	33	1.0	52	176	12	0.20	0.13	1.7	0
Yellow with chocolate frosting:																		
Piece, 1/16 of cake	69	23	245	2	11	3.3	38	39	1	23	1.2	123	192	30	0.05	0.14	0.6	0
Cheesecake:																		
Piece, 1/12 of cake	92	46	280	5	18	10.6	170	26	2	52	0.4	90	204	69	0.03	0.12	0.4	5
Cookies made with enriched flour:																		
Brownies with nuts:																		
Commercial, with frosting, 1-1/2 by 1-3/4 by 7/8 in. 1 brownie	25	13	100	1	4	1.1	14	16	1	13	0.6	50	59	18	0.08	0.07	0.3	Tr
Chocolate chip:																		
Commercial, 2-1/4 in. diam., 3/8 in. thick 4 cookies	42	4	180	2	9	3.1	5	28	1	13	0.8	68	140	15	0.10	0.23	1.0	Tr
From refrigerated dough, 2-1/4 in. diam., 3/8 in. thick 4 cookies	48	5	225	2	11	3.2	22	32	1	13	1.0	62	173	8	0.06	0.10	0.9	0
Oatmeal with raisins, 2-5/8 in. diam., 1/4 in. thick 4 cookies	52	4	245	3	10	1.7	2	36	2	18	1.1	90	148	12	0.09	0.08	1.0	0
Peanut butter cookie, from home recipe, 2-5/8 in. diam.25 4 cookies	48	3	245	4	14	2.1	0	28	1	21	1.1	110	142	5	0.07	0.07	1.9	0
Sandwich type (chocolate or vanilla), 1-3/4 in. diam., 3/8 in. thick 4 cookies	40	2	195	2	8	1.7	0	29	1	12	1.4	66	189	0	0.09	0.07	0.8	0
Sugar cookie, from refrigerated dough, 2-1/2 in. diam., 1/4 in. thick 4 cookies	48	4	235	2	12	2.8	29	31	Tr	50	0.9	33	261	11	0.09	0.06	1.1	0
Vanilla wafers, 1-3/4 in. diam., 1/4 in. thick 10 cookies	40	4	185	2	7	1.4	25	29	8	16	0.8	50	150	14	0.07	0.10	1.0	0
Corn chips 1 oz. package	28	1	155	2	9	1.3	0	16	1	35	0.5	52	233	11	0.04	0.05	0.4	1
Cornmeal:																		
Degermed, enriched:																		
Dry form 1 cup	138	12	500	11	2	0.3	0	108	10	8	5.9	166	1	61	0.61	0.36	4.8	0
Cooked 1 cup	240	88	120	3	Tr	0.1	0	26	4	2	1.4	38	0	14	0.14	0.10	1.2	0
Crackers:39																		
Cheese:																		
Plain, 1 in. square 10 crackers	10	4	50	1	3	0.9	6	6	Tr	11	0.3	17	112	5	0.05	0.04	0.4	0
Sandwich type (peanut butter) 1 sandwich	8	3	40	1	2	0.4	1	5	Tr	7	0.3	17	90	Tr	0.04	0.03	0.6	0
Graham, plain, 2-1/2 in. square 2 crackers	14	5	60	1	1	0.4	0	11	Tr	6	0.4	36	86	0	0.02	0.03	0.6	0
Saltines40 4 crackers	12	4	50	1	1	0.3	4	9	Tr	3	0.5	17	165	0	0.06	0.05	0.6	0
Snack-type, standard 1 round cracker	3	3	15	Tr	1	0.1	0	2	Tr	3	0.1	4	30	Tr	0.01	0.01	0.1	0
Wheat, thin 4 crackers	8	3	35	1	1	0.7	0	5	1	3	0.3	17	69	Tr	0.04	0.03	0.4	0
Croissants, made with enriched flour, 4-1/2 by 4 by 1-3/4 in. 1 croissant	57	22	235	5	12	6.7	13	27	1	20	2.1	68	452	13	0.17	0.13	1.3	0
Danish pastry, made with enriched flour:																		
Plain without fruit or nuts:																		
Round piece, about 4-1/4 in. diam., 1 in. high 1 pastry	57	27	220	4	12	2.3	49	26	Tr	60	1.1	53	218	17	0.16	0.17	1.4	Tr
Fruit, round piece 1 pastry	65	30	235	4	13	2.3	56	28	0	17	1.3	57	233	11	0.16	0.14	1.4	Tr
Doughnuts, made with enriched flour:																		
Cake type, plain, 3-1/4 in. diam., 1 in. high 1 doughnut	50	21	210	3	12	1.9	20	24	1	22	1.0	58	192	5	0.12	0.12	1.1	Tr
Yeast-leavened, glazed, 3-3/4 in. diam., 1-1/4 in. high 1 doughnut	60	27	235	4	13	3.5	21	26	1	17	1.4	64	222	Tr	0.28	0.12	1.8	0

(A)	(B)	(C)	(D)	(E)	(F)	(G)	(H)	(I)	(J)	(K)	(L)	(M)	(N)	(O)	(P)	(Q)	(R)	(S)
English muffins, plain, enriched	1 muffin	57	42	140	5	1	0.1	0	27	2	96	1.7	331	378	0	0.26	0.19	2.2	0
French toast, from home recipe	1 slice	65	53	155	6	7	2.0	112	17	Tr	72	1.3	86	257	32	0.12	0.16	1.0	Tr
Macaroni, enriched, cooked (cut lengths, elbows, shells):																		
Firm stage (hot)	1 cup	130	64	190	7	1	0.1	0	39	2	14	2.1	103	1	0	0.23	0.13	1.8	0
Muffins made with enriched flour, 2-1/2 in. diam., 1-1/2 in. high:																		
From home recipe:																		
Blueberry[25]	1 muffin	45	37	135	3	5	1.1	19	20	7	54	0.9	47	198	9	0.10	0.11	0.9	1
Bran[36]	1 muffin	45	35	125	3	6	1.2	24	19	3	60	1.4	99	189	30	0.11	0.13	1.3	3
From commercial mix (egg and water added):																		
Blueberry	1 muffin	45	33	140	3	5	0.7	45	22	1	15	0.9	54	225	11	0.10	0.17	1.1	Tr
Bran	1 muffin	45	28	140	3	4	1.1	28	24	4	27	1.7	50	385	14	0.08	0.12	1.9	0
Corn	1 muffin	45	30	145	3	6	1.3	42	22	2	30	1.3	31	291	16	0.09	0.09	0.8	Tr
Noodles (egg noodles), enriched, cooked	1 cup	160	70	200	7	2	0.5	50	37	2	16	2.6	70	3	34	0.22	0.13	1.9	0
Noodles, chow mein, canned	1 cup	45	11	220	6	11	2.0	5	26	2	14	0.4	33	450	0	0.05	0.03	0.6	0
Pancakes, 4 in. diam.:																		
Buckwheat, from mix (with buckwheat and enriched flours), egg and milk added	1 pancake	27	58	55	2	2	0.5	20	6	1	59	0.4	66	125	17	0.04	0.05	0.2	Tr
Plain:																		
From mix (with enriched flour), egg, milk, and oil added	1 pancake	27	54	60	2	2	0.1	16	8	Tr	36	0.7	43	160	7	0.09	0.12	0.8	Tr
Piecrust, made with enriched flour and vegetable shortening, baked:																		
From home recipe, 9 in. diam.	1 pie shell	180	15	900	11	60	15.5	0	79	3	25	4.5	90	1,100	0	0.54	0.40	5.0	0
From mix, 9 in. diam.	Piecrust for 2-crust pie	320	19	1,485	20	93	27.6	0	141	6	131	9.3	179	2,602	0	1.06	0.80	9.9	0
Pies, piecrust made with enriched flour, vegetable shortening, 9 in. diam.:																		
Apple:																		
Piece, 1/6 of pie	1 piece	158	48	405	3	18	3.3	0	60	3	13	1.6	126	476	5	0.17	0.13	1.6	2
Blueberry:																		
Piece, 1/6 of pie	1 piece	158	51	380	4	17	4.6	0	55	2	17	2.1	158	423	14	0.17	0.14	1.7	6
Cherry:																		
Piece, 1/6 of pie	1 piece	158	47	410	4	18	4.7	0	61	2	22	1.6	166	480	70	0.19	0.14	1.6	0
Creme:																		
Piece, 1/6 of pie	1 piece	152	43	455	3	23	7.4	8	59	0	46	1.1	133	369	65	0.06	0.15	1.1	0
Custard:																		
Piece, 1/6 of pie	1 piece	152	58	330	9	17	4.2	169	36	2	146	1.5	208	436	96	0.14	0.32	0.9	0
Lemon meringue:																		
Piece, 1/6 of pie	1 piece	140	47	355	5	14	2.2	143	53	2	20	1.4	70	395	66	0.10	0.14	0.8	4
Peach:																		
Piece, 1/6 of pie	1 piece	158	48	405	4	17	4.4	0	60	2	16	1.9	235	423	115	0.17	0.16	2.4	5
Pecan:																		
Piece, 1/6 of pie	1 piece	138	20	575	7	32	5.2	95	71	5	65	4.6	170	305	54	0.30	0.17	1.1	0
Pumpkin:																		
Piece, 1/6 of pie	1 piece	152	59	320	6	17	4.2	109	37	6	78	1.4	243	325	416	0.14	0.21	1.2	0
Pies, fried:																		
Apple	1 pie	85	43	255	2	14	6.5	14	31	2	12	0.9	42	326	3	0.09	0.06	1.0	1
Cherry	1 pie	85	42	250	2	14	2.0	13	32	2	11	0.7	61	371	19	0.06	0.06	0.6	1
Popcorn, popped:																		
Air-popped, unsalted	1 cup	8	4	30	1	Tr	Tr	0	6	1	1	0.2	20	Tr	1	0.03	0.01	0.2	0
Popped in vegetable oil, salted	1 cup	11	3	55	1	3	0.5	0	6	1	3	0.3	19	86	2	0.01	0.02	0.1	0
Sugar syrup coated	1 cup	35	4	135	2	1	1.3	0	30	2	2	0.5	90	Tr	3	0.13	0.02	0.4	0
Pretzels, made with enriched flour:																		
Twisted, dutch, 2-3/4 by 2-5/8 in.	1 pretzel	16	3	65	2	1	0.1	0	13	Tr	4	0.3	16	258	0	0.05	0.04	0.7	0
Twisted, thin, 3-1/4 by 2-1/4 by 1/4 in.	10 pretzels	60	3	240	6	2	0.4	0	48	2	16	1.2	61	966	0	0.19	0.15	2.6	0
Rice:																		
Brown, cooked, served hot	1 cup	195	70	230	5	1	0.4	0	50	4	23	1.0	137	0	0	0.18	0.04	2.7	0
White, enriched:																		
Commercial varieties, all types:																		
Cooked, served hot	1 cup	205	73	225	4	Tr	0.2	0	50	1	21	1.8	57	0	0	0.23	0.02	2.1	0
Instant, ready-to-serve, hot	1 cup	165	73	180	4	0	0.1	0	40	1	5	1.3	0	0	0	0.21	0.02	1.7	0

Nutritive Value of Foods – Continued
(Tr indicates nutrient present in trace amount.)

Nutrients in Indicated Quantity

Item No. — Foods, approximate measures, units, and weight (weight of edible portion only) (A)	(B)	Grams	Water (C) Percent	Food energy (D) Calories	Protein (E) Grams	Fat (F) Grams	Saturated fat (G) Grams	Cholesterol (H) Milligrams	Carbohydrate (I) Grams	Dietary fiber (J) Grams	Calcium (K) Milligrams	Iron (L) Milligrams	Potassium (M) Milligrams	Sodium (N) Milligrams	Vitamin A (O) Micrograms	Thiamin (P) Milligrams	Riboflavin (Q) Milligrams	Niacin (R) Milligrams	Vitamin C (S) Milligrams
Rolls, enriched:																			
Commercial:																			
Dinner, 2-1/2 in. diam., 2 in. high	1 roll	28	32	85	2	2	0.7	Tr	14	1	33	0.8	36	155	Tr	0.14	0.09	1.1	Tr
Frankfurter and hamburger (8 per 11-1/2 oz. pkg.)	1 roll	40	34	115	3	2	0.5	Tr	20	1	54	1.2	56	241	Tr	0.20	0.13	1.6	Tr
Hard, 3-3/4 in. diam., 2 in. high	1 roll	50	25	155	5	2	0.3	Tr	30	1	24	1.4	49	313	0	0.20	0.12	1.7	0
Hoagie or submarine, 11-1/2 by 3 by 2-1/2 in.	1 roll	135	31	400	11	8	0.9	Tr	72	4	100	3.8	128	683	0	0.54	0.33	4.5	0
Spaghetti, enriched, cooked:																			
Firm stage, "al dente," served hot	1 cup	130	64	190	7	1	0.1	0	39	2	14	2.0	103	1	0	0.23	0.13	1.8	0
Toaster pastries	1 pastry	54	13	210	2	6	0.8	0	38	1	104	2.2	91	248	52	0.17	0.18	2.3	4
Tortillas, corn	1 tortilla	30	45	65	2	1	0.1	0	13	2	42	0.6	43	1	8	0.05	0.03	0.4	0
Waffles, made with enriched flour, 7 in. diam.:																			
From mix, egg and milk added	1 waffle	75	42	205	7	8	1.7	59	27	1	179	1.2	146	515	49	0.14	0.23	0.9	Tr
Wheat flours:																			
All-purpose or family flour, enriched:																			
Sifted, spooned	1 cup	115	12	420	12	1	0.2	0	88	3	18	5.1	109	2	0	0.73	0.46	6.1	0
Cake or pastry flour, enriched, sifted, spooned	1 cup	96	12	350	7	1	0.1	0	76	2	16	4.2	91	2	0	0.58	0.38	5.1	0
Self-rising, enriched, unsifted, spooned	1 cup	125	12	440	12	1	0.2	0	93	3	331	5.5	113	1,349	0	0.80	0.50	6.6	0
Whole-wheat, from hard wheats, stirred	1 cup	120	12	400	16	2	0.4	0	85	15	49	5.2	444	4	0	0.66	0.14	5.2	0
Legumes, Nuts, and Seeds																			
Almonds, shelled:																			
Slivered, packed	1 cup	135	4	795	27	70	6.7	0	28	13	359	4.9	988	15	0	0.28	1.05	4.5	1
Beans, dry:																			
Cooked, drained:																			
Lima	1 cup	190	64	260	16	1	0.2	0	49	14	55	5.9	1,163	4	0	0.25	0.11	1.3	0
Canned, solids and liquid:																			
White with:																			
Pork and tomato sauce	1 cup	255	71	310	16	7	1	10	48	12	138	4.6	536	1,181	33	0.20	0.08	1.5	5
Red kidney	1 cup	255	76	230	15	1	Tr	0	42	5	74	4.6	673	968	1	0.13	0.10	1.5	0
Black-eyed peas, dry, cooked (with residual cooking liquid)	1 cup	250	80	190	13	1	0.2	0	35	12	43	3.3	573	20	3	0.40	0.10	1.0	0
Brazil nuts, shelled	1 oz.	28	3	185	4	19	4.6	0	4	2	50	1.0	170	1	Tr	0.28	0.03	0.5	Tr
Carob flour	1 cup	140	3	255	6	Tr	0.1	0	126	41	390	5.7	1,275	24	Tr	0.07	0.07	2.2	Tr
Cashew nuts, salted:																			
Dry roasted	1 cup	137	2	785	21	63	12.5	0	45	4	62	8.2	774	877[41]	0	0.27	0.27	1.9	0
Roasted in oil	1 cup	130	4	750	21	63	12.4	0	37	4	53	5.3	689	814[42]	0	0.55	0.23	2.3	0
Chestnuts, European (Italian), roasted, shelled	1 cup	143	40	350	5	3	0.6	0	76	9	41	1.3	847	3	3	0.35	0.25	1.9	37
Chick-peas, cooked, drained	1 cup	163	60	270	15	4	0.4	0	45	8	80	4.9	475	11	Tr	0.18	0.09	0.9	0
Coconut:																			
Dried, sweetened, shredded	1 cup	93	13	470	3	33	29.3	0	44	13	14	1.8	313	244	0	0.03	0.02	0.4	1
Filberts (hazelnuts), chopped	1 cup	115	5	725	15	72	5.3	0	18	9	216	3.8	512	3	8	0.58	0.13	1.3	1
	1 oz.	28	5	180	4	18	1.3	0	4	2	53	0.9	126	1	2	0.14	0.03	0.3	Tr
Lentils, dry, cooked	1 cup	200	72	215	16	1	0.1	0	38	5	50	4.2	498	26	4	0.14	0.12	1.2	Tr
Macadamia nuts, roasted in oil, salted	1 cup	134	2	960	10	103	15.3	0	17	12	60	2.4	441	348[43]	1	0.29	0.15	2.7	0
Mixed nuts, with peanuts, salted:																			
Dry roasted	1 oz.	28	2	170	5	15	3.1	0	7	3	20	1.0	169	190[44]	Tr	0.06	0.06	1.3	0
Roasted in oil	1 oz.	28	2	175	5	16	4.0	0	6	3	31	0.9	165	185[44]	1	0.14	0.06	1.4	0
Peanuts, roasted in oil, salted	1 cup	145	2	840	39	71	9.8	0	27	10	125	2.8	1,019	626[45]	0	0.42	0.15	21.5	0
Peanut butter	1 tbsp.	16	1	95	5	8	1.5	0	3	1	5	0.3	110	75	0	0.02	0.02	2.2	0
Peas, split, dry, cooked	1 cup	200	70	230	16	1	0.2	0	42	6	22	3.4	592	26	8	0.30	0.18	1.8	0
Pecans, halves	1 cup	108	5	720	8	73	5.8	0	20	5	39	2.3	423	1	14	0.92	0.14	1.0	2
	1 oz.	28	4	190	2	19	1.5	0	5	1	10	0.6	111	Tr	4	0.24	0.04	0.3	1
Pistachio nuts, dried, shelled	1 oz.	28	4	165	6	14	1.7	0	7	3	38	1.9	310	2	7	0.23	0.05	0.3	Tr

(A)	(B)	(C)	(D)	(E)	(F)	(G)	(H)	(I)	(J)	(K)	(L)	(M)	(N)	(O)	(P)	(Q)	(R)	(S)
Refried beans, canned	1 cup	290	72	295	18	3	1.0	0	51	14	141	5.1	1,141	1,228	0	0.14	0.16	1.4	17
Sesame seeds, dry, hulled	1 tbsp.	8	5	45	2	4	2.9	0	1	3	11	0.6	33	3	1	0.06	0.01	0.4	0
Soy products:																		
Tofu, piece 2-1/2 by 2-3/4 by 1 in.	1 piece	120	85	85	9	5	0.9	0	3	1	108	2.3	50	8	0	0.07	0.04	0.1	0
Sunflower seeds, dry, hulled	1 oz.	28	5	160	6	14	1.9	0	5	2	33	1.9	195	1	1	0.65	0.07	1.3	Tr
Walnuts:																		
Black, chopped	1 cup	125	4	760	30	71	4.5	0	15	6	73	3.8	655	1	37	0.27	0.14	0.9	Tr
English or Persian, pieces or chips	1 cup	120	4	770	17	74	6.7	0	22	5	113	2.9	602	12	15	0.46	0.18	1.3	4
Meat and Meat Products																		
Beef, cooked:[46]																		
Cuts braised, simmered, or pot roasted:																		
Relatively fat such as chuck blade:																		
Lean and fat, piece, 2-1/2 by 2-1/2 by 3/4 in.	3 oz.	85	43	325	22	26	11.6	87	0	0	11	2.5	163	53	Tr	0.06	0.19	2.0	0
Relatively lean, such as bottom round:																		
Lean and fat, piece, 4-1/8 by 2-1/4 by 1/2 in.	3 oz.	85	54	220	25	13	3.6	81	0	0	5	2.8	248	43	Tr	0.06	0.21	3.3	0
Ground beef, broiled, patty, 3 by 5/8 in.:																		
Lean	3 oz.	85	56	230	21	16	7.0	74	0	0	9	1.8	256	65	Tr	0.04	0.18	4.4	0
Regular	3 oz.	85	54	245	20	18	7.9	76	0	0	9	2.1	248	70	Tr	0.03	0.16	4.9	0
Liver, fried, slice, 6-1/2 by 2-3/8 by 3/8 in.[47]	3 oz.	85	56	185	23	7	3.0	410	7	0	9	5.3	309	90	[48]g,120	0.18	3.52	12.3	23
Roast, oven cooked, no liquid added:																		
Relatively fat, such as rib:																		
Lean and fat, 2 pieces, 4-1/8 by 2-1/4 by 1/4 in.	3 oz.	85	46	315	19	26	14.3	72	0	0	8	2.0	246	54	Tr	0.06	0.16	3.1	0
Relatively lean, such as eye of round:																		
Lean and fat, 2 pieces, 2-1/2 by 2-1/2 by 3/8 in.	3 oz.	85	57	205	23	12	6.2	62	0	0	5	1.6	308	50	Tr	0.07	0.14	3.0	0
Steak:																		
Sirloin, broiled:																		
Lean and fat, piece, 2-1/2 by 2-1/2 by 3/4 in.	3 oz.	85	53	240	23	15	8.7	77	0	0	9	2.6	306	53	Tr	0.10	0.23	3.3	0
Beef, canned, corned	3 oz.	85	59	185	22	10	7.0	80	0	0	17	3.7	51	802	Tr	0.02	0.20	2.9	0
Beef, dried, chipped	2.5 oz.	72	48	145	24	4	0.5	46	0	0	14	2.3	142	3,053	Tr	0.05	0.23	2.7	0
Lamb, cooked:																		
Chops, (3 per lb. with bone):																		
Lean and fat	2.2 oz.	63	44	220	20	15	3.5	77	0	0	16	1.5	195	46	Tr	0.04	0.16	4.4	0
Leg, roasted:																		
Lean and fat, 2 pieces, 4-1/8 by 2-1/4 by 1/4 in.	3 oz.	85	59	205	22	13	7.8	78	0	0	8	1.7	273	57	Tr	0.09	0.24	5.5	0
Rib, roasted:																		
Lean and fat, 3 pieces, 2-1/2 by 2-1/2 by 1/4 in.	3 oz.	85	47	315	18	26	14.5	77	0	0	19	1.4	224	60	Tr	0.08	0.18	5.5	0
Pork, cured, cooked:																		
Bacon:																		
Regular	3 medium slices	19	13	110	6	9	3.3	16	Tr	0	2	0.3	92	303	0	0.13	0.05	1.4	6
Canadian-style	2 slices	46	62	85	11	4	1.3	27	1	0	5	0.4	179	711	0	0.38	0.09	3.2	10
Ham, light cure, roasted:																		
Lean and fat, 2 pieces, 4-1/8 by 2-1/4 by 1/4 in.	3 oz.	85	58	205	18	14	6.8	53	0	0	6	0.7	243	1,009	0	0.51	0.19	3.8	0
Ham, canned, roasted, 2 pieces, 4-1/8 by 2-1/4 by 1/4 in.	3 oz.	85	67	140	18	7	3.2	35	Tr	0	6	0.9	298	908	0	0.82	0.21	4.3	[49]19
Luncheon meat:																		
Canned, spiced or unspiced, slice, 3 by 2 by 1/2 in.	2 slices	42	52	140	5	13	4.6	26	1	0	3	0.3	90	541	0	0.15	0.08	1.3	Tr
Cooked ham (8 slices per 8 oz. pkg.):																		
Regular	2 slices	57	65	105	10	6	1.9	32	2	0	4	0.6	189	751	0	0.49	0.14	3.0	[49]16
Extra lean	2 slices	57	71	75	11	3	0.9	27	1	0	4	0.4	200	815	0	0.53	0.13	2.8	[49]15
Pork, fresh, cooked:																		
Chop, loin (cut 3 per lb. with bone):																		
Broiled:																		
Lean and fat	3.1 oz.	87	50	275	24	19	4.6	84	0	0	3	0.7	312	61	3	0.87	0.24	4.3	Tr
Ham (leg), roasted:																		
Lean and fat, piece, 2-1/2 by 2-1/2 by 3/4 in.	3 oz	85	53	250	21	18	0.7	79	0	0	5	0.9	280	50	2	0.54	0.27	3.9	Tr
Rib, roasted:																		
Lean and fat, piece, 2-1/2 by 3/4 in.	3 oz.	85	51	270	21	20	6.7	69	0	0	9	0.8	313	37	3	0.50	0.24	4.2	Tr
Shoulder cut, braised:																		
Lean and fat, 3 pieces, 2-1/2 by 2-1/2 by 1/4 in.	3 oz.	85	47	295	23	22	9.6	93	0	0	6	1.4	286	75	3	0.46	0.26	4.4	Tr
Sausages																		
Bologna, slice (8 per 8 oz. pkg.)	2 slices	57	54	180	7	16	3.2	31	2	0	7	0.9	103	581	0	0.10	0.08	1.5	[49]12
Braunschweiger, slice (6 per 6 oz. pkg.)	2 slices	57	48	205	8	18	3.1	89	2	0	5	5.3	113	652	2,405	0.14	0.87	4.8	[49]6

Nutritive Value of Foods – Continued
(Tr indicates nutrient present in trace amount.)

Nutrients in Indicated Quantity

Item No. / Foods, approximate measures, units, and weight (weight of edible portion only) (A)	(B)	Grams	Water Percent (C)	Food energy Calories (D)	Protein Grams (E)	Fat Grams (F)	Saturated fat Grams (G)	Cholesterol Milligrams (H)	Carbohydrate Grams (I)	Dietary fiber Grams (J)	Calcium Milligrams (K)	Iron Milligrams (L)	Potassium Milligrams (M)	Sodium Milligrams (N)	Vitamin A Micrograms (O)	Thiamin Milligrams (P)	Riboflavin Milligrams (Q)	Niacin Milligrams (R)	Vitamin C Milligrams (S)
Brown and serve (10-11 per 8 oz. pkg.), browned	1 link	13	45	50	2	5	1.7	Tr	Tr	0	1	0.1	25	105	0	0.05	0.02	0.4	0
Frankfurter (10 per 1 lb. pkg.), cooked (reheated)	1 frankfurter	45	54	145	5	13	4.9	23	1	0	5	0.5	75	504	0	0.09	0.05	1.2	49[12]
Salami:																			
Dry type, slice (12 per 4 oz. pkg.)	2 slices	20	35	85	5	7	2.5	16	1	0	2	0.3	76	372	0	0.12	0.06	1.0	495
Sandwich spread (pork, beef)	1 tbsp.	15	60	35	1	3	0.9	6	2	Tr	2	0.1	17	152	1	0.03	0.02	0.3	0
Veal, medium fat, cooked, bone removed:																			
Cutlet, 4-1/8 by 2-1/4 by 1/2 in., braised or broiled	3 oz.	85	60	185	23	9	7.6	109	0	0	9	0.8	258	56	Tr	0.06	0.21	4.6	0
Rib, 2 pieces, 4-1/8 by 2-1/4 by 1/4 in., roasted	3 oz.	85	55	230	23	14	6.1	109	0	0	10	0.7	259	57	Tr	0.11	0.26	6.6	0

Mixed Dishes and Fast Foods

Item No. / Foods (A)	(B)	Grams	Water Percent (C)	Food energy Calories (D)	Protein Grams (E)	Fat Grams (F)	Saturated fat Grams (G)	Cholesterol Milligrams (H)	Carbohydrate Grams (I)	Dietary fiber Grams (J)	Calcium Milligrams (K)	Iron Milligrams (L)	Potassium Milligrams (M)	Sodium Milligrams (N)	Vitamin A Micrograms (O)	Thiamin Milligrams (P)	Riboflavin Milligrams (Q)	Niacin Milligrams (R)	Vitamin C Milligrams (S)
Mixed dishes:																			
Beef and vegetable stew, from home recipe	1 cup	245	82	220	16	11	4.9	71	15	2	29	2.9	613	292	568	0.15	0.17	4.7	17
Beef potpie, from home recipe, baked, piece, 1/3 of 9 in. diam. pie[51]	1 piece	210	55	515	21	30	8.4	42	39	3	29	3.8	334	596	517	0.29	0.29	4.8	6
Chicken a la king, cooked, from home recipe	1 cup	245	68	470	27	34	12.7	221	12	1	127	2.5	404	760	272	0.10	0.42	5.4	12
Chicken chow mein:																			
Canned	1 cup	250	89	95	7	Tr	0.0	8	18	2	45	1.3	418	725	28	0.05	0.10	1.0	13
From home recipe	1 cup	255	72	340	19	16	3.4	28	31	4	82	4.3	594	1,354	15	0.08	0.18	3.3	8
Chop suey with beef and pork, from home recipe	1 cup	250	75	300	26	17	5.7	68	13	4	60	4.8	425	1,053	60	0.28	0.38	5.0	33
Macaroni (enriched) and cheese:																			
Canned[52]	1 cup	240	80	230	9	10	4.2	24	26	1	199	1.0	139	730	72	0.12	0.24	1.0	Tr
From home recipe[38]	1 cup	200	58	430	17	22	8.9	44	40	1	362	1.8	240	1,086	232	0.20	0.40	1.8	1
Spaghetti (enriched) in tomato sauce with cheese:																			
Canned	1 cup	250	80	190	6	2	0.0	3	39	2	40	2.8	303	955	120	0.35	0.28	4.5	10
From home recipe	1 cup	250	77	260	9	9	2.0	8	37	2	80	2.3	408	955	140	0.25	0.18	2.3	13
Spaghetti (enriched) with meatballs and tomato sauce:																			
Canned	1 cup	250	78	260	12	10	2.1	23	29	6	53	3.3	245	1,220	100	0.15	0.18	2.3	5
From home recipe	1 cup	248	70	330	19	12	3.3	89	39	8	124	3.7	665	1,009	159	0.25	0.30	4.0	22
Fast food entrees:																			
Cheeseburger:																			
Regular	1 sandwich	112	46	300	15	15	6.7	44	28	0	135	2.3	219	672	65	0.26	0.24	3.7	1
4 oz. patty	1 sandwich	194	46	525	30	31	10.2	104	40	0	236	4.5	407	1,224	128	0.33	0.48	7.4	3
Chicken, fried. See Poultry and Poultry Products.																			
Enchilada	1 enchilada	230	72	235	20	16	15.0	19	24	0	322	11.0	2,180	4,451	352	0.18	0.26	Tr	Tr
English muffin, egg, cheese, and bacon	1 sandwich	138	49	360	18	18	8.6	213	31	1	197	3.1	201	832	160	0.46	0.50	3.7	1
Fish sandwich:																			
Regular, with cheese	1 sandwich	140	43	420	16	23	6.2	56	39	Tr	132	1.8	274	667	25	0.32	0.26	3.3	2
Large, without cheese	1 sandwich	170	48	470	18	27	5.6	91	41	Tr	61	2.2	375	621	15	0.35	0.23	3.5	1
Hamburger:																			
Regular	1 sandwich	98	46	245	12	11	3.2	32	28	0	56	2.2	202	463	14	0.23	0.24	3.8	1
4 oz. patty	1 sandwich	174	50	445	25	21	9.7	71	38	0	75	4.8	404	763	28	0.38	0.38	7.8	1
Pizza, cheese, 1/8 of 15 in. diam. pizza[51]	1 slice	120	46	290	15	9	2.9	56	39	2	220	1.6	230	699	106	0.34	0.29	4.2	2
Taco	1 taco	81	55	195	9	11	4.6	21	15	1	109	1.2	263	456	57	0.09	0.07	1.4	1

Poultry and Poultry Products

Item No. / Foods (A)	(B)	Grams	Water Percent (C)	Food energy Calories (D)	Protein Grams (E)	Fat Grams (F)	Saturated fat Grams (G)	Cholesterol Milligrams (H)	Carbohydrate Grams (I)	Dietary fiber Grams (J)	Calcium Milligrams (K)	Iron Milligrams (L)	Potassium Milligrams (M)	Sodium Milligrams (N)	Vitamin A Micrograms (O)	Thiamin Milligrams (P)	Riboflavin Milligrams (Q)	Niacin Milligrams (R)	Vitamin C Milligrams (S)
Chicken:																			
Fried, flesh, with skin:[53]																			
Batter dipped:																			
Breast, 1/2 breast (5.6 oz. with bones)	4.9 oz.	140	52	365	35	18	4.9	119	13	Tr	28	1.8	281	385	28	0.16	0.20	14.7	0

(A)	(B)	(C)	(D)	(E)	(F)	(G)	(H)	(I)	(J)	(K)	(L)	(M)	(N)	(O)	(P)	(Q)	(R)	(S)
Drumstick (3.4 oz. with bones)	2.5 oz.	53	195	16	11	3.0	62	6	Tr	12	1.0	134	194	19	0.08	0.15	3.7	0
Roasted, flesh only:																		
Breast, 1/2 breast (4.2 oz. with bones and skin)	3.0 oz.	65	140	27	3	0.9	73	0	0	13	0.9	220	64	5	0.06	0.10	11.8	0
Drumstick, (2.9 oz. with bones and skin)	1.6 oz.	67	75	12	2	1.4	41	0	0	5	0.6	108	42	8	0.03	0.10	2.7	0
Chicken liver, cooked	1 liver	68	30	5	1	1.6	126	Tr	0	3	1.7	28	10	983	0.03	0.35	0.9	3
Duck, roasted, flesh only	1/2 duck	64	445	52	25	9.2	197	0	0	27	6.0	557	144	51	0.57	1.04	11.3	0
Turkey, roasted, flesh only:																		
Dark meat, piece, 2-1/2 by 1-5/8 by 1/4 in.	4 pieces	63	160	24	6	4.0	72	0	0	27	2.0	246	67	0	0.05	0.21	3.1	0
Light meat, piece, 4 by 2 by 1/4 in.	2 pieces	66	135	25	3	2.7	59	0	0	16	1.1	259	54	0	0.05	0.11	5.8	0
Poultry food products:																		
Chicken:																		
Canned, boneless	5 oz.	69	235	31	11	3.1	88	0	0	20	2.2	196	714	48	0.02	0.18	9.0	3
Frankfurter (10 per 1-lb. pkg.)	1 frankfurter	58	115	6	9	2.5	45	3	0	43	0.9	38	616	17	0.03	0.05	1.4	0
Roll, light (6 slices per 6 oz. pkg.)	2 slices	69	90	11	4	1.1	28	1	0	24	0.6	129	331	14	0.04	0.07	3.0	0
Turkey:																		
Gravy and turkey, frozen	5 oz. package	85	95	8	4	1.0	26	7	Tr	20	1.3	87	787	18	0.03	0.18	2.6	0
Loaf, breast meat (8 slices per 6 oz. pkg.)	2 slices	72	45	10	1	0.5	17	0	0	3	0.2	118	608	0	0.02	0.05	3.5	54
Patties, breaded, battered, fried (2.25 oz.)	1 patty	50	180	9	12	2.7	40	10	Tr	9	1.4	176	512	7	0.06	0.12	1.5	0
Roast, boneless, frozen, seasoned, light and dark meat, cooked	3 oz.	68	130	18	5	2.2	45	3	0	4	1.4	253	578	0	0.04	0.14	5.3	0

Soups, Sauces, and Gravies

(A)	(B)	(C)	(D)	(E)	(F)	(G)	(H)	(I)	(J)	(K)	(L)	(M)	(N)	(O)	(P)	(Q)	(R)	(S)
Soups:																		
Canned, condensed:																		
Prepared with equal volume of milk:																		
Clam chowder, New England	1 cup	85	165	9	7	2.9	22	17	1	186	1.5	300	992	40	0.07	0.24	1.0	3
Cream of chicken	1 cup	85	190	7	11	4.6	27	15	Tr	181	0.7	273	1,047	94	0.07	0.26	0.9	1
Cream of mushroom	1 cup	85	205	6	14	5.1	20	15	1	179	0.6	270	1,076	37	0.08	0.28	0.9	2
Tomato	1 cup	85	160	6	6	2.9	17	22	1	159	1.8	449	932	109	0.13	0.25	1.5	68
Prepared with equal volume of water:																		
Bean with bacon	1 cup	84	170	8	6	1.5	3	23	9	81	2.0	402	951	89	0.09	0.03	0.6	2
Beef broth, bouillon, consommé	1 cup	98	15	3	1	0.3	Tr	Tr	0	14	0.4	130	782	0	Tr	0.05	1.9	0
Beef noodle	1 cup	92	85	5	3	1.1	5	9	1	15	1.1	100	952	63	0.07	0.06	1.1	Tr
Chicken noodle	1 cup	92	75	4	2	0.7	7	9	Tr	17	0.8	55	1,106	71	0.05	0.06	1.4	Tr
Chicken rice	1 cup	94	60	4	2	0.5	7	7	1	17	0.7	101	815	66	0.02	0.02	1.1	Tr
Clam chowder, Manhattan	1 cup	90	80	4	2	0.4	2	12	1	34	1.9	261	1,808	92	0.06	0.05	1.3	3
Pea, green	1 cup	83	165	9	3	1.8	0	27	5	28	2.0	190	988	20	0.11	0.07	1.2	2
Vegetable beef	1 cup	92	80	6	2	0.9	5	10	Tr	17	1.1	173	956	189	0.04	0.05	1.0	2
Vegetarian	1 cup	92	70	2	2	0.3	0	12	Tr	22	1.1	210	822	301	0.05	0.05	0.9	1
Dehydrated:																		
Prepared with water:																		
Chicken noodle	1 pkt. (6 fl. oz.)	94	40	2	1	0.3	2	6	Tr	24	0.4	23	957	5	0.05	0.04	0.7	Tr
Tomato vegetable	1 pkt. (6 fl. oz.)	94	40	1	1	0.4	0	8	1	6	0.5	78	856	14	0.04	0.03	0.6	5
Sauces:																		
From dry mix:																		
Cheese, prepared with milk	1 cup	77	305	16	17	9.3	53	23	1	569	0.3	552	1,565	117	0.15	0.56	0.3	2
From home recipe:																		
White sauce, medium[55]	1 cup	73	395	10	30	6.4	32	24	Tr	292	0.9	381	888	340	0.15	0.43	0.8	2
Ready to serve:																		
Barbecue	1 tbsp.	81	10	Tr	Tr	Tr	0	2	Tr	3	0.1	28	130	14	Tr	Tr	0.1	1
Soy	1 tbsp.	68	10	2	0	Tr	0	2	0	3	0.5	64	1,029	0	0.01	0.02	0.6	0
Gravies:																		
Canned:																		
Beef	1 cup	87	125	9	5	2.7	7	11	1	14	1.6	189	117	0	0.07	0.08	1.5	0
Chicken	1 cup	85	190	5	14	3.4	5	13	Tr	48	1.1	259	1,373	264	0.04	0.10	1.1	0
Mushroom	1 cup	89	120	3	6	0.8	0	13	Tr	17	1.6	252	1,357	0	0.08	0.15	1.6	0
From dry mix:																		
Brown	1 cup	91	80	3	2	0.8	2	14	Tr	66	0.2	61	1,147	0	0.04	0.09	0.9	0
Chicken	1 cup	91	85	3	2	0.5	3	14	Tr	39	0.3	62	1,134	0	0.05	0.15	0.8	3

Sugars and Sweets

(A)	(B)	(C)	(D)	(E)	(F)	(G)	(H)	(I)	(J)	(K)	(L)	(M)	(N)	(O)	(P)	(Q)	(R)	(S)
Candy:																		
Caramels, plain or chocolate	1 oz.	8	115	1	3	3	1.9	22	Tr	42	0.4	54	64	Tr	0.01	0.05	0.1	Tr

Nutritive Value of Foods – Continued
(Tr indicates nutrient present in trace amount.)

Item No. (A)	Foods, approximate measures, units, and weight (weight of edible portion only) (B)	Weight Grams	Water (C) Percent	Food energy (D) Calories	Protein (E) Grams	Fat (F) Grams	Saturated fat (G) Grams	Cholesterol (H) mg	Carbohydrate (I) Grams	Dietary fiber (J) Grams	Calcium (K) mg	Iron (L) mg	Potassium (M) mg	Sodium (N) mg	Vitamin A (O) mcg	Thiamin (P) mg	Riboflavin (Q) mg	Niacin (R) mg	Vitamin C (S) mg
	Chocolate:																		
	Milk, plain	28	1	145	2	9	5.2	6	16	1	50	0.4	96	23	10	0.02	0.10	0.1	Tr
	Milk, with almonds	28	2	150	3	10	4.8	5	15	2	65	0.5	125	23	8	0.02	0.12	0.2	Tr
	Milk, with peanuts	28	1	155	4	11	3.4	5	13	2	49	0.4	138	19	8	0.07	0.07	1.4	Tr
	Milk, with rice cereal	28	2	140	2	7	4.5	6	18	1	48	0.2	100	46	8	0.01	0.08	0.1	Tr
	Semisweet, small pieces (60 per oz.)	170	1	860	7	61	29.8	0	97	10	51	5.8	593	24	3	0.10	0.14	0.9	Tr
	Sweet (dark)	28	1	150	1	10	5.9	1	16	2	7	0.6	86	5	Tr	0.01	0.04	0.1	Tr
	Fudge, chocolate, plain	28	8	115	Tr	3	1.5	1	21	Tr	22	0.3	42	54	Tr	0.01	0.03	0.1	Tr
	Gum drops	28	12	100	Tr	Tr	0.0	0	25	0	2	0.1	1	10	0	0.00	Tr	Tr	0
	Hard	28	1	110	0	Tr	0.0	0	28	0	Tr	0.1	1	7	0	0.00	0.00	0.0	0
	Jelly beans	28	6	105	Tr	Tr	0.0	0	26	0	1	0.3	11	7	0	0.00	Tr	Tr	0
	Marshmallows	28	17	90	1	0	0.0	0	23	Tr	1	0.5	2	25	0	0.00	Tr	Tr	0
	Custard, baked	265	77	305	14	15	6.2	278	29	0	297	1.1	387	209	146	0.11	0.50	0.3	1
	Gelatin dessert prepared with gelatin dessert powder and water	120	84	70	2	0	0.0	0	17	0	2	Tr	Tr	55	0	0.00	0.00	0.0	0
	Honey, strained or extracted	339	17	1,030	1	0	0.0	0	279	Tr	17	1.7	173	17	0	0.02	0.14	1.0	3
	Honey, strained or extracted	21	17	65	Tr	0	0.0	0	17	Tr	1	0.1	11	1	0	Tr	0.01	0.1	Tr
	Jams and preserves	20	29	55	Tr	Tr	0.0	0	14	Tr	4	0.2	18	2	Tr	Tr	0.01	Tr	Tr
	Jellies	18	28	50	Tr	Tr	Tr	0	13	Tr	2	0.1	16	5	Tr	Tr	0.01	Tr	1
	Popsicle, 3 fl. oz. size	95	80	70	0	0	0.0	0	18	0	0	Tr	4	11	0	0.00	0.00	0.0	0
	Puddings:																		
	Canned:																		
	Chocolate	142	68	205	3	11	1.0	1	30	1	74	1.2	254	285	31	0.04	0.17	0.6	Tr
	Vanilla	142	69	220	2	10	0.8	1	33	Tr	79	0.2	155	305	Tr	0.03	0.12	0.6	Tr
	Dry mix, prepared with whole milk:																		
	Chocolate: Instant	130	71	155	4	4	2.4	14	27	2	130	0.3	176	440	33	0.04	0.18	0.1	1
	Rice	132	73	155	4	4	2.3	15	27	1	133	0.5	165	140	33	0.10	0.18	0.6	1
	Vanilla: Instant	130	73	150	4	4	2.3	15	27	Tr	129	0.1	164	375	33	0.04	0.17	0.1	1
	Sugars:																		
	Brown, pressed down	220	2	820	0	0	0.0	0	212	0	187	4.8	757	97	0	0.02	0.07	0.2	0
	White: Granulated	200	1	770	0	0	0.0	0	199	0	Tr	Tr	Tr	Tr	0	0.00	0.00	0.0	0
	Granulated	12	1	45	0	0	0.0	0	12	0	Tr	Tr	Tr	Tr	0	0.00	0.00	0.0	0
	Powdered, sifted, spooned into cup	100	1	385	0	0	0.0	0	99	0	Tr	Tr	4	Tr	0	0.00	0.00	0.0	0
	Syrups:																		
	Chocolate-flavored syrup or topping: Thin type	38	37	85	1	Tr	0.2	0	21	1	6	0.8	85	36	Tr	0.02	0.08	0.1	0
	Fudge type	38	25	125	2	5	2.2	0	22	Tr	38	0.5	82	42	13	0.04	0.08	0.8	0
	Table syrup (corn and maple)	42	25	122	0	0	0.0	0	32	0	1	Tr	7	19	0	0.02	0.07	0.2	0
	Vegetables and Vegetable Products																		
	Alfalfa seeds, sprouted, raw	33	91	10	1	Tr	Tr	0	1	1	11	0.3	26	2	5	0.03	0.04	0.2	3
	Asparagus, green: Cooked, drained: From raw: Cuts and tips	180	92	45	5	1	0.2	0	8	4	43	1.2	558	7	149	0.18	0.22	1.9	49
	From frozen: Cuts and tips	180	91	50	5	1	0.2	0	9	4	41	1.2	392	7	147	0.12	0.19	1.9	44
	Bamboo shoots, canned, drained	131	94	25	2	1	0.1	0	4	3	10	0.4	105	9	1	0.03	0.03	0.2	1

(A)	(B)	(C)	(D)	(E)	(F)	(G)	(H)	(I)	(J)	(K)	(L)	(M)	(N)	(O)	(P)	(Q)	(R)	(S)
Beans:																		
Lima, immature seeds, frozen, cooked, drained:																		
Thick-seeded types (Ford-hooks)	1 cup	74	170	10	1	0.2	0	32	12	37	2.3	694	90	32	0.13	0.10	1.8	22
Snap:																		
Cooked, drained:																		
From raw (cut and French style)	1 cup	89	45	2	Tr	Tr	0	10	4	58	1.6	374	4	[57]83	0.09	0.12	0.8	12
From frozen (cut)	1 cup	92	35	2	Tr	Tr	0	8	4	61	1.1	151	18	[58]71	0.06	0.10	0.6	11
Canned, drained solids (cut)	1 cup	93	25	2	Tr	Tr	0	6	2	35	1.2	147	[59]339	[60]47	0.02	0.08	0.3	6
Beets:																		
Canned, drained solids, diced or sliced	1 cup	91	55	2	Tr	Tr	0	12	4	26	3.1	252	[61]466	2	0.02	0.07	0.3	7
Beet greens, leaves and stems, cooked, drained	1 cup	89	40	4	Tr	Tr	0	8	4	164	2.7	1,309	347	734	0.17	0.42	0.7	36
Broccoli:																		
Cooked, drained:																		
From raw:																		
Spears, cut into 1/2 in. pieces	1 cup	90	45	5	Tr	Tr	0	9	2	177	1.8	253	17	218	0.13	0.32	1.2	97
From frozen:																		
Chopped	1 cup	91	50	6	Tr	Tr	0	10	5	94	1.1	333	44	350	0.10	0.15	0.8	74
Brussels sprouts, cooked, drained:																		
From frozen	1 cup	87	65	6	1	0.2	0	13	6	37	1.1	504	36	91	0.16	0.18	0.8	71
Cabbage, common varieties:																		
Raw, coarsely shredded or sliced	1 cup	93	15	1	Tr	Tr	0	4	1	33	0.4	172	13	9	0.04	0.02	0.2	33
Cooked, drained	1 cup	94	30	1	Tr	0.1	0	7	4	50	0.6	308	29	13	0.09	0.08	0.3	36
Cabbage, red, raw, coarsely shredded or sliced	1 cup	92	20	1	Tr	Tr	0	4	2	36	0.3	144	8	3	0.04	0.02	0.2	40
Carrots:																		
Raw, without crowns and tips, scraped:																		
Whole, 7-1/2 by 1-1/8 in., or strips, 2-1/2 to 3 in. long	1 carrot or 18 strips	88	30	1	Tr	Tr	0	7	2	19	0.4	233	25	2,025	0.07	0.04	0.7	7
Cooked, sliced, drained:																		
From frozen	1 cup	90	55	2	Tr	Tr	0	12	6	41	0.7	231	86	2,585	0.04	0.05	0.6	4
Cauliflower:																		
Raw, (flowerets)	1 cup	92	25	2	Tr	Tr	0	5	2	29	0.6	355	15	2	0.08	0.06	0.6	72
Cooked, drained:																		
From frozen (flowerets)	1 cup	94	35	3	Tr	Tr	0	7	4	31	0.7	250	32	4	0.07	0.10	0.6	56
Celery, pascal type, raw:																		
Stalk, large outer, 8 by 1-1/2 in. (at root end)	1 stalk	95	5	Tr	Tr	Tr	0	1	1	14	0.2	114	35	5	0.01	0.01	0.1	3
Collards, cooked, drained:																		
From frozen (chopped)	1 cup	88	60	5	1	0.2	0	12	6	357	1.9	427	85	1,017	0.08	0.20	1.1	45
Corn, sweet:																		
Cooked, drained:																		
From raw, ear 5 by 1-3/4 in.	1 ear	70	85	3	1	0.2	0	19	2	2	0.5	192	13	[63]17	0.17	0.06	1.2	5
From frozen:																		
Ear, trimmed to about 3-1/2 in. long	1 ear	73	60	2	Tr	0.1	0	14	2	2	0.4	158	3	[63]13	0.11	0.04	1.0	3
Kernels	1 cup	76	135	5	Tr	Tr	0	34	4	3	0.5	229	8	[63]41	0.11	0.12	2.1	4
Canned:																		
Cream style	1 cup	79	185	4	1	0.2	0	46	4	8	1.0	343	[64]730	[63]25	0.06	0.14	2.5	12
Whole kernel, vacuum pack	1 cup	77	165	5	1	0.2	0	41	4	11	0.9	391	[65]571	[63]51	0.09	0.15	2.5	17
Cucumber, with peel, slices, 1/8 in. thick (large, 2-1/8 in. diam.; small, 1-3/4 in. diam.)	6 large or 8 small slices	96	5	Tr	Tr	Tr	0	1	Tr	4	0.1	42	1	1	0.01	0.01	0.1	1
Eggplant, cooked, steamed	1 cup	92	25	1	Tr	Tr	0	6	4	6	0.3	238	3	6	0.07	0.02	0.6	1
Kale, cooked, drained:																		
From frozen, chopped	1 cup	91	40	4	1	Tr	0	7	2	179	1.2	417	20	826	0.06	0.15	0.9	33
Lettuce, raw:																		
Butterhead, as Boston types:																		
Head, 5 in. diam.	1 head	96	20	2	Tr	Tr	0	4	4	52	0.5	419	8	158	0.10	0.10	0.5	13
Crisphead, as iceberg:																		
Head, 6 in. diam.	1 head	96	70	5	1	Tr	0	11	4	102	2.7	852	49	178	0.25	0.16	1.0	21
Wedge, 1/4 of head	1 wedge	96	20	1	Tr	Tr	0	3	1	26	0.7	213	12	45	0.06	0.04	0.3	5
Pieces, chopped or shredded	1 cup	96	5	1	Tr	Tr	0	1	1	10	0.3	87	5	18	0.03	0.02	0.1	2
Mushrooms:																		
Raw, sliced or chopped	1 cup	92	20	1	Tr	Tr	0	3	Tr	4	0.9	259	3	0	0.07	0.31	2.9	2
Canned, drained solids	1 cup	91	35	3	Tr	Tr	0	8	4	17	1.2	201	663	0	0.13	0.03	2.5	0

Nutritive Value of Foods – Continued
(Tr indicates nutrient present in trace amount.)

Item No. Foods (A)	Foods, approximate measures, units, and weight (weight of edible portion only) (B)	Water (C) Percent	Food energy (D) Calories	Protein (E) Grams	Fat (F) Grams	Saturated fat (G) Grams	Cholesterol (H) Milligrams	Carbohydrate (I) Grams	Dietary fiber (J) Grams	Calcium (K) Milligrams	Iron (L) Milligrams	Potassium (M) Milligrams	Sodium (N) Milligrams	Vitamin A (O) Micrograms	Thiamin (P) Milligrams	Riboflavin (Q) Milligrams	Niacin (R) Milligrams	Vitamin C (S) Milligrams
Onions:																		
Raw:																		
Chopped	1 cup	91	55	2	Tr	Tr	0	12	3	40	0.6	248	3	0	0.10	0.02	0.2	13
Cooked (whole or sliced), drained	1 cup	92	60	2	Tr	Tr	0	13	2	57	0.4	319	17	0	0.09	0.02	0.2	12
Onion rings, breaded, par-fried, frozen, prepared	2 rings	29	80	1	5	1.7	0	8	Tr	6	0.3	26	75	5	0.06	0.03	0.7	Tr
Parsley:																		
Freeze-dried	1 tbsp.	2	Tr	Tr	Tr	Tr	0	Tr	1	1	0.2	25	2	25	Tr	0.01	Tr	1
Peas, edible pod, cooked, drained	1 cup	89	65	5	Tr	0.1	0	11	4	67	3.2	384	6	21	0.20	0.12	0.09	77
Peas, green:																		
Canned, drained solids	1 cup	82	115	8	1	0.2	0	21	6	34	1.6	294	[66]372	131	0.21	0.13	1.2	16
Frozen, cooked, drained	1 cup	80	125	8	Tr	Tr	0	23	8	38	2.5	269	139	107	0.45	0.16	2.4	16
Peppers:																		
Hot chili, raw	1 pepper	88	20	1	Tr	Tr	0	4	1	8	0.5	153	3	[67]484	0.04	0.04	0.4	109
Sweet (about 5 per lb., whole), stem and seeds removed:																		
Raw	1 pepper	93	20	1	Tr	Tr	0	4	1	4	0.9	144	2	[68]39	0.06	0.04	0.4	[69]95
Potatoes, cooked:																		
Baked (about 2 per lb., raw):																		
With skin	1 potato	71	220	5	Tr	0.1	0	51	5	20	2.7	844	16	0	0.22	0.07	3.3	26
Flesh only	1 potato	75	145	3	Tr	Tr	0	34	2	8	0.5	610	8	0	0.16	0.03	2.2	20
Boiled (about 3 per lb., raw):																		
Peeled after boiling	1 potato	77	120	3	Tr	Tr	0	27	2	7	0.4	515	5	0	0.14	0.03	2.0	18
French fried, strip, 2 to 3-1/2 in. long, frozen:																		
Oven heated	10 strips	53	110	2	4	3.8	0	17	1	5	0.7	229	16	0	0.06	0.02	1.2	5
Fried in vegetable oil	10 strips	38	160	2	8	2.5	0	20	2	10	0.4	366	108	0	0.09	0.01	1.6	5
Potato products, prepared:																		
Au gratin:																		
From dry mix	1 cup	79	230	6	10	6.4	12	31	4	203	0.8	537	1,076	76	0.05	0.20	2.3	8
Hashed brown, from frozen	1 cup	56	340	5	18	7.0	0	44	3	23	2.4	680	53	0	0.17	0.03	3.8	10
Mashed:																		
From home recipe:																		
Milk and margarine added	1 cup	76	225	4	9	2.2	4	35	4	55	0.5	607	620	42	0.18	0.08	2.3	13
Potato chips	10 chips	3	105	1	7	3.1	0	10	1	5	0.2	260	94	0	0.03	Tr	0.8	8
Pumpkin:																		
Canned	1 cup	90	85	3	1	0.4	0	20	6	64	3.4	505	12	5,404	0.06	0.13	0.9	10
Radishes, raw, stem ends, rootlets cut off	4 radishes	95	5	Tr	Tr	Tr	0	1	Tr	4	0.1	42	4	Tr	Tr	0.01	0.1	4
Spinach:																		
Raw, chopped	1 cup	92	10	2	Tr	Tr	0	2	2	54	1.5	307	43	369	0.04	0.10	0.4	15
Cooked, drained:																		
From frozen (leaf)	1 cup	90	55	6	Tr	Tr	0	10	4	277	2.9	566	163	1,479	0.11	0.32	0.8	23
Canned, drained solids	1 cup	92	50	6	1	0.2	0	7	6	272	4.9	740	[72]683	1,878	0.03	0.30	0.8	31
Squash, cooked:																		
Summer (all varieties), sliced, drained	1 cup	94	35	2	1	0.2	0	8	2	49	0.6	346	2	52	0.08	0.07	0.9	10
Winter (all varieties), baked, cubes	1 cup	89	80	2	1	0.3	0	18	6	29	0.7	896	2	729	0.17	0.05	1.4	20
Sweet potatoes:																		
Cooked (raw, 5 by 2 in.; about 2-1/2 per lb.):																		
Baked in skin, peeled	1 potato	73	115	2	Tr	Tr	0	28	4	32	0.5	397	11	2,488	0.08	0.14	0.7	28
Candied, 2-1/2 by 2 in. piece	1 piece	67	145	1	3	1.4	8	29	2	27	1.2	198	74	440	0.02	0.04	0.4	7
Canned:																		
Vacuum pack, piece 2-3/4 by 1 in.	1 piece	76	35	1	Tr	Tr	0	8	1	9	0.4	125	21	319	0.01	0.02	0.3	11
Tomatoes:																		
Raw, 2-3/5 in. diam. (3 per 12 oz. pkg.)	1 tomato	94	25	1	Tr	Tr	0	5	1	9	0.6	255	10	139	0.07	0.06	0.7	22
Canned, solids and liquid	1 cup	94	50	2	1	0.1	0	10	2	62	1.5	530	[73]391	145	0.11	0.07	1.8	36

Nutrients in Indicated Quantity

(A)	(B)	(C)	(D)	(E)	(F)	(G)	(H)	(I)	(J)	(K)	(L)	(M)	(N)	(O)	(P)	(Q)	(R)	(S)
Tomato juice, canned	1 cup	244	94	40	2	Tr	Tr	0	10	1	22	1.4	74881	136	0.11	0.08	1.6	45
Tomato products, canned:																		
Paste	1 cup	262	74	220	10	2	0.3	0	49	11	92	7.8	75170	647	0.41	0.50	8.4	111
Puree	1 cup	250	87	105	4	Tr	Tr	0	25	6	38	2.3	7650	340	0.18	0.14	4.3	88
Sauce	1 cup	245	89	75	3	Tr	Tr	0	18	3	34	1.9	771,482	240	0.16	0.14	2.8	32
Turnip greens, cooked, drained:																		
From frozen (chopped)	1 cup	164	90	50	5	1	0.2	0	8	7	249	3.2	25	1,308	0.09	0.12	0.8	36
Vegetable juice cocktail, canned	1 cup	242	94	45	2	Tr	Tr	0	11	1	27	1.0	883	283	0.10	0.07	1.8	67
Vegetables, mixed:																		
Canned, drained solids	1 cup	163	87	75	4	Tr	Tr	0	15	3	44	1.7	243	1,899	0.08	0.08	0.9	8
Frozen, cooked, drained	1 cup	182	83	105	5	Tr	Tr	0	24	5	46	1.5	308	778	0.13	0.22	1.5	6
Water chestnuts, canned	1 cup	140	86	70	1	Tr	Tr	0	17	1	6	1.2	165	11	0.02	0.03	0.5	2

[1]Value not determined.
[2]Mineral content varies depending on water source.
[3]Blend of aspartame and saccharin; if only sodium saccharin is used, sodium is 75 mg; if only aspartame is used, sodium is 23 mg.
[4]With added ascorbic acid.
[5]Vitamin A value is largely from beta-carotene used for coloring.
[6]Yields 1 qt. of fluid milk when reconstituted according to package directions.
[7]With added vitamin A.
[8]Carbohydrate content varies widely because of amount of sugar added and amount and solids content of added flavoring. Consult the label if more precise values for carbohydrate and calories are needed.
[9]For salted butter; unsalted butter contains 12 mg sodium per stick, 2 mg per tbsp., or 1 mg per pat.
[10]Values for vitamin A are year-round average.
[11]For salted margarine.
[12]Based on average vitamin A content of fortified margarine. Federal specifications for fortified margarine require a minimum of 15,000 IU per pound.
[14]Dipped in egg, milk, and breadcrumbs; fried in vegetable shortening.
[15]If bones are discarded, value for calcium will be greatly reduced.
[16]Dipped in egg, breadcrumbs, and flour; fried in vegetable shortening.
[18]Sodium bisulfite used to preserve color; unsulfited product would contain less sodium.
[19]Also applies to pasteurized apple cider.
[20]Without added ascorbic acid. For value with added ascorbic acid, refer to label.
[21]With added ascorbic acid.
[22]For white grapefruit; pink grapefruit have about 310 IU or 31 RE.
[23]Sodium benzoate and sodium bisulfite added as preservatives.
[24]Egg bagels have 44 mg cholesterol and 22 IU or 7 RE vitamin A per bagel.
[25]Made with vegetable shortening.
[27]Nutrient added.
[28]Cooked without salt. If salt is added according to label recommendations, sodium content is 540 mg.
[29]For white corn grits. Cooked yellow grits contain 145 IU or 14 RE.
[30]Value based on label declaration for added nutrients.
[31]For regular and instant cereal. For quick cereal, phosphorus is 102 mg and sodium is 142 mg.
[32]Cooked without salt. If salt is added according to label recommendations, sodium content is 390 mg.
[33]Cooked without salt. If salt is added according to label recommendations, sodium content is 324 mg.
[34]Cooked without salt. If salt is added according to label recommendations, sodium content is 374 mg.
[35]Excepting angel food cake, cakes were made from mixes containing vegetable shortening and frostings were made with margarine.
[36]Made with vegetable oil.

[37]Cake made with vegetable shortening; frosting with margarine.
[38]Made with margarine.
[39]Crackers made with enriched flour except for rye wafers and whole-wheat wafers.
[40]Made with lard.
[41]Cashews without salt contain 21 mg sodium per cup or 4 mg per oz.
[42]Cashews without salt contain 22 mg sodium per cup or 5 mg per oz.
[43]Macadamia nuts without salt contain 9 mg sodium per cup or 2 mg per oz.
[44]Mixed nuts without salt contain 3 mg sodium per oz.
[45]Peanuts without salt contain 22 mg sodium per cup or 4 mg per oz.
[46]Outer layer of fat was removed to within approximately 1/2 inch of the lean. Deposits of fat within the cut were removed.
[47]Fried in vegetable shortening.
[48]Value varies widely.
[49]Contains added sodium ascorbate. If sodium ascorbate is not added, ascorbic acid content is negligible.
[51]Crust made with vegetable shortening and enriched flour.
[52]Made with corn oil.
[53]Fried in vegetable shortening.
[54]If sodium ascorbate is added, product contains 11 mg ascorbic acid.
[55]Made with enriched flour, margarine, and whole milk.
[57]For green varieties; yellow varieties contain 101 IU or 10 RE.
[59]For regular pack; special dietary pack contains 3 mg sodium.
[60]For green varieties; yellow varieties contain 142 IU or 14 RE.
[61]For regular pack; special dietary pack contains 78 mg sodium.
[63]For yellow varieties; white varieties contain only a trace of vitamin A.
[64]For regular pack; special dietary pack contains 8 mg sodium.
[65]For regular pack; special dietary pack contains 6 mg sodium.
[66]For regular pack; special dietary pack contains 3 mg sodium.
[67]For red peppers; green peppers contain 350 IU or 35 RE.
[68]For green peppers; red peppers contain 4,220 IU or 422 RE.
[69]For green peppers; red peppers contain 141 mg ascorbic acid.
[72]With added salt; if none is added, sodium content is 58 mg.
[73]For regular pack; special dietary pack contains 31 mg sodium.
[74]With added salt; if none is added, sodium content is 24 mg.
[75]With no added salt; if salt is added, sodium content is 2,070 mg.
[76]With no added salt; if salt is added, sodium content is 998 mg.
[77]With salt added.

Appendix E

Exchange Lists for Meal Planning

The Food Lists

The following chart shows the amount of nutrients in 1 serving from each list.

Food List	Carbohydrate (grams)	Protein (grams)	Fat (grams)	Calories
Carbohydrates				
Starch: breads, cereals and grains; starchy vegetables; crackers, snacks; and beans, peas, and lentils	15	0–3	0–1	80
Fruits	15	—	—	60
Milk				
Fat-free, low-fat, 1%	12	8	0–3	100
Reduced-fat, 2%	12	8	5	120
Whole	12	8	8	160
Sweets, Desserts, and Other Carbohydrates	15	varies	varies	varies
Nonstarchy Vegetables	5	2	—	25
Meat and Meat Substitutes				
Lean	—	7	0–3	45
Medium-fat	—	7	4–7	75
High-fat	—	7	8+	100
Plant-based proteins	varies	7	varies	varies
Fats	—	—	5	45

* = More than 3 grams of dietary fiber per serving.

♦ = Extra fat, or prepared with added fat.

‡ = 480 milligrams or more of sodium per serving; 600 milligrams or more of sodium per serving (for combination or fast-food main dishes/meals).

Starch

Cereals, grains, pasta, breads, crackers, snacks, starchy vegetables, and cooked beans, peas, and lentils are starches. In general, 1 starch is

- ½ cup of cooked cereal, grain, or starchy vegetable
- ⅓ cup of cooked rice or pasta
- 1 oz. of a bread product, such as 1 slice of bread
- ¾ oz. to 1 oz. of most snack foods (some snack foods may also have extra fat)

Bread

Food	Serving Size
Bagel, large (about 4 oz) . . . . ¼ (1 oz)	
♦ Biscuit, 2½ inches across. .1	
* Bread, reduced-calorie. . . . . 2 slices (1½ oz)	
Bread, white, whole-grain, pumpernickel, rye, unfrosted raisin . . . . 1 slice (1 oz)	
Chapatti, small, 6 inches across 1	
♦ Cornbread, 1¾-inch cube. . . . . 1 (1½ oz)	
English muffin. . . . . ½	
Hot dog bun or hamburger bun . . . . ½ (1 oz)	
Naan, 8 inches by 2 inches . . . . ¼	
Pancake, 4 inches across, ¼-inch thick. 1	
Pita, 6 inches across . . . . ½	
Roll, plain, small . . . . .1 (1 oz)	
♦ Stuffing, bread . . . . ⅓ cup	
♦ Taco shell, 5 inches across 2	
Tortilla, corn, 6 inches across 1	
Tortilla, flour, 6 inches across. 1	
Tortilla, flour, 10 inches across. . . . . ⅓ tortilla	
♦ Waffle, 4-inch square or 4 inches across. 1	

Cereals and Grains

Food	Serving Size
Barley, cooked . . . . ⅓ cup	
* Bran, dry, oat . . . . ¼ cup	
* Bran, dry, wheat . . . . ½ cup	
* Bulgur (cooked) . . . . ½ cup	
* Bran cereal. . . . . ½ cup	
Cereal, cooked (oats, oatmeal) . . . . ½ cup	
Cereal, puffed. . . . . 1½ cups	
Cereal, shredded wheat, plain . . . . ½ cup	
Cereal, sugar-coated . . . . ½ cup	
Cereal, unsweetened, ready-to-eat . . . . ¾ cup	
Couscous . . . . ⅓ cup	
Granola, low-fat . . . . ¼ cup	
♦ Granola, regular . . . . ¼ cup	
Grits, cooked . . . . ½ cup	
Kasha . . . . ½ cup	
Millet, cooked . . . . ⅓ cup	
Muesli. . . . . ¼ cup	
Pasta, cooked. . . . . ⅓ cup	
Polenta, cooked . . . . ⅓ cup	
Quinoa, cooked . . . . ⅓ cup	
Rice, white or brown, cooked . . . . ⅓ cup	
Tabbouleh (tabouli), prepared . . . . ½ cup	
Wheat germ, dry. . . . . 3 Tbsp	
Wild rice, cooked . . . . ½ cup	

Tip: An open handful is equal to about 1 cup or 1 oz to 2 oz of snack food.

Starchy Vegetables

Food	Serving Size
Cassava . . . . ⅓ cup	
Corn . . . . ½ cup	
Corn on cob, large . . . . ½ cob (5 oz)	
* Hominy, canned . . . . ¾ cup	
* Mixed vegetables with corn, peas, or pasta. . . . 1 cup	
* Parsnips . . . . ½ cup	
* Peas, green . . . . ½ cup	
Plantain, ripe. . . . . ⅓ cup	
Potato, baked with skin. . . . . ¼ large (3 oz)	
Potato, boiled, all kinds . . . ½ cup or ½ medium (3 oz)	
♦ Potato, mashed, with milk and fat . . . . ½ cup	
Potato, French fried (oven-baked) . . . . . . 1 cup (2 oz)	
* Pumpkin, canned, no sugar added . . . . 1 cup	
Spaghetti/pasta sauce . . . . ½ cup	
* Squash, winter (acorn, butternut). . . . . 1 cup	
* Succotash. . . . . ½ cup	
Yam, sweet potato, plain . . . . ½ cup	

Note: Restaurant-style French fries are on the **Fast Foods** list.

Crackers and Snacks

Food	Serving Size
Animal crackers 8	
♦ Crackers, round, butter-type 6	
Crackers, saltine-type 6	
♦ Crackers, sandwich-style, cheese or peanut butter filling. 3	
♦ Crackers, whole-wheat regular . . . . 2–5 (¾ oz)	
* Crackers, whole-wheat lower fat or crispbreads . . . . 2–5 (¾ oz)	
Graham cracker, 2½ inch square. 3	
Matzoh . . . . ¾ oz	
Melba toast, about 2-inch by 4-inch piece . . . 4 pieces	
Oyster crackers 20	
*♦ Popcorn, with butter. 3 cups	
* Popcorn, no fat added . . . . 3 cups	
* Popcorn, lower fat. . . . . 3 cups	
Pretzels. . . . . ¾ oz	
Rice cakes, 4 inches across. 2	
Snack chips, fat-free or baked (tortilla, potato), baked pita chips. . . . . 15–20 (¾ oz)	
♦ Snack chips, regular (tortilla, potato) . . . . 9–13 (¾ oz)	

Note: For other snacks, see the **Sweets, Desserts, and Other Carbohydrates** list.

Beans, Peas, and Lentils

The choices on this list count as 1 starch + 1 lean meat.

Food	Serving Size
★ Baked beans	⅓ cup
★ Beans, cooked (black, garbanzo, kidney, lima, navy, pinto, white)	½ cup
★ Lentils, cooked (brown, green, yellow)	½ cup
★ Peas, cooked (black-eyed, split)	½ cup
★‡ Refried beans, canned	½ cup

Note: Beans, peas, and lentils are also found on the **Meat and Meat Substitutes** list.

Fruits

Fresh, frozen, canned, and dried fruits and fruit juices are on this list. In general, 1 fruit choice is
- ½ cup of canned or fresh fruit or unsweetened fruit juice
- 1 small fresh fruit (4 oz)
- 2 tablespoons of dried fruit

Fruit

The weight listed includes skin, core, seeds, and rind.

Food	Serving Size
Apple, unpeeled, small	1 (4 oz)
Apples, dried	4 rings
Applesauce, unsweetened	½ cup
Apricots, canned	½ cup
Apricots, dried	8 halves
★ Apricots, fresh	4 whole (5½ oz)
Banana, extra small	1 (4 oz)
★ Blackberries	¾ cup
Blueberries	¾ cup
Cantaloupe, small	⅓ melon or 1 cup cubed (11 oz)
Cherries, sweet, canned	½ cup
Cherries, sweet, fresh	12 (3 oz)
Dates	3
Dried fruits (blueberries, cherries, cranberries, mixed fruit, raisins)	2 Tbsp
Figs, dried	1½
Figs, fresh	1½ large or 2 medium (3½ oz)
Fruit cocktail	½ cup
Grapefruit, large	½ (11 oz)
Grapefruit, sections, canned	¾ cup
Grapes, small	17 (3 oz)
Honeydew melon	1 slice or 1 cup cubed (10 oz)
★ Kiwi	1 (3½ oz)
Mandarin oranges, canned	¾ cup
Mango, small	½ fruit (5½ oz) or ½ cup
Nectarine, small	1 (5 oz)
★ Orange, small	1 (6½ oz)
Papaya	½ fruit or 1 cup cubed (8 oz)
Peaches, canned	½ cup
Peaches, fresh, medium	1 (6 oz)
Pears, canned	½ cup
Pears, fresh, large	½ (4 oz)
Pineapple, canned	½ cup
Pineapple, fresh	¾ cup
Plums, canned	½ cup
Plums, dried (prunes)	3
Plums, small	2 (5 oz)
★ Raspberries	1 cup
★ Strawberries	1¼ cup whole berries
★ Tangerines, small	2 (8 oz)
Watermelon	1 slice or 1¼ cups cubes (13½ oz)

Fruit Juice

Food	Serving Size
Apple juice/cider	½ cup
Fruit juice blends, 100% juice	⅓ cup
Grape juice	⅓ cup
Grapefruit juice	½ cup
Orange juice	½ cup
Pineapple juice	½ cup
Prune juice	⅓ cup

Milk

Different types of milk and milk products are on this list. However, 2 types of milk products are found in other lists:
- Cheeses are on the **Meat and Meat Substitutes** list (because they are rich in protein)
- Cream and other dairy fats are on the **Fats** list

	Carbohydrate (grams)	Protein (grams)	Fat (grams)	Calories
Fat-free (skim)/low-fat (1%)	12	8	0–3	100
Reduced-fat (2%)	12	8	5	120
Whole	12	8	8	160

Milk and Yogurts

Food	Serving Size	Count As
Fat-free (skim) or low-fat (1%)		
Milk, buttermilk, acidophilus milk, Lactaid	1 cup	1 fat-free milk
Evaporated milk	½ cup	1 fat-free milk
Yogurt, plain or flavored with an artificial sweetener	⅔ cup (6 oz)	1 fat-free milk
Reduced-fat (2%)		
Milk, acidophilus milk, kefir, Lactaid	1 cup	1 reduced-fat milk
Yogurt, plain	⅔ cup (6 oz)	1 reduced-fat milk
Whole		
Milk, buttermilk, goat's milk	1 cup	1 whole milk
Evaporated milk	½ cup	1 whole milk
Yogurt, plain	1 cup (8 oz)	1 whole milk

Dairy-Like Foods

Food	Serving Size	Count As
Chocolate milk, fat-free	1 cup	1 fat-free milk + 1 carbohydrate
Chocolate milk, whole	1 cup	1 whole milk + 1 carbohydrate
Eggnog, whole milk	½ cup	1 carbohydrate + 2 fats
Rice drink, flavored, low-fat	1 cup	2 carbohydrates
Rice drink, plain, fat-free	1 cup	1 carbohydrate
Smoothies, flavored, regular	10 oz	1 fat-free milk + 2½ carbohydrates
Soy milk, light	1 cup	1 carbohydrate + ½ fat
Soy milk, regular, plain	1 cup	1 carbohydrate + 1 fat
Yogurt, and juice blends	1 cup	1 fat-free milk + 1 carbohydrate
Yogurt, low-carbohydrate (less than 6 grams carbohydrate per serving)	⅔ cup (6 oz)	½ fat-free milk
Yogurt, with fruit, low-fat	⅔ cup (6 oz)	1 fat-free milk + 1 carbohydrate

Note: Coconut milk is on the **Fats** list.

Sweets, Desserts, and Other Carbohydrates

Foods on this list have added sugars or fat. However, you can substitute food choices from this list for other carbohydrate-containing foods (such as those found on the **Starch**, **Fruits**, or **Milk** lists) in your meal plan.

Beverages, Soda, and Energy/Sports Drinks

Food	Serving Size	Count As
Cranberry juice cocktail	½ cup	1 carbohydrate
Energy drink	1 can (8.3 oz)	2 carbohydrates
Fruit drink or lemonade	1 cup (8 oz)	2 carbohydrates
Hot chocolate, regular	1 envelope added to 8 oz water	1 carbohydrate + 1 fat
Hot chocolate, sugar-free or light	1 envelope added to 8 oz water	1 carbohydrate
Soft drink (soda), regular	1 can (12 oz)	2½ carbohydrates
Sports drink	1 cup (8 oz)	1 carbohydrate

Brownies, Cake, Cookies, Gelatin, Pie, and Pudding

Food	Serving Size	Count As
Brownies, small, unfrosted	1¼ inch square, ⅞ inch high (about 1 oz)	1 carbohydrate + 1 fat
Cake, angel food, unfrosted	1/12 of cake (about 2 oz)	2 carbohydrates
Cake, frosted	2-inch square (about 2 oz)	2 carbohydrates + 1 fat
Cake, unfrosted	2-inch square (about 1 oz)	1 carbohydrate + 1 fat

Cookies, chocolate chip	2 cookies (2¼ inches across)	1 carbohydrate + 2 fats
Cookies, gingersnap	3 cookies	1 carbohydrate
Cookies, sandwich, with crème filling	2 small (about ⅔ oz)	1 carbohydrate + 1 fat
Cookies, sugar-free	3 small or 1 large (¾–1 oz)	1 carbohydrate + 1–2 fats
Cookies, vanilla wafer	5 cookies	1 carbohydrate + 1 fat
Cupcake, frosted	1 small (about 1¾ oz)	2 carbohydrates + 1–1½ fats
Fruit cobbler	½ cup (3½ oz)	3 carbohydrates + 1 fat
Gelatin, regular	½ cup	1 carbohydrate
Pie, commercially prepared fruit, 2 crusts	⅙ of 8-inch pie	3 carbohydrates + 2 fats
Pie, pumpkin or custard	⅛ of 8-inch pie	1½ carbohydrates + 1½ fats
Pudding, regular (made with reduced-fat milk)	½ cup	2 carbohydrates
Pudding, sugar-free or sugar- and fat-free (made with fat-free milk)	½ cup	1 carbohydrate

Candy, Spreads, Sweets, Sweeteners, Syrups, and Toppings

Food	Serving Size	Count As
Candy bar, chocolate/peanut	2 "fun size" bars (1 oz)	1½ carbohydrates + 1½ fats
Candy, hard	3 pieces	1 carbohydrate
Chocolate "kisses"	5 pieces	1 carbohydrate + 1 fat
Coffee creamer, dry, flavored	4 tsp.	½ carbohydrate + ½ fat
Coffee creamer, liquid, flavored	2 Tbsp	1 carbohydrate
Fruit snacks, chewy (pureed fruit concentrate)	1 roll (¾ oz)	1 carbohydrate
Fruit spreads, 100% fruit	1½ Tbsp	1 carbohydrate
Honey	1 Tbsp	1 carbohydrate
Jam or jelly, regular	1 Tbsp	1 carbohydrate
Sugar	1 Tbsp	1 carbohydrate
Syrup, chocolate	2 Tbsp	2 carbohydrates
Syrup, light (pancake syrup)	2 Tbsp	1 carbohydrate
Syrup, regular (pancake type)	1 Tbsp	1 carbohydrate

Condiments and Sauces

Food	Serving Size	Count As
Barbecue sauce	3 Tbsp	1 carbohydrate
Cranberry sauce, jellied	¼ cup	1½ carbohydrates
‡ Gravy, canned or bottled	½ cup	½ carbohydrate + ½ fat
Salad dressing, fat-free, low-fat, cream-based	3 Tbsp	1 carbohydrate
Sweet and sour sauce	3 Tbsp	1 carbohydrate

Note: You can also check the **Fats** list and **Free Foods** list for other condiments.

Doughnuts, Muffins, Pastries, and Sweet Breads

Food	Serving Size	Count As
Banana nut bread	1-inch slice (2 oz)	2 carbohydrates + 1 fat
Doughnut, cake, plain	1 medium (1½ oz)	1½ carbohydrates + 2 fats
Doughnut, yeast type, glazed	3¾ inches across (2 oz)	2 carbohydrates + 2 fats
Muffin (4 oz)	¼ muffin (1 oz)	1 carbohydrate + ½ fat
Sweet roll or Danish	1 (2½ oz)	2½ carbohydrates + 2 fats

Frozen Bars, Frozen Desserts, Frozen Yogurt, and Ice Cream

Food	Serving Size	Count As
Frozen pops	1	½ carbohydrate
Fruit juice bars, frozen, 100% juice	1 bar (3 oz)	1 carbohydrate
Ice cream, fat-free	½ cup	1½ carbohydrates
Ice cream, light	½ cup	1 carbohydrate + 1 fat

Ice cream, no sugar added . . . . ½ cup . . . . 1 carbohydrate + 1 fat

Ice cream, regular . . . . ½ cup . . . . 1 carbohydrate + 2 fats

Sherbet, sorbet. . . . . ½ cup . . . . .2 carbohydrates

Yogurt, frozen, fat-free . . . . ⅓ cup . . . . 1 carbohydrate

Yogurt, frozen, regular . . . . ½ cup . . . . 1 carbohydrate + 0–1 fat

Granola Bars, Meal Replacement Bars/Shakes, and Trail Mix

Food	Serving Size	Count As
Granola or snack bar, regular or low-fat.	1 bar (1 oz).	1½ carbohydrates
Meal replacement bar.	1 bar (1⅓ oz)	1½ carbohydrates + 0–1 fat
Meal replacement bar.	1 bar (2 oz).	2 carbohydrates + 1 fat
Meal replacement shake, reduced calorie	1 can (10–11 oz).	1½ carbohydrates + 0–1 fat
Trail mix, candy/nut-based	1 oz	1 carbohydrate + 2 fats
Trail mix, dried fruit-based	1 oz	1 carbohydrate + 1 fat

Nonstarchy Vegetables

Vegetable choices include vegetables in this **Nonstarchy Vegetables** list and the **Starch Vegetables** list found within the **Starch** list. Vegetables with small amounts of carbohydrate and calories are on the **Nonstarchy Vegetables** list. Vegetables contain important nutrients. Try to eat at least 2 to 3 nonstarchy vegetable choices each day (as well as choices from the Starchy Vegetables list). In general, 1 nonstarchy vegetable choice is

- ½ cup of cooked vegetables or juice
- 1 cup of raw vegetables

If you eat 3 cups or more of raw vegetables or 1½ cups of cooked nonstarchy vegetables in a meal, count them as 1 carbohydrate choice.

Nonstarchy Vegetables

Amaranth or Chinese spinach

Artichoke

Artichoke hearts

Asparagus

Baby corn

Bamboo shoots

Bean sprouts

Beans (green, wax, Italian)

Beets

‡ Borscht

Broccoli

* Brussels sprouts

Cabbage (green, bok choy, Chinese)

* Carrots

Cauliflower

Celery

* Chayote

Coleslaw, packaged, no dressing

Cucumber

Daikon

Eggplant

Gourds (bitter, bottle, luffa, bitter melon)

Green onions or scallions

Greens (collard, kale, mustard, turnip)

Hearts of palm

Jicama

Kohlrabi

Leeks

Mixed vegetables (without corn, peas, or pasta)

Mung bean sprouts

Mushrooms, all kinds, fresh

Okra

Onions

Pea pods

* Peppers (all varieties)

Radishes

Rutabaga

‡ Sauerkraut

Soybean sprouts

Spinach

Squash (summer, crookneck, zucchini)

Sugar snap peas

* Swiss chard

Tomato

Tomatoes, canned

‡ Tomato sauce

‡ Tomato/vegetable juice

Turnips

Water chestnuts

Yard-long beans

Note: Salad greens (like chicory, endive, escarole, lettuce, romaine, arugula, radicchio, watercress) are on the **Free Foods** list.

Meat and Meat Substitutes

Meat and meat substitutes are rich in protein. Foods from this list are divided into 4 groups based on the amount of fat they contain. These groups are lean meat, medium-fat meat, high-fat meat, and plant-based proteins. The following chart shows you what one choice includes.

	Carbohydrate (grams)	Protein (grams)	Fat (grams)	Calories
Lean meat	—	7	0–3	45
Medium-fat meat	—	7	4–7	75
High-fat meat	—	7	8+	100
Plant-based protein	varies	7	varies	varies

Lean Meats and Meat Substitutes
Food   **Serving Size**

Beef: Select or Choice grades trimmed
   of fat: ground round, roast (chuck, rib,
   rump), round, sirloin, steak (cubed, flank,
   porterhouse, T-bone), tenderloin . . . . 1 oz
‡ Beef jerky . . . . .½ oz
Cheeses with 3 grams of fat or less per oz . . . . . 1 oz
Cottage cheese . . . . .¼ cup
Egg substitutes, plain . . . . .¼ cup
Egg whites 2
Fish, fresh or frozen, plain: catfish, cod,
   flounder, haddock, halibut, orange roughy,
   salmon, tilapia, trout, tuna . . . . 1 oz
‡ Fish, smoked: herring or salmon (lox) . . . . 1 oz
Game: buffalo, ostrich, rabbit, venison . . . . 1 oz
‡ Hot dog with 3 grams of fat or less per oz
   (8 hot dogs per 14 oz package)
   Note: May be high in carbohydrate. 1
Lamb: chop, leg, or roast . . . . 1 oz
Organ meats: heart, kidney, liver
   Note: May be high in cholesterol. . . . . 1 oz
Oysters, fresh or frozen . . . . .6 medium
‡ Pork, lean, Canadian bacon. . . . . 1 oz
Pork, lean, rib or loin chop/roast, ham, tenderloin. . . 1 oz
Poultry, without skin: chicken, Cornish hen,
   domestic duck or goose (well-drained of fat),
   turkey . . . . 1 oz
Processed sandwich meats with 3 grams of fat
   or less per oz: chipped beef, deli thin-sliced
   meats, turkey ham, turkey kielbasa, turkey
   pastrami . . . . 1 oz
Salmon, canned . . . . 1 oz
Sardines, canned . . . . .2 small
‡ Sausage with 3 grams of fat or less per oz . . . . . 1 oz
Shellfish: clams, crab, imitation shellfish,
   lobster, scallops, shrimp . . . . 1 oz

Tuna, canned in water or oil, drained . . . . 1 oz
Veal: loin chop, roast . . . . 1 oz

‡ = 480 milligrams or more of sodium per serving
   (based on the sodium content of a typical 3-oz
   serving of meat, unless ½ oz to 2 oz is the normal
   serving size).

Medium-Fat Meat and Meat Substitutes
Food   **Serving Size**

Beef: corned beef, ground beef, meatloaf,
   Prime grades trimmed of fat (prime rib),
   short ribs, tongue . . . . 1 oz
Cheeses with 4–7 grams of fat per oz: feta,
   mozzarella, pasteurized processed cheese
   spread, reduced-fat cheeses, string. . . . . 1 oz
Egg
   Note: High in cholesterol, so limit to 3 per week 1
Fish, any fried type. . . . . 1 oz
Lamb: ground, rib roast . . . . 1 oz
Pork: cutlet, shoulder roast . . . . 1 oz
Poultry: chicken with skin; dove, pheasant,
   wild duck, or goose; fried chicken;
   ground turkey . . . . 1 oz
Ricotta cheese . . . . .2 oz (¼ cup)
‡ Sausage with 4–7 grams of fat per oz . . . . 1 oz
Veal, cutlet (no breading) . . . . 1 oz

High-Fat Meat and Meat Substitutes

These foods are high in saturated fat, cholesterol, and calories and may raise blood cholesterol levels if eaten on a regular basis. Try to eat 3 or fewer servings from this group per week.
Food   **Serving Size**

‡ Bacon, pork . . . . 2 slices (16 slices per lb or
                                                1 oz each, before cooking)
‡ Bacon, turkey . . . 3 slices (1/2 oz each before cooking)

Cheese, regular: American, bleu, brie, cheddar,
   hard goat, Monterey jack, queso, and Swiss . . . 1 oz
◆‡ Hot dog: beef, pork, or combination
   (10 per 1 lb-sized package) 1
‡ Hot dog: turkey or chicken
   (10 per 1 lb-sized package) 1

Pork: ground, sausage, spareribs . . . . 1 oz
Processed sandwich meats with 8 grams of fat or
   more per oz: bologna, hard salami, pastrami . . . 1 oz
‡ Sausage with 8 grams fat or more per oz:
   bratwurst, chorizo, Italian, knockwurst,
   Polish, smoked, summer . . . . 1 oz

Plant-Based Proteins

Because carbohydrate content varies among plant-based proteins, you should read the food label. A carbohydrate choice has 15 grams of carbohydrate and about 70 calories.

Food	Serving Size	Count As
"Bacon" strips, soy-based	3 strips	1 medium-fat meat
* Baked beans	⅓ cup	1 starch + 1 lean meat
* Beans, cooked: black, garbanzo, kidney, lima, navy, pinto, white	½ cup	1 starch + 1 lean meat
* "Beef" or "sausage" crumbles, soy-based	2 oz	½ carbohydrate + 1 lean meat
"Chicken" nuggets, soy-based	2 nuggets (1½ oz)	½ carbohydrate + 1 medium-fat meat
* Edamame	½ cup	½ carbohydrate + 1 lean meat
Falafel (spiced chickpea and wheat patties)	3 patties (about 2 inches across)	1 carbohydrate + 1 high-fat meat
Hot dog, soy-based	1 (1½ oz)	½ carbohydrate + 1 lean meat
* Hummus	⅓ cup	1 carbohydrate + 1 high-fat meat
* Lentils, brown, green, or yellow	½ cup	1 carbohydrate + 1 lean meat
* Meatless burger, soy-based	3 oz	½ carbohydrate + 2 lean meats
* Meatless burger, vegetable- and starch-based	1 patty (about 2½ oz)	1 carbohydrate + 2 lean meats
Nut spreads: almond butter, cashew butter, peanut butter, soy nut butter	1 Tbsp	1 high-fat meat
* Peas, cooked: black-eyed and split peas	½ cup	1 starch + 1 lean meat
*‡ Refried beans, canned	½ cup	1 starch + 1 lean meat
"Sausage" patties, soy-based	1 (1½ oz)	1 medium-fat meat
Soy nuts, unsalted	¾ oz	½ carbohydrate + 1 medium-fat meat
Tempeh	¾ cup	1 medium-fat meat
Tofu	4 oz (½ cup)	1 medium-fat meat
Tofu, light	4 oz (½ cup)	1 lean meat

Note: Beans, peas, and lentils are also found on the **Starch** list. Nut butters in smaller amounts are found in the **Fats** list.

Fats

Fats and oils have mixtures of unsaturated (polyunsaturated and monounsaturated) and saturated fats. Foods on the **Fats** list are grouped together based on the major type of fat they contain. In general, 1 fat choice equals:

- 1 teaspoon of regular margarine, vegetable oil, or butter
- 1 tablespoon of regular salad dressing

Unsaturated Fats—Monounsaturated Fats

Food	Serving Size
Avocado, medium	2 Tbsp (1 oz)

Nut butters (*trans* fat-free): almond butter, cashew butter, peanut butter (smooth or crunchy) . . . . 1½ tsp
Nuts, almonds . . . . .6 nuts
Nuts, Brazil. . . . . .2 nuts
Nuts, cashews . . . . .6 nuts
Nuts, filberts (hazelnuts) . . . . .5 nuts
Nuts, macadamia . . . . .3 nuts
Nuts, mixed (50% peanuts) . . . . .6 nuts
Nuts, peanuts . . . . .10 nuts
Nuts, pecans . . . . 4 halves
Nuts, pistachios . . . . .16 nuts
Oil: canola, olive, peanut . . . . .1 tsp
Olives, black (ripe) . . . . 8 large
Olives, green, stuffed . . . . 10 large

Unsaturated Fats—Polyunsaturated Fats

Food	Serving Size
Margarine: lower-fat spread (30%–50% vegetable oil, *trans* fat-free)	1 Tbsp
Margarine: stick, tub (*trans* fat-free), or squeeze (*trans* fat-free)	1 tsp
Mayonnaise, reduced-fat	1 Tbsp
Mayonnaise, regular	1 tsp
Mayonnaise-style salad dressing, reduced-fat	1 Tbsp
Mayonnaise-style salad dressing, regular	2 tsp
Nuts, Pignolia (pine nuts)	1 Tbsp
Nuts, walnuts, English	4 halves
Oil: corn, cottonseed, flaxseed, grape seed, safflower, soybean, sunflower	1 tsp
Oil: made from soybean and canola oil—Enova	1 tsp
Plant stanol esters, light	1 Tbsp
Plant stanol esters, regular	2 tsp
‡ Salad dressing, reduced-fat *Note: May be high in carbohydrate*	2 Tbsp
‡ Salad dressing, regular	1 Tbsp
Seeds, flaxseed, whole	1 Tbsp
Seeds, pumpkin, sunflower	1 Tbsp
Seeds, sesame seeds	1 Tbsp
Tahini or sesame paste	2 tsp

Saturated Fats

Food	Serving Size
Bacon, cooked, regular or turkey	1 slice
Butter, reduced-fat	1 Tbsp
Butter, stick	1 tsp
Butter, whipped	2 tsp
Butter blends made with oil, reduced-fat or light	1 Tbsp
Butter blends made with oil, regular	1½ tsp
Chitterlings, boiled	2 Tbsp (½ oz)
Coconut, sweetened, shredded	2 Tbsp
Coconut milk, light	⅓ cup
Coconut milk, regular	1½ Tbsp
Cream, half and half	2 Tbsp
Cream, heavy	1 Tbsp
Cream, light	1½ Tbsp
Cream, whipped	2 Tbsp
Cream, whipped, pressurized	¼ cup
Cream cheese, reduced-fat	1½ Tbsp (¾ oz)
Cream cheese, regular	1 Tbsp (½ oz)
Lard	1 tsp
Oil: coconut, palm, palm kernel	1 tsp
Salt pork	¼ oz
Shortening, solid	1 tsp
Sour cream, reduced-fat or light	3 Tbsp
Sour cream, regular	2 Tbsp

Free Foods

A "free" food is any food or drink choice that has less than 20 calories and 5 grams or less of carbohydrate per serving.

- Most foods on this list should be limited to 3 servings (as listed here) per day. Spread out the servings throughout the day. If you eat all 3 servings at once, it could raise blood glucose level.
- Food and drink choices listed here without a serving size can be eaten whenever you like.

Low-Carbohydrate Foods

Food	Serving Size
Cabbage, raw	½ cup
Candy, hard (regular or sugar-free)	1 piece
Carrots, cauliflower, or green beans, cooked	¼ cup
Cranberries, sweetened with sugar substitute	½ cup
Cucumber, sliced	½ cup
Gelatin, dessert, sugar-free	
Gelatin, unflavored	
Gum	
Jam or jelly, light or no sugar added	2 tsp
Rhubarb, sweetened with sugar substitute	½ cup
Salad greens	
Sugar substitutes (artificial sweeteners)	
Syrup, sugar-free	2 Tbsp

Modified-Fat Foods with Carbohydrate

Food	Serving Size
Cream cheese, fat-free	1 Tbsp (½ oz)
Creamers, nondairy, liquid	1 Tbsp
Creamers, nondairy, powdered	2 tsp
Margarine spread, fat-free	1 Tbsp
Margarine spread, reduced-fat	1 tsp
Mayonnaise, fat-free	1 Tbsp
Mayonnaise, reduced-fat	1 tsp
Mayonnaise-style salad dressing, fat-free	1 Tbsp
Mayonnaise-style salad dressing, reduced-fat	1 tsp
Salad dressing, fat-free or low-fat	1 Tbsp
Salad dressing, fat-free, Italian	2 Tbsp
Sour cream, fat-free or reduced fat	1 Tbsp
Whipped topping, light or fat-free	2 Tbsp
Whipped topping, regular	1 Tbsp

Condiments

Food	Serving Size
Barbecue sauce	2 tsp
Catsup (ketchup)	1 Tbsp
Honey mustard	1 Tbsp
Horseradish	
Lemon juice	
Miso	1½ tsp

Mustard

Parmesan cheese, freshly grated . . . . 1 Tbsp

Pickle relish . . . . 1 Tbsp

‡ Pickles, dill . . . . 1½ medium

Pickles, sweet, bread and butter . . . . 2 slices

Pickles, sweet, gherkin. . . . . .¾ oz

Salsa. . . . . .¼ cup

‡ Soy sauce, light or regular . . . . 1 Tbsp

Sweet and sour sauce .2 tsp

Sweet chili sauce . . . . .2 tsp

Taco sauce. . . . . 1 Tbsp

Vinegar

Yogurt, any type . . . . 2 Tbsp

Drinks/Mixes

The foods on this list without a serving size listed can be consumed in any moderate amount.

‡ Bouillon, broth, consommé

Bouillon or broth, low-sodium

Carbonated or mineral water

Club soda

Cocoa powder, unsweetened (1 Tbsp)

Coffee, unsweetened or with sugar substitute

Diet soft drinks, sugar-free

Drink mixes, sugar-free

Tea, unsweetened or with sugar substitute

Tonic water, diet

Water

Water, flavored, carbohydrate free

Seasonings

Any food on this list can be consumed in any moderate amount.

Flavoring extracts (for example, vanilla, almond, peppermint)

Garlic

Herbs, fresh or dried

Nonstick cooking spray

Pimento

Spices

Hot pepper sauce

Wine, used in cooking

Worcestershire sauce

Note: Be careful with seasonings that contain sodium or are salts, such as garlic salt, celery salt, and lemon pepper.

Combination Foods

Many of the foods you eat are mixed together in various combinations, such as casseroles. These "combination" foods do not fit into any one choice list. This is a list of choices for some typical combination foods. This list will help you fit these foods into your meal plan. Ask your registered dietitian for nutrient information about other combination foods you would like to eat, including your own recipes. A carbohydrate choice has 15 grams of carbohydrate and about 70 calories.

Entrees

Food	Serving Size	Count As
‡ Casserole type (tuna noodle, lasagna, spaghetti with meatballs, chili with beans, macaroni and cheese)	1 cup (8 oz)	2 carbohydrates + 2 medium-fat meats
‡ Stews (beef/other meats and vegetables)	1 cup (8 oz)	1 carbohydrate + 1 medium-fat meat + 0–3 fats
Tuna salad or chicken salad	½ cup (3½ oz)	½ carbohydrate + 2 lean meats + 1 fat

‡ = 600 milligrams or more of sodium per serving (for combination food main dishes/meals).

Frozen Meals/Entrees

Food	Serving Size	Count As
*‡ Burrito (beef and bean)	1 (5 oz)	3 carbohydrates + 1 lean meat + 2 fats
‡ Dinner-type meal	generally 14–17 oz	3 carbohydrates + 3 medium-fat meats + 3 fats
‡ Entrée or meal with less than 340 calories	about 8–11 oz	2–3 carbohydrates + 1–2 lean meats
‡ Pizza, cheese/vegetarian, thin crust	¼ of a 12-inch (4½–5 oz)	2 carbohydrates + 2 medium-fat meats
‡ Pizza, meat topping, thin crust	¼ of a 12-inch (5 oz)	2 carbohydrates + 2 medium-fat meats + 1½ fats
‡Pocket sandwich	1 (4½ oz)	3 carbohydrates + 1 lean meat + 1–2 fats
‡Pot pie	1 (7 oz)	2½ carbohydrates + 1 medium-fat meat + 3 fats

Salads (Deli-Style)

Food	Serving Size	Count As
Coleslaw	½ cup	1 carbohydrate + 1½ fats
Macaroni/pasta salad	½ cup	2 carbohydrates + 3 fats
‡ Potato salad	½ cup	1½–2 carbohydrates + 1–2 fats

* = More than 3 grams of dietary fiber per serving.

♦ = Extra fat, or prepared with added fat.

‡ = 600 milligrams or more of sodium per serving (for combination food main dishes/meals).

Soups

Food	Serving Size	Count As
‡ Bean, lentil, or split pea	1 cup	1 carbohydrate + 1 lean meat
‡ Chowder (made with milk)	1 cup (8 oz)	1 carbohydrate + 1 lean meat + 1½ fats
‡ Cream (made with water)	1 cup (8 oz)	1 carbohydrate + 1 fat
‡ Instant	6 oz prepared	1 carbohydrate
‡ Instant with beans or lentils	8 oz prepared	2½ carbohydrates + 1 lean meat
‡ Miso soup	1 cup	½ carbohydrate + 1 fat
‡ Ramen noodle	1 cup	2 carbohydrates + 2 fats
Rice (congee)	1 cup	1 carbohydrate
‡ Tomato (made with water)	1 cup (8 oz)	1 carbohydrate
‡ Vegetable beef, chicken noodle, or other broth-type	1 cup (8 oz)	1 carbohydrate

Fast Foods

The choices in the **Fast Foods** list are not specific fast food meals or items, but are estimates based on popular foods. You can get specific nutrition information for almost every fast food or restaurant chain. Ask the restaurant or check its website for nutrition information about your favorite fast foods. A carbohydrate choice has 15 grams of carbohydrate and about 70 calories.

Breakfast Sandwiches

Food	Serving Size	Count As
‡ Egg, cheese, meat, English muffin	1 sandwich	2 carbohydrates + 2 medium-fat meats
‡ Sausage biscuit sandwich	1 sandwich	2 carbohydrates + 2 high-fat meats + 3½ fats

Main Dishes/Entrees

Food	Serving Size	Count As
*‡ Burrito (beef and beans)	1 (about 8 oz)	3 carbohydrates + 3 medium-fat meats + 3 fats
‡ Chicken breast, breaded and fried	1 (about 5 oz)	1 carbohydrate + 4 medium-fat meats
Chicken drumstick, breaded and fried	1 (about 2 oz)	2 medium-fat meats
‡ Chicken nuggets	6 (about 3½ oz)	1 carbohydrate + 2 medium-fat meats + 1 fat
‡ Chicken thigh, breaded and fried	1 (about 4 oz)	½ carbohydrate + 3 medium-fat meats + 1½ fats
‡ Chicken wings, hot	6 (5 oz)	5 medium-fat meats + 1½ fats

Asian

Food	Serving Size	Count As
‡ Beef/chicken/shrimp with vegetables in sauce	1 cup (about 5 oz)	1 carbohydrate + 1 lean meat + 1 fat
‡ Egg roll, meat	1 (about 3 oz)	1 carbohydrate + 1 lean meat + 1 fat
Fried rice, meatless	½ cup	1½ carbohydrates + 1½ fats
‡ Meat and sweet sauce (orange chicken)	1 cup	3 carbohydrates + 3 medium-fat meats + 2 fats
*‡ Noodles and vegetables in sauce (chow mein, lo mein)	1 cup	2 carbohydrates + 1 fat

Pizza

Food	Serving Size	Count As
‡ Pizza, cheese, pepperoni, regular crust	⅛ of a 14-inch (about 4 oz)	2½ carbohydrates + 1 medium-fat meat + 1½ fats
‡ Pizza, cheese/vegetarian, thin crust	¼ of a 12-inch (about 6 oz)	2½ carbohydrates + 2 medium-fat meats + 1½ fats

* = More than 3 grams of dietary fiber per serving.

♦ = Extra fat, or prepared with added fat.

‡ = 600 milligrams or more of sodium per serving (for fast-food main dishes/meals).

Sandwiches

Food	Serving Size	Count As
‡ Chicken sandwich, grilled	1	3 carbohydrates + 4 lean meats
‡ Chicken sandwich, crispy	1	3½ carbohydrates + 3 medium-fat meats + 1 fat
Fish sandwich with tartar sauce	1	2½ carbohydrates + 2 medium-fat meats + 2 fats
‡ Hamburger, large with cheese	1	2½ carbohydrates + 4 medium-fat meats + 1 fat
Hamburger, regular	1	2 carbohydrates + 1 medium-fat meat + 1 fat
‡ Hot dog with bun	1	1 carbohydrate + 1 high-fat meat + 1 fat
‡ Submarine sandwich, less than 6 grams fat	6-inch sub	3 carbohydrates + 2 lean meats
‡ Submarine sandwich, regular	6-inch sub	3½ carbohydrates + 2 medium-fat meats + 1 fat
Taco, hard or soft shell (meat and cheese)	1 small	1 carbohydrate + 1 medium-fat meat + 1½ fats

Salads

Food	Serving Size	Count As
*‡ Salad, main dish (grilled chicken type, no dressing or croutons)	salad	1 carbohydrate + 4 lean meats
Salad, side (no dressing or cheese)	small (about 5 oz)	1 vegetable

Sides/Appetizers

Food	Serving Size	Count As
♦ French fries, restaurant style	small	3 carbohydrates + 3 fats
♦ French fries	medium	4 carbohydrates + 4 fats
♦ French fries	large	5 carbohydrates + 6 fats
‡ Nachos with cheese	small (about 4½ oz)	2½ carbohydrates + 4 fats
‡ Onion rings	1 serving (about 3 oz)	2½ carbohydrates + 3 fats

Desserts

Food	Serving Size	Count As
Milkshake, any flavor	12 oz	6 carbohydrates + 2 fats
Soft-serve ice cream cone	1 small	2½ carbohydrates + 1 fat

Note: See the **Starch** list and **Sweets, Desserts, and Other Carbohydrates** list for foods such as bagels and muffins.

Appendix F

Body Mass Index-for-Age Percentiles

2 to 20 years: Boys
Body mass index-for-age percentiles

NAME _____

RECORD # _____

Weight Status Category	Percentile Range
Underweight	Less than the 5th percentile
Healthy weight	5th percentile to less than the 85th percentile
Overweight	85th to less than the 95th percentile
Obese	Equal to or greater than the 95th percentile

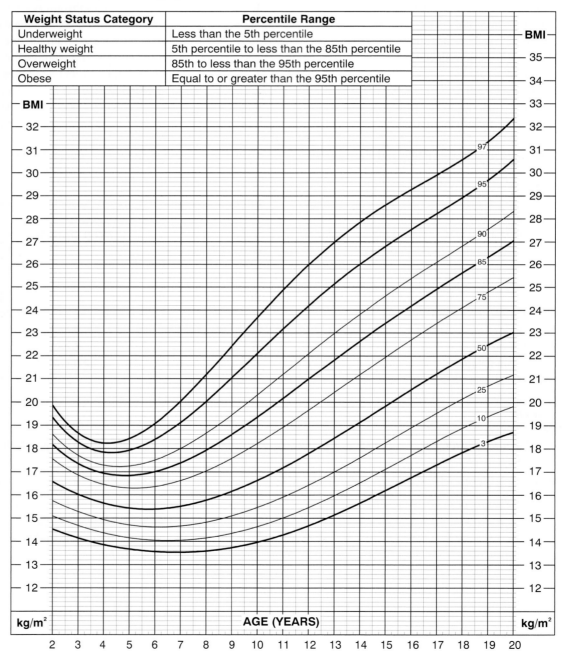

Published May 30, 2000 (modified 10/16/00).
SOURCE: Developed by the National Center for Health Statistics in collaboration with
the National Center for Chronic Disease Prevention and Health Promotion (2000).
http://www.cdc.gov/growthcharts

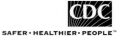

SAFER · HEALTHIER · PEOPLE™

2 to 20 years: Girls
Body mass index-for-age percentiles

NAME _____

RECORD # _____

Weight Status Category	Percentile Range
Underweight	Less than the 5th percentile
Healthy weight	5th percentile to less than the 85th percentile
Overweight	85th to less than the 95th percentile
Obese	Equal to or greater than the 95th percentile

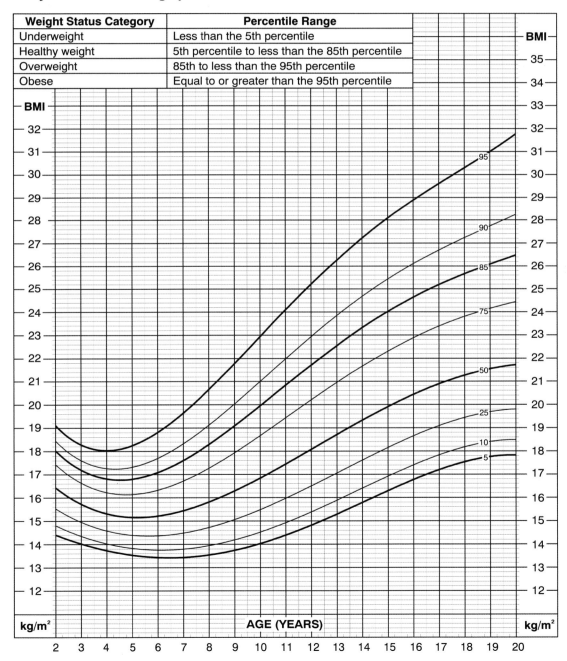

Published May 30, 2000 (modified 10/16/00).
SOURCE: Developed by the National Center for Health Statistics in collaboration with
the National Center for Chronic Disease Prevention and Health Promotion (2000).
http://www.cdc.gov/growthcharts

CDC

SAFER · HEALTHIER · PEOPLE™

Glossary

A

absorption. The passage of nutrients from the digestive tract into the circulatory or lymphatic system. (3)

acid. A compound that has a pH lower than 7. (9)

acid-base balance. The maintenance of the correct level of acidity of a body fluid. (7)

addiction. A psychological or physical dependence on a drug. (19)

Adequate Intake (AI). A reference value that is used when there is insufficient scientific evidence to determine an EAR. (4)

adipose tissue. Tissue in which the body stores lipids. (6)

adolescence. The period of life between childhood and adulthood. (11)

aerobic activity. An activity that uses large muscles and is done at a moderate, steady pace for fairly long periods. The heart and lungs are able to meet the muscles' oxygen needs throughout an aerobic activity. (15)

agility. The ability to change body position with speed and control. (15)

alcoholism. An addiction to alcohol. (19)

amenorrhea. An abnormal cessation of menstrual periods. (9)

amino acid. One of the building blocks of protein molecules. (7)

amphetamine. A stimulant drug. (19)

anabolic steroid. An artificial hormone used to build a more muscular body. (19)

anaerobic activity. An activity in which the muscles are using oxygen faster than the heart and lungs can deliver it. (15)

anorexia nervosa. An eating disorder characterized by the person refusing to maintain a minimal normal body weight and an intense fear of weight gain that leads to self-starvation. (14)

antibody. A protein made by the immune system to defend the body against infection and disease. (7)

antidepressant. A drug that alters the nervous system and relieves depression. (14)

antioxidant. A substance that reacts with free radicals (unstable single oxygen molecules) to protect other substances from harmful effects of the free radicals. (8)

aseptic packaging. A food packaging process that involves packing sterile food in sterile containers within a sterile atmosphere. (2)

assertiveness. A person's boldness to express what he or she thinks and feels in a way that does not offend others. (17)

atherosclerosis. Hardened and narrowed arteries caused by plaque deposits. (6)

ATP (adenosine triphosphate). The storage form of energy in the body. (3)

B

bacteria. Single-celled microorganisms that live in soil, water, and the bodies of plants and animals. (20)

balance. The ability to keep the body in an upright position while standing still or moving. (15)

basal metabolic rate (BMR). The rate at which the body uses energy for basal metabolism. (12)

basal metabolism. The amount of energy required to support the operation of all internal body systems except digestion. (12)

base. A compound that has a pH greater than 7. (9)

beriberi. The thiamin deficiency disease, which is characterized by weakness, loss of appetite, irritability, poor arm and leg coordination, and a tingling throughout the body. (8)

bile. A digestive juice produced by the liver to aid fat digestion. (3)

binge-eating disorder. An eating disorder that involves repeatedly eating very large amounts of food without a follow-up behavior to prevent weight gain. (14)

bingeing. Uncontrollable eating of huge amounts of food in a relatively short period of time. (14)

bioelectrical impedance. A process that measures body fat by measuring the body's resistance to a low-energy electrical current. (12)

biofeedback. A technique of focusing on involuntary bodily processes, such as breathing and pulse rate, in order to control them. (18)

blood lipid profile. A medical test that measures the amounts of cholesterol, triglycerides, HDL, and LDL in the blood. (6)

body composition. The proportion of lean body tissue to fat tissue in the body. (12)

body mass index (BMI). A calculation of body weight and height used to define underweight, healthy weight, overweight, and obesity. (12)

budget. A spending plan that outlines how to use sources of income to meet various fixed and flexible expenses. (21)

buffer. A compound that can counteract an excess of acid or base in a fluid. (7)

bulimia nervosa. An eating disorder that involves uncontrollable eating of huge amounts of food followed by an inappropriate behavior to prevent weight gain. (14)

burnout. A lack of energy and motivation to work toward goals. (17)

C

calorie density. The concentration of energy in a food. (12)

cancer. A disease in which abnormal cells grow out of control. (6)

carbohydrate loading. A technique used by endurance athletes to trick the muscles into storing more glycogen for extra energy. (16)

carbohydrates. One of the six classes of nutrients that includes sugars, starches, and fibers. Carbohydrates are the body's main source of energy. (5)

cardiorespiratory fitness. The body's ability to take in adequate amounts of oxygen and carry it efficiently through the blood to body cells. (15)

cholesterol. A white, waxy lipid made by the body that is part of every cell. Cholesterol is also found in foods of animal origin. (6)

chylomicron. A ball of triglycerides thinly coated with cholesterol, phospholipids, and proteins formed to carry absorbed dietary fat to body cells. (6)

chyme. A mixture of gastric juices and food formed in the stomach during digestion. (3)

cirrhosis. A liver disease in which liver cells die, causing the liver to lose its ability to work. (19)

coagulation. The blood clotting process that stops bleeding. (8)

coenzyme. A nonprotein compound (usually a vitamin) that combines with an inactive enzyme to form an active enzyme system. (8)

cofactor. A substance that acts with enzymes to increase enzyme activity. (9)

collagen. A protein substance in the connective tissue that holds cells together. (8)

communication. The sending of a message from one source to another. (17)

comparison shopping. Assessing prices and quality of similar products to choose those that best meet a consumer's needs and price range. (22)

complementary proteins. Two or more incomplete protein sources that can be combined to provide all the indispensable amino acids. (7)

complete protein. A protein that contains all the indispensable amino acids. (7)

complex carbohydrate. A polysaccharide. Starch and fiber are complex carbohydrates. (5)

compromise. A solution to a problem that blends ideas from two differing parties. (17)

conflict. Disagreement. (17)

congenital disability. A condition existing from birth that limits a person's ability to use his or her body or mind. (11)

congregate meal. A group meal. (21)

constipation. A condition that occurs when the feces become massed and hard in the large intestine, making expulsion infrequent. (3)

consumer. Someone who buys and uses products and services. (22)

contaminant. An undesirable substance that unintentionally gets into food. (20)

convenience food. A food item that is purchased partially or completely prepared. (21)

coordination. The ability to integrate the use of two or more parts of the body. (15)

coronary heart disease (CHD). Disease of the heart and blood vessels. Atherosclerosis and hypertension are the two most common forms of CHD. (6)

crash diet. A weight-loss plan that provides fewer than 1,200 calories per day. (13)

cretinism. Severe mental retardation and dwarfed physical features of an infant caused by the mother's iodine deficiency during pregnancy. (9)

cross-contamination. The transfer of harmful bacteria from either an object or a food to another food. (20)

culture. The beliefs and social customs of a group of people. (2)

D

daily hassles. Minor stressors that produce tension. (18)

Daily Values. Recommended nutrient intakes, which are based on daily calorie needs, used as references on food labels. (4)

deficiency disease. A sickness caused by a lack of an essential nutrient. (7)

dehydration. A state in which the body contains a lower than normal amount of body fluids. (10)

denaturation. A change in shape that happens to protein molecules when they are exposed to heat, acids, bases, salts of heavy metals, or alcohol. (7)

dental caries. Tooth decay. (5)

depressant. A drug that decreases the activity of the central nervous system. (19)

designer drug. A lab-created imitation of an illegal drug. (19)

diabetes mellitus. A lack of or an inability to use the hormone insulin, which results in a buildup of glucose in the bloodstream. (5)

diagnosis. The identification of a disease. (1)

diarrhea. Frequent expulsion of watery feces. (3)

diet. All the foods and beverages a person consumes. (1)

dietary fiber. The nondigestible carbohydrates and lignins that make up the tough, fibrous cell walls of plants. (5)

Dietary Guidelines for Americans. A document developed by the United States Departments of Agriculture and Health and Human Services that provides information and advice to promote health through improved nutrition and physical activity for Americans two years and older, including those at increased risk of chronic disease. (4)

Dietary Reference Intakes (DRI). Reference values for nutrients and food components that can be used to plan and assess diets for healthy people. (4)

digestion. The process by which the body breaks down food, and the nutrients in food, into simpler parts for use in growth, repair, and maintenance. (3)

disaccharide. A carbohydrate made up of two sugar units. Sucrose, lactose, and maltose are the disaccharides. (5)

dispensable amino acids. The amino acids the body can make for itself, also called nonessential amino acids. (7)

distress. Harmful stress. (18)

diuretic. A substance that increases urine production. (10)

diverticulosis. A disorder in which many abnormal pouches form in the intestinal wall. (3)

drug. Any substance other than food or water that changes the way the body or mind operates. (19)

drug abuse. The deliberate use of a drug or chemical substance for other than medical reasons and in such a way that the person's health or ability to function is threatened. (19)

drug misuse. Unintentionally using a medicine in a manner that could cause harm to the individual. (19)

E

eating disorder. An abnormal eating pattern that focuses on body weight and food issues, which can have life threatening consequences. (14)

emulsifier. A substance, such as a phospholipid, that can mix with water and fat. (6)

endurance athlete. An athlete involved in a sport, such as marathon bicycling or distance swimming, that requires sustained muscle efforts for several hours at a time. (16)

energy. The ability to do work. (12)

enriched food. A food that has had vitamins and minerals added back that were lost in the refining process. (8)

environmental contaminant. A substance released into the air or water by industrial plants. (20)

environmental cue. An event or situation around a person that triggers him or her to eat. (13)

environmental quality. The state of the physical world a person is exposed to, including the condition of water, air, and food. (1)

enzyme. A complex protein produced by cells to speed a specific chemical reaction in the body. (3)

epithelial cells. The surface cells that line the outside of the body, cover the eyes, and line the passages of the lungs, intestines, and reproductive tract. (8)

ergogenic aids. Any substances designed to enhance strength and endurance. (19)

erythrocyte hemolysis. A vitamin E deficiency condition that is sometimes seen in premature babies and is characterized by broken red blood cells, resulting in weakness and listlessness. (8)

essential fatty acid. A fatty acid needed by the body for normal growth and development that cannot be made by the body and, therefore, must be supplied by the diet. (6)

Estimated Average Requirement (EAR). A nutrient recommendation estimated to meet the needs of 50 percent of the people in a defined group. (4)

Estimated Energy Requirement (EER). The average calories needed to maintain energy balance in a healthy person of a certain age, gender, weight, height, and level of physical activity. (12)

ethnic food. A food that is typical of a given racial, national, or religious culture. (2)

Exchange Lists for Meal Planning. A system for planning healthy meals or special diets that classifies foods into groups of similar nutrient and caloric content. (4)

extracellular water. The water outside the cells. (10)

F

fad diet. An eating plan that is popular for a short time because it promises rapid weight loss. (13)

fasting. Refraining from consuming most or all sources of calories. (13)

fat replacer. An ingredient used in food products to replace some or all of the fat typically found in those products. (6)

fat-soluble vitamin. A vitamin, specifically vitamin A, D, E, or K, that dissolves in fats. (8)

fatty acid. An organic compound made up of a chain of carbon atoms to which hydrogen atoms are attached and having an acid group at one end. (6)

feces. Solid wastes that result from digestion. (3)

female athlete triad. A set of three related medical problems—disordered eating, amenorrhea, and osteoporosis—common among female athletes. (14)

fetal alcohol syndrome (FAS). A set of symptoms that can occur in a newborn whose mother drinks alcohol while pregnant. (11)

fetus. A developing human from nine weeks after conception until birth. (11)

fight or flight response. Physical reactions to stress that happen as the body gathers its resources to conquer danger or escape to safety. (18)

flexibility. The ability to move body joints through a full range of motion. (15)

fluorosis. A spotty discoloration of teeth caused by high fluoride intake. (9)

food additive. A substance added to food products to cause desired changes in the products. (22)

food allergy. A reaction of the immune system to certain proteins found in foods. (3)

food biotechnology. The use of knowledge of plant science and genetics to develop plants and animals with specific desirable traits while eliminating traits that are not wanted. (2)

foodborne illness. A disease transmitted by food. (20)

food diary. A record of the kinds and amounts of all foods and beverages consumed for a given time. (4)

food-drug interaction. A physical or chemical effect a drug has on a food or a food has on a drug. (19)

food intolerance. An unpleasant reaction to a food that does not cause an immune system response. (3)

food irradiation. The treatment of approved foods with ionizing energy to improve food safety and extend shelf life. (22)

food norm. Typical standard or pattern related to food and eating behaviors. (2)

food processing. Any procedure performed on food to prepare it for consumers. (22)

food taboo. A social custom that prohibits the use of certain edible resources as food. (2)

fortified food. A food that has one or more nutrients added during processing. (8)

fortified water. Water that has been enhanced with specific nutrients or supplements intended to aid or improve health or energy outcomes. (10)

free radical. A highly reactive, unstable single oxygen molecule, which can generate a harmful chain reaction that can damage tissue. (8)

functional fiber. The isolated, nondigestible carbohydrates that have beneficial effects in human health. (5)

functional food. A food to which ingredients have been added, such as fiber, to provide health benefits beyond basic nutrition. (5)

fungi. An organism that can vary greatly in size and structure and is classified as a plant, such as mold and yeast. (20)

G

gallstones. Small crystals that form from bile in the gallbladder. (3)

gastric juices. A mixture of hydrochloric acid, digestive enzymes, and mucus produced by the stomach that helps digest food. (3)

gastrointestinal (GI) tract. A muscular tube leading from the mouth to the anus through which food passes as it is digested. (3)

generally recognized as safe (GRAS) list. A list prepared by the U.S. Food and Drug Administration of substances that have proved to be safe to use in food processing. (22)

generic drug. A drug available under its generic name. (19)

generic product. An unbranded product, which can be identified by plain, simple packaging. (22)

glucose. A monosaccharide that circulates in the bloodstream and serves as the body's source of energy. (5)

glycemic index (GI). A measure of the speed at which various carbohydrates are digested into glucose, absorbed, and enter the bloodstream. (5)

glycogen. The body's storage form of glucose. (5)

goiter. An enlargement of the thyroid gland. (9)

growth spurt. A period of rapid physical growth. (11)

H

habit. A routine behavior that is often difficult to break. (13)

hallucinogen. A drug that causes the mind to create images that do not really exist. (19)

hazard analysis critical control point (HACCP) system. A food safety procedure that identifies the steps at which a food product is at risk of biological, chemical, or physical contamination and creates a plan to minimize or eliminate the risk. (20)

healthy body weight. Body weight specific to gender, height, and body frame size that is associated with health and longevity. (12)

heart attack. The death of heart tissue caused by blockage of an artery carrying nutrients and oxygen to that tissue. (6)

heartburn. A burning pain in the middle of the chest caused by stomach acid flowing back into the esophagus. (3)

heart rate. The number of times the heart beats per minute. (15)

hemoglobin. An iron-containing protein that helps red blood cells carry oxygen from the lungs to cells throughout the body and carbon dioxide from body tissues back to the lungs for excretion. (9)

high-density lipoprotein (HDL). A lipoprotein that picks up cholesterol from around the body and transfers it to other lipoproteins for transport back to the liver for removal from the body. (6)

holistic medicine. An approach to health care that focuses on all aspects of patient care—physical, mental, and social. (1)

hormone. A chemical produced in the body and released into the bloodstream to regulate specific body processes. (5)

hydrogenation. The process of breaking the double carbon bonds in unsaturated fatty acids and adding hydrogen to make the fatty acid more saturated. (6)

hygiene. Practices that promote good health. (20)

hypertension. Abnormally high blood pressure; an excess force on the walls of the arteries as blood is pumped from the heart. (6)

hypoglycemia. A low blood glucose level. (5)

hypothesis. A suggested answer to a scientific question, which can be tested and verified. (1)

I

illegal drug. A drug that is unlawful to buy or use. (19)

impulse buying. Making unplanned purchases. (22)

incomplete protein. A protein that is missing or short in one or more of the indispensable amino acids. (7)

indigestion. A difficulty in digesting food. (3)

indispensable amino acids. The nine amino acids the body is unable to make, also called essential amino acids. (7)

infant. A child in the first year of life. (11)

inhalant. A substance that is inhaled for its mind-numbing effects. (19)

insulin. A hormone secreted by the pancreas to regulate blood glucose level. (5)

intracellular water. The water inside body cells. (10)

iron-deficiency anemia. A condition in which the number of red blood cells declines, causing the blood to have a decreased ability to carry oxygen to body tissues. (9)

K

ketone bodies. Compounds formed from fatty acids the nervous system can use for energy when carbohydrates are not available. (12)

ketosis. An abnormal buildup of ketone bodies in the bloodstream. (12)

kilocalorie. The unit used to measure the energy value of food. (3)

kosher food. Foods prepared according to Jewish dietary laws. (2)

kwashiorkor. A protein deficiency disease. (7)

L

lactation. The production of breast milk by a mother's body following the birth of a baby. (11)

lactic acid. A product formed in the muscles as the result of the incomplete breakdown of glucose during anaerobic activity. (16)

lactose intolerance. An inability to digest lactose, the main carbohydrate in milk, due to a lack of the digestive enzyme lactase. (5)

lecithin. A phospholipid made by the liver and found in many foods. (6)

legume. A plant that has a special ability to capture nitrogen from the air and transfer it to protein-rich seeds. (7)

life-change events. Major stressors, such as death, divorce, and legal problems that can greatly alter a person's lifestyle. (18)

life cycle. A series of stages through which people pass between birth and death. (11)

life expectancy. The average length of life of people living in the same environment. (1)

lipid. A group of compounds that includes triglycerides (fats and oils), phospholipids (lecithin), and sterols (cholesterol). (6)

lipoprotein. Fat droplets coated by proteins so they can be transported in the bloodstream. (6)

low-birthweight baby. A baby that weighs less than 5½ pounds (2,500 g) at birth. (11)

low-density lipoprotein (LDL). A lipoprotein that carries cholesterol made by the liver through the bloodstream to body cells. (6)

lubricant. A substance that reduces friction between surfaces. (10)

M

macromineral. Mineral required in the diet in an amount of 100 or more milligrams per day. (9)

marasmus. A wasting disease caused by a lack of calories and protein. (7)

mastication. Chewing. (3)

maximum heart rate. The highest speed at which the heart muscle is able to contract. (15)

meal management. Using resources to meet nutritional needs through food selection and preparation. (21)

medicine. A drug used to treat an ailment or improve a disabling condition. (19)

menopause. The time in a woman's life when menstruation ends due to a decrease in production of the hormone estrogen. (9)

mental health. The way a person feels about himself or herself, life, and the world. (1)

metabolism. All the chemical changes that occur as cells produce energy and materials needed to sustain life. (3)

micromineral. Mineral required in the diet in an amount of less than 100 milligrams per day. (9)

microorganism. A living being so small it can be seen only under a microscope. (20)

minerals. An inorganic element needed in small amounts as a nutrient to perform various functions in the body. (9)

monosaccharide. A carbohydrate made up of single sugar units. Glucose, fructose, and galactose are the monosaccharides. (5)

monounsaturated fatty acid. A fatty acid that has only one double bond between carbon atoms in a carbon atom chain. (6)

muscular endurance. The ability to use a group of muscles over and over without getting tired. (15)

myoglobin. An iron-containing protein that carries oxygen and carbon dioxide in muscle tissue. (9)

MyPlate. The USDA's new food guidance system based on the *Dietary Guidelines for Americans*. (MyPlate replaced MyPyramid.) (4)

N

narcotic. A drug that brings on sleep, relieves pain, or dulls the senses. (19)

national brand. A brand that is distributed and advertised throughout the country by a major company. (22)

negative stress. Stress that can reduce a person's effectiveness by causing him or her to be fearful and perform poorly. (18)

night blindness. A condition in which the cells in the eyes adjust slowly to dim light, causing night vision to become poor. (8)

nitrogen balance. A comparison of the nitrogen a person consumes with the nitrogen he or she excretes. (7)

nonverbal communication. The sending of a message from one source to another without the use of words. (17)

nutrient. A basic component of food that nourishes the body. (1)

nutrient dense. Foods and beverages that provide vitamins, minerals, and other substances that may have positive health effects, but supply relatively few calories. (4)

nutrition. The sum of the processes by which a person takes in and uses food substances. (1)

O

obese. Describes an adult with a body mass index of 30 or more. (12)

omega-3 fatty acids. A certain type of polyunsaturated fatty acids found in fish oils and shown to have a positive effect on heart health. (6)

opiate. A narcotic drug, such as codeine, morphine, opium, or heroin, made from the opium poppy. (19)

optimum health. A state of wellness characterized by peak physical, mental, and social well-being. (1)

organic food. A food produced without the use of synthetic fertilizers, pesticides, antibiotics, herbicides, or growth hormones. (22)

osmosis. The movement of water across a semipermeable membrane to equalize the solution concentrations of mineral particles on each side of the membrane. (9)

osteomalacia. A vitamin D deficiency disease in adults that causes the bones to become misshapen. (8)

osteoporosis. A condition in which bones become porous and fragile due to a loss of minerals. (9)

outpatient treatment. Medical care that does not require a hospital stay. (14)

overdose. Taking an unsafe quantity of a drug. (19)

over-the-counter (OTC) drug. A legal drug that can be bought without a prescription written by a physician. (19)

overweight. Describes an adult with a body mass index of 25 to 29.9. (12)

P

parasite. An organism that lives off another organism, which is called a host. (20)

pathogen. Organism that causes foodborne illness, such as bacteria, parasites, viruses, and fungi. (20)

peer pressure. The influence people in a person's age and social group have on his or her behavior. (1)

pellagra. The niacin deficiency disease, which is characterized by diarrhea and dermatitis and can lead to dementia and death. (8)

peristalsis. A series of squeezing actions by the muscles in the gastrointestinal tract that helps move food through the tract. (3)

pernicious anemia. A deficiency disease caused by an inability to absorb vitamin B12, which is characterized by fatigue; weakness; a red, painful tongue; and a tingling or burning in the skin. (8)

pesticide residue. Chemical pesticide particles left in food after it is prepared for consumption. (20)

pH. A term used to express a substance's acidity or alkalinity as measured on a scale from 0 (extreme acid) to 14 (extreme base). (9)

phospholipids. A class of lipids that have a phosphorus-containing compound in their chemical structures, which allows them to combine with both fat and water to form emulsions. (6)

Physical Activity Guidelines for Americans. A set of recommendations that specify amounts and types of exercise individuals at different stages of the life cycle should do to achieve health benefits. (4, 15)

physical fitness. A state in which all body systems function together efficiently. (15)

physical health. The fitness of the body. (1)

phytochemicals. Health-enhancing nonnutrient compounds in plant foods that are active in the body at the cellular level. (8)

pica. The craving for and ingestion of nonfood materials such as clay, soil, or chalk. (11)

placebo effect. A change in a person's condition that is not a result of treatment given, but of the individual's belief that the treatment is working. (8)

placenta. An organ that forms inside the uterus during pregnancy in which blood vessels from the mother and the fetus are entwined, enabling the transfer of materials carried in the blood. (11)

plaque. A buildup of fatty compounds made up largely of cholesterol that form on the inside walls of arteries. (6)

polysaccharide. A carbohydrate made up of many sugar units that are linked in straight or branched chains. (5)

polyunsaturated fatty acid. A fatty acid that has two or more double bonds between carbon atoms in a carbon atom chain. (6)

positive stress. Stress that motivates a person to accomplish challenging goals. (18)

posture. The position of the body when standing or sitting. (15)

power. The ability to do maximum work in a short time. (15)

prebiotics. The nondigestible food ingredients that stimulate the growth of good microorganisms in the colon. (8)

premature baby. A baby born before the 37th week of pregnancy. (11)

premature death. Death that occurs due to lifestyle behaviors that lead to a fatal accident or the formation of an avoidable disease. (1)

prescription drug. A medicine that can only be obtained from a pharmacy with a written order from a doctor. (19)

proactive. Taking steps in advance to deal with anticipated situations. (17)

probiotics. The "good" microorganisms found in foods that help to counterbalance the "bad" microorganisms in your intestinal tract. (8)

progressive muscle relaxation. A relaxation technique that involves slowly tensing and then relaxing different groups of muscles. (18)

protein. An energy-yielding nutrient composed of carbon, hydrogen, oxygen, and nitrogen. (7)

protein-energy malnutrition (PEM). A condition caused by a lack of calories and proteins in the diet. (7)

protozoa. Single-celled animals. (20)

provitamin. A compound the body can convert to the active form of a vitamin. (8)

psychoactive drug. A drug that affects the central nervous system. (19)

puberty. The time during which a person develops sexual maturity. (11)

purging. Clearing food from the digestive system. (14)

Q

quality of life. A person's satisfaction with his or her looks, lifestyle, and responses to daily events. (1)

R

rancid. Describes a fat in which the fatty acid molecules have combined with oxygen, causing them to break down, which makes the fat spoil and gives it an unpleasant smell and taste. (6)

reactant. A substance that enters into a chemical reaction and is changed by it. (10)

reaction time. The amount of time it takes to respond to a signal once the signal is received. (15)

Recommended Dietary Allowance (RDA). The average daily intake of a nutrient required to meet the needs of most (97 to 98 percent) healthy individuals. RDAs are based on EAR. (4)

recovery. The phase after exercise when glycogen stores are replenished to pre-exercise levels. (16)

reduction. The process of cooking a liquid with the intent of losing volume through evaporation in order to concentrate the flavors and thicken the liquid. (21)

refined sugar. A carbohydrate sweetener that is separated from its natural source for use as a food additive. (5)

relationship. A connection a person forms with another person. (17)

resting heart rate. The speed at which a person's heart muscle contracts when he or she is sitting quietly. (15)

resting metabolic rate (RMR). A method used to measure the body's resting energy expenditure, which can be used interchangeably with basal metabolic rate (BMR). (12)

rickets. A deficiency disease in children caused by a lack of vitamin D and characterized by soft, misshapen bones. (8)

risk factor. A characteristic or behavior that influences a person's chance of being injured or getting a disease. (1)

S

sanitation. Maintaining clean conditions to help prevent disease. (20)

satiety. The feeling of fullness a person has after eating food. (5)

saturated fatty acid. A fatty acid that has no double bonds in its chemical structure and, therefore, carries a full load of hydrogen atoms. (6)

scientific method. The process researchers use to find answers to their questions. (1)

scurvy. The vitamin C deficiency disease, characterized by tiredness, weakness, shortness of breath, aching bones and muscles, swollen and bleeding gums, lack of appetite, slow healing of wounds, and tiny bruises on the skin. (8)

secondhand smoke. The smoke released into the air by someone smoking that is inhaled by another individual as he or she breathes. (19)

sedentary activity. An activity that requires much sitting or little movement. (12)

self-actualization. A person's belief that he or she is doing his or her best to reach full human potential. (17)

self-concept. The idea a person has about himself or herself. (17)

self-esteem. The worth or value a person assigns himself or herself. (17)

self-talk. A person's internal conversations about himself or herself and the situations he or she faces. (18)

serving size. The amount of a food item customarily eaten at one time. (22)

side effect. A reaction caused by a drug that differs from the drug's desired effect. (19)

simple carbohydrate. A monosaccharide or disaccharide. (5)

skinfold test. A test in which a caliper is used to measure the thickness of a fold of skin to estimate how much of the thickness is due to subcutaneous fat. (12)

smokeless tobacco. Tobacco products that are not intended to be smoked, such as chewing tobacco or snuff. (19)

social development. Learning how to get along with others. (17)

social health. The way a person gets along with other people. (1)

SoFAS. Foods and beverages that are high in solid fats and/or added sugars. (4)

solvent. A liquid in which substances can be dissolved. (10)

soul food. Traditional food of the African American ethnic group. (2)

speed. The quickness with which a person is able to complete a motion. (15)

staple food. A food that supplies a large portion of the calories people need to maintain health. (2)

starch. A polysaccharide that is the storage form of energy in plants. (5)

status food. A food that has a social impact on others. (2)

sterols. A class of lipids that have a complex molecular structure, including some hormones, vitamin D, and cholesterol. (6)

stimulant. A kind of psychoactive drug that speeds up the nervous system. (19)

store brand. A brand that is sold in only specific chains of food stores. (22)

strength. The ability of the muscles to move objects. (15)

stress. The inner agitation a person feels when he or she is exposed to change. (1)

stressor. A source of stress. (18)

stroke. The death of brain tissue caused by blockage of an artery carrying nutrients and oxygen to that tissue. (6)

subcutaneous fat. Fat that lies underneath the skin. (12)

sugars. A collective term used to refer to all the monosaccharides and disaccharides. (5)

supplement. A concentrated source of a nutrient, usually in pill, liquid, or powder form. (5)

support system. A group of people who can provide a person with physical help and emotional comfort. (18)

T

target heart rate zone. The range of heartbeats per minute at which the heart muscle receives the best workout; 60 to 90 percent of maximum heart rate. (15)

technology. The application of a certain body of knowledge. (2)

theory. A principle that tries to explain something that happens in nature. (1)

thermic effect of food. The energy required to complete the processes of digestion, absorption, and metabolism. (12)

thyroxine. A hormone produced by the thyroid gland that helps control metabolism. (9)

toddler. A child between one and three years of age. (11)

Tolerable Upper Intake Level (UL). The maximum level of ongoing daily intake for a nutrient that is unlikely to cause harm to most people in the defined group. (4)

tolerance. The ability of the body and mind to become less responsive to a drug. (19)

total fiber. The sum of dietary and functional fibers. (5)

toxicity. A poisonous condition. (8)

toxin. Poison. (20)

trans fatty acid. An unsaturated fatty acid that has had hydrogen added to convert it to a solid fat. (6)

triglycerides. The major type of fat found in foods and in the body. Triglycerides consist of three fatty acids attached to glycerol. (6)

trimester. A span of about 13 to 14 weeks that represents one-third of the pregnancy period in humans. (11)

U

ulcer. An open sore in the lining of the stomach or small intestine caused by a bacterium. (3)

underweight. Describes an adult with a body mass index below 18.5. (12)

unit price. A product's cost per standard unit of weight or volume. (22)

unsaturated fatty acid. A fatty acid that has at least one double bond between two carbon atoms in a carbon atom chain and, therefore, is missing at least two hydrogen atoms. (6)

V

value. A belief or attitude that is important to an individual. (2)

vegetarianism. The practice of eating a diet consisting entirely or largely of plant foods. (7)

verbal communication. The sending of a message from one source to another through the use of words. (17)

very low-density lipoprotein (VLDL). A lipoprotein that carries triglycerides and cholesterol made by the liver through the bloodstream to body cells. (6)

villi. Tiny, fingerlike projections that cover the wall of the small intestine. (3)

virus. A disease-causing agent that is the smallest type of life-form. (20)

vitamin. An organic compound needed in tiny amounts as a nutrient to regulate body processes. (8)

W

water intoxication. A rare condition caused by drinking too much water and consuming too few electrolytes. (10)

water-soluble vitamin. A vitamin, specifically vitamin C or one of the B-complex vitamins, that dissolves in water. (8)

weight cycling. A lifelong pattern of weight gain and loss. (13)

weight management. Attaining healthy weight and keeping it throughout life. (13)

wellness. The state of being in good health. (1)

withdrawal. Symptoms experienced by a person who stops taking a drug to which he or she is addicted. (19)

Index